BIOLOGICAL
and BIOMEDICAL
COATINGS
HANDBOOK

Applications

BIOLOGICAL
and BIOMEDICAL
COATINGS
HANDBOOK

Applications

Edited by
Sam Zhang

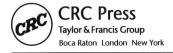

CRC Press
Taylor & Francis Group
Boca Raton London New York

CRC Press is an imprint of the
Taylor & Francis Group, an **informa** business

CRC Press
Taylor & Francis Group
6000 Broken Sound Parkway NW, Suite 300
Boca Raton, FL 33487-2742

First issued in paperback 2018

© 2011 by Taylor and Francis Group, LLC
CRC Press is an imprint of Taylor & Francis Group, an Informa business

No claim to original U.S. Government works

ISBN-13: 978-1-4398-4996-5 (hbk)
ISBN-13: 978-1-138-11439-5 (pbk)

Visit the Taylor & Francis Web site at
http://www.taylorandfrancis.com

and the CRC Press Web site at
http://www.crcpress.com

Contents

Series Preface vii
Preface.. ix
Editor... xi
Contributors.. xiii

1 Sol–Gel Derived Hydroxyapatite Coatings on Metallic Implants:
  Characterization, *In Vitro* and *In Vivo* Analysis 1
  Wang Yongsheng

2 Amorphous Carbon Coatings for Biological Applications 45
  Soon-Eng Ong and Sam Zhang

3 Biomedical Applications of Carbon-Based Materials............................. 111
  Subbiah Alwarappan, Shree R. Singh, and Ashok Kumar

4 Impedance Spectroscopy on Carbon-Based Materials for Biological
  Application.. 135
  Haitao Ye and Shi Su

5 Control of Drug Release from Coatings: Theories and Methodologies ... 195
  Lei Shang, Sam Zhang, Subbu S. Venkatraman, and Hejun Du

6 Release-Controlled Coatings 259
  James Zhenggui Tang and Nicholas P. Rhodes

7 Orthopedic and Dental Implant Surfaces and Coatings...................... 301
  Racquel Z. LeGeros, Paulo G. Coelho, David Holmes, Fred Dimaano, and John P. LeGeros

8 Piezoelectric Zinc Oxide and Aluminum Nitride Films for Microfluidic
  and Biosensing Applications... 335
  Yong Qing Fu, J. K. Luo, A. J. Flewitt, A. J. Walton, M. P. Y. Desmulliez, and W. I. Milne

9 Medical Applications of Sputter-Deposited Shape Memory Alloy Thin Films 381
  Yong Qing Fu, Wei Min Huang, and Shuichi Miyazaki

10 Bioactive Coatings for Implanted Devices 471
  Subbu Venkatraman, Xia Yun, Huang Yingying, Debasish Mondal, and Liu Kerh Lin

Index.. 491

Series Preface

Advances in Materials Science and Engineering

Series Statement

Materials form the foundation of technologies that govern our everyday life, from housing and household appliances to handheld phones, drug delivery systems, airplanes, and satellites. Development of new and increasingly tailored materials is key to further advancing important applications with the potential to dramatically enhance and enrich our experiences.

The *Advances in Materials Science and Engineering* series by CRC Press/Taylor & Francis is designed to help meet new and exciting challenges in Materials Science and Engineering disciplines. The books and monographs in the series are based on cutting-edge research and development, and thus are up-to-date with new discoveries, new understanding, and new insights in all aspects of materials development, including processing and characterization and applications in metallurgy, bulk or surface engineering, interfaces, thin films, coatings, and composites, just to name a few.

The series aims at delivering an authoritative information source to readers in academia, research institutes, and industry. The Publisher and its Series Editor are fully aware of the importance of Materials Science and Engineering as the foundation for many other disciplines of knowledge. As such, the team is committed to making this series the most comprehensive and accurate literary source to serve the whole materials world and the associated fields.

As Series Editor, I'd like to thank all authors and editors of the books in this series for their noble contributions to the advancement of Materials Science and Engineering and to the advancement of humankind.

Sam Zhang

Preface

As the clock of history ticks into the twenty-first century, "life sciences" has become one of the buzzwords of the time. Various nanotechnologies are mobilized to serve this field, the field of understanding life, the field of prevention of disease and cure, the field of enhancing quality of life. This two-volume handbook, *Biological and Biomedical Coatings*, comes at the right time to help meet these needs.

Volume 1 has nine chapters focusing on process and characterization of biological and biomedical coatings through sol–gel method, thermal spraying, hydrothermal and physical or chemical vapor deposition, and so forth. These chapters are "Bone-Like Mineral and Organically Modified Bone-Like Mineral Coatings," "Synthesis and Characterization of Hydroxyapatite Nanocoatings by Sol–Gel Method for Clinical Applications," "Hydroxyapatite and Other Biomedical Coatings by Electrophoretic Deposition," "Thermal Sprayed Bioceramic Coatings: Nanostructured Hydroxyapatite (HA) and HA-Based Composites," "Nanostructured Titania Coatings for Biological Applications: Fabrication and Characterization," "Hydrothermal Crystallization with Microstructural Self-Healing Effect on Mechanical and Failure Behaviors of Plasma-Sprayed Hydroxyapatite Coatings," "Bioceramic Coating on Titanium by Physical and Chemical Vapor Deposition," "Coating of Material Surfaces with Layer-by-Layer Assembled Polyelectrolyte Films," and "Bioactive Glass-Based Coatings and Modified Surfaces: Strategies for the Manufacture, Testing, and Clinical Applications for Regenerative Medicine."

Volume 2 contains 10 chapters centering on coating applications in the medical field such as implant and implanted devices, drug release, biosensing, and so forth. These chapters are "Sol–Gel Derived Hydroxyapatite Coatings on Metallic Implants: Characterization, *In Vitro* and *In Vivo* Analysis," "Amorphous Carbon Coatings for Biological Applications," "Biomedical Applications of Carbon-Based Materials," "Impedance Spectroscopy on Carbon-Based Materials," "Control of Drug Release from Coatings: Theories and Methodologies," "Release-Controlled Coatings," "Orthopedic and Dental Implant Surfaces and Coatings," "Piezoelectric Zinc Oxide and Aluminum Nitride Films for Microfluidic and Biosensing Applications," "Medical Applications of Sputter-Deposited Shape Memory Alloy Thin Films," and "Bioactive Coatings for Implanted Devices."

A striking feature of these handbooks is the consideration of both novice and experts: the chapters are written in such a way that, for newcomers in the relevant field, the handbooks serve as an introduction and a stepping stone for them to enter the field with less confusion, whereas for experts, the books provide up-to-date information through figures, tables, and images that will assist their research. I sincerely hope this aim is achieved.

The chapter authors come from different regions all over the globe: Australia, China, France, Hong Kong, Japan, Singapore, Taiwan, the United Kingdom, and the United States. As top researchers in the forefront of their relevant research fields, naturally they all are very busy. As the editor of these volumes, I am very grateful that they all made a special effort to ensure timely response and progress of their respective chapters. I am extremely indebted to many people who accepted my request and acted as reviewers for all the chapters. Since these volumes aim to cater to both novice and experts, the chapters are inevitably lengthy; many were more than 100 pages in the manuscript stage. To ensure the highest quality, close to 50 reviewers (at least two and sometimes three per chapter) painstakingly went through the chapters and came out with sincere and frank criticism and modification suggestions that helped make the chapters what they are today. I would like to take this opportunity to say a big "thank you" to all of them. Last but not least, I would like to register my gratitude to many CRC Press staff, especially Ms. Allison Shatkin, Miss Kari A. Budyk, and Miss Andrea Dale at Taylor & Francis Group for the invaluable assistance they have rendered to me throughout the entire endeavor, which made the smooth publication of these volumes a reality.

Sam Zhang

Editor

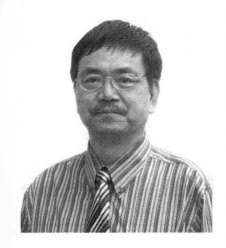

Sam Zhang Shanyong, better known as **Sam Zhang**, received his B. Eng. in Materials in 1982 from Northeastern University (Shenyang, China), his M. Eng. in Materials in 1984 from the Central Iron and Steel Research Institute (Beijing, China), and his Ph.D. in Ceramics in 1991 from the University of Wisconsin–Madison (Madison, WI). He has been a full professor since 2006 at the School of Mechanical and Aerospace Engineering, Nanyang Technological University, Singapore.

Professor Zhang serves as editor-in-chief for *Nanoscience and Nanotechnology Letters* (United States) and principal editor for *Journal of Materials Research* (United States), among his other editorial involvements in international journals. Much of his career has been devoted to processing and characterization of thin films and coatings—from hard coatings to biological coatings and from electronic thin films to energy films and coatings—for the past almost 20 years. He has authored/coauthored more than 200 peer-reviewed papers (published in international journals) and 15 book chapters, and guest-edited 11 journal volumes in *Surface and Coatings Technology, Thin Solid Films*, etc. Including this handbook, so far he has published seven books: *CRC Handbook of Nanocomposite Films and Coatings*: Vol. 1, *Nanocomposite Films and Coatings: Mechanical Properties*, Vol. 2, *Nanocomposite Films and Coatings: Functional Properties*, Vol. 3, *Organic Nanostructured Film Devices and Coatings for Clean Energy*, and *Advanced Characterization Techniques* (Sam Zhang, Lin Li, Ashok Kumar, CRC Press Taylor & Francis Group, 2008), *Nanocomposite Films and Coatings—Processing, Properties and Performance* (edited by Sam Zhang and Nasar Ali, Imperial College Press, UK, 2007), and this *Biological and Biomedical Coatings Handbook* two-volume set (CRC Press Taylor & Francis Group): *Biological and Biomedical Coatings Handbook: Processing and Characterization* (vol. 1) and *Biological and Biomedical Coatings Handbook: Applications* (vol. 2).

Professor Zhang is currently serving as president of the Thin Films Society, and is a fellow of the Institute of Materials, Minerals, and Mining (UK); an honorary professor of the Institute of Solid State Physics, Chinese Academy of Sciences; guest professor at Zhejiang University and Harbin Institute of Technology; and distinguished professor at the Central Iron and Steel Research Institute. He was featured in the first edition of *Who's Who in Engineering Singapore* (2007), and featured in the 26th and 27th editions of *Who's Who in the World* (2009 and 2010, respectively). Since 1998, he has been frequently invited to deliver plenary keynote lectures at international conferences including those held in Japan, the United States, France, Spain, Germany, China, Portugal, New Zealand, Russia, etc. He is also frequently invited by industries and universities to conduct short courses and workshops in Singapore, Malaysia, Portugal, the United States, and China.

Professor Zhang has been actively involved in organizing international conferences: 11 conferences as chairman, 13 conferences as member of the organizing committee, and six conferences as member of the scientific committee. The "Thin Films" conference series

(International Conference on Technological Advances of Thin Films & Surface Coatings), initiated and chaired by Professor Zhang, has grown from its inauguration in 2002 with 70 attendees to 800 strong since 2008. The Thin Films conference series has been a biannual focus in the field of films and coatings in the world.

Professor Zhang served as consultant to a city government in China and to industrial organizations in China and Singapore. He also served in numerous research evaluation/ advisory panels in Singapore, Israel, Estonia, China, Brunei, and Japan.

Other details of Professor Zhang's research and publications are easily accessible at his personal Web site, http://www.ntu.edu.sg/home/msyzhang.

Contributors

Subbiah Alwarappan
Nanomaterials and Nanomanufacturing
 Research Center
University of South Florida
Tampa, Florida

P. G. Coelho
Department of Biomaterials and
 Biomimetics
New York University College of Dentistry
New York, New York

M. P. Y. Desmulliez
School of Engineering and Physical
 Sciences
Institute of Integrated Systems
Heriot-Watt University
Edinburgh, United Kingdom

F. Dimaano
Stryker Orthopaedics
Mahwah, New Jersey

Hejun Du
School of Mechanical and Aerospace
 Engineering
Nanyang Technological University
Singapore

A. J. Flewitt
Department of Engineering
University of Cambridge
Cambridge, United Kingdom

Yong Qing Fu
Thin Film Centre
University of the West of Scotland
Paisley, United Kingdom

D. Holmes
Department of Biomaterials and
 Biomimetics
New York University College of Dentistry
New York, New York

W. M. Huang
School of Mechanical and Aerospace
 Engineering
Nanyang Technological University
Singapore

Ashok Kumar
Nanomaterials and Nanomanufacturing
 Research Center
University of South Florida
Tampa, Florida

J. P. LeGeros
Department of Biomaterials and
 Biomimetics
New York University College of Dentistry
New York, New York

R. Z. LeGeros
Department of Biomaterials and
 Biomimetics
New York University College of Dentistry
New York, New York

Liu Kerh Lin
School of Materials Science and
 Engineering
Nanyang Technological University
Singapore

J. K. Luo
Centre for Material Research and Innovation
University of Bolton
Bolton, United Kingdom

W. I. Milne
Department of Engineering
University of Cambridge
Cambridge, United Kingdom

S. Miyazaki
Institute of Materials Science
University of Tsukuba
Tsukuba, Japan

Debasish Mondal
School of Materials Science and
    Engineering
Nanyang Technological University
Singapore

Soon-Eng Ong
Temasek Laboratories
Nanyang Technological University
Singapore

Nicholas P. Rhodes
Division of Clinical Engineering
School of Clinical Sciences
University of Liverpool
Liverpool, United Kingdom

Lei Shang
School of Mechanical and Aerospace
    Engineering
Nanyang Technological University
Singapore

Shree R. Singh
Department of Biological Sciences
Alabama State University
Montgomery, Alabama

Shi Su
Electronic Engineering, School of
    Engineering and Applied Science
Aston University
Birmingham, United Kingdom

Subbu S. Venkatraman
School of Materials Science and
    Engineering
Nanyang Technological University
Singapore

A. J. Walton
Scottish Microelectronics Centre
School of Engineering
Institute of Integrated Systems
University of Edinburgh
Edinburgh, United Kingdom

Yongsheng Wang
School of Mechanical and Aerospace
    Engineering
Nanyang Technological University
Singapore

Haitao Ye
Electronic Engineering
School of Engineering and Applied Science
Aston University
Birmingham, United Kingdom

Huang Yingying
School of Materials Science and
    Engineering
Nanyang Technological University
Singapore

Xia Yun
School of Materials Science and
    Engineering
Nanyang Technological University
Singapore

Sam Zhang
School of Mechanical and Aerospace
    Engineering
Nanyang Technological University
Singapore

James Zhenggui Tang
School of Applied Sciences
University of Wolverhampton
Wolverhampton, United Kingdom

1

Sol–Gel Derived Hydroxyapatite Coatings on Metallic Implants: Characterization, In Vitro *and* In Vivo *Analysis*

Wang Yongsheng

CONTENTS

Introduction 1
HA and HA Coating 3
Sol–Gel Derived HA Coating 6
   Brief Introduction of the Sol–Gel Technique 6
   Metallic Substrates 6
   Precursors for Sol–Gel Derived HA Coating...7
   Chemical and Physical Properties of Sol–Gel Derived HA Coating......................8
      Phase Composition...8
      Surface Chemistry and Composition 10
      Surface Morphology...12
      Interfacial Analysis...13
   Mechanical Properties of Sol–Gel Derived HA Coating..14
      Pull-Out Tensile Adhesion Strength and Interfacial Shear Strength..............14
      Evaluation of Interfacial Shear Strength 17
      Scratch Test..18
      Toughness of Sol–Gel Derived HA Coating 19
      Residual Stress Measurement...19
   In Vitro Assay 22
      Dissolution Behavior..22
      In Vitro Test in Acellular Simulated Body Fluid...25
      Cell Response to HA Coating 27
   In Vivo Animal Trial...30
Recent Trends Related to Sol–Gel Derived HA Coatings..32
References..33

Introduction

In modern society, the rapid development of biomedical engineering has provided considerable improvement on human quality of life. Biomaterials, as the main part of biomedical engineering, have attracted more and more attention regarding replacing a part or certain function of the body in a safe, reliable, economic, and physiologically acceptable manner

(Bronzino 2000). A vast array of manmade biomaterials, including metals, polymers, ceramics, and composites, have been widely developed during the past 90 years for the requirements of clinical applications. Each biomaterial has its own advantages and disadvantages for a specific application (Ratner et al. 1996; Smallman and Bishop 1998). In other words, the selection of a biomaterial for a specified case depends on the particular repair or replacement situation and the properties of related biomaterials. Herein, this chapter is limited to some issues related to load-bearing implants, such as hip joint replacement and teeth roots repair. The demands for these kind of load-bearing implants have increased enormously in the current industrial era due to increased injuries caused by accidents and the improvement of social awareness about the right of existence. According to the American Academy of Orthopedic Surgeons, for example, more than 120,000 total hip replacement operations are performed each year (Marsha, Leonard, and Randall 2000). As such, the development of reliable high-performance implants is greatly meaningful and valuable.

Many kinds of materials have been developed, including metals and alloys, polymers, ceramics, and composites, and are widely used in biomedical fields. However, no matter what the source, biomaterials must meet several criteria to perform successfully as load-bearing implants in orthopedic and dental applications (Hench 1998; Poitout 2004). First of all, they must be biocompatible, or able to function *in vivo* without eliciting any intolerable response in the body, either locally or systemically. On the other hand, those appropriate biomaterials must be able to withstand the often hostile environment of the body, and show better properties, such as resistance to corrosion and degradation, such that the body environment does not adversely affect material performance over the implant's intended performance lifetime. Furthermore, adequate mechanical properties, such as tensile/compressive strength, elastic modulus, and fatigue endurance, are also critical criteria for the selection of biomaterials to be used as devices intended to replace or reinforce load-bearing skeletal structures. In addition, they must be capable of reproducible fabrication to the highest standards of quality control at, of course, a reasonable cost. Biomaterials that meet these criteria are fundamental to the practice of orthopedic surgery and to ensuring the success of implantation.

Among all the suggested biomaterials, metallic biomaterials, such as Co–Cr–Mo alloys and titanium alloys, may be the most preferred selection for load-bearing implants due to their excellent mechanical properties (Table 1.1). However, all these metallic

TABLE 1.1

Mechanical Properties of Bone and Some Biomaterials

Types of Materials	Young's Modulus (GPa)	Ultimate Tensile Strength (MPa)	Tensile Elongation Rate (%)	Fracture Toughness (MPa m$^{1/2}$)
Alumina	420	282–551	<1	3–5.4
Hydroxyapatite (3% porosity)	7–13	38–48	–	3.7–5.5
Stainless steel	200	1000	10	100
Co–Cr alloys	230	450–1300	10–30	100
Ti–Al–V and c.p. Ti	100–140	500–1150	15–25	80
Mg and Mg alloys	41–45	225	–	–
PMMA	2.8	55	8	1.19
Cortical bone	3.8–11.7	82–114	–	2–12

Source: Leyens, C., Peters, M., *Titanium and Titanium Alloys: Fundamentals and Applications*, Wiley-VCH, Weinheim, 2003; Smallman, R.E., Bishop, R.J., *Modern Physical Metallurgy and Materials Engineering-Science, Process, Application*, Elsevier, 1998; Friedrich, H.E., Mordike, B.L., *Magnesium Technology*, Springer-Velag, Berlin, Germany, 2006; Ben-Nissan, B., Pezzotti, G., *Biomaterials*, 25, 20, 4971–4975, 2004. With permission.

biomaterials are bioinert and would release some undesired metal ions caused by corrosion in the human body's biological environment. Of the bioceramics, alumina, calcium phosphate, and bioglass in use are mainly because of their superior biocompatibility and bioactivity. However, their poor mechanical properties (e.g., tensile strength and fracture toughness) are serious design limitations for these materials when used in load-bearing implants (Table 1.1). Polymers, including polymethyl methacrylate (PMMA), polyethylene, polyurethane, etc., are widely used in plastic surgery, cardiovascular surgery, and other soft tissue surgery due to their properties of resilience and malleability, which are not at all suitable for load-bearing implants. Therefore, none of the three kinds of above-mentioned biomaterials meet all the requirements of implants for hard tissue repair and/ or replacement.

However, in view of the advantages and disadvantages of each kind of biomaterial, an advisable and practicable solution is to develop bioceramic-coated metallic implants. It is believed that such kinds of implants can do well in combining the desired biological properties of bioceramics and the excellent mechanical properties of metallic substrates. The bioceramic coating can also protect the metallic substrate from corrosion and serve as a barrier for the possible release of toxic metal ions into the human body. Among all these bioceramics, hydroxyapatite (HA) is the most suitable candidate to be used as a coating on the surface of metallic implants due to its chemical and biological similarity to human hard tissues (Boretoes and Eden 1984). HA coating cannot only improve the rate of osseointegration, but can also establish a high bone–implant interfacial strength by forming strong chemical bonds with the surrounding tissues (Vedantam and Ruddlesdin 1996; Roop, Kumar, and Wang 2002).

HA and HA Coating

HA is the main mineral component of human hard tissues (mainly bones and teeth), and provides storage for the control of calcium uptake and release for the human body (Aoki 1994). HA belongs to a class of calcium phosphate-based bioceramics with a chemical formula of $Ca_{10}(PO_4)_6(OH)_2$. The word "hydroxyapatite" consists of "hydroxyl" ion and "apatite," which is the mineral name. The stoichiometric Ca/P molar ratio is 1.67, and the calculated density is about 3.219 g/cm³. HA crystallite possesses a hexagonal structure with the unit cell dimensions of: $a = b = 0.9432$ nm and $c = 0.6881$ nm (Hench and Wilson 1993; Kay, Young, and Posner 1964). The atomic structure of HA projected along the c-axis on the basal plane is shown in Figure 1.1.

It is well known that HA can be used as bone substitutes in orthopedics and dental treatment due to its biocompatibility and osteoconductive properties (Boretoes and Eden 1984). In order to meet the clinical requirements of different applications, HA has been developed well to be fabricated into different forms, such as particulates (solid, porous, or even hollow particles) in different sizes, blocks, and coatings (Wang et al. 2009). As for load-bearing implants, bulk HA seems not suitable because of the limitation of its mechanical properties (Hench and Wilson 1993; Bronzino 2000). There is a wide variation in the reported mechanical properties of synthesized HA, which strongly depended on the process applied with the HA sample preparation. For example, the compressive strength of synthesized HA ranges from 294 to 917 MPa (Park 1984). Other related mechanical properties are listed in Table 1.1. The mechanical properties of HA strongly influence their

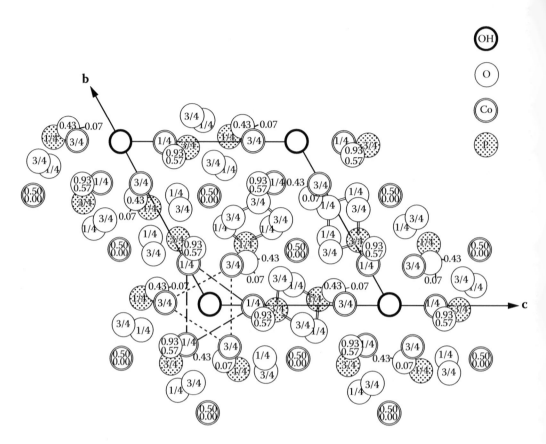

FIGURE 1.1
Crystal structure of hydroxyapatite, viewed along *c*-axis. (From Kay et al., *Nature*, 204, 4963, 1050–1052, 1964. With permission.)

applications as implants. Therefore, the application of bulk HA as load-bearing implants is inevitably impracticable because of its poor fracture toughness (too brittle).

The most interesting property of HA in bone repair is its attractive bioactivity and strong ability to form direct chemical bonds with surrounding tissues. Therefore, HA-coated metallic implants could integrate the bioactivity of HA and the mechanical properties of metallic substrates for an ideal combination. Many techniques have been developed for the fabrication of HA coatings onto metallic implant surfaces. Commonly used methods include pulsed laser deposition (PLD) or laser ablation (Koch et al. 2007; Bao et al. 2005; Arias et al. 2003), hot isostatic pressing (HIP) (Onoki and Hashida 2006; Fu, Batchelor, and Khor 1998), thermal spraying techniques, including plasma spraying (Wang, Lu et al. 2007; Yan, Leng, and Weng 2003; Gu, Khor, and Cheang 2003), flame spraying (Cheang and Khor 1995; Oguchi et al. 1992), and high-velocity oxy-fuel combustion spraying (HVOF) (Lima et al. 2005; Khor et al. 2003), electrophoretic deposition (Wei et al. 2001; Xiao and Liu 2006), biomimetic coating (Reiner and Gotman 2009; Bharati, Sinha, and Basu 2005), sputtering coating (Pichugin et al. 2008; Ding 2003), and the sol–gel method (Haddow, James, and Van Noort 1999; Ak Azem and Cakir 2009; Avés et al. 2009). Each method has its own advantages and disadvantages in the coating properties, such as coating chemistry, phase composition, crystallinity, and mechanical properties, as well as biological properties. A comparison of these coating techniques is summarized in Table 1.2. Among all these

TABLE 1.2

Comparison of Different Methods for HA Coating Preparation

	Method	Coating Thickness	Advantages	Disadvantages	References
High temperature deposition techniques	Pulsed laser deposition	<5 μm	Coating crystalline and amorphous; dense or porous; active atmosphere conditions	Expensive, time-consuming, multiphase coating including α-TCP, β-TCP, TTCP besides HA and amorphous HA	(Koh et al. 2007; Bao et al. 2005; Arias et al. 2003; Katto et al. 2002)
	Hot isostatic pressing	0.2–2.0 mm	Produces dense coatings	Cannot coat complex substrates; high temperature required; thermal expansion mismatch; elastic property differences; expensive	(Onoki and Hashida 2006; Fu, Batchelor, and Khor 1998)
	Thermal spraying	30–200 μm	High deposition rates; can obtain various coating thickness and can be used for complex substrate shapes; low cost	High temperature induces decomposition; rapid cooling produces amorphous coatings	(Wang, Lu et al. 2007; Yan, Leng, and Weng 2003; Gu, Khor, and Cheang 2003; Cheang and Khor 1995; Oguchi et al. 1992; Lima et al. 2005; Khor et al. 2003)
Low temperature deposition techniques	Electrophoretic deposition	0.1–2.0 mm	Rapid deposition rates; can coat complex substrates	Non-uniform thickness; impurity; poor biological fixation to the metal substrates	(Wei et al. 2001; Xiao and Liu 2006; Ma, Liang et al. 2003; Stoch et al. 2001)
	Biomimetic coating	<30 μm	Low processing temperatures; can form bonelike apatite; can coat complex shapes; can incorporate bone growth stimulating factors	Time-consuming; requires replenishment and a constant pH of simulated body fluid	(Reiner and Gotman 2009; Bharati, Sinha, and Basu 2005; Barrere et al. 2001; Rigo et al. 2004)
	Sputter coating	<3 μm	Uniform coating thickness on flat substrates; dense coating	Ca/P ratio of the coating is higher than that of synthetic HA if RF magnetron sputtering is used; expensive; time consuming; producing amorphous coatings	(Pichugin et al. 2008; Ding 2003; Nelea et al. 2003; Nieh, Jankowsk, and Koike 2001; Cooley et al. 1992)
	Sol–gel method	<1 μm	Low processing temperature; can coat complex shapes, can obtain very thin coatings; higher purity and homogeneity; low cost	Some processes require controlled atmosphere and high sintering temperature	(Haddow, James, and Van Noort 1999; Ak Azem and Cakir 2009; Avés et al. 2009; Duran et al. 2004; Tkalcec et al. 2001; Montenero et al. 2000; Gross et al. 1998; Kim et al. 2005)

Source: Y. Yang et al., *Biomaterials*, 26, 3, 327–337, 2005. With permission.

coating techniques, the sol–gel method is commonly used for its advantages of composition homogeneity, low cost, and ease in operation (Zhang et al. 2006).

Sol–Gel Derived HA Coating

Brief Introduction of the Sol–Gel Technique

The sol–gel process is a chemical synthesis method generally used for the preparation of ceramics, glasses, and composites at much lower temperatures than other traditional methods, such as hot pressing and sintering (Hench and Wilson 1993). The use of the sol–gel method can be traced back to as early as the mid-1800s, and a fast-growing development of sol–gel applications has been achieved within the past three decades (Gupta and Kumar 2008; Wang and Bierwagen 2009). In the sol–gel process, the solution system involves a transition from a liquid "sol" into solid "gel" phase. The starting materials used in the preparation of "sol" are usually inorganic metal salts or metal organic compounds such as metal alkoxides. After a certain process with the sol (e.g., the coating of "sol" onto a substrate), followed by drying to remove residual organics and heat treatment, the "gel" is converted into dense materials (Klein 1988). Since the design of the sol–gel system and related sol–gel process can be controlled easily, this method has been employed to produce various products of desired sizes, shapes, and formats (e.g., particle, fiber, coating, bulk). The main advantages and important features of the sol–gel method can be summarized as (Wang and Bierwagen 2009; Klein 1988):

- Increased homogeneity due to the mixing at the molecular level
- Reduced processing temperature, frequently close to room temperature
- Substrate/mold shape-independent, since liquid precursors are used (such that complex shapes of products can be successfully fabricated)
- Easy mixing for multicomponent systems
- Use of different chemical routes (precursor selection)
- Possibility of producing materials with special properties (e.g., composition, crystallinity, morphology, and even composites)
- Low cost and easy operation

Today, sol–gel technology is widely used in the development of catalyst (Blum, Avnir, and Schumann 1999), nanomaterials (Răileanu et al. 2009), chemical sensors (Lin and Brown 1997), biosensors (Pastor et al. 2010), and electrochemical devices in diverse scientific and engineering fields, including the ceramic industry (Klein 1988), optical engineering (Gvishi et al. 1997), biomedical field (Gupta and Kumar 2008), and electronic industry (Dulay et al. 2002). Sol–gel technology shows great potential for the development of novel materials and devices in a broad range of applications.

Metallic Substrates

Because of the preliminary requirement of biocompatibility for a biomaterial, the number of metallic materials that can be considered for implants is limited. Metals and alloys used in clinical applications mainly include stainless steel, Co–Ni–Cr alloy, cast and wrought Co–Cr–Mo alloy, commercially pure titanium (c.p. titanium), and titanium alloy (Ratner et al. 1996). Compared with other metals and alloys, however, c.p. titanium and titanium alloy–Ti6Al4V have been used as implant materials only for a short time. They have been widely used in clinical application and have a great potential prospect for medical applications due to their good biocompatibility, superior mechanical properties, and corrosion resistance (Leyens and Peters 2003). In the case of other metals as implants, the accumulation of toxic metal ions caused by dissolution and corrosion in the body's physiological environment often leads to severe pathological problems (Jaffe and Scott 1996). Furthermore, in comparison with cobalt chromium alloys, titanium and its alloy demonstrate a 33% increase in bonding strength to HA coating *in vitro*. Moreover, concerning the costs of semiproducts, Ti and its alloys belong to the same groups as stainless steel, whereas Co–Cr alloys are more expensive (Leyens and Peters 2003). Thus, titanium and its alloys with their favorable properties are more preferable for medical applications compared to other metallic materials.

Recently, magnesium and magnesium alloys, as the lightweight metals (density $\sim 1.75 \text{g}/\text{cm}^3$), have been proposed as biodegradable implants for orthopedic and trauma surgery due to their outstanding biocompatibility, biodegradability, and mechanical properties (Witte 2010; Friedrich and Mordike 2006). According to Wolff's law, Mg alloys are most preferred because of the similarity of Young's modulus between Mg alloys and human bones (cf. Table 1.1). Such kind of similarity can effectively avoid the stress shielding effect, leading to enhanced stimulation of new bone growth and remodeling (Zberg, Uggowitzer, and Löffler 2009). Noticeably, because of the bioresorbable characteristic, Mg alloy-based implants are strongly expected as biodegradable implants (e.g., coronary stent) rather than the permanent ones. Therefore, it is still questionable for Mg alloys to be used as load-bearing implants for hard tissue repair or replacement.

Precursors for Sol–Gel Derived HA Coating

Theoretically, any precursor able to form reactive inorganic monomers or oligomers can be used for sol–gel process to synthesize the corresponding inorganic products. However, in order to obtain sol–gel derived coatings with the desired quality, the selection of related precursors (as well as the designed sols) should satisfy some basic requirements (Klein 1988; Gupta and Kumar 2008):

(1) Must be soluble in the selected reaction media and reactive enough to participate in the gel forming process.

(2) The precursors should be stable (do not produce any unwanted by-product).

(3) The sols containing precursors should have certain viscosity and can wet the substrate well to produce an overall homogeneous deposited layer.

(4) Uniform and long-term stability of the sols is possible.

(5) Easy removal of unused ions or organic groups to obtain a coating with pure phase and uniform surface morphology.

A number of calcium and phosphate precursors have been employed for sol–gel synthesis of HA coatings on metallic implant surfaces at a low temperature. An overview of different calcium and phosphate precursors commonly used for the preparation of HA coatings is listed in Table 1.3. Due to the difference in chemical activity of different precursors, the temperature required to produce the apatite structure depends largely on the chemical

TABLE 1.3

Overview of Different Calcium and Phosphate Precursors for Preparation of HA Coatings

Calcium Precursor	Phosphate Precursor	References
Calcium nitrate tetrahydrate $(Ca(NO_3)_2 \cdot 4H_2O)$	Diphosphorous pentoxide (P_2O_5); Ammonium hydrogen phosphate $((NH_4)_2HPO_4)$; Ammonium dihydrogen phosphate; Triethyl phosphite; Triethyl phosphate (TEP); Phosphoric acid (H_3PO_4); n-Butyl acid phosphate (n-BAP); Triethyl phosphate	(Weng, Han et al. 2003; Montenero et al. 2000; Hsieh, Perng, and Chin 2002; You, Oh, and Kim 2001; Cavalli et al. 2001; Liu, Yang, and Troczynski 2002; Kim et al. 2004; Manso, Ogueta et al. 2002; Manso, Langlet et al. 2002; Hwang et al. 2000; Wang, Chen, and Wang 2009; Gan and Pilliar 2004; Weng and Baptista 1998)
Calcium acetate monohydrate $(Ca(OA-c)_2 \cdot H_2O)$	Diethyl hydrogen-phosphonate $((C_2H_5)_2HPO)$;	(Ben-Nissan, Milev, and Vago 2004; Balamurugan, Kannan, and Rajeswari 2002)
Calcium diethoxide	Triethyl phosphite; Diethyl hydrogen-phosphonate $((C_2H_5)_2HPO)$; Phosphoric acid (H_3PO_4)	(Ben-Nissan, Milev, and Vago 2004; Haddow, James, and Van Noort 1999; Chai and Ben-Nissan 1999)
Calcium hydroxide $(Ca(OH)_2)$	2-Ethylhexyl-phosphate	(Metikos-Hukovic et al. 2003; Tkalcec et al. 2001)

nature of the precursors (Haddow, James, and Van Noort 1996; Liu, Troczynski, and Tseng 2001). With the use of different precursors and processing conditions, the expected properties (chemical composition, phase components, crystallinity, thickness, morphology, porosity, etc.) of these HA coatings can be successfully achieved and well controlled.

Chemical and Physical Properties of Sol–Gel Derived HA Coating

Phase Composition

According to the processing temperature, all coating methods can be classified into two groups, low-temperature and high-temperature deposition techniques, as shown in Table 1.2. Even though the sol–gel method is classified into the low-temperature group, almost all the HA coatings prepared with this method must be treated with an essential sintering or heat treatment step at an elevated temperature. (Generally, the temperature is lower than 1000°C.) (Chen et al. 2005). Such a heat treatment process is usually required to remove the unwanted chemical components (to obtain the final HA coating) or to increase the coating crystallinity. However, the following decomposition reactions may also occur during the heat treatment (Ogiso, Yamashita, and Matsumoto 1998; Senamaud et al. 1997):

$$Ca_{10}(PO_4)_6(OH)_2 \rightarrow 2Ca_3(PO_4)_2 + Ca_4(PO_4)_2O + H_2O\uparrow$$

$$Ca_{10}(PO_4)_6(OH)_2 \rightarrow 3Ca_3(PO_4)_2 + CaO + H_2O\uparrow$$

Generally, the final coating is a pure HA coating or with a small amount of impurity phases, such as CaO, and/or TCP, OCP, carbonated HA, $CaCO_3$ (Montenero et al. 2000; Hsieh, Perng, and Chin 2002; Wang, Chen, and Wang 2009; Weng and Baptista 1998). Figure 1.2 shows a typical HA phase with small amount β-TCP (less than 5%) of sol–gel

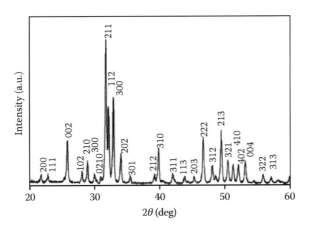

FIGURE 1.2
Phase composition of sol–gel derived HA coatings on Ti6Al4V substrate after calcination at 900°C. (From Montenero et al., *Journal of Materials Science*, 35, 11, 2791–2797, 2000. With permission.)

derived HA coatings on Ti6Al4V after being calcined at 900°C by using $Ca(NO_3)_2 \bullet 4H_2O$ and $(NH_4)_2HPO_4$ as corresponding precursors (Montenero et al. 2000).

On the other hand, the phase purity and the degree of crystallinity of sol–gel derived HA coatings is reported to depend on the kind of precursors used for the preparation of HA coatings (Haddow, James, and Van Noort 1996). For instance, Gan and Pilliar (2004) pointed out that the HA coating prepared with an organic route (precursors: calcium nitrate tetrahydrate and triethyl phosphite) possesses higher crystallinity than that obtained with an inorganic route (precursors: $Ca(NO_3)_2 \bullet 4H_2O$ and ammonium dihydrogen phosphate). Moreover, besides the selection of temperature, some other factors, including time of heat treatment, heating rate, and surrounding atmosphere, are also quite important to control the final phase composition and crystallinity (Chen et al. 1997; Wang, Chen, and Wang 2009; Hsieh, Perng, and Chin 2002). For instance, water molecules in the firing atmosphere could promote HA crystallization, whereas in a dry atmosphere TCP and TTCP are more stable than HA in a higher temperature (Chen et al. 1997). Comparatively, the phase composition of HA coatings produced by the sol–gel method is simpler than those coatings obtained by using high temperature deposition methods, which usually contain a certain amount of other impure phases, such as amorphous hydroxyapatite (ACP), oxyapatite, tricalcium phosphate (TCP), tetracalcium phosphate (TTCP), and calcium oxide (CaO) (Ong et al. 2006; Yan, Leng, and Weng 2003; Lima et al. 2005).

No matter the impure phases, all have crucial effects on the performance of coated implants, especially on the dissolution behavior of the coatings (Sun et al. 2001; You, Oh, and Kim 2001; Yang, Kim, and Ong 2005). All of the others' phases in the coating have larger solubility than that of HA (Ducheyne, Radin, and King 1993; Wang, Lu et al. 2007; Khor et al. 2003). Although the faster dissolution produces a supersaturated environment, which allows physiologically produced HA to precipitate on the coating and enhance the bone ingrowth, it also leads to the serious resorption or degradation of the coatings, and even to the failure of the implants (Cheng, Zhang, and Weng 2007; Kim, Kim, and Knowles 2005). On the other hand, the impure phase, CaO, has no biocompatibility and dissolves significantly faster than TCP. Thus, it is a detrimental phase that should be avoided (Wang, Chen et al. 2008; Sun et al. 2001). As such, both the purity and the crystallinity of the coating should be strictly controlled in order to obtain the expected effective HA coating layers.

The smaller amount of other phases, the higher degree of crystallinity, and the lower the dissolution rate, the better the performance of the implants, and vice versa. Thereby, from the viewpoint of phase purity, the sol–gel method is preferred in depositing the expected HA coatings on metallic substrates.

X-ray diffraction (XRD) is a powerful, nondestructive analysis tool and has been widely used as a means of determining the phase composition and crystallinity of the HA coatings. That is, it estimates the percentage of crystallinity and identifies the secondary phases generated during the preparation of HA coatings from the relative peak intensity of different phases (Löbmann 2007). The new phases can be identified from the plot of the intensity vs. 2θ, or from the lattice parameter change determined by XRD results. Also, other analytical techniques, such as differential thermal analysis (DTA)/differential scanning calorimetry (DSC), Fourier transform infrared spectroscopy (FTIR), can help in this analysis.

Surface Chemistry and Composition

The surface chemistry of sol–gel derived HA coatings, as one of the most significant factors for the coating in a clinical application, has received considerable attention because of its dominant role in osseointegration (Hench and Wilson 1993; Kačiulis et al. 1998). X-ray photoelectron spectroscopy (XPS) or electron spectroscopy for chemical analysis (ESCA) is the most famous technique for the analysis of surface chemistry, since it can detect all elements except hydrogen and helium with high sensitivity even for the trace amount of contaminants in the materials (Briggs and 2003; Brundle, Evans, and Wilson 1992). XPS is an important analytical tool in the area of coatings/thin films, and it can provide useful information, including compositions (elements), chemical states, and coating thickness. Based on the survey and narrow scan, the possible elements can be accurately ascertained since each element has its own characteristic binding energy. The chemical state (valence) or bonding information of each element can be determined through the shift of corresponding peak position (binding energy).

There are two main properties of concern regarding surface chemistry: the composition of the HA coating and the chemical status of the elements existing in the HA coating (Kačiulis et al. 1999). As for the composition of HA coatings, it is mainly the three elements of Ca, P, and O and their concentration (commonly described as Ca/P and O/Ca molar or weight ratio). The Ca/P and O/Ca peak ratios can help distinguish and quantify different Ca/P phases in the mixtures. With respect to the stoichiometry of the HA coatings, the Ca/P ratios for the sol–gel samples were in good agreement with the stoichiometric values compared with other coating techniques (Massaro et al. 2001; Metikos-Hukovic et al. 2003). However, as Haddow, James, and Van Noort (1996) have pointed out, the Ca/P ratio could have a great difference in response to different precursors selected. For example, the Ca/P ratio was 1.46 for the inorganic-route precursors and 2.10 for the organic-route precursors in the work of Gan and Pilliar (2004). All these changes on the Ca/P ratio can be demonstrated by other analytical methods, such as XRD and FTIR. As for the chemical states analysis, it is becoming more and more important in the biological development. Each element has the "fingerprint" characteristics that can be determined by some analytical techniques (Kačiulis et al. 1998). According to the analysis, some new phases can be determined. For HA coatings, many studies have been done on this point. Generally, Ca2p (or Ca2p$_{1/2}$ and Ca2p$_{3/2}$), P2p, and O1s are the most studied for determining the chemical properties of the coating. For example, in Figure 1.3, the O1s peaks of the HA coatings deposited by different methods are presented (Massaro et al. 2001). As indicated, peak 1 is the characteristic O1s peak in HA structure with a binding energy of 531.4eV; peak 2 is

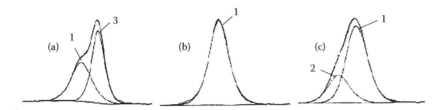

FIGURE 1.3
O1s spectra (XPS) of HA coatings prepared by different methods ([a] sol–gel coating; [b] sputtered coating; [c] plasma-sprayed coating). Peak 1 is the characteristic O1s peak in HA structure with a binding energy of 531.4eV; peak 2 is attributed to the O1s in adsorbed water; peak 3 is the O1s coming from TiO_2. (From Massaro et al., *Journal of Biomedical Materials Research*, 58, 6, 651–657, 2001. With permission.)

attributed to the O1s in adsorbed water, whereas peak 3 is the O1s coming from TiO_2. As such, according to the binding energy of a specified element, it is quite easy to find out what kind of phase/compound of this element is in. Table 1.4 summarizes the binding energy levels of core elements in some calcium-containing salts. Importantly, based on the XPS analysis (especially the narrow scan screening), the determination of trace elements in the coating is critical for the investigation and evaluation of new biomaterials (Kačiulis et al. 1999).

Surface chemistry and composition can also be analyzed by FTIR. The FTIR technique is rapid and nondestructive, requires no vacuum, and is applicable to samples of any dimension and even to those with curvature (Kazarian et al. 2004). The chemically specific information contained in the unique "fingerprint" region of the IR spectrum allows one to distinguish different chemical groups and even different materials. In HA, compound groupings, such as hydroxyl bands (OH groups), carbonate bands (CO_3 groups), and phosphate bands (PO_4 groups), are usually quantified by FTIR (Stoch et al. 2005; Vijayalakshmi, Prabakaran, and Rajeswari 2008). Crystalline HA generates two characteristic OH bands at about 3570 and 630 cm^{-1} (Weng and Baptista 1999; Stoch et al. 2000). Sometimes they are absent in FTIR spectra, and some authors attribute this missing OH modes to a perturbation of hydroxyl stretching and bending modes on the apatite surface by the hydrogen

TABLE 1.4

XPS Binding Energy Values of Main Elements in Some Calcium-Containing Salts

Phase	Binding Energy (eV)			
	Ca $2p_{1/2}$	Ca $2p_{3/2}$	P 2p	O 1s
HA	351.0–351.2	347.2–347.5	133.3–133.5	531.3–531.6
α-TCP[a]	350.7	347.2	133.3	531.0
β-TCP[a]	350.6	347.0	133.1	530.9
ACP[a]	350.6	347.1	133.1	531.1
$CaCO_3$[b]	350.1	346.5	–	533.9 (O_I)
				535.6 (O_{II})

Source: Amrah-Bouali et al., *Biomaterials*, 15, 4, 269–272, 1994; Lu et al., *Anal. Chem.*, 72, 13, 2886–2894, 2000; Chusuei, C.C., *Anal. Chem.*, 71, 1, 149–153, 1999; Yan et al., *Biomaterials*, 24, 15, 2585–2592, 2003; Battistoni et al., *Surf. Interface Anal.*, 29, 11, 773–781, 2000. With permission.
[a] Peak positions are calibrated by setting the adventitious C1s to 284.7eV.
[b] Powder form in calcite phase.

bonding of water molecules to the surface OH ions. The adsorbed water yields a broad band in the 3000–3500 cm^{-1} range and at about 1650 cm^{-1} (Stoch et al. 1999).

The phosphate group has a T_d symmetry resulting in four internal modes' being IR active: v_3 asymmetric stretching mode of vibration characterized by a strong, complex band in 1000–1150 cm^{-1} range and a medium intensity band at about 963 cm^{-1} due to v_1 symmetric stretching vibration (Tkalcec et al. 2001). The v_4 bending vibration of PO$_4$ is characterized by bands located at 560–610 cm^{-1}. A weak band at 430–463 cm^{-1} corresponds to v_2 bending vibration (Stoch et al. 1999).

The FTIR spectrum is very sensitive to the carbonate (CO$_3^{2-}$) group; even a very small amount of carbonate can be detected. Generally, carbonate can be incorporated into the HA structure by replacing the OH group (type A substitution) or by replacing PO$_4$ groups (type B substitution) (Stoch et al. 1999). The presence of CO$_3^{2-}$ as well as its position can be well determined by FTIR: type A substitutions have a singlet band at ~880 cm^{-1} (out-of-plane deformation, $v2$) and a doublet band at about 1450 and 1545 cm^{-1} (asymmetric stretching vibration, $v3$); the co-occurrence of CO$_3^{2-}$ absorption peaks recorded at 873 cm^{-1} ($v2$), 1412 and 1465 cm^{-1} ($v3$) indicates the incorporation of CO$_3^{2-}$ groups into HA lattice structure through the B-type substitution (Tkalcec et al. 2001).

Along with FTIR, Raman spectroscopy (RS) is another powerful analytical technique for the determination of molecular vibrations. The vibration activity is different in FTIR and RS due to the symmetry dependence of some chemical groups. In other words, some vibrations are both FTIR and RS active, but others are only FTIR or RS active. Therefore, complementary detailed information about the molecular vibrations could be well characterized by combing the FTIR and RS analysis. A detailed report about the application of RS in characterizing HA samples can be found in some related references (Mihály et al. 2009; Silva and Sombra 2004).

Surface Morphology

Surface morphology is another important coating characteristic that influences its performance. Surface morphology of the HA coating also affects the dissolution and bone apposition on the coating or bone ingrowth, because the coating surface, once implanted, is directly in contact with the bone and body fluid, thus playing a major role in the formation and maintenance of tissue integrity (Ben-Nissan, Milev, and Vago 2004). Scanning electron microscopy (SEM) and atomic force microscopy (AFM) are the most widely used techniques to characterize the surface morphology of HA coatings in practice.

In sol–gel technology, the solvent can be evaporated to leave a solid with a certain level of fine porosity. So, generally, according to the process characteristics of sol–gel technique, it is a common phenomenon that the sol–gel derived HA coating is a homogeneous, but rough with micro pores (about a few hundred microns) and even micro cracks (Massaro et al. 2001; Montenero et al. 2000). Figure 1.4 shows a typical SEM micrograph (Figure 1.4a, precursors: Ca(NO$_3$)$_2$•4H$_2$O and P$_2$O$_5$) and AFM image (Figure 1.4b, precursors: Ca(NO$_3$)$_2$•4H$_2$O and (NH$_4$)$_2$HPO$_4$)) about the surface morphology of sol–gel derived HA coating on the titanium and titanium alloy substrates. The coating looks quite uniform with a certain degree of porosity. The surface morphology of sol–gel derived HA coatings can be controlled by sol–gel parameters, such as different precursors (Guo and Li 2004; Gan and Pilliar 2004), post heat treatment (Hwang et al. 2000), the addition of chemical additives (Weng, Han et al. 2003), and surface roughness of the substrates as well as the thickness of the coating (You, Oh, and Kim 2001). Therefore, a customized surface morphology can be obtained according to the different requirements in practical application.

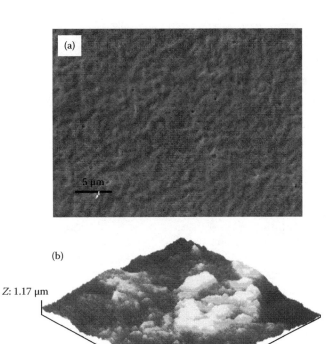

FIGURE 1.4
Surface morphology of sol–gel derived HA coating on Ti and Ti-alloy substrates: (a) SEM micrograph; (b) AFM image. (From *Massaro et al., Journal of Biomedical Materials Research*, 35, 11, 2791–2797, 2000. With permission.) The surface is uniform with certain degree of porosity.

Interfacial Analysis

Interfacial failure is reported to be one of the most predominate failure modes of HA-coated implants (Cheng et al. 2005). Generally, the interfacial adhesion of a sol–gel derived coating–substrate system comes from two aspects: the mechanical interlock and the chemical bonding. As for the mechanical interlock, surface pretreatment of metallic substrate is commonly applied, such as surface polishing and chemical treatment (Balakrishnan et al. 2007). However, it is believed that the contribution of mechanical interlock to adhesion is quite limited. The formation of certain chemical bonds at/near the coating substrate is strongly desired to improve the adhesion properties. Interfacial analysis (usually, the distribution of elements at/near the interface between the coating and substrate) is always carried out to provide the necessary bonding information about adhesion property. Time-of-flight secondary ion mass spectrometry (ToF-SIMS) (Cheng et al. 2005), glow discharge optical emission spectroscopy (GDOES) (Qi et al. 2008), and electron dispersive x-ray spectroscopy (EDS/EDX) (Zhang et al. 2006) are commonly used techniques for determining element distribution near the coating–substrate interface.

As a typical result, Figure 1.5 shows the SIMS composition depth profiles analysis of a sol–gel derived HA coating on Ti6Al4V substrate (precursors: $Ca(NO_3)_2 \cdot 4H_2O$ and P_2O_5). According to the distribution of the concerned elements along the cross section (i.e., Ca, O, P, and Ti), the cross section can be divided into three regions at/near the interface: the substrate (Rs) region, the transitional region (Rt), and the coating region (Rc). The transitional

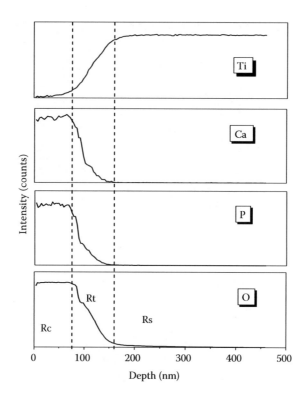

FIGURE 1.5

SIMS composition depth profile analysis of HA–Ti6Al4V interface. Three regions can be divided for cross sections: coating region (Rc), a transitional region (Rt), and substrate region (Rs). Within the transitional region, Ca and P concentrations decrease drastically from the coating toward the substrate, while the O concentration decrease gradually toward the substrate; Ti concentration increases gradually from transitional region to the substrate.

region (Rt) has a thickness of about 85 nm, and within the transitional region, the Ca and P concentrations decrease drastically toward the substrate, whereas O element decreases gradually from the coating region (Rc) to the substrate region (Rs), and the concentration of Ti element increases gradually from the transitional region (Rt) to the substrate region (Rs). It can be speculated from the existence of the transitional region and the distribution of the elements along the cross section that certain Ti–P–Ca–O compounds have formed at/near the interface (Montenero et al. 2000; Hsieh, Perng, and Chin 2002).

Mechanical Properties of Sol–Gel Derived HA Coating

Pull-Out Tensile Adhesion Strength and Interfacial Shear Strength

In view of the successful implantation as well as long-term stable performance, mechanical properties are important for HA-coated metallic implants. Among all the mechanical properties required, adhesion strength (or bonding strength) between the coating and metallic substrate is the most important property for those load-bearing implants. Two kinds of pull-out based methods are widely used to evaluate the adhesion strength: uniaxial pull-out tensile test method (as shown in Figure 1.6a) for the determination of tensile adhesion strength and shear pull-out test (Figure 1.6b) for the measurement of shear adhesion strength (Zhang et al. 2008; Ma, Wong et al. 2003; Implants for Surgery-

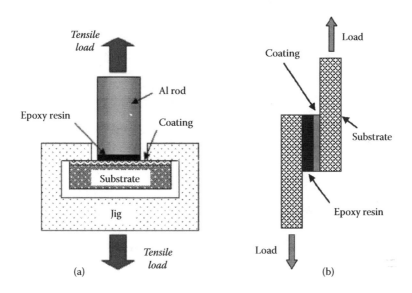

FIGURE 1.6
Schematic diagrams of pull-out testing methods for assessing of adhesion strength: (a) tensile adhesion strength test (from Zhang et al., *Thin Solid Films*, 516, 16, 5162–5167, 2008; with permission); (b) shear adhesion strength test.

Hydroxyapatite—Part 4: Determination of Coating Adhesion Strength 2002). Both of these two methods are tested using epoxy or super glues to fix the coating onto the counterpart. Accordingly, the bonding strength will be highly influenced by many factors, such as the uniformity of the epoxy layer, penetration depth of the glues, porosity and thickness of the coating, and alignment of the applied force. Therefore, it could be imagined that a wide range (large deviation) of adhesion strengths would be obtained, even for the coatings deposited with the same deposition method. According to the documented results, the adhesion strengths of HA coatings on metallic substrates prepared with different deposition techniques were summarized in Table 1.5. As stipulated by ISO standards (ISO13779), the recommended bonding strength (pull-out tensile test) should be not less than 15 MPa (Implants for Surgery-Hydroxyapatite—Part 2: Coatings of Hydroxyapatite 2000). The sol–gel method is thus acceptable for the preparation of HA coatings from the standpoint of adhesion (cf. Table 1.5).

More importantly, the adhesion strength after *in vitro* or even after *in vivo* tests is quite crucial in estimating the survivability of HA coating on implant surfaces. As reported, *in vivo* studies suggested that the failure of plasma sprayed HA-coated metallic implants mainly occurs at the coating–substrate interface, and the failure probability at this interface increased with the period of implantation because the strength of the coating–bone interface tends to increase with more healing time (Sun et al. 2001; Albrektsson 1998). Such degradation of adhesion is generally attributed to the dissolution behaviors related to the coating properties (e.g., impurity phases [TCP, CaO, etc.], crystallinity, cracks) (Lima et al. 2005), which would impair the mechanical properties (especially, adhesion strength) of the coating. Detailed description and discussion about the adhesion properties after *in vitro* and/or *in vivo* tests can be found in some related reports (Aksakal, Gavgali, and Dikici 2009; Zhang et al. 2008; Kim et al. 2005; Albrektsson 1998).

Noticeably, cohesion failure (failure within the coating layer) was always observed in those pull-out based tests (Figure 1.7), indicating that the obtained results are not the actual

TABLE 1.5

Adhesion Strength of HA Coatings Deposited with Different Deposition Methods

	Pulsed laser Deposition	Hot Isostatic Pressing	Thermal Spraying	Electrophoretic Deposition	Biomimetic Coating	Sputter Coating	Sol-Gel Method
Tensile adhesion strength (MPa)	30–58	–	10–60	<14	<15	>60	15–60
Shear adhesion strength (MPa)	–	4.0–5.5	11–26.8	8–23	<9.5	–	<17
References	(Wang et al. 1997; Garcia-Sanz et al. 1997)	(Onoki and Hashida 2006)	(Li, Khor, and Cheang 2002; Ding et al. 2001; Gu, Khor, and Cheang 2003; Yang, Chang, and Lee 2003; Li, Khor, and Cheang 2002; Kweh, Khor, and Cheang 2000)	(Han et al. 2001; Xiao and Liu 2006; Wei et al. 2001)	(Ma, Wong et al. 2003; Pena et al. 2006)	(Ding, Ju, and Lin 1999; Ding 2003)	(Balamurugan et al. 2006; Kim et al. 2004; Hsieh, Perng, and Chin 2002)

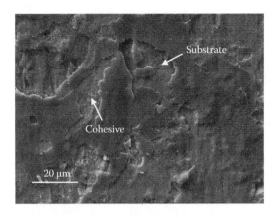

FIGURE 1.7
Typical fracture surface of fluoridated HA coatings after pull-out tensile test: a mixed failure mode is commonly observed, which consists of adhesion failure occurring at the coating–substrate interface, cohesion failure occurring within the coating, and gluing failure occurring at the epoxy-coating interface. (From Zhang et al., *Thin Solid Films*, 516, 16, 5162–5167, 2008. With permission.)

adhesion strengths between the coating and substrate (Zhang et al. 2008). In other words, those pull-out based testing methods are highly influenced by the coating characteristics and infiltration of epoxy, resulting in limited information about the adhesion properties at the coating–substrate interface. Therefore, other evaluation techniques/methods (e.g., scratch test) are necessary to get a sound evaluation of adhesion properties.

Evaluation of Interfacial Shear Strength

Generally, for bioceramic-coated, load-bearing implants, the adhesion behaviors of coating–substrate interface can be roughly classified into tensile and shear adhesion. Therefore, besides the tensile strength, the interfacial shear strength also serves as a crucial factor for those implants used as tooth root and hip joint replacement. Although certain quantitative evaluations have been done with the commonly used pull-out shear test, in viewing the intrinsic drawbacks of the "pull-out test," those obtained shear strength should be the "cohesive shear strength" rather than the "interfacial shear strength" (Li, Khor, and Cheang 2002). However, the shear lag strain approach described by Agrawal and Raj (Agrawal and Raj 1989, 1990), which utilizes the regular crack patterns obtained through the designed tests, appears useful and relatively straightforward for the determination of interfacial shear strength. Basically, this method relies on the development of transverse crack patterns in a brittle coating when the relatively ductile supporting substrate is plastically deformed under an applied uniaxial load. This crack behavior can be adequately described by a shear-lag analysis that directly relates crack density to the load transfer capabilities of the interface, and this shear lag theory predicts the establishment of a steady state of constant crack density observed at relatively high strain levels. For a coating of thickness t, the interfacial shear strength $\tau_{\max}$ can be determined by a simplified expression (Agrawal and Raj 1989):

$$\tau_{\max} = \sigma_f \frac{\pi t}{1.5\lambda}$$

where λ is the average steady-state crack spacing and σ_f is the tensile strength of the film (i.e., the coating). σ_f can be determined experimentally by measuring the maximum elastic strain, ε_f, of the coating (at which the initial formation of cracks is detected):

$$\sigma_f = \varepsilon_f E_f$$

where E_f is the Young's modulus of the coating.

The interfacial shear strength evaluated with the shear lag strain method are reported to be at least an order of magnitude greater than the pull-out shear strengths reported for plasma-sprayed and high-velocity oxy-fuel sprayed HA (Li, Khor, and Cheang 2002; Brossa et al. 1994; Gan, Wang, and Pilliar 2005). On the other hand, the reported interfacial shear strength between the coating surface and surrounding tissues *in vivo* was about 16.65 MPa after a 24-implantation (Yang et al. 1997). Therefore, from the standpoint of interfacial shear strength, sol–gel derived HA coatings appear quite promising for long-term load-bearing implants. However, it should be noted that the determination of interfacial shear strength using the shear lag analysis requires a limited film thickness, hence the low transverse residual stress within the coating.

Scratch Test

The scratch test is generally accepted as one of the simple and popular methods in assessing the adhesion properties of coating–substrate interface (Arias et al. 2003; Zhang et al. 2006). Basically, it is carried out by drawing a diamond tip over the coating surface to produce a scratch. The applied normal load is increased linearly until a critical load is reached at which the adhesion failure is induced at the coating–substrate interface. Thus, the critical load can be taken as a semiquantitative measurement of the coating–substrate adhesion strength, and the failure mode can provide further qualitative information upon the coating–substrate interface (Zhang et al. 2006). Figure 1.8 shows a typical scanning scratch

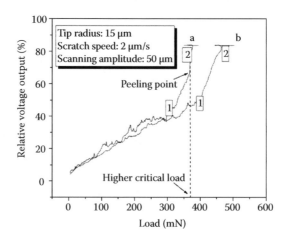

FIGURE 1.8
Coefficient of friction in terms of relative output voltage as a function of normal load in the scratch test of sol–gel derived coating: (a) HA coating, (b) fluoridated HA coating. At point 1, the indenter starts to plough into the coating, resulting in a steeper increase in coefficient of friction; at point 2, the indenter completely peels off the coating and scratches onto the substrate causing an abrupt increase in friction. (From Zhang et al., *Surface and Coatings Technology*, 200, 22–23 Spec. Iss., 6350–6354, 2006. With permission.)

curve of sol–gel derived HA and fluoridated HA coatings. The curves indicate a good adhesion between the coating and substrate, and reveal that the coating–substrate interfacial failure mode changes from brittle to ductile with fluorine ion were incorporated into the HA lattice structure (Zhang et al. 2006). That is to say, the scratch test can provide a lot of remarkable information about the coating–substrate interface, even though some of the data are just qualitative. Therefore, by considering the features of the pull-out tensile test, shear lag strain method, and scratch test, the combination of these three testing methods could be more helpful in getting a comprehensive understanding of the coating–substrate adhesion properties.

Toughness of Sol–Gel Derived HA Coating

Fracture toughness serves as a decisive factor in evaluating the functionality of coated implants and determines the level to which the material can be stressed in the presence of cracks, or equivalently, the magnitude of cracking that can be tolerated at a specific stress level. Regarding the interfacial fracture toughness of HA-coated Ti6Al4V implants, Filliaggi, Coombs, and Pilliar (1991) used a short bar chevron notch test and obtained the K_{IC} values of 0.6–1.41 MPa m$^{1/2}$. By using a single-edge notch-bend test, Tsui, Doyle, and Clyne (1998) reported some similar values of K_{IC} of about 0.28–1.1 MPa m$^{1/2}$. In addition, an indentation based method was also employed by Li, Khor, and Cheang (2002), and the corresponding value was reported as 0.48 MPa m$^{1/2}$ for K_{IC}.

However, for HA coatings prepared with the sol–gel method, indentation-based energy analysis method is preferred due to the limitation of the thickness of HA coating. Theoretically, the energy approach examines the energy difference before and after the cracking, which is responsible for the fracture of the coating. The energy difference would then be the energy release in the through-thickness cracking in the coating. The energy release can be obtained from a "step" that would be observed in the load–displacement curve for the indentation. Therefore, based on the energy difference before and after the crack generation, the fracture toughness of the coating can be determined as (Li, Diao, and Bhushan 1997):

$$K_{IC} = \left[\frac{\Delta U}{t} \frac{E_f}{2\pi C_R \left(1 - v_f^2\right)} \right]$$

where v_f is the Poisson's ratio of the coating, $2\pi C_R$ is the crack length in the coating plane, t and E_f are the coating thickness and elastic modulus, respectively, and ΔU is the strain energy difference before and after cracking. Figure 1.9 displays a typical load–displacement curve of indentation together with the corresponding SEM micrograph, which can be used readily for toughness evaluation of the HA coating (Zhang et al. 2008).

Residual Stress Measurement

Residual stress is inherently induced in any coating deposited by a method with a high temperature process due to the differences in the thermal properties between the coating and the substrate. Residual stress in the coating might vary with coating thickness, deposition parameters, etc. Therefore, both tensile and compressive residual stresses have been

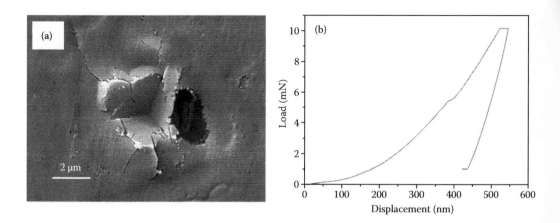

FIGURE 1.9
(a) SEM micrograph of nanoindentation of sol–gel derived HA coating and (b) its corresponding load–displacement curve.

reported with different values. For instance, tensile residual stresses of 200–450 and 20–40 MPa were reported by Brown, Turner, and Reiter (1994) and Tsui, Doyle, and Clyne (1998), respectively. In contrast, a compressive residual stress of about 35–78 MPa was reported by Yang, Chang, and Lee (2003), and Yang and Chang (2005). The differences may result from the coating preparation method and process, as well as the method employed for the measurement of residual stress.

Considerable efforts have been made in recent years to understand and measure the residual stresses developed during the preparation of HA coatings (Tsui, Doyle, and Clyne 1998; Yang and Chang 2005). Popular among the various methods is the XRD method, which is a nondestructive and simple technique for residual stress measurement. However, since this method is based on the shift of the peaks in XRD patterns, the use of this method is limited by some factors of the coating, such as surface roughness, phase composition, and especially the doping of some expected ions. Considering the intrinsic characteristic of residual stress, a "wafer curvature method" was developed to evaluate residual stress, especially for sol–gel derived coatings (Watanabe et al. 2002; Xie and Hawthorne 2003): on a relatively thin substrate, the residual stress distributed in the coating layer will cause the substrate to bend, and the induced curvature for the coated substrate depends on the force, the elastic properties, and the thickness for both substrate and coating. By measuring the curvature difference before and after the removal of the coating (Δk), the residual stress, σ_R, in the coating, can be calculated:

$$\sigma_R = \frac{\Delta k E_f \left[h^2 + \left(E_s h_T^3\right)/(E_f h) + (E_t h^3)/(E_s h_T) + h_T^2 + 3(h + h_T)^2 \right]}{6(h + h_T)(1 - v_S)}$$

where h_T is the total thickness of the substrate plus coating, h is the coating thickness, v_S is the Poisson's ratio of the substrate, and E_S and E_f are the Young's modulus of the substrate and the coating, respectively. Detailed description about the curvature measurement has been reported by Xie and Hawthorne (2003). Figure 1.10 depicts the typical profiles of measured curvatures for sol–gel derived fluoridated HA coatings (Zhang et al. 2007). A larger

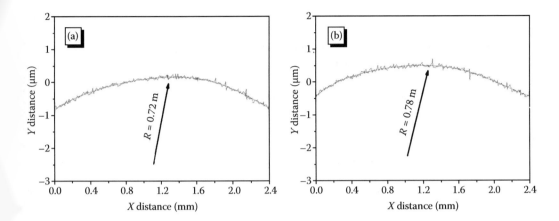

FIGURE 1.10
Typical profilometry results of measured curvatures for sol–gel derived fluoridated HA coating: (a) before removing the coating and (b) after removing the coating. The reduction of curvature caused by the removal of fluoridated HA coatings indicates a tensile residual stress existing in the coatings. (From Zhang et al., *Engineering Fracture Mechanics*, 74, 12, 1884–1893, 2007. With permission.)

curvature radius after removing the coating indicates a tensile residual stress existed in the coating.

A great number of possible parameters can cause residual stresses, depending on the deposition technique. Structure-related residual stress results from the following three aspects: thermal stress, growth-induced stress, and structural mismatch-induced (including lattice distortion) stress (Zhang et al. 2004). In a sol–gel deposition process, the thermal stress comes from the drying and firing process coupled with the difference in the coefficient of thermal expansion (CTE) between the coating and the substrate, the growth-induced stress comes from the coating shrinkage driven by capillary stresses during the drying and firing process, and the structural mismatch-induced stress comes from the difference in crystal structure between the coating and the substrate as well as the lattice distortion within the coating as a result of defects or incorporation of foreign molecules or molecule groups. Mainly, thermal stress, σ_{Rt}, always contributes more to the total residual stress in the coating, and it can be calculated by (Watanabe et al. 2002):

$$\sigma_{Rt} = \frac{\Delta\alpha\Delta T E_f}{1 - v_S}$$

where $\Delta\alpha$ is the difference of CTE between the interested coating and the metallic substrate and ΔT is the temperature variation during drying or firing. For example, CTE of HA is 15×10^{-6}/K, whereas that of Ti6Al4V substrate is about 8.9×10^{-6}/K (Zhang et al. 2006). Thereafter, the residual stress caused by thermal mismatch between HA coating and Ti6Al4V substrate should be tensile.

The presence of residual stress in the coating serves as an important influencing factor in determining the durability of the coated implants. Previous work has demonstrated that the existence of residual stress in HA coatings can alter the concentration of supernatant species in solution: tensile residual stresses enhancing dissolution and compressive residual stress impeding dissolution (Han, Xu, and Lu 2001; Yang and Chang 2001). In addition, tensile residual stress will promote multiple cracking of the coating, and the compressive residual stress can weaken the bonding and bonding strength at the coating–substrate interface. Therefore, since both the tensile and compressive residual stresses exert detrimental influences on HA-coated implants, it is desirable to produce coatings on metallic implants without any unexpected residual stress.

In Vitro Assay

It is well known that any biomaterial must be thoroughly evaluated to determine its biocompatibility/bioactivity and whether it functions appropriately in actual biomedical applications. Generally, two kinds of evaluation techniques are employed for such purposes: *in vitro* (in a glass tube) and *in vivo* (in a living organism) tests. Although *in vivo* tests are the most direct and reliable evaluation methods for biomaterials, their results are normally difficult to obtain and interpret due to a lack of animal sources and the complexity of different cellular responses. (During *in vivo* tests, the cells that migrate to the implant surface contain different cell lineage, and the final results are demonstrated by the fact that the progeny of these cells may form a variety of tissue types adjacent to the implant.) (Boyan et al. 2001). *In vitro* testing can provide more rapid and relatively inexpensive data compared with *in vivo* testing. Moreover, *in vitro* testing can provide useful initial screening of materials and can aid in understanding the performance of a material *in vivo*. These valuable insights could also help to determine whether an implant/device needs further evaluation in expensive *in vivo* experimental models and minimize the amount of animals required in *in vivo* testing (Ratner et al. 1996). *In vitro* tests of biomaterials can be carried out in any cell-free or cell-containing environment to study their biocompatibility and bioactivity. In particular, cell-free solutions allow the study of chemical and mineralogical changes of the material under conditions that simulate the physiological interactions between the material surface and the surrounding tissues.

Dissolution Behavior

A prerequisite for any implant used in orthopedic or dental treatment is permanent fixation to the surrounding tissues with no intervening gaps or fibrous tissues (Vedantam and Ruddlesdin 1996). According to the *in vivo* and *in vitro* studies as well as more than a decade's clinical practice with HA-coated prostheses, there is general agreement that the originally desired benefits of HA coatings, that is, earlier fixation and stability with more bone ingrowth or outgrowth, can be achieved. However, doubts still exist concerning the durability of the fixation (Greenspan 1999). One of the most important events occurring at the bone–implant interface is the resorption of the HA coatings, also called degradation or coating loss (Bloebaum et al. 1994; Dalton and Cook 1995). Although some resorption or dissolution is, of course, essential to trigger bone–implant bonding, the fast resorption could lead to disintegration of the coating, with rapid loss of the bonding strength between it and the substrates, resulting in delamination, the production of particles, and loss of mechanical fixation. It is reported that a decrease as high as 31.6% was observed for plasma-sprayed HA coatings after only 2 weeks' immersion in SBF (Gu, Khor, and Cheang 2003). Other studies have shown resorption of HA coatings up to 2 years after implantation and a complete loss of a 60-μm-thick HA coating after 4 years (Sun et al. 2001). Aebli et al. (2003) carried out a histological study of a proximally HA-coated femoral component and found that the HA coating had completely degraded after 9.5 years' implantation.

Generally, the dissolution behavior of HA coatings are investigated in some Ca^{2+} ion free simulated physiological saline solution, such as Tris-buffered physiological saline solution (TPS) (Wang, Zhang et al. 2007) or citric acid-modified phosphate buffer solution (CPBS) (Weng, Zhang et al. 2003). Two competitive processes are commonly used to describe the surface reactions during the dissolution progress, dissolution and reprecipitation (Dorozhkin 1997). For HA coating, the dissolution/reprecipitation process can be described as:

$$Ca_{10}(PO_4)_6(OH)_2 \Leftrightarrow 10Ca^{2+} + 6PO_4^{3-} + 2OH^-$$

If the dissolution process is predominant, the coating will be dissolved continuously until a thermodynamic equilibrium is established for these two concurrent processes, and vice versa. Therefore, after incubating the coatings in the testing solutions, they will inevitably be dissolved quickly at first in such an unsaturated environment, and a thin Nernst layer will be formed in the solution near to the coating surface, which results in a certain reduction of coating dissolution rate.

The degradation of HA coating is strongly influenced by the coating phase composition (phase purity and crystallinity). Accordingly, using different solubilities of CaPs, the *in vivo* degradation rates of CaPs can be predicated and follow the order of (Yang, Kim, and Ong 2005; Ducheyne, Radin, and King 1993):

$$ACP \gg TTCP \approx \alpha\text{-}TCP > DCPD > DCP > OCP > \beta\text{-}TCP \gg HA$$

where ACP denotes amorphous calcium phosphate, TTCP is tetracalcium phosphate, α-TCP id α-tricalcium phosphate, DCPD is dicalcium phosphate dehydrate, DCP is dicalcium phosphate, OCP is octocalcium phosphate, and β-TCP is β-tricalcium phosphate.

Therefore, the presence of ACP (related to crystallinity) or other impurity phase (e.g., TCP) can cause a higher degradation rate at the initial stage after the immersion of HA-coated implants into the testing solution, followed by a "constant rate" dissolution of the remaining coating (Figure 1.11).

On the other hand, it is well known that actual human body fluid contains various kinds of organic components (such as carbohydrates and proteins), and these organic components are thought to exert certain influences on the degradation of HA coating (Dorozhkin, Dorozhkina, and Epple 2003; Liu et al. 2003). As a typical result, Figure 1.11 indicates the dissolution behaviors of sol–gel derived HA coating in glucose-modified TPS solution and in albumin-containing TPS solution. The results indicate that the addition of glucose has no significant influence on dissolution behaviors of FHA coatings in comparison with the tests in TPS. However, in comparison with the testing in TPS or G-TPS, the presence of albumin results in a significantly higher Ca^{2+} concentration released in the solution during the whole testing period.

Moreover, residual stress may affect the thermodynamics of dissolution behaviors by altering the chemical potential of the coatings. For those stress-free coatings, the unit free energy change of an equilibrium status, ΔG^0, can be described as (Han, Xu, and Lu 2001; Sergo, Sbaizero, and Clarke 1997):

$$\Delta G^0 = -RT \ln K_{sp}$$

where R is the gas constant, T is the temperature, and K_{sp} is the solubility product of the corresponding coating. If the constraint of a stress-free solid is removed and a stress, σ_{ss},

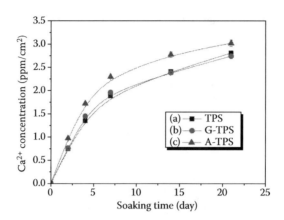

FIGURE 1.11
Dissolution behavior of sol–gel derived HA coatings in different testing conditions: (a) Tris-buffered physiological saline solution (TPS), (b) glucose-modified TPS (G-TPS), and (c) albumin-containing TPS (A-TPS).

is applied, such as a residual, the system is no longer in equilibrium because the chemical potential of the coatings is altered by an amount proportional to the stress, namely, $\sigma_{ss}\Omega/3$ per unit volume. (Ω is the unit volume of the species under consideration.) As a result, according to the thermodynamic analysis, with the presence of residual stress, additional free energy for the dissolution equilibrium becomes available in the form of elastic strain energy stored in the coatings, and the new equilibrium condition is represented by an altered value of the solubility product, K_{sp}^{σ}:

$$\Delta G^0 - \frac{\sigma_{ss}\Omega}{3} = -RT \ln K_{sp}^{\sigma}$$

The negative sign implies that a compressive residual stress will hinder, whereas a tensile residual stress will enhance the dissolution. Therefore, the ratio of the solubility product under different stresses (e.g., σ_1 and σ_2) is:

$$\frac{K_{sp}^{\sigma_1}}{K_{sp}^{\sigma_2}} = \exp\left[\left(\sigma_1 - \sigma_2\right)\frac{\Omega}{3RT}\right]$$

This expression can be used to estimate the change of solubility product owing to the presence of different residual stresses. Therefore, if the residual stresses in the sol–gel derived HA coatings are tensile stresses, a higher dissolution rate would be observed than the stress-free coatings correspondingly.

All in all, even though the mass loss caused by dissolution is somehow detrimental to the adhesion, it is still believed that the initial dissolution behaviors are quite beneficial to the healing process as well as the long-term successful osteointegration (Martini et al. 2003). First, the initial fast dissolution of the coating will result in a local super saturated environment (e.g., Ca^{2+}), which is more favorable for the nucleation and growth of bonelike apatite, speeding up the formation of chemical bonds between the implant and surrounding tissues. On the other hand, a rough implant surface appears to be favorable for cell attachment and particularly suitable for primary implant stability as compared to a smooth implant surface. HA coatings with controllable degradation rate are much desired and can be realized by altering the phase composition, doping of other ions (F^-, Mg^{2+}, Zn^{2+}, etc.) (Cai et al. 2009; Wang, Sam et al. 2007; Miao et al. 2005), and controlling the residual stress.

In Vitro Test in Acellular Simulated Body Fluid

Currently, Simulated Body Fluid (SBF), which was first developed by Kokubo et al. in 1991, has been routinely used as an effective *in vitro* testing method to predict the *in vivo* bone bioactivity of various biomaterials (Kokubo and Takadama 2006). The development of SBF is based on the concept that the essential requirement for an artificial material to bond to living bone is the formation of bonelike apatite on its surface when implanted into the living body. The acellular SBF has similar inorganic ion concentrations to those of human blood plasma (as shown in Table 1.6) and can reproduce the formation process of bonelike apatite on biomaterials *in vitro*. Furthermore, this test can be used for the determination of the number of animals used during *in vivo* testing, as well as the duration of animal experiments. For a material to be bioactive *in vivo*, it must possess the capability to induce bonelike apatite formation on its surface in SBF. Many studies have been done on HA-coated metallic implants in SBF, which verified the intrinsic bioactivity of HA to be used as coatings (Gu, Khor, and Cheang 2003; Nagarajan, Raman, and Rajendran 2010; Stoch et al. 2005). On the other hand, the response of HA coatings in SBF was observed to be highly affected by coating phase composition, crystallinity, morphology, etc. (Ducheyne, Radin, and King 1993; Khor et al. 2003), and the precipitation rate of bonelike apatite was directly dependent on the Ca^{2+} ion concentration in the SBF at the vicinity of the coating surface (Lee et al. 2005; Montenero et al. 2000). As mentioned above, besides the HA phase, there also exists some other phases, including TCP, TTCP, and CaO, which possess higher solubilities than that of the HA phase. Therefore, in SBF testing, the dissolution of such impure phases will accelerate the precipitation rate of bonelike apatite through significantly enhancing the Ca^{2+} ion concentration at a localized area near to the implant surface (Gu, Khor, and Cheang 2003; Khor et al. 2003). To some extent, this indicates that the existence of impure phases in HA coating could improve the bioactivity of HA-coated metallic implants.

However, actual body fluid contains not only the inorganic components, but also various kinds of organic components (Table 1.6), and the organic components would exert noticeable influence on the implants (Dorozhkin, Dorozhkina, and Epple 2003; Wang, Sam et al. 2007). Therefore, it is unwise to neglect the influences of organic components in *in vitro* tests. Jaou et al. (2000) and Balint et al. (2001) reported that although sugar and/or glucose have a minor influence on crystallization of HA, they significantly inhibit the crystallization process of fluoridated apatite (FA). This effect was attributed to the formation of nonstoichiometric apatite in the presence of sugar. The inhibition effects of carbohydrates on the bone mineralization were also reported by other researchers (Pearce, Hancock, and Gallagher 1984; Balint et al. 2001). Dorozhkin, Dorozhkina, and Epple (2003) concluded that glucose exhibited negligible influence on crystallization of calcium phosphate based on *in vitro* tests with the glucose-modified SBF solution. On effects of proteins, extensive investigations have been done on CaP biomaterials, especially on HA (Luo and Andrade 1998; Xie, Riley, and Chittur 2001). It has been reported that plasma proteins would adsorb immediately on the surface of HA after it was implanted *in vivo*, and the initial cellular

TABLE 1.6

Chemical Composition of Human Blood Plasma Compared to Ion Concentration of Kokubo's SBF

	Inorganic Ion Concentration (mM)							Organic Composition (mg/dL)			
	Ca^{2+}	HPO_4^{2-}	Na^+	Cl^-	Mg^{2+}	K^+	HCO_3^-	SO_4^{2-}	Albumin	Globulin	Fibrinogen	Glucose
Blood plasma	2.5	1	142	103	1.5	5	27	0.5	3300–4000	880–3530	340–430	100
Kokubo's C-SBF	2.5	1	142	148	1.5	5	4.2	0.5	–	–	–	–

Source: Wang et al., *Materials Science and Engineering C*, 27, 2, 244–250, 2007. With permission.

response was partly dependent on the proteins adsorbed by the implant surfaces (Bender et al. 2000). The first protein layer adsorbed on the implant surface affects the cellular adhesion, differentiation, and production of extracellular matrix production (Combes and Rey 2002; Ducheyne and Qiu 1999). It also affects dissolution (Bender et al. 2000), nucleation, and crystal growth of HA as well as the final fixation between the implant and surrounding tissues (Xie, Riley, and Chittur 2001). Albumin is usually selected for this kind of study due to its high concentration in blood plasma, favorable diffusion coefficient, and ability to bind other ions and molecules (Jenney and Anderson 2000). It has been reported that albumin could slow down the nucleation rate and growth rate of new bonelike apatite in albumin-containing SBF.

Cell Response to HA Coating

Cell culture methods have been used to evaluate the biological compatibility of a material for more than two decades. Investigations on cell responses to materials can provide more details of understanding cell–materials interactions and can aid in establishing actual biological responses to artificial materials (Knabe et al. 2000). Because HA-coated metallic implants are used for hard tissue replacement/repairing, *in vitro* models using osteoblastic cells are essential and valuable tools for the initial assessment of candidate implants. Osteoblastic cells, which arise from pluripotential mesenchymal stem cells, have a set of distinguishing characteristics that include the ability to synthesize osteoid or bone matrix and to mineralize the osteoid to get the calcified bone (Aubin et al. 1995). Since then, osteoblastic cell lines are commonly employed for *in vitro* cellular assessments of hard tissue implants.

Initial Cell Attachment on HA-Coated Implant

The fixation of implants to bone is based on the process of osteointegration, which leads to direct apposition of mature living bone onto the implant surface (Menezes et al. 2003; Dorota et al. 2005). Since that osteointegration process is strictly mediated by osteoblastic cells, the fate of such implants is thus determined by the response of cells to the material's surface. Therefore, the implant should create favorable conditions for osteoblast attachment, spreading, growth, differentiation, and functionalization. Virtually, in a physiological environment, all implant surfaces become immediately coated with a 1- to 10-nm-thick adsorbed protein layer before cells can adhere to the material (Kasemo 1998; Tengvall 2003). The rapid adsorption of proteins effectively translates the structure and composition of the foreign surface into a biological language, which is also a response to the following host responses (Wilson et al. 2005). As such, when the cells arrive at the implant surface, they can only "see" a protein-covered surface. Those adsorbed proteins offer necessary binding sites to those anchorage-dependent cells, leading to the initial cell attachment onto the surface of biomaterials. For anchorage-dependent cells (e.g., osteoblastic cells), initial cell attachment and spreading are crucial prerequisites in determination of long-term viability of cells on the implant surface, involving DNA synthesis and cell growth (cell proliferation), differentiation, mineralization, and successful osseointegration (Folkman and Moscona 1978; Baxter et al. 2002). Therefore, a quick attachment of a certain amount of osteoblastic cells and the following rapid cell spreading are strongly expected.

Figure 1.12 shows the typical morphological change sequences of osteoblastic cell (MG63) spreading on sol–gel derived HA coatings during the first 4 h of incubation (Wang, Zhang et al. 2008). The process of cell attachment and spreading can be described by the following steps: (1) adsorption of proteins on coating surface (surface roughness plays a positive

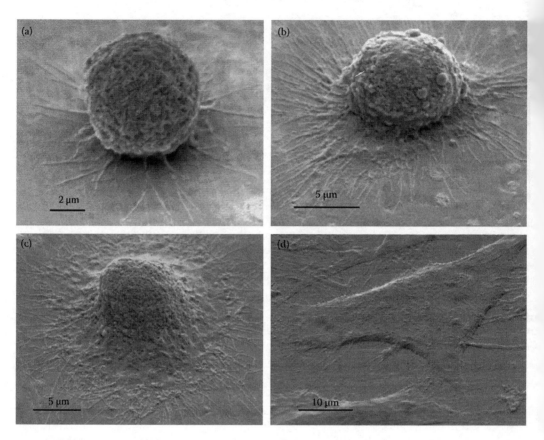

FIGURE 1.12
Morphological changes of osteoblastic cells after incubating on HA coatings for up to 4 h: (a) 0.5 h, (b) 1 h, (c) 2 h, (d) 4 h. The process of initial cell attachment and spreading can be described as the following continuous steps: contact and attachment of cells (a), centrifugal growth of filopodia (b), cytoplasma spreading (c), and cell flattening (d). (From Wang et al., *Journal of Biomedical Materials Research Part A*, 84, 3, 769–776, 2008. With permission.)

role); (2) contact and attachment of cells onto the protein layer (surface roughness does not have an effect unless very rough—a difference of more than a few microns); (3) centrifugal growth of filopodia; (4) cytoplasma spreading; and finally (5) cell flattening. It should be emphasized that these different stages are not discretely separable but are different phases of a contiguous progress. Recognition and studies of these different morphological events during initial cell adhesion and spreading on HA-coated implants would be of great value in understanding the behavior of osteoblastic cells *in vitro* and *in vivo*.

Cell Morphology

Along with the initial cell attachment and spreading, further cell spreading and the corresponding morphology also should be investigated in order to evaluate cell viability on the coating surface (Folkman and Moscona 1978). Figure 1.13 shows typical SEM micrographs of MG63 cells after a culture duration of 3 days on sol–gel derived HA coating surface. All cells spread well and grew favorably throughout the coating surface (Figure 1.13a). Under higher magnification (Figure 1.13b), the cells are seen flattened and attached tightly on coating surface with their filopodium and lamellipodium, suggesting good cell viability

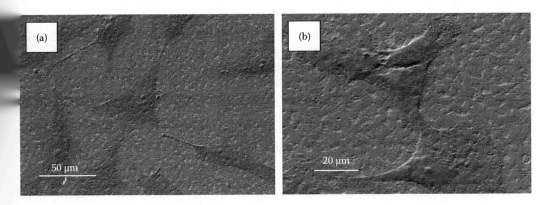

FIGURE 1.13
Morphology of MG63 cell after 3 days on sol–gel derived HA coating at (a) low magnification and (b) high magnification. All cells spread well and grow favorably throughout the coating surface, suggesting good cell viability of the HA coating. (From Wang et al., *Materials Science and Engineering C*, 27, 2, 244–250, 2007. With permission.)

on the fabricated HA coating (Wang, Zhang et al. 2007). As reported, the well-spread cells on the fabricated HA coating surface are believed to be favorable for the following DNA synthesis and cell growth.

Cell Proliferation and Differentiation

Following the initial cell attachment and spreading, those well-spread cells will step into the stages of proliferation and functionalization. Roughly, the progress from an initially attached osteoblastic cell to well-differentiated mature osteoblast (osteocyte) can be divided into three stages: proliferation, differentiation or extracellular matrix synthesis and maturation, and mineralization (Stein and Lian 1993).

During the first several days following cell attachment and spreading, cells try to reproduce, and an active cell proliferation is directly reflected by the exponential increase of cell number as well as the deposition of type I collagen. On the other hand, several genes related to cell cycle (e.g., histone) and cell growth (e.g., c-*myc*, c-*fos*, and c-*jun*) are actively expressed and can be used to monitor those mitotic activities (Stein and Lian 1993). Commonly, cell proliferation (increase in cell number) is directly monitored through the following two quantitative methods: cell counting under a microscope (with a hemocytometer) and MTT assay (Kim et al. 2005; Wang, Zhang et al. 2007). These two methods are much easier than other protein- or gene-based methods. Noticeably, the variation in cell numbers is sometimes employed to assess and screen the cytotoxicity of a biomaterial (cell viability). Roughly, a decrease in cell number during the culture span reveals a cytotoxic environment caused by the biomaterial, or the material itself is toxic to the cells.

Immediately after the down-regulation of proliferation, cell phenotypes associated with osteoblastic cell differentiation can be detected, indicating that the cells step into the differentiation stage (Stein and Lian 1993). The most frequently used markers of osteoblast differentiation are alkaline phosphatase (ALP), and osteocalcin (OC). As an early differentiation marker, ALP is an enzyme associated with calcification. This is an early marker of osteoblastic cell differentiation because activity is greatest just before mineralization actually begins. It is reported that an enhanced expression of this enzyme is apparently needed just before the onset of matrix mineralization, providing localized enrichment of inorganic phosphate, one of the components of apatite (the mineral phase of bone) (Boyan et al. 2001; Kartsogiannis and Ng 2004). High levels of bone ALP are usually detected in both preosteoblasts (osteoblastic cells) and osteoblasts *in vivo* and in differentiating osteoblastic cells *in vitro*. Along with ALP, OC, known as a late marker of cell differentiation, is a small molecular weight protein (5.7 kDa) produced by osteoblasts and has the ability to chelate Ca^{2+} to form bone minerals (Stein and Lian 1993; Gerstenfeld et al. 1987). For this reason, it is a particularly effective marker of a well-differentiated osteoblastic cell. Generally, once mineralization is initiated, ALP will decrease, whereas osteocalcin accumulation continues, reflecting an expression related to deposition of mineral for the latter.

As one of calcium phosphate ceramics, sintered HA has been well established as a bioactive material that enhances osteoblastic cell viability and osteointegration with host bone (Hench 1991; Greenspan 1999). Those valuable biological properties are well maintained when HA is used as coatings on metallic implants. In comparison with those bioinert metallic implants, many studies reported that the fabricated HA coatings on their surface not only can help to stimulate cell growth and DNA synthesis, but also can enhance the ALP and OC activities and the mineralization of extracellular matrix (Massaro et al. 2001; Yang, Kim, and Ong 2005; Li et al. 2005). However, these desired biological properties of HA coatings are highly dependent on coating surface roughness. Lee et al. (2002) investigated the cell responses to HA coatings with different roughness values (R_a), 0.67 and 10.37 µm, and concluded that the smoother surface was more favorable for cell attachment than the rougher one. Moreover, Kim et al. (2005) reported that the higher surface roughness ($R_a = 0.84$ µm) could significantly enhance the number of attached cells compared with the lower surface roughness ($R_a = 0.22$ µm), but there was no significant difference regarding cell proliferation and differentiation. An enhanced effect on cell differentiation activities and the formation of bone nodules was observed in other researchers' studies (Li et al. 2005; Perizzolo et al. 2001; Borsari et al. 2005).

On the other hand, several other studies also indicated that the behavior of cultured osteoblastic cells are affected by the crystallinity and phase composition of the prepared HA coatings (Yang, Kim, and Ong 2005). Kim et al. (2005) claimed that on the coatings with higher crystallinity (>76%), the cells attached and proliferated well and expressed ALP and OC to a higher degree as compared to the poorly crystallized coatings (~43% crystallinity). Chou, Marek, and Wagner (1999) reported that the lower crystalline coatings with some other impure phases (CaO, TCP, etc.) were favorable to cell attachment but exerted inhibiting effects on cell proliferation due to the elevated medium pH value caused by the dissolution of the impure phase. However, other studies illustrated insignificant influences on cell attachment, proliferation, and differentiation or mineralization with respect to different crystallinity and/or phase compositions (Siebers et al. 2006).

Although it is commonly accepted that the HA coatings could improve the *in vitro* biological properties for those metallic implants, there still exist some inconsistent or even conflicting viewpoints regarding the influences of coating properties on cell responses. Considering those differences in coating preparation, experimental setup, testing methods, etc., it is hard to judge which one is more acceptable.

In Vivo Animal Trial

Practically speaking, the goal of *in vivo* animal trial of implants or devices is to determine and predict whether such implants/devices possess potential harm to the human body by evaluations under conditions simulating clinical end-use applications (Anderson 2001). *In vivo* models allow the direct evaluation of toxicity of a biomaterial and the efficacy of a biomaterial as implant/device within a therapeutic application. Therefore, those osteointegration (the close apposition of bone to implant surface) examinations during *in vivo* studies are essential for further analysis about the effect of the implant on the expression of osteoblast phenotype and even for future clinical application.

Histological analysis of HA-coated implants has shown that bone ingrowth with osseous integration occurs as early as 10 days following implantation (Furlong and Osborn 1991). Thereby, HA coating could provide the crucial initial fixation requirement for the success of an implant. Furthermore, a histomorphometric study by Moroni et al. (1994) comparing the percentage of bone bonding to plasma sprayed HA-coated and uncoated implants in dogs revealed a significant increase in bone amount in the HA-coated implants. They also showed enhancement of bone-to-pin osseointegration and interfacial strength in HA-coated pins as compared to uncoated pins in a sheep study (Moroni et al. 1998). Figure 1.14 shows the typical histological micrograph on the enhancing effect of HA coating on bone–implant fixation (Hirai et al. 2004): after 4 weeks' implantation in the transfemoral drill hole on a rat, the area of the new bone of the cross-sectional implants was 0.108 mm^2 for sol–gel HA-coated titanium and only 0.087 mm^2 for uncoated samples. That is to say, the implant with HA coating had comparatively higher bone apposition ability than the uncoated implant. Similar results have been reported in other studies (Ramires et al. 2003; Gerber et al. 2003; You, Yeo et al. 2005).

Along with the histological analysis, extensive investigations have been conducted on the bonding strength of HA-coated implants during *in vivo* animal trials. For instance, in the studies of Oonishi et al. (1989), the adhesion strength between the implant and bone was ~0.53 and ~1.35 MPa for uncoated and HA-coated implants, respectively, at 2 weeks after implantation, whereas those bonding strengths increased to ~7.5 and ~14.15 MPa at 6 weeks, correspondingly. Other short-term *in vivo* trials also elucidated the similar trend regarding the bone-implant bonding property (Yang, Lin et al. 1997; Chang et al. 1997; Dalton et al. 1995). Essentially, it is revealed that those rapid and positive responses of HA coatings *in vivo* benefit significantly from the fast dissolution of related impure phases (e.g., amorphous phase, TCP), which results in an increase in Ca^{2+} and PO$_4^{3-}$ ion concentrations in local areas around the implant–bone interface. Nevertheless, from the viewpoint of long-term stability, whether the loss of HA coating could maintain such a desired bonding strength between the implant and surrounding tissue is questioned.

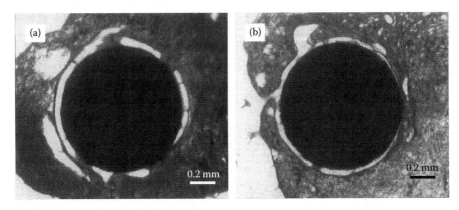

FIGURE 1.14
Histological sections of the nondecalcified sections after 4 weeks' implantation in a transfemoral drill hole on a male Wister rat: (a) sol–gel coated titanium, (b) uncoated titanium. The area of the bone of the cross-sectional implants was 0.108 mm^2 for sol–gel HA-coated titanium and 0.087 mm^2 for uncoated titanium. (From Hirai et al., *Journal of the American Ceramic Society*, 87, 1, 29–34, 2004. With permission.)

Recent Trends Related to Sol–Gel Derived HA Coatings

Even though previous studies on HA-coated metallic implants have shown good fixation to the host bones and increased bone ingrowth into the implants, there are still many concerns about the application of HA coatings, especially the related long-term stability of HA coating (Greenspan 1999). One of the most serious concerns raised is the resorption or degradation of HA coating in a biological environment. Faster resorption or degradation rate is likely to result in faster and stronger fixation in the initial stage of implantation, but could also lead to disintegration of the coating, including rapid loss of interface bonding strength of the coating–substrate and implant-surrounding tissue, delamination of HA coating, etc. (Bloebaum et al. 1994). Hence, the stability and integrity of the coating on metallic implants should be carefully considered prior to any clinical application. By contrast, a controlled resorption or degradation rate may allow the surrounding bone the opportunity to replace the resorbed coating at the similar rate and achieve the desired long-term stability.

Unfortunately, particles or particulates, as the products of HA degradation, may cause severe damage or complications to the bone–implant system. It is reported that the HA particles can be resorbed by macrophages if their size is sufficiently small compared to the macrophages (approximately 30 μm) (Mullermai, Voigt, and Gross 1990). When a macrophage phagocytizes the particles, the cells release cytokines, prostaglandins, and collagenases almost immediately. If the particles do not dissolve within the life span of the macrophage, more macrophages will accumulate at the site in response to the release of cytokines to digest the dead macrophages and those undissolved HA particulates. As well, particles larger than a macrophage (>30 μm), will not be digested by macrophages and will probably become engulfed by a giant cell. The excessive cellular reaction to HA particulates and the stimulation of a foreign-body response could lead to a decrease in local pH value, which disrupts the bone remodeling process, causing the dissolution/resorption of both HA coating and bone (Gross, Walsh, and Swarts 2004). Additional problems could arise if particulate debris travels to the implant–bone interface, producing third-body wear and component loosening/failure. Morscher, Hefti, and Aebi (1998) investigated six revisions of HA-coated implants follow-up over 10 years after successful primary implantation. They found that HA granules had embedded in all of the examined implants, and as high as 66.7% of them had loosened and 50% of them showed severe osteolysis of the proximal femur.

Understanding that the essential issue of the above problems is the high rate of biodegradation, a possible solution has been proposed: fabrication of macro- and micro-textured porous surfaces to overcome the problems of dissolution and micromotion. Overgaard et al. (1998) compared the influences of different surface textures (microporous and grit-blasted) of plasma sprayed HA-coated implants on the mechanical fixation, bone ingrowth, bone remodeling, and gap healing after implanting the implants in dogs for 16 weeks. It was concluded that the microporous HA-coated surface could provide better fixation for both interfaces of coating–substrate and implant-surround tissues. What's more, more new bone was generated on the microporous HA-coated implants to replace and/or compensate the resorption of HA coating, suggesting a possible long-term fixation for this kind of implant. However, this kind of HA coating commonly possesses a larger thickness, which could cause the potential risk of generating large particulate debris. Another possible way is the incorporation of F^- into HA lattice structure through the $F^- \leftrightarrow OH^-$ exchange to form a fluoridated HA coating ($Ca_{10}(PO_4)_6F_x(OH)_{2-x}$, where x is the degree of fluoridation: $x = 0$, pure HA; $x = 2$, pure FA; $0 < x < 2$, fluoridated hydroxyapatite [FHA]). Considering the advantages of the sol–gel method (cf. Section 1.3.1), preliminary studies on fluoridated HA coatings have been successfully produced using the sol–gel method on titanium alloy substrates (Zhang et al. 2006). The incorporation of F^- cannot only reduce the degradation rate of the coating, but also benefit the interfacial adhesion properties of the coating–substrate. Fluoridate HA coatings have since attracted much attention as a promising replacement for pure HA because fluoridated HA demonstrates significant resistance to biodegradation.

On the other hand, it is well known that human bone contains certain trace elements, such as K^+, Na^+, Mg^{2+}, Zn^{2+}, Cl^-, F^-, etc., and these trace elements exert crucial influences on bone metabolism through promoting biocatalytic reactions and/or controlling some related metabolic processes (Hench and Wilson 1993; Aoki 1994). As such, some efforts have been made to incorporate some of these trace elements into the HA structure to improve further related properties of pure HA (to mimic the actual composition of human bones). Besides F^-, Mg^{2+} and Zn^{2+} are the two most promising ions to improve the bioactivity of pure HA coating (Qi et al. 2008; Köseoğlu et al. 2009; Chung et al. 2006). However, those Mg- and Zn-incorporated HA coatings always possess higher solubility than that of pure HA coating. Recalling the feature of an ideal coating, short-term rapid degradation (bioactivity) and long-term dissolution-resistance (stability), codoping of (Mg^{2+}, F^-) or (Zn^{2+}, F^-) are accordingly proposed (Miao et al. 2005). In addition, biphasic coatings of β-TCP/FHA and functional graded multilayered coatings are also possible ways to achieve the combination of bioactivity and stability (Cheng, Zhang, and Weng 2006).

In summary, HA-coated metallic implants are attracting the highest interest for hard tissue repair/replacement, since these kinds of implants can combine the advantages of both materials: the bioactivity of HA and the excellent mechanical properties of metallic substrates. The sol–gel technique is the most preferred method for preparing HA coatings due to its distinguishing characteristics (e.g., ability for tailoring chemical compositions, improved homogeneity at the molecular level, ability to produce uniform coating, low cost, and easy operation). More HA-base high-performance coatings are expected to be produced using the sol–gel method in order to satisfy the requirement of bioimplants.

References

Aebli, N., J. Krebs, D. Schwenke, H. Stich, P. Schawalder, and J. C. Theis. 2003. Degradation of hydroxyapatite coating on a well-functioning femoral component. *Journal of Bone and Joint Surgery-British Volume* 85B (4):499–503.

Agrawal, D. C., and R. Raj. 1989. Measurement of the ultimate shear—strength of a metal ceramic interface. *Acta Metallurgica* 37 (4):1265–1270.

Agrawal, D. C., and R. Raj. 1990. Ultimate shear strengths of copper silica and nickel silica interfaces. *Materials Science and Engineering A Structural Materials Properties Microstructure and Processing* 126:125–131.

Ak Azem, F., and A. Cakir. 2009. Synthesis of HAP coating on galvanostatically treated stainless steel substrates by sol–gel method. *Journal of Sol–Gel Science and Technology* 51 (2):190–197.

Aksakal, B., M. Gavgali, and B. Dikici. 2009. The effect of coating thickness on corrosion resistance of hydroxyapatite coated Ti6Al4V and 316L SS omplants. *Journal of Materials Engineering and Performance* 1–6.

Albrektsson, T. 1998. Hydroxyapatite-coated implants: A case against their use. *Journal of Oral and Maxillofacial Surgery* 56 (11):1312–1326.

Amrah-Bouali, S., C. Rey, A. Lebugle, and D. Bernache. 1994. Surface modifications of hydroxyapatite ceramics in aqueous media. *Biomaterials* 15 (4):269–272.

Anderson, J. M. 2001. Biological responses to materials. *Annual Review of Materials Research* 31:81–110.

Aoki, Hideki. 1994. *Medical Applications of Hydroxyapatite*. Toyoko: Ishiyaku Euroamerica.

Arias, J. L., M. B. Mayor, J. Pou, Y. Leng, B. Leon, and M. Perez Amor. 2003. Micro- and nano-testing of calcium phosphate coatings produced by pulsed laser deposition. *Biomaterials* 24 (20):3403–3408.

Aubin, J. E., F. Liu, L. Malaval, and A. K. Gupta. 1995. Osteoblast and chondroblast differentiation. *Bone* 17 (2):S77–S83.

Avés, E. P., G. F. Estévez, M. S. Sader, J. C. G. Sierra, J. C. L. Yurell, I. N. Bastos, and G. D. A. Soares. 2009. Hydroxyapatite coating by sol–gel on Ti–6Al–4V alloy as drug carrier. *Journal of Materials Science: Materials in Medicine* 20 (2):543–547.

Balakrishnan, A., B. C. Lee, T. N. Kim, and B. B. Panigrahi. 2007. Hydroxyapatite coatings on NaOH treated Ti–6Al–4V alloy using sol–gel precursor. *Materials Science and Technology* 23 (8):1005–1007.

Balamurugan, A., G. Balossier, S. Kannan, and S. Rajeswari. 2006. Elaboration of sol–gel derived apatite films on surgical grade stainless steel for biomedical applications. *Materials Letters* 60 (17–18):2288–2293.

Balamurugan, A., S. Kannan, and S. Rajeswari. 2002. Bioactive sol–gel hydroxyapatite surface for biomedical applications—in vitro study. *Trends in Biomaterials and Artificial Organs* 16:18.

Balint, E., P. Szabo, C. F. Marshall, and S. M. Sprague. 2001. Glucose-induced inhibition of in vitro bone mineralization. *Bone* 28:21–28.

Bao, Q. H., C. Z. Chen, D. G. Wang, Q. M. Ji, and T. Q. Lei. 2005. Pulsed laser deposition and its current research status in preparing hydroxyapatite thin films. *Applied Surface Science* 252 (5):1538–1544.

Barrere, F., P. Layrolle, C. A. van Blitterswijk, and K. de Groot. 2001. Biomimetic coatings on titanium: a crystal growth study of octacalcium phosphate. *Journal of Materials Science Materials in Medicine* 12 (6):529–534.

Battistoni, C., M. P. Casaletto, G. M. Ingo, S. Kaciulis, G. Mattogno, and L. Pandolfi. 2000. Surface characterization of biocompatible hydroxyapatite coatings. *Surface and Interface Analysis* 29 (11):773–781.

Baxter, L. C., V. Frauchiger, M. Textor, I. Gwynn, and R. G. Richards. 2002. Fibroblast and osteoblast adhesion and morphology on calcium phosphate surfaces. *European Cells and Materials* 4:1–17.

Ben-Nissan, B., A. Milev, and R. Vago. 2004. Morphology of sol–gel derived nano-coated coralline hydroxyapatite. *Biomaterials* 25 (20):4971–4975.

Ben-Nissan, B., and G. Pezzotti. 2004. Bioceramics: An introduction In *Engineering Materials for Biomedical Applications*, ed S. H. Teoh. Hackensack, NJ: World Scientific.

Bender, S. A., J. D. Bumgardner, M. D. Roach, K. Bessho, and J. L. Ong. 2000. Effect of protein on the dissolution of HA coatings. *Biomaterials* 21 (3):299–305.

Bharati, S., M. K. Sinha, and D. Basu. 2005. Hydroxyapatite coating by biomimetic method on titanium alloy using concentrated SBF. *Bulletin of Materials Science* 28 (6):617–621.

Bloebaum, R. D., D. Beeks, L. D. Dorr, C. G. Savory, J. A. Dupont, and A. A. Hofmann. 1994. Complications with hydroxyapatite particulate separation in total hip-arthroplasty. *Clinical Orthopaedics and Related Research* (298):19–26.

Blum, J., D. Avnir, and H. Schumann. 1999. Sol–gel encapsulated transition-metal catalysts. *CHEMTECH* 29 (2):32–38.

Boretoes, J. W., and M. Eden. 1984. *Contemporary Biomaterials—Material and Host Response, Clinical Applications, New Technology and Legal Aspects*. New Jersey: William Andrew Publishing.

Borsari, V., G. Giavaresi, P. Torricelli, A. Salito, R. Chiesa, L. Chiusoli, A. Volpert, L. Rimondini, R. Giardino. 2005. Physical characterization of different-roughness titanium surfaces, with and without hydroxyapatite coating, and their effect on human osteoblast-like cells. *Journal of Biomedical Materials Research Part B* 75B (2):359–368.

Boyan, B. D., C. H. Lohmann, D. D. Dean, V. L. Sylvia, D. L. Cochran, and Z. Schwartz. 2001. Mechanisms involved in osteoblast response to implant surface morphology. *Annual Review of Materials Research* 31:357–371.

Briggs, D., and J. T. Grant. 2003. *Surface Analysis by Auger and X-ray Photoelectron Spectroscopy.* Trowbridge, UK: IM Publications.

Bronzino, J. D. 2000. *The Biomedical Engineering Handbook,* 2nd edn. Boca Raton, FL: CRC Press.

Brossa, F., A. Cigada, R. Chiesa, L. Paracchini, and C. Consonni. 1994. Postdeposition treatment effects on hydroxyapatite vacuum plasma spray coatings. *Journal of Materials Science—Materials in Medicine* 5 (12):855–857.

Brown, S. R., I. G. Turner, and H. Reiter. 1994. Residual stress measurement in thermal sprayed hydroxyapatite coatings. *Journal of Materials Science: Materials in Medicine* 5 (9–10):756–759.

Brundle, C. R., C. A. Evans Jr., and S. Wilson. 1992. *Encyclopedia of Materials Characterization-Surface, Interface, Thin film.* Boston, MA: Butterworth-Heinemann.

Cai, Y., S. Zhang, X. Zeng, Y. Wang, M. Qian, and W. Weng. 2009. Improvement of bioactivity with magnesium and fluorine ions incorporated hydroxyapatite coatings via sol–gel deposition on Ti6Al4V alloys. *Thin Solid Films* 517 (17):5347–5351.

Cavalli, M., G. Gnappi, A. Montenero, D. Bersani, P. P. Lottici, S. Kaciulis, G. Mattogno, and M. Fini. 2001. Hydroxy- and fluorapatite films on Ti alloy substrates: Sol–gel preparation and characterization. *Journal of Materials Science* 36 (13):3253–3260.

Chai, C. S., and B. Ben-Nissan. 1999. Bioactive nanocrystalline sol–gel hydroxyapatite coatings. *Journal of Materials Science: Materials in Medicine* 10 (8):465–469.

Chang, C. K., J. S. Wu, D.L. Mao, and C. X. Ding. 2001. Mechanical and histological evaluations of hydroxyapatite-coated and noncoated Ti6Al4V implants in tibia bone. *Journal of Biomedical Materials Research* 56 (1):17–23.

Cheang, P., and K. A. Khor. 1995. Thermal spraying of hydroxyapatite (HA) coatings: Effects of powder feedstock. *Journal of Materials Processing Technology* 48 (1–4):429–436.

Chen, J., W. Tong, Y. Cao, J. Feng, and X. Zhang. 1997. Effect of atmosphere on phase transformation in plasma-sprayed hydroxyapatite coatings during heat treatment. *Journal of Biomedical Materials Research* 34 (1):15–20.

Chen, Y., C. Gan, T. Zhang, G. Yu, P. Bai, and A. Kaplan. 2005. Laser-surface-alloyed carbon nanotubes reinforced hydroxyapatite composite coatings. *Applied Physics Letters* 86:251905.

Cheng, K., S. Zhang, and W. Weng. 2006. Sol–gel prepared β-TCP/FHA biphasic coatings. *Thin Solid Films* 515 (1):135–140.

Cheng, K., S. Zhang, and W. Weng. 2007. Surface characterization of colloidal-sol gel derived biphasic HA/FA coatings. *Journal of Materials Science: Materials in Medicine* 18 (10):2011–2015.

Cheng, K., S. Zhang, W. Weng, and X. Zeng. 2005. The interfacial study of sol–gel-derived fluoridated hydroxyapatite coatings. *Surface and Coatings Technology* 198 (1–3 Spec. Iss.):242–246.

Chou, L., B. Marek, and W. R. Wagner. 1999. Effects of hydroxylapatite coating crystallinity on biosolubility, cell attachment efficiency and proliferation in vitro. *Biomaterials* 20 (10):977–985.

Chung, R. J., M. F. Hsieh, C. W. Huang, L. H. Perng, H. W. Wen, and T. S. Chin. 2006. Antimicrobial effects and human gingival biocompatibility of hydroxyapatite sol–gel coatings. *Journal of Biomedical Materials Research B* 76 (1):169–178.

Chusuei, C. C. 1999. Calcium phosphate phase identification using XPS and time-of-flight cluster SIMS. *Analytical Chemistry* 71 (1):149–153.

Combes, C., and C. Rey. 2002. Adsorption of proteins and calcium phosphate materials bioactivity. *Biomaterials* 23 (13):2817–2823.

Cooley, D. R., A. F. Vandellen, J. O. Burgess, and A. S. Windeler. 1992. The advantages of coated titanium implants prepared by radiofrequency sputtering from hydroxyapatite. *Journal of Prosthetic Dentistry* 67 (1):93–100.

Dalton, J. E., and S. D. Cook. 1995. In vivo mechanical and histological characteristics of HA-coated implants vary with coating vendor. *Journal of Biomedical Materials Research* 29 (2):239–245.

Ding, S. J. 2003. Properties and immersion behavior of magnetron-sputtered multi-layered hydroxyapatite/titanium composite coatings. *Biomaterials* 24 (23):4233–4238.

Ding, S. J., C. P. Ju, and J. H. C. Lin. 1999. Characterization of hydroxyapatite and titanium coatings sputtered on Ti–6Al–4V substrate. *Journal of Biomedical Materials Research* 44 (3):266–279.

Ding, S. J., Y. M. Su, C. P. Ju, and J. H. Chern Lin. 2001. Structure and immersion behavior of plasma-sprayed apatite-matrix coatings. *Biomaterials* 22 (8):833–845.

Dorota, K. M., L. S. Malgorzata, M. Mazur, and J. Komender. 2005. Osteogenic cell contact with bio-materials influences phenotype expression. *Cell and Tissue Banking* 6:55–64.

Dorozhkin, S. V. 1997. Surface reactions of apatite dissolution. *Journal of Colloid and Interface Science* 191 (2):489–497.

Dorozhkin, S. V., E. I. Dorozhkina, and M. Epple. 2003. Precipitation of carbonate apatite from a revised simulated body fluid in the presence of glucose. *Journal of Applied Biomaterials and Biomechanics* 1:200–207.

Ducheyne, P., S. Radin, and L. King. 1993. The effect of calcium-phosphate ceramic composition and structure on in vitro behavior: 1. Dissolution. *Journal of Biomedical Materials Research* 27 (1):25–34.

Ducheyne, P., and Q. Qiu. 1999. Bioactive ceramics: The effect of surface reactivity on bone formation and bone cell function. *Biomaterials* 20 (23–24):2287–2303.

Dulay, M. T., J. P. Quirino, B. D. Bennett, and R. N. Zare. 2002. Bonded-phase photopolymerized sol–gel monoliths for reversed phase capillary electrochromatography. *Journal of Separation Science* 25 (1–2):3–9.

Duran, A., A. Conde, A. G. Coedo, T. Dorado, C. Garcia, and S. Cere. 2004. Sol–gel coatings for protection and bioactivation of metals used in orthopaedic devices. *Journal of Materials Chemistry* 14 (14):2282–2290.

Filiaggi, M. J., N. A. Coombs, and R. M. Pilliar. 1991. Characterization of the interface in the plasma-sprayed HA coating/Ti–6Al–4V implant system. *Journal of Biomedical Materials Research* 25 (10):1211–1229.

Folkman, J., and A. Moscona. 1978. Role of cell shape in growth control. *Nature* 273 (5661):345–349.

Friedrich, H. E., and B. L. Mordike. 2006. *Magnesium Technology*. Berlin, Germany: Springer-Velag.

Fu, Y. Q., A. W. Batchelor, and K. A. Khor. 1998. Hot isostatic pressing of hydroxyapatite coating for improved fretting wear resistance. *Journal of Materials Science Letters* 17 (20):1695–1696.

Furlong, R. J., and J. F. Osborn. 1991. Fixation of hip prostheses by hydroxyapatite ceramic coatings. *Journal of Bone and Joint Surgery—British Volume* 73 (5):741–745.

Gan, L., and R. Pilliar. 2004. Calcium phosphate sol–gel-derived thin films on porous-surfaced implants for enhanced osteoconductivity: Part I. Synthesis and characterization. *Biomaterials* 25 (22):5303–5312.

Gan, L., J. Wang, and R. M. Pilliar. 2005. Evaluating interface strength of calcium phosphate sol–gel-derived thin films to Ti6Al4 V substrate. *Biomaterials* 26 (2):189–196.

Garcia-Sanz, F. J., M. B. Mayor, J. L. Arias, J. Pou, B. Leon, and M. Perez-Amor. 1997. Hydroxyapatite coatings: A comparative study between plasma-spray and pulsed laser deposition techniques. *Journal of Materials Science: Materials in Medicine* 8 (12):861–865.

Gerber, T., T. Traykova, K. O. Henkel, and V. Bienengraeber. 2003. Development and in vivo test of sol–gel derived bone grafting materials. *Journal of Sol–Gel Science and Technology* 26 (1–3):1173–1178.

Gerstenfeld, L. C., S. D. Chipman, J. Glowacki, and J. B. Lian. 1987. Expression of differentiated function by mineralizing cultures of chicken osteoblasts. *Developmental Biology* 122 (1):49–60.

Greenspan, D. C. 1999. Bioactive ceramic implant materials. *Current Opinion in Solid State & Materials Science* 4 (4):389–393.

Gross, K. A., C. S. Chai, G. S. K. Kannangara, B. Ben-Nissan, and L. Hanley. 1998. Thin hydroxyapatite coatings via sol–gel synthesis. *Journal of Materials Science: Materials in Medicine* 9 (12):839–843.

Gross, K. A., W. Walsh, and E. Swarts. 2004. Analysis of retrieved hydroxyapatite-coated hip prostheses. *Journal of Thermal Spray Technology* 13 (2):190–199.

Gu, Y. W., K. A. Khor, and P. Cheang. 2003. In vitro studies of plasma-sprayed hydroxyapatite/Ti–6Al–4V composite coatings in simulated body fluid (SBF). *Biomaterials* 24 (9):1603–1611.

Guo, L., and H. Li. 2004. Fabrication and characterization of thin nano-hydroxyapatite coatings on titanium. *Surface and Coatings Technology* 185 (2–3):268–274.

Gupta, R., and A. Kumar. 2008. Bioactive materials for biomedical applications using sol–gel technology. *Biomedical Materials* 3 (3).

Gvishi, R., U. Narang, G. Ruland, D. N. Kumar, and P. N. Prasad. 1997. Novel, organically doped, sol–gel-derived materials for photonics: multiphasic nanostructured composite monoliths and optical fibers. *Applied Organometallic Chemistry* 11 (2):107–127.

Haddow, D. B., P. F. James, and R. Van Noort. 1996. Characterization of sol–gel surfaces for biomedical applications. *Journal of Materials Science: Materials in Medicine* 7 (5):255–260.

Haddow, D. B., P. F. James, and R. Van Noort. 1999. Sol–gel derived calcium phosphate coatings for biomedical applications. *Journal of Sol–Gel Science and Technology* 13 (1–3):261–265.

Han, Y., K. W. Xu, and J. Lu. 2001. Dissolution response of hydroxyapatite coatings to residual stresses. *Journal of Biomedical Materials Research* 55 (4):596–602.

Han, Y., T. Fu, J. Lu, and K. Xu. 2001. Characterization and stability of hydroxyapatite coatings prepared by an electrodeposition and alkaline-treatment process. *Journal of Biomedical Materials Research* 54 (1):96–101.

Hench, L. L. 1998. Biomaterials: a forecast for the future. *Biomaterials* 19 (16):1419–1423.

Hench, L. L., and J. Wilson. 1993. *An Introduction to Bioceramics*. Singapore: World Scientific.

Hench, L. L. 1991. Bioceramics—from concept to clinic. *Journal of the American Ceramic Society* 74:1487–1510.

Hirai, S., K. Nishinaka, K. Shimakage, M. Uo, and F. Watari. 2004. Hydroxyapatite coating on titanium substrate by the sol–gel process. *Journal of the American Ceramic Society* 87 (1):29–34.

Hsieh, M. F., L. H. Perng, and T. S. Chin. 2002. Hydroxyapatite coating on Ti6Al4V alloy using a sol–gel derived precursor. *Materials Chemistry and Physics* 74 (3):245–250.

Hwang, K., J. Song, B. Kang, and Y. Park. 2000. Sol–gel derived hydroxyapatite films on alumina substrates. *Surface and Coatings Technology* 123 (2–3):252–255.

Implants for Surgery-Hydroxyapatite—Part 2: Coatings of Hydroxyapatite. 2000. In *British Standard, BS ISO 13779-2*.

Implants for Surgery-Hydroxyapatite—Part 4: Determination of Coating Adhesion Strength 2002. In *British Standard, BS ISO 13779-4*.

Jaffe, W. L., and D. F. Scott. 1996. Total hip arthroplasty with hydroxyapatite-coated prostheses. *Journal of Bone and Joint Surgery-American Volume* 78A (12):1918–1934.

Jaou, W., M. B. Hachimi, T. Koutit, J. L. Lacout, and M. Ferhat. 2000. Effects of calcium phosphate on the reaction of reducing sugars in an alkaline medium. *Materials Research Bulletin* 35:1419–1427.

Jenney, C. R., and J. M. Anderson. 2000. Adsorbed serum proteins responsible for surface dependent human macrophage behavior. *Journal of Biomedical Materials Research* 49 (4):435–447.

Kačiulis, S., G. Mattogno, A. Napoli, E. Bemporad, F. Ferrari, A. Montenero, and G. Gnappi. 1998. Surface analysis of biocompatible coatings on titanium. *Journal of Electron Spectroscopy and Related Phenomena* 95 (1):61–69.

Kačiulis, S., G. Mattogno, L. Pandolfi, M. Cavalli, G. Gnappi, and A. Montenero. 1999. XPS study of apatite-based coatings prepared by sol–gel technique. *Applied Surface Science* 151 (1):1–5.

Kartsogiannis, V., and K. W. Ng. 2004. Cell lines and primary cell cultures in the study of bone cell biology. *Molecular and Cellular Endocrinology* 228:79–102.

Kasemo, B. 1998. Biological surface science. *Current Opinion in Solid State and Materials Science* 3 (5):451–459.

Katto, M., M. Nakamura, T. Tanaka, and T. Nakayama. 2002. Hydroxyapatite coatings deposited by laser-assisted laser ablation method. *Applied Surface Science* 197:768–771.

Kay, M. I., R. A. Young, and A. S. Posner. 1964. Crystal structure of hydroxyapatite. *Nature* 204 (4963):1050–1052.

Kazarian, S. G., K. L. A. Chan, V. Maquet, and A. R. Boccaccini. 2004. Characterisation of bioactive and resorbable polylactide/Bioglass® composites by FTIR spectroscopic imaging. *Biomaterials* 25 (18):3931–3938.

Khor, K. A., H. Li, P. Cheang, and S. Y. Boey. 2003. In vitro behavior of HVOF sprayed calcium phosphate splats and coatings. *Biomaterials* 24 (5):723–735.

Kim, H. W., H. E. Kim, and J. C. Knowles. 2005. Improvement of hydroxyapatite sol–gel coating on titanium with ammonium hydroxide addition. *Journal of the American Ceramic Society* 88 (1):154–159.

Kim, H. W., H. E. Kim, V. Salih, and J. C. Knowles. 2005. Hydroxyapatite and titania sol–gel composite coatings on titanium for hard tissue implants; mechanical and in vitro biological performance. *Journal of Biomedical Materials Research—Part B Applied Biomaterials* 72 (1):1–8.

Kim, H. W., H. E. Kim, V. Salih, and J. C. Knowles. 2005. Sol–gel-modified titanium with hydroxyapatite thin films and effect on osteoblast-like cell responses. *Journal of Biomedical Materials Research A* 74 (3):294–305.

Kim, H. W., Y. H. Koh, L. H. Li, S. Lee, and H. E. Kim. 2004. Hydroxyapatite coating on titanium substrate with titania buffer layer processed by sol–gel method. *Biomaterials* 25 (13):2533–2538.

Klein, L. C. 1988. *Sol–Gel Technology for Thin Films, Fibers, Preforms, Electronics, and Specialty Shapes.* Park Ridge, NJ: Noyes Publications.

Knabe, C., F. C. M. Driessens, J. A. Planell, R. Gildenhaar, G. Berger, D. Reif, R. Fitzner, R. J. Radlanski, and U. Gross. 2000. Evaluation of calcium phosphates and experimental calcium phosphate bone cements using osteogenic cultures. *Journal of Biomedical Materials Research* 52 (3):498–508.

Koch, C. F., S. Johnson, D. Kumar, M. Jelinek, D. B. Chrisey, A. Doraiswamy, C. Jin, R. J. Narayan, and I. N. Mihailescu. 2007. Pulsed laser deposition of hydroxyapatite thin films. *Materials Science and Engineering C* 27 (3):484–494.

Kokubo, T., and H. Takadama. 2006. How useful is SBF in predicting in vivo bone bioactivity? *Biomaterials* 27 (15):2907–2915.

Köseoğlu, N. C., A. Büyükaksoy, M. H. Aslan, and A. Y. Oral. 2009. Effects of Mg doping on sol–gel derived nanocrystalline hydroxyapatite thin film. *Materials Science and Technology* 25 (6):799–804.

Kweh, S. W. K., K. A. Khor, and P. Cheang. 2000. Plasma-sprayed hydroxyapatite (HA) coatings with flame-spheroidized feedstock: microstructure and mechanical properties. *Biomaterials* 21 (12):1223–1234.

Lee, Y. P., C. K. Wang, T. H. Huang, Ch. C. Chen, C. T. Kao, and S. J. Ding. 2005. In vitro characterization of postheat-treated plasma-sprayed hydroxyapatite coatings. *Surface and Coatings Technology* 197 (2–3):367–374.

Lee, T. M., R. S. Tsai, E. Chang, C. Y. Yang, and M. R. Yang. 2002. The cell attachment and morphology of neonatal rat calvarial osteoblasts on the surface of Ti–6Al–4V and plasma-sprayed HA coating: Effect of surface roughness and serum contents. *Journal of Materials Science-Materials in Medicine* 13 (4):341–350.

Leyens, C., and M. Peters. 2003. *Titanium and Titanium Alloys: Fundamentals and Applications.* Weinheim: Wiley-VCH.

Li, H., K. A. Khor, and P. Cheang. 2002. Properties of heat-treated calcium phosphate coatings deposited by high-velocity oxy-fuel (HVOF) spray. *Biomaterials* 23 (10):2105–2112.

Li, H., K. A. Khor, and P. Cheang. 2002. Titanium dioxide reinforced hydroxyapatite coatings deposited by high velocity oxy-fuel (HVOF) spray. *Biomaterials* 23 (1):85–91.

Li, H., K. A. Khor, and P. Cheang. 2002. Young's modulus and fracture toughness determination of high velocity oxy-fuel-sprayed bioceramic coatings. *Surface and Coatings Technology* 155 (1):21–32.

Li, L. H., H. W. Kim, S. H. Lee, Y. M. Kong, and H. E. Kim. 2005. Biocompatibility of titanium implants modified by microarc oxidation and hydroxyapatite coating. *Journal of Biomedical Materials Research A* 73 (1):48–54.

Li, X. D., D. F. Diao, and B. Bhushan. 1997. Fracture mechanisms of thin amorphous carbon films in nanoindentation. *Acta Materialia* 45 (11):4453–4461.

Lima, R. S., K. A. Khor, H. Li, P. Cheang, and B. R. Marple. 2005. HVOF spraying of nanostructured hydroxyapatite for biomedical applications. *Materials Science and Engineering. A, Structural Materials: Properties, Microstructure, and Processing* 396 (1–2):181–187.

Lin, J., and C. W. Brown. 1997. Sol–gel glass as a matrix for chemical and biochemical sensing. *Trends in Analytical Chemistry* 16 (4):200–211.

Liu, D. M., T. Troczynski, and W. J. Tseng. 2001. Water-based sol–gel synthesis of hydroxyapatite: Process development. *Biomaterials* 22 (13):1721–1730.

Liu, D. M., Q. Yang, and T. Troczynski. 2002. Sol–gel hydroxyapatite coatings on stainless steel substrates. *Biomaterials* 23 (3):691–698.

Liu, Y., E. B. Hunziker, N. X. Randall, K. de Groot, and P. Layrolle. 2003. Proteins incorporated into biomimetically prepared calcium phosphate coatings modulate their mechanical strength and dissolution rate. *Biomaterials* 24 (1):65–70.

Löbmann, P. 2007. From sol–gel processing to bio-inspired materials synthesis. *Current Nanoscience* 3 (4):306–328.

Lu, H. B., C. T. Campbell, D. J. Graham, and B. D. Ratner. 2000. Surface characterization of hydroxyapatite and related calcium phosphates by XPS and TOF-SIMS. *Analytical Chemistry* 72 (13):2886–2894.

Luo, Q., and J. D. Andrade. 1998. Cooperative adsorption of proteins onto hydroxyapatite. *Journal of Colloidal and Interface Science* 200 (1):104–113.

Ma, J., C. H. Liang, L. B. Kong, and C. Wang. 2003. Colloidal characterization and electrophoretic deposition of hydroxyapatite on titanium substrate. *Journal of Materials Science—Materials in Medicine* 14 (9):797–801.

Ma, J., H. F. Wong, L. B. Kong, and K. W. Peng. 2003. Biomimetic processing of nanocrystallite bioactive apatite coating on titanium. *Nanotechnology* 14 (6):619–623.

Manso, M., M. Langlet, C. Jiménez, and J. M. Martínez-Duart. 2002. Microstructural study of aerosol–gel derived hydroxyapatite coatings. *Biomolecular Engineering* 19 (2–6):63–66.

Manso, M., S. Ogueta, P. Herrero-Fernández, L. Vázquez, M. Langlet, and J. P. García-Ruiz. 2002. Biological evaluation of aerosol–gel-derived hydroxyapatite coatings with human mesenchymal stem cells. *Biomaterials* 23 (19):3985–3990.

Marsha, N. S., T. Leonard, and A. Randall. 2000. Special feature: consistency in postoperative education programs following total hip replacement. *Topics in Geriatric Rehabilitation* 15 (4):68–76.

Martini, D., M. Fini, M. Franchi, V. De Pasquale, B. Bacchelli, M. Gamberini, A. Tinti, P. Taddei, G. Giavaresi, and V. Ottani. 2003. Detachment of titanium and fluorohydroxyapatite particles in unloaded endosseous implants. *Biomaterials* 24 (7):1309–1316.

Massaro, C., M. A. Baker, F. Cosentino, P. A. Ramires, S. Klose, and E. Milella. 2001. Surface and biological evaluation of hydroxyapatite-based coatings on titanium deposited by different techniques. *Journal of Biomedical Materials Research* 58 (6):651–657.

Menezes, G. C., C. N. Elias, M. Attias, and F. C. Silva-Filho. 2003. Osteoblast adhesion onto titanium dental implants. *Acta Microscopica* 12 (1):13–20.

Metikos-Hukovic, M., E. Tkalcec, A. Kwokal, and J. Piljac. 2003. An in vitro study of Ti and Ti-alloys coated with sol–gel derived hydroxyapatite coatings. *Surface & Coatings Technology* 165 (1):40–50.

Miao, S., W. Weng, K. Cheng, P. Du, G. Shen, G. Han, and S. Zhang. 2005. Sol–gel preparation of Zn-doped fluoridated hydroxyapatite films. *Surface and Coatings Technology* 198 (1–3):223–226.

Mihály, J., V. Gombás, A. Afishah, and J. Mink. 2009. FT-Raman investigation of human dental enamel surfaces. *Journal of Raman Spectroscopy* 40 (8):898–902.

Montenero, A., G. Gnappi, F. Ferrari, M. Cesari, E. Salvioli, L. Mattogno, S. Kaciulis, and M. Fini. 2000. Sol–gel derived hydroxyapatite coatings on titanium substrate. *Journal of Materials Science* 35 (11):2791–2797.

Moroni, A., V. L. Caja, C. Sabato, E. L. Egger, F. Gottsauner-Wolf, and E. Y. S. Chao. 1994. Bone ingrowth analysis and interface evaluation of hydroxyapatite coated versus uncoated titanium porous bone implants. *Journal of Materials Science: Materials in Medicine* 5 (6–7):411–416.

Moroni, A., S. Toksvig-Larsen, M. C. Maltarello, L. Orienti, S. Stea, and S. Giannini. 1998. A comparison of hydroxyapatite-coated, titanium-coated, and uncoated tapered external-fixation pins: An in vivo study in sheep. *Journal of Bone and Joint Surgery Series A* 80 (4):547–554.

Morscher, E. W., A. Hefti, and U. Aebi. 1998. Severe osteolysis after third-body wear due to hydroxyapatite particles from acetabular cup coating. *Journal of Bone and Joint Surgery-British Volume* 80B (2):267–272.

Mullermai, C. M., C. Voigt, and U. Gross. 1990. Incorporation and degradation of hydroxyapatite implants of different surface-roughness and surface-structure in bone. *Scanning Microscopy* 4 (3):613–624.

Nagarajan, S., V. Raman, and N. Rajendran. 2010. Synthesis and electrochemical characterization of porous niobium oxide coated 316L SS for orthopedic applications. *Materials Chemistry and Physics* 119 (3):363–366.

Nelea, V., C. Morosanu, M. Iliescu, and I. N. Mihailescu. 2003. Microstructure and mechanical properties of hydroxyapatite thin films grown by RF magnetron sputtering. *Surface & Coatings Technology* 173 (2–3):315–322.

Nieh, T. G., A. F. Jankowski, and J. Koike. 2001. Processing and characterization of hydroxyapatite coatings on titanium produced by magnetron sputtering. *Journal of Materials Research* 16 (11):3238–3245.

Ogiso, M., Y. Yamashita, and T. Matsumoto. 1998. Differences in microstructural characteristics of dense HA and HA coating. *Journal of Biomedical Materials Research* 41 (2):296–303.

Oguchi, H., K. Ishikawa, S. Ojima, Y. Hirayama, K. Seto, and G. Eguchi. 1992. Evaluation of a high-velocity flame-spraying technique for hydroxyapatite. *Biomaterials* 13 (7):471–477.

Ong, J. L., M. Appleford, S. Oh, Y. Yang, W. H. Chen, J. D. Bumgardner, and W. O. Haggard. 2006. The characterization and development of bioactive hydroxyapatite coatings. *JOM* 58 (7):67–69.

Onoki, T., and T. Hashida. 2006. New method for hydroxyapatite coating of titanium by the hydrothermal hot isostatic pressing technique. *Surface & Coatings Technology* 200 (24):6801–6807.

Oonishi, H., M. Yamamoto, H. Ishimaru, E. Tsuji, S. Kushitani, M. Aono, and Y. Ukon. 1989. The effect of hydroxyapatite coating on bone-growth into porous titanium-alloy implants. *Journal of Bone and Joint Surgery-British Volume* 71 (2):213–216.

Overgaard, S., M. Lind, H. Glerup, C. Bünger, and K. Søballe. 1998. Porous-coated versus grit-blasted surface texture of hydroxyapatite-coated implants during controlled micromotion: mechanical and histomorphometric results. *Journal of Arthroplasty* 13 (4):449–458.

Park, J. B. 1984. *Biomaterials Science and Engineering*. New York, NY: Plenum Publishing Corporation.

Pastor, I., A. Salinas-Castillo, R. Esquembre, R. Mallavia, and C. R. Mateo. 2010. Multienzymatic system immobilization in sol–gel slides: fluorescent superoxide biosensors development. *Biosensors and Bioelectronics* 25 (6):1526–1529.

Pearce, E. I. F., E. M. Hancock, and I. H. C. Gallagher. 1984. The effect of fluorhydroxyapatite in experimental human dental plaque on its pH, acid production and soluble calcium, phosphate and fluride levels following glucose challenge. *Archives of Oral Biology* 29:521–527.

Pena, J., I. Izquierdo-Barba, A. Martinez, and M. Vallet-Regi. 2006. New method to obtain chitosan/apatite materials at room temperature. *Solid State Sciences* 8 (5):513–519.

Perizzolo, D., W. R. Lacefield, and D. M. Brunette. 2001. Interaction between topography and coating in the formation of bone nodules in culture for hydroxyapatite- and titanium-coated micromachined surfaces. *Journal of Biomedical Materials Research* 56 (4):494–503.

Pichugin, V. F., R. A. Surmenev, E. V. Shesterikov, M. A. Ryabtseva, E. V. Eshenko, S. I. Tverdokhlebov, O. Prymak, and M. Epple. 2008. The preparation of calcium phosphate coatings on titanium and nickel-titanium by rf-magnetron-sputtered deposition: composition, structure and micromechanical properties. *Surface and Coatings Technology* 202 (16):3913–3920.

Poitout, D. G. 2004. *Biomechanics and Biomaterials in Orthopedics*. London: Springer.

Qi, G., S. Zhang, K. A. Khor, W. Weng, X. Zeng, and C. Liu. 2008. An interfacial study of sol–gel-derived magnesium apatite coatings on Ti6Al4V substrates. *Thin Solid Films* 516 (16):5172–5175.

Răileanu, M., M. Crişan, N. Drăgan, D. Crişan, A. Galtayries, A. Brăileanu, A. Ianculescu, V. S. Teodorescu, I. Niţoi, and M. Anastasescu. 2009. Sol–gel doped TiO_2 nanomaterials: a comparative study. *Journal of Sol–Gel Science and Technology* 51 (3):315–329.

Ramires, P. A., A. Wennerberg, C. B. Johansson, F. Cosentino, S. Tundo, and E. Milella. 2003. Biological behavior of sol–gel coated dental implants. *Journal of Materials Science: Materials in Medicine* 14 (6):539–545.

Ratner, B. D., A. S. Hoffman, F. J. Schoen, and J. E. Lemons. 1996. *Biomaterials Science—An Introduction to Materials in Medicine*. San Diego, CA: Academic Press.

Reiner, T., and I. Gotman. 2009. Biomimetic calcium phosphate coating on Ti wires versus flat substrates: structure and mechanism of formation. *Journal of Materials Science: Materials in Medicine*:1–9.

Rigo, E. C. S., A. O. Boschi, M. Yoshimoto, S. Allegrini, B. Konig, and M. J. Carbonari. 2004. Evaluation in vitro and in vivo of biomimetic hydroxyapatite coated on titanium dental implants. *Materials Science & Engineering C-Biomimetic and Supramolecular Systems* 24 (5):647–651.

Roop Kumar, R., and M. Wang. 2002. Functionally graded bioactive coatings of hydroxyapatite/titanium oxide composite system. *Materials Letters* 55 (3):133–137.

Senamaud, N., D. Bernache-Assollant, E. Champion, M. Heughebaert, and C. Rey. 1997. Calcination and sintering of hydroxyfluorapatite powders. *Solid State Ionics* 101:1357–1362.

Sergo, Valter, Orfeo Sbaizero, and David R. Clarke. 1997. Mechanical and chemical consequences of the residual stresses in plasma sprayed hydroxyapatite coatings. *Biomaterials* 18 (6):477–482.

Siebers, M. C., X. F. Walboomers, S. C. G. Leeuwenburgh, J. G. C. Wolke, and J. A. Jansen. 2006. The influence of the crystallinity of electrostatic spray deposition-derived coatings on osteoblast-like cell behavior, in vitro. *Journal of Biomedical Materials Research-Part A* 78A (2):258–267

Silva, C. C., and A. S. B. Sombra. 2004. Raman spectroscopy measurements of hydroxyapatite obtained by mechanical alloying. *Journal of Physics and Chemistry of Solids* 65 (5):1031–1033.

Smallman, R. E., and R. J. Bishop. 1998. *Modern Physical Metallurgy and Materials Engineering-Science, Process, Application*. Woburn, MA: Elsevier.

Stein, G. S., and J. B. Lian. 1993. Molecular mechanisms mediating proliferation differentiation inter-relationships during progressive development of the osteoblast phenotype. *Endocrine Reviews* 14 (4):424–442.

Stoch, A., A. Brozek, G. Kmita, J. Stoch, W. Jastrzebski, and A. Rakowska. 2001. Electrophoretic coating of hydroxyapatite on titanium implants. *Journal of Molecular Structure* 596:191–200.

Stoch, A., W. Jastrzębski, A. Brozek, J. Stoch, J. Szaraniec, B. Trybalska, and G. Kmita. 2000. FTIR absorption–reflection study of biomimetic growth of phosphates on titanium implants. *Journal of Molecular Structure* 555:375–382.

Stoch, A., W. Jastrzębski, A. Brozek, B. Trybalska, M. Cichocińska, and E. Szarawara. 1999. FTIR monitoring of the growth of the carbonate containing apatite layers from simulated and natural body fluids. *Journal of Molecular Structure* 511–512:287–294.

Stoch, A., W. Jastrzzębski, E. Długoń, W. Lejda, B. Trybalska, G. J. Stoch, and A. Adamczyk. 2005. Sol–gel derived hydroxyapatite coatings on titanium and its alloy Ti6Al4V. *Journal of Molecular Structure* 744–747 (Spec. Iss.):633–640.

Sun, L., C. C. Berndt, K. A. Gross, and A. Kucuk. 2001. Material fundamentals and clinical performance of plasma-sprayed hydroxyapatite coatings: a review. *Journal of Biomedical Materials Research* 58 (5):570–592.

Tengvall, P. 2003. How surface interact with the biological environment. *Bio-implant Interface: Improving Biomaterials and Tissue Reactions*. CRC Press, New York, USA.

Tkalcec, E., M. Sauer, R. Nonninger, and H. Schmidt. 2001. Sol–gel-derived hydroxyapatite powders and coatings. *Journal of Materials Science* 36 (21):5253–5263.

Tsui, Y. C., C. Doyle, and T. W. Clyne. 1998. Plasma sprayed hydroxyapatite coatings on titanium substrates Part 1: Mechanical properties and residual stress levels. *Biomaterials* 19 (22):2015–2029.

Vedantam, R., and C. Ruddlesdin. 1996. The fully hydroxyapatite-coated total hip implant—Clinical and roentgenographic results. *Journal of Arthroplasty* 11 (5):534–542.

Vijayalakshmi, U., K. Prabakaran, and S. Rajeswari. 2008. Preparation and characterization of sol–gel hydroxyapatite and its electrochemical evaluation for biomedical applications. *Journal of Biomedical Materials Research A* 87 (3):739–749.

Wang, A. J., Y. P. Lu, C. Z. Chen, and R. X. Sun. 2007. Effect of plasma spraying parameters on the sprayed hydroxyapatite coating. *Surface Review and Letters* 14 (2):179–184.

Wang, C. K., J. H. C. Lin, C. P. Ju, H. C. Ong, and R. P. H. Chang. 1997. Structural characterization of pulsed laser-deposited hydroxyapatite film on titanium substrate. *Biomaterials* 18 (20):1331–1338.

Wang, D., and G. P. Bierwagen. 2009. Sol–gel coatings on metals for corrosion protection. *Progress in Organic Coatings* 64 (4):327–338.

Wang, D., C. Chen, T. He, and T. Lei. 2008. Hydroxyapatite coating on Ti6Al4V alloy by a sol–gel method. *Journal of Materials Science: Materials in Medicine* 19 (6):2281–2286.

Wang, H., C. Z. Chen, and D. G. Wang. 2009. Effect of heating rate on structure of HA coating prepared by sol–gel. *Surface Engineering* 25 (2):131–135.

Wang, Y., M. S. Hassan, P. Gunawan, R. Lau, X. Wang, and R. Xu. 2009. Polyelectrolyte mediated formation of hydroxyapatite microspheres of controlled size and hierarchical structure. *Journal of Colloid and Interface Science* 339 (1):69–77.

Wang, Y., S. Zhang, X. Zeng, C. Kui, Q. Min, and W. Weng. 2007. In vitro behavior of fluoridated hydroxyapatite coatings in organic-containing simulated body fluid. *Materials Science and Engineering C* 27 (2):244–250.

Wang, Y., S. Zhang, X. Zeng, L. M. Lwin, A. K. Khiam, and M. Qian. 2008. Initial attachment of osteoblastic cells onto sol–gel derived fluoridated hydroxyapatite coatings. *Journal of Biomedical Materials Research Part A* 84 (3):769–776.

Wang, Y., S. Zhang, X. Zeng, L. L. Ma, W. Weng, W. Yan, and M. Qian. 2007. Osteoblastic cell response on fluoridated hydroxyapatite coatings. *Acta Biomaterialia* 3 (2):191–197.

Watanabe, M., D. R. Mumm, S. Chiras, and A. G. Evans. 2002. Measurement of the residual stress in a Pt–aluminide bond coat. *Scripta Materialia* 46 (1):67–70.

Wei, M., A. J. Ruys, B. K. Milthorpe, C. C. Sorrell, and J. H. Evans. 2001. Electrophoretic deposition of hydroxyapatite coatings on metal substrates: A nanoparticulate dual-coating approach. *Journal of Sol–Gel Science and Technology* 21 (1–2):39–48.

Weng, W., and J. L. Baptista. 1998. Sol–gel derived porous hydroxyapatite coatings. *Journal of Materials Science: Materials in Medicine* 9 (3):159–163.

Weng, W., and J. L. Baptista. 1999. Preparation and characterization of hydroxyapatite coatings on Ti6Al4V alloy by a sol–gel method. *Journal of the American Ceramic Society* 82 (1):27–32.

Weng, W., G. Han, P. Du, and G. Shen. 2003. The effect of citric acid addition on sol–gel preparation of apatite films. *Materials Chemistry and Physics* 77 (2):578–582.

Weng, W., S. Zhang, K. Cheng, H. Qu, P. Du, G. Shen, J. Yuan, and G. Han. 2003. Sol–gel preparation of bioactive apatite films. *Surface and Coatings Technology* 167 (2–3):292–296.

Wilson, C. J., R. E. Clegg, D. I. Leavesley, and M. J. Pearcy. 2005. Mediation of biomaterial–cell interaction by adsorbed proteins: a review. *Tissue Engineering* 11 (1–2):1–18.

Witte, F. 2010. The history of biodegradable magnesium implants: a review. *Acta Biomaterialia* 6 (5): 1680–1692.

Xiao, X. F., and R. F. Liu. 2006. Effect of suspension stability on electrophoretic deposition of hydroxyapatite coatings. *Materials Letters* 60 (21–22):2627–2632.

Xie, J., C. Riley, and K. Chittur. 2001. Effect of albumin on brushite transformation to hydroxyapatite. *Journal of Biomedical Materials Research* 57 (3):357–365.

Xie, Y., and H. M. Hawthorne. 2003. Measuring the adhesion of sol–gel derived coatings to a ductile substrate by an indentation-based method. *Surface & Coatings Technology* 172 (1):42–50.

Yan, L., Y. Leng, and L. T. Weng. 2003. Characterization of chemical inhomogeneity in plasma-sprayed hydroxyapatite coatings. *Biomaterials* 24 (15):2585–2592.

Yang, C. Y., R. M. Lin, B. C. Wang, T. M. Lee, E. Chang, Y. S. Hang, and P. Q. Chen. 1997. In vitro and in vivo mechanical evaluations of plasma-sprayed hydroxyapatite coatings on titanium implants: the effect of coating characteristics. *Journal of Biomedical Materials Research* 37 (3):335–345.

Yang, Y. C., E. Chang, and S. Y. Lee. 2003. Mechanical properties and Young's modulus of plasma-sprayed hydroxyapatite coating on Ti substrate in simulated body fluid. *Journal of Biomedical Materials Research Part A* 67A (3):886–899.

Yang, Y. C., and E. Chang. 2001. Influence of residual stress on bonding strength and fracture of plasma-sprayed hydroxyapatite coatings on Ti–6Al–4V substrate. *Biomaterials* 22 (13):1827–1836.

Yang, Y. C., and E. Chang. 2005. Measurements of residual stresses in plasma-sprayed hydroxyapatite coatings on titanium alloy. *Surface and Coatings Technology* 190 (1):122–131.

Yang, Y., K.-H. Kim, and J. L. Ong. 2005. A review on calcium phosphate coatings produced using a sputtering process—an alternative to plasma spraying. *Biomaterials* 26 (3):327–337.

You, C. K., S. Oh, and S. Kim. 2001. Influences of heating condition and substrate-surface roughness on the characteristics of sol–gel-derived hydroxyapatite coatings. *Journal of Sol–Gel Science and Technology* 21 (1–2):49–54.

You, C., I. S. Yeo, M. D. Kim, T. K. Eom, J. Y. Lee, and S. Kim. 2005. Characterization and in vivo evaluation of calcium phosphate coated cp-titanium by dip-spin method. *Current Applied Physics* 5 (5):501–506.

Zberg, B., P. J. Uggowitzer, and J. F. Löffler. 2009. MgZnCa glasses without clinically observable hydrogen evolution for biodegradable implants. *Nature Materials* 8 (11):887–891.

Zhang, S., D. Sun, Y. Q. Fu, H. J. Du, and Q. Zhang. 2004. Effect of sputtering target power density on topography and residual stress during growth of nanocomposite nc-TiN/a-SiNx thin films. *Diamond and Related Materials* 13 (10):1777–1784.

Zhang, S., Y. S. Wang, X. T. Zeng, K. Cheng, M. Qian, D. E. Sun, W. J. Weng, and W. Y. Chia. 2007. Evaluation of interfacial shear strength and residual stress of sol–gel derived fluoridated hydroxyapatite coatings on Ti6Al4V substrates. *Engineering Fracture Mechanics* 74 (12):1884–1893.

Zhang, S., Y. S. Wang, X. T. Zeng, K. A. Khor, Wenjian Weng, and D. E. Sun. 2008. Evaluation of adhesion strength and toughness of fluoridated hydroxyapatite coatings. *Thin Solid Films* 516 (16):5162–5167.

Zhang, S., Z. Xianting, W. Yongsheng, C. Kui, and W. Wenjian. 2006. Adhesion strength of sol–gel derived fluoridated hydroxyapatite coatings. *Surface and Coatings Technology* 200 (22–23 Spec. Iss.):6350–6354.

2

Amorphous Carbon Coatings for Biological Applications

Soon-Eng Ong and Sam Zhang

CONTENTS

Introduction—The Material..45
    Bonding in Amorphous Carbon...46
    Amorphous Carbon Growth Mechanism...46
    Bonding Characterization of Amorphous Carbon 52
        X-ray Photoelectron Spectroscopy 52
        Raman Spectroscopy 52
    Determination of Surface Energetics...55
        Concept of Surface Energy 55
        Surface Tension Component 57
    Remarks 59
Hemocompatibility 59
    Hydrogenated and Unhydrogenated Amorphous Carbon 61
    Effects of Doping 66
    Effects of Post-Deposition Treatment 71
Cytocompatibility 76
    Endothelials...77
    Macrophages...81
    Fibroblasts 82
    Osteoblasts 85
    Other Cells...88
    In Vivo Studies...90
Antibacterial Behavior..92
Biomedical Applications 95
    Orthopedic Implants...95
    Coronary Stent...97
    Other Biomedical Applications 98
Summary 99
References...100

Introduction—The Material

Since the first fabrication of amorphous carbon (a-C) in 1971 [1], the material has been largely studied and utilized as passivation or protective coatings. The material is known to have superior mechanical properties, such as high hardness, low stiction, low friction coefficient, and low surface roughness. The material also has good chemical and biological properties, such as resistance to chemical corrosion and biocompatibility, and thus has attracted the attention of researchers around the world on studying and developing it for biological and biomedical applications.

Before discussing the various biological/biomedical studies done over the years, it is important to have an understanding on the material itself. In this section, the material, amorphous carbon, and some useful ways of characterizing it will be covered. In addition, an introduction on how to determine its surface characteristics will be briefly discussed.

Bonding in Amorphous Carbon

Amorphous carbon contains both sp^3 and sp^2 bonded carbon (refer to Figure 2.1). It is also called "diamond-like carbon." In the sp^3 configuration, as with diamond, a carbon atom's four valence electrons are each assigned to a tetrahedrally directed sp^3 orbital with an angle of 109.5° from each other, which makes a strong σ bond to an adjacent atom. In the sp^2 configuration, as in graphite, three of the four valence electrons enter trigonally directed sp^2 orbitals equally separated by an angle of 120°, which form σ bonds in a plane. The fourth electron of the sp^2 atom lies in a π orbital, normal to the σ bonding plane. This π orbital forms a weaker π bond with a π orbital on one or more neighboring atoms.

Amorphous carbon bonding structures and electronic properties have been widely studied using ab initio molecular dynamics of the first principles. Both sp^2-rich a-C [2] and sp^3-rich a-C (sp^3 fraction > ~80% is popularly known as the tetrahedral amorphous carbon or ta-C) [3] models were studied. Results have shown an increase in sp^2 hybridizations when the temperature is increased. It is therefore apparent that in order to fabricate high-quality amorphous carbon with properties that are near diamond (high sp^3 bondings), the synthesis process should be carried out at room temperature or lower.

Amorphous Carbon Growth Mechanism

Lifshitz et al. [4,5] used the Auger analysis of the depth profiles of medium energy carbon ions incident on nickel substrates to show that the growth was subsurface and denoted the process as "subplantation" (low-energy subsurface implantation). This process advances as follows:

(a) Penetration

Penetration of the impinging species into the subsurface layers of the substrate, with the penetration depth and distribution depending on the mass and energy

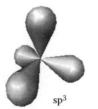
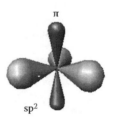

FIGURE 2.1
sp^3 and sp^2 hybridized bonding of carbon.

of the impinging species and nature of the target material. Some of the impinging species may be backscattered and will not contribute to the net film growth.

(b) Stopping

Stopping of the energetic species via three energy-loss mechanisms: atomic displacements, phonon excitations, and electron excitations. (The latter two phenomena are sometimes collectively referred to as "thermal spikes.")

(c) Site occupation

The possible initial sites the impinging atoms occupy after being stopped are determined by the host matrix that serves as a "mold" for the structure of the growing film. Hyperthermal species trapped in a site may occupy another during further impingement of energetic species, either due to collisions or recrystallization induced by compositional changes during deposition.

(d) Phase formation

The increase in concentration of the penetrating species in the host matrix results in the formation of an inclusion of a new phase, accompanied by the outward expansion of the substrate layer (internal subsurface growth).

(e) Surface composition

During the early stages of film growth, the surface is mainly composed of substrate atoms due to the subsurface penetration of the impinging particles. These substrate surface atoms are gradually sputtered and/or diluted by ion-mixing mechanisms until a surface consisting of only projectile species evolves.

(f) Film structure

Several factors determine the phase and structure of the film: (1) the "mold" effect of the host matrix that determines the possible site occupancies of the penetrating species and places constraints on initial evolution of the new phase; (2) preferential displacement of atoms with low displacement energies leaving atoms with high displacement energies in their more stable positions; (3) diffusion rates of vacancies and interstitials created in the deposition process. When the temperature is sufficiently low, the interstitials are immobile, and their concentration increases with fluence until an athermal spontaneous transformation to a new phase occurs.

(g) Sputtering

The surface features of the evolving film and the efficiency of the deposition process depend on the sputtering yield of both substrate and trapped atoms by the impinging ions. Low sputtering yield is essential for efficient deposition and is necessarily less than unity for net film growth to occur at all.

(h) Film evolution

Evolution of a pure film from hyperthermal species impinging on a substrate consisting of atoms different from that of the bombarding species is feasible only when collisional ion-mixing and diffusion processes are small enough so as to allow evolution of a pure layer. Therefore, the "deposition" process has two stages: (1) initial "heterodeposition" followed by evolution into a pure layer as described in (a)–(e) and (2) "homodeposition" of energetic species adding to the pure film.

Lifshitz et al. [4,5] proposed that the sp^3 sites accumulate via preferential displacement of sp^2 sites. Moller [6] modeled preferential displacement in more detail and proposed that the sp^2 and sp^3 atoms would be displaced at certain rates into interstitial sites and then fall back at similar rates into sp^2 and sp^3 sites. The fraction of sp^3 sites increases if there is a preferential displacement of sp^2 atoms. However, this model arose from some early estimates of the displacement threshold in graphite and diamond of 25 and 80 eV, respectively. The more recent direct measurements find similar values for graphite (35 eV) and diamond (37–47 eV) [7,8], so preferential displacement is unlikely.

McKenzie et al. [9] noted that sp^2 bonded graphite occupies 50% more volume than sp^3 bonded diamond. This leads to the phase diagram of diamond and graphite shown in Figure 2.2, with diamond stable at a higher pressure above the Berman–Simon curve, and therefore it stabilizes the high-pressure diamond-like phase.

Robertson [10,11] proposed that subplantation would create a metastable increase in density, causing the local bonding to change into sp^3. Preferential displacement is not required, as only the subsurface growth in a restricted volume is needed to get sp^3 bonding.

A number of numerical and analytical simulations substantiate the basic idea of the subplantation model [12–14]. The unsolved problem is in the details of the relaxation process, which suppresses sp^3 bonding at higher ion energies and higher deposition temperatures.

In the following, the atomic scale processes will be discussed using Robertson's data [10,11,15]. In the energy range of 10–1000 eV, the carbon ions have a range of a few nm, and their energies are lost mainly by elastic collisions with the substrate atoms (nuclear stopping). The cross section of the collisions decreases as the energy is raised due to the repulsive part of the interatomic potential. Therefore, an ion of low energy incident on a surface sees an impenetrable wall of touching spheres. At a higher energy, the atomic radii decrease, so the interstices of the substrate are relatively wider. At some energy, the ion can pass through an interstice and so penetrate the surface layer. This ion energy is termed the penetration threshold, E_p.

The displacement threshold, E_d, is the minimum energy of an incident ion needed to displace an atom from a bonded site and create a permanent vacancy-interstitial pair. The ions when entering the surface must also overcome the substrate's surface binding energy, E_B. Thus, the net penetration threshold for free ions is:

$$E_p \approx E_d + E_B \tag{2.1}$$

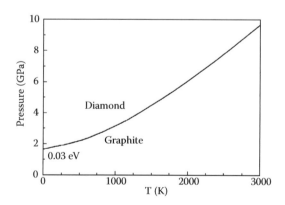

FIGURE 2.2
Berman–Simon P–T phase diagram for carbon. (Reprinted with permission from Robertson, J., *Mater. Sci. Eng. R*, 37, 129, 2002.)

Considering carbon ions incident on an amorphous carbon surface [11], a low energy ion will not have enough energy to penetrate the surface, so it will just stick on the surface and remain in its lowest energy state, which is sp^2. If the ion energy is greater than E_p, then it will have a probability to penetrate the surface and enter a subsurface interstitial site. This will cause an increase in local density, and so the local bonding will reform around that atom according to the new density. Robertson assumed that, in the highly energetic conditions of ion bombardment existing during film growth, atomic hybridizations will adjust easily to changes in the local density and become more sp^2 if the density is low and more sp^3 if the density is high.

When the ion energy increases, the ion range increases as well, hence the ion can penetrate deeper into the substrate. A rather small fraction of this energy is used to penetrate the surface, and another fraction of about 30% is dissipated in atom displacements [16]. The ion must dissipate the rest of this energy ultimately as phonons. This whole process consists of three stages: (a) a collisional stage of 10^{-13} s, (b) a thermalization stage of 10^{-12} s, and (c) a relaxation stage of 10^{-10} s. Process (b) and/or (c) allow the excess density to relax to zero and cause a loss of sp^3 bonding at higher ion energies.

Referring to Figure 2.3, consider an incident beam of flux F with a fraction ϕ of energetic ions of energy E_i. The nonenergetic fraction of the atoms or ions $(1 - f\phi)$ will just stick on the outer surface, while some of the penetrating ions will relax back to the surface. This flux is proportional to a driving force, the fraction of interstitials below the surface, n.

In the steady state, the fraction of the ions remaining at the interstitial sites to give densification is $n = f\phi - \beta n$, where β is a constant. This gives:

$$n = \frac{f\phi}{1 + \beta} \tag{2.2}$$

A fraction n of the beam becomes subplanted inside the film, and a fraction $(1 - n)$ is left on the surface as sp^2 sites. The subplanted fraction creates a density increment of:

$$\frac{\Delta\rho}{\rho} = \frac{n}{1 - n} \tag{2.3}$$

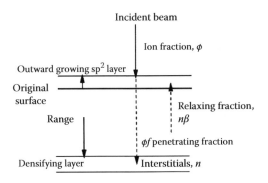

FIGURE 2.3
Schematic diagram of densification by subplantation. A fraction of incident ions penetrates the film and densifies it, and the remainders end up on the surface to give thickness growth. (Reprinted with permission from Robertson, J., *Mater. Sci. Eng. R*, 37, 129, 2002.)

which gives:

$$\frac{\Delta\rho}{\rho} = \frac{f\phi}{1 - f\phi + \beta} \tag{2.4}$$

where ρ is the density of sp^2 carbon and $\Delta\rho$ is the density increase.

Figure 2.4 shows that penetration can occur in two ways, either directly or indirectly by knock-on. Knock-on penetrations only occur for the case of ion-assisted deposition.

The first numerical models assumed that relaxation occurs in the thermal spike stage of $\sim 10^{-12}$ s [10,11]. This will give a relaxation rate of $\beta \approx 0.016(E_i/E_0)^{5/3}$, where E_0 is the diffusion activation energy, and so:

$$\frac{\Delta\rho}{\rho} = \frac{f\phi}{1 - f\phi + 0.016\left(E_i/E_0\right)^{5/3}} \tag{2.5}$$

The thermal spike model proposes that all the excess energy of the ion is converted to thermal energy at a point or along the ion trajectory. Then the energy diffuses outward by thermal diffusion, creating an expanding front in which all atoms inside the front have a similar thermal energy, by equipartition. The temperature profile of a spherical spike is:

$$T\left(r,t\right) = \frac{Q}{c\left[4\pi Dt\right]^{3/2}} \exp\left(-\frac{r^2}{4Dt}\right) \tag{2.6}$$

where r is the distance from the impact, t the time from the impact, D the thermal diffusivity, and c the thermal capacity of the carbon. Q is the ion energy E_i minus that lost in displacements [17]. Taking $Q \approx E_i$ for now, Robertson assumed that the thermal spike allows

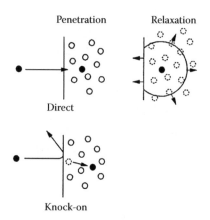

FIGURE 2.4
Schematic of basic processes in subplantation: direct penetration, penetration by knock-on of a surface atom, and relaxation of a densified region. (Reprinted with permission from Robertson, J., *Mater. Sci. Eng. R*, 37, 129, 2002.)

atoms to diffuse back to the surface to relax the density to a lower, stable sp² density. He also assumed that relaxation occurs by thermally activated diffusion at a rate of:

$$v = v_0 \exp\left(-\frac{E_0}{kT}\right) \tag{2.7}$$

where E_0 is the activation energy for atomic diffusion. The total number of hops of all the atoms within one spike is the integral over the spike volume and time:

$$\beta = \int_{r_1}^{\infty} 4\pi n_0 r^2 \int_{t_1}^{\infty} v \exp\left(-\frac{E_0}{kT(r,t)}\right) dt\,dr \tag{2.8}$$

where k is Boltzmann's constant, n_0 the atomic number density, v_0 the phonon frequency, r_1 the minimum radius of the spike, and t_1 the minimum time of the spike. It is useful to put everything in dimensionless atomic units, with an atomic radius a. Robertson defines reduced distances $r' = r/a$, times $t' = v_0 t$, and a reduced temperature $\tau = kT/E_0$. The heat capacity per atom is $3k$, so $c = 9k/4\pi a^3$, $D \approx v_0 a^2$, and $n_0 = 3/4\pi a^3$. Integration over t' is carried out, and the integral over r' is converted to one over τ to give:

$$\beta = \int_{\tau_1}^{\tau_2} \tau^{-8/3} \exp\left(-\frac{1}{\tau}\right) d\tau \tag{2.9}$$

In the limits $\tau_1 \to 0$ and $\tau_2 \to \infty$ this gives:

$$\beta = 0.016p\left(\frac{E_i}{E_0}\right)^{5/3} \tag{2.10}$$

where p is a dimensionless constant of order 1. All the other quantities cancel out. This is the equation used in Equation 2.5.

Equation 2.5 gives a good representation of the variation of density or sp³ fraction with energy for tetrahedal-amorphous carbon (ta-C) deposited by filtered cathodic vacuum arc (FCVA) [11,18] with $E_0 = 3.1$ eV. The increasing sp³ fraction at lower ion energy is controlled by the penetration probability f, and the decline in sp³ fraction at high ion energy is controlled by the relaxation.

Despite this superficial agreement between theory and experiment, this model of deposition is still deficient. There are many faults with the thermal spike concept when applied to carbon deposition. A thermal spike is only truly valid for much heavier ions and higher ion energies, where the energy loss rate per distance (stopping power) is much higher, so the energy density is greater [19,20]. In carbon, energy equipartition does not really hold, so the spike volume consists of a few excited atoms among much less excited atoms.

A satisfactory model of growth must account for

- The transition temperature to sp² bonding, being 400–500 K [21,22], despite the temperature in a thermal spike's being 10⁶ K
- The variation of the transition temperature for sp³ formation with ion energy [21].
- The variation of transition temperature with instantaneous growth rate [17,23]

Bonding Characterization of Amorphous Carbon

X-ray Photoelectron Spectroscopy

X-ray photoelectron spectroscopy (XPS) is a technique used to investigate the composition of deposited films by ionizing surface atoms and measuring the energy of ejected photoelectrons. The method requires the sample of interest to be bombarded with low energy x-rays, produced from an aluminum or magnesium source, with an energy of hv, where h is Planck's constant (6.62×10^{-34} Js) and v is the frequency (Hz) of the radiation. These x-rays cause electrons to be ejected from either a valence or inner core electron shell. The kinetic energy of the electron, KE, is given by $KE = hv - BE$, where BE is the binding energy of the atom. If the energy of the ejected photoelectrons were measured, its binding energy, which is the energy required to remove the electron from its atom, can be calculated. Some important facts about the sample under investigation can be learned from the binding energy: (1) the elements from which it is made, (2) the relative quantity of each element, (3) the chemical state of the elements present, and (4) the lateral and depth distributions (profiles).

The change in chemical state (interatomic bonding) will cause a shift in the binding energy. In a-C, there are two main hybridizations, namely sp^3 diamond and sp^2 graphite (as discussed in Section 2.1.1). Since both are formed by bondings of carbon atoms, the chemical shift between that of sp^3 and sp^2 is small. That is, the binding energy of the two as determined from XPS will be relatively close to each other. Therefore, there will be a superpositioning of the C 1s core level peak due to the contribution of the two hybridized carbons. The peak of amorphous carbon is thus broadened. In order to determine the contribution of each hybridized carbon in the film, the C 1s peak can be deconvoluted. It was found that the full-width at half-maximum of both the sp^3 peak and the sp^2 peak tend to be wider than those from pure diamond and graphite [24]. This is attributed to the environment within the a-C film with mixed sp^2 and sp^3 bondings. A deconvoluted C 1s peak is shown in Figure 2.5. This regime for the approximation of the sp^2 and sp^3 concentration in the a-C is widely used [24–27].

Raman Spectroscopy

Raman spectroscopy is widely used, being a routine, nondestructive way to characterize the structural quality of amorphous carbons. The Raman effect is possible because of the

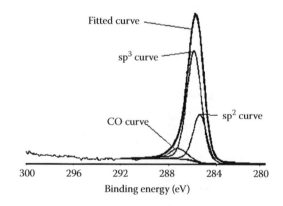

FIGURE 2.5
Example of fits of C 1s peak from an XPS spectrum. (Reprinted with permission from Filik et al., *Diamond Rel. Mater.*, 12, 974, 2003.)

strain dependence of the electronic polarizability. It is the light scattering by the change in polarizability due to lattice vibration. The difference in energy between the incident photon and the Raman scattered photon is equal to the energy of a vibration of the scattering molecule. A plot of intensity of scattered light versus energy difference (or shift) is a Raman spectrum.

The Raman spectra of diamond, graphite, and some disordered carbons are compared in Figure 2.6. Diamond has a single Raman active mode at 1332 cm^{-1}, which is a zone-center mode of T_{2g} symmetry. Single crystal graphite has a single Raman active mode, which is the zone-center mode at 1581 cm^{-1} of E_{2g} symmetry labeled "G" for "graphite." The zone-center optical modes in graphite can be decomposed into irreducible representation [28,29]:

$$\Gamma = 2B_{2g} + 2E_{2g} + A_{2u} + E_{1u} \tag{2.11}$$

The A_{2u} and E_{1u} modes are infrared active, the B_{2g} modes are optically inactive, and the E_{2g} modes are Raman active. The symmetry of the E modes restricts the motion of the carbon atoms. The two different E_g modes occur because adjacent planes can vibrate in phase or with opposite phase [28,29]. The two in-plane Raman active E_{2g} modes are found to occur at frequencies of 1581 cm^{-1} (E_{2g2}) and 42 cm^{-1} (E_{2g1}). The peak at 1581 cm^{-1} from the Raman active zone-center mode of graphite, assigned to the C–C stretching mode [28,29], is also referred to as the G peak. When the long-range order of the graphite is disrupted (disordered graphite), a second peak appears at about 1355 cm^{-1} referred to as the D peak ("D" for "disorder"). The D peak is associated with in-plane vibrations and results from structural imperfections. The Raman spectra of most disordered carbons remain dominated

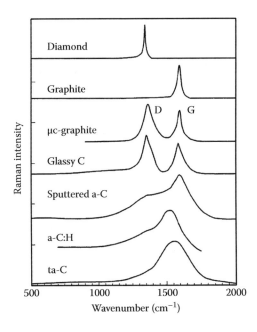

FIGURE 2.6
Comparison of typical Raman spectra of carbons. (Reprinted with permission from Robertson, J., *Mater. Sci. Eng. R*, 37, 129, 2002.)

by these two G and D modes of graphite, even when the carbons do not have particular graphitic ordering [30].

The G mode of graphite at 1581 cm^{-1} has E_{2g} symmetry, and it involves the in-plane bond-stretching motion of pairs of carbon sp^2 atoms. This mode does not require the presence of six fold rings, and so it can occur at all sp^2 sites, not only in rings. It is always in the range between 1500 and 1630 cm^{-1}. The D peak around 1355 cm^{-1} is a breathing mode of A_{1g} symmetry. This mode is forbidden in perfect graphite and only becomes active in the presence of disorder. And its peak intensity is connected to the presence of six fold aromatic rings [30].

Figure 2.7 shows the various factors that can shift the G and D peaks in either direction and alter their relative intensity.

Ferrari and Robertson [30] found that the Raman spectra of all disordered carbons can be classified within a three-stage model of increasing disorder. The Raman spectrum is considered to depend on

1. Clustering of the sp^2 phase
2. Bond disorder
3. Presence of sp^2 rings or chains
4. The sp^3/sp^2 ratio

The above factors act as competing forces on the shape of the Raman spectra, as shown in Figure 2.7. Ferrari and Robertson [30] defined an amorphitization trajectory ranging from graphite to ta-C consisting of three stages:

1. Graphite → nanocrystalline graphite
2. Nanocrystalline graphite → a-C
3. a-C → ta-C

Stage 1 corresponds to the progressive reduction in grain size of ordered graphite layers, while keeping aromatic rings. As the grain size decreases, phonon confinement causes the

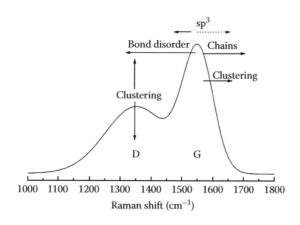

FIGURE 2.7
Schematic of the factors affecting position and heights of Raman G and D peaks of noncrystalline carbons. (Reprinted with permission from Robertson, J., *Mater. Sci. Eng. R*, 37, 129, 2002.)

phonons to disperse upward from 1581 cm^{-1}, so this causes an up-shift of the G peak to ~1600 cm^{-1}. The D mode is forbidden in an ideal graphitic layer, but the disorder causes it to appear.

In Stage 2, defects are progressively introduced into the graphite layer, causing disordering and the loss of aromatic bonding, but with a purely sp^2 network. The disordering and loss of aromatic bonding weaken the bonds, thus causing the G peak to shift downward to ~1510 cm^{-1}. The number of ordered rings now decreases, and I$_D$ starts to decrease. The intensity of the G peak remains unchanged as it is only related to bond stretching of sp^2 pairs. The I$_D$/I$_G$ decreases with increasing amorphization. The end of Stage 2 corresponds to a completely disordered, almost fully sp^2-bonded a-C consisting of distorted six fold rings or rings of other orders (maximum 20% sp^3). A typical example is sputtered a-C [31,32].

In Stage 3, when passing from a-C to ta-c, the sp^3 content rises from ~10–20% to ~85%. This changes the sp^2 configuration from mainly rings to short chains [30]. The bond length of the chains (olefins) is shorter than that of the rings, so they have higher vibrational frequencies. Therefore, the G peak increases from ~1510 to ~1570 cm^{-1}. The D-peak is absent in curve fit, and the G-peak skew falls to almost zero (more symmetric) at high sp^3 content [33].

Determination of Surface Energetics

The interaction between biological entities, such as cells or proteins, is very much affected by the contacting amorphous carbon surface properties. Subsequent sections have numerous works discussing this. Here, a brief introduction on the concept of surface energy and the means to their determination will be discussed. More comprehensive coverage of the topic can be found elsewhere [34].

Concept of Surface Energy

The ability of a liquid to wet a solid surface depends on the surface energies of the solid–vapor interface, the liquid–vapor interface, and the solid–liquid interface. The surface energy across an interface is a measure of the energy required to form a unit area of new surface at the interface. The intermolecular bonds or cohesive forces between the molecules of a liquid cause surface tension. There is usually an attraction between the liquid and another substance when they are brought into contact. The adhesive forces between the liquid and the second substance will compete against the cohesive forces of the liquid. Liquids with weak cohesive bonds and a strong attraction to the other material will tend to spread over the material. Liquids with strong cohesive bonds and weaker adhesive forces will tend to bead up and form a droplet when in contact with another material.

The definition of "surface energy" is the work required to increase the surface area of a substance by unit area. Surface energy derives from the unsatisfied bonding potential of molecules at a surface, giving rise to "free energy." This is unlike the molecules within a material which have less energy because they are interacting with like molecules in all directions. Molecules at the surface will try to reduce this free energy by interacting with molecules in an adjacent phase. The free energy per unit area is termed the surface energy for solids, and the surface tension in liquids when one of the bulk phases is a gas. On the other hand, when both phases are condensed (e.g., solid–solid, solid–liquid, and immiscible liquid–liquid interfaces), the free energy per unit area of the interface is called the "interfacial energy."

Surface energy is also related with surface hydrophobicity. Whereas surface energy describes interactions with a range of materials, surface hydrophobicity describes these interactions with water only. Since water has a high capacity for bonding, a material of high surface energy (i.e., high bonding potential) can have more interactions with water and consequently will be more hydrophilic. Therefore, hydrophobicity generally decreases as surface energy increases. Hydrophilic surfaces such as glass have high surface energies, whereas hydrophobic surfaces such as polytetrafluoroethylene (PTFE) or polystyrene have low surface energies.

The determination of solid–vapor (γ_{sv}) and solid–liquid (γ_{sl}) interfacial tensions is important in a wide range of problems in pure and applied sciences. Due to the immerse difficulties involved in the direct measurement of surface tension when a solid phase is involved, indirect approaches are usually required. Several approaches have been used to estimate solid surface tensions, but among these methods, contact angle measurements are believed to be the simplest.

Contact angle can be measured by establishing the tangent (angle) of a liquid drop with a solid surface at the base. The possibility of estimating solid surface energies from contact angles relies on a relation that has been recognized by Young [35]. The contact angle of a liquid drop on a solid surface is defined by the equilibrium of the drop under the action of three interfacial tensions (Figure 2.8): solid–vapor, γ_{sv}, solid–liquid, γ_{sl}, and liquid–vapor, γ_{lv}. This equilibrium relation is known as Young's equation:

$$\gamma_{lv} \cos \theta_Y = \gamma_{sv} - \gamma_{sl} \tag{2.12}$$

where θ_Y is the Young contact angle, or the measured contact angle.

The calculation of the solid surface tension γ_{sv} from the contact angle of a liquid of surface tension γ_{lv} begins with Young's equation. Of the four parameters in Young's equation, only θ and γ_{lv} are readily measurable. θ, of course, can be determined during the test, and γ_{lv} can be determined and calculated using the pendant drop method by fitting the shape of the suspended droplet (in a captured video image) to the Young–Laplace equation, which relates the interfacial tension to drop shape:

$$\Delta P = \gamma \left(\frac{1}{R_1} + \frac{1}{R_2} \right) \tag{2.13}$$

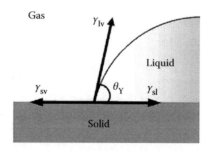

FIGURE 2.8
Contact angle and respective interfacial tensions component of a liquid sample.

where ΔP = interfacial pressure difference in a column of fluid of density ρ and height h, $\Delta P = \rho g h$ and g is the acceleration due to gravity (9.8 m/s²). γ = interfacial tension (γ_{lv}), R_1, R_2 = surface's radii of curvature of the drop.

Therefore, there are only two unknown parameters in Young's equation. An obvious approach is to solve for the two unknowns simultaneously from the two simultaneous equations generated by two test liquids (each with its own γ_{lv} value and θ generated). However, the problem with this approach is the γ_{ls}, which is a function of the liquid's own γ_{lv} and the solid's γ_{sv}. That is to say, the γ_{ls} value should be different when two liquids are used, and hence cannot be determined simultaneously. So a more appropriate method is to combine the equations from the surface tension component approaches (γ_{sv} is the sum of different surface tension components, e.g., dispersive or polar components) with Young's equation and then solve simultaneously the equations generated by using two or three liquids. If deionized water (which is polar in nature) is used, diiodomethane (which is dispersive) can be a supplementary liquid to be used, as the γ_{lv} and θ values are more prominently differentiated from that of deionized water.

Surface Tension Component

Fowkes

The approach of surface tension components was pioneered by Fowkes [36]. The total surface tension can be expressed as a sum of different surface tension components, each of which arises due to a specific type of intermolecular force:

$$\gamma = \gamma^d + \gamma^h + \gamma^{di} + \times\times\times \tag{2.14}$$

where γ, γ^d, γ^h, and γ^{di} are, respectively, the total surface tension, dispersive surface tension component, and surface tension components due to hydrogen and dipole–dipole bonding. Equation 2.14 is often rearranged into:

$$\gamma = \gamma^d + \gamma^n \tag{2.15}$$

where the total surface tension γ is a sum of only the dispersive γ^d and nondispersive γ^n surface tension components. The former arises from molecular interaction due to London forces; the latter is from all the other interactions due to non-London forces. A geometric mean relationship was postulated both of the solid–liquid and liquid–liquid interfacial tensions:

$$\gamma_{12} = \gamma_1 + \gamma_2 - 2\sqrt{\gamma_1^d \gamma_2^d} \tag{2.16}$$

For solid–liquid systems, combining Equation 2.16 with Young's Equation 2.12 yields:

$$\gamma_1 \cos\theta_Y = 2\sqrt{\gamma_s^d \gamma_1^d} - \gamma_1 \tag{2.17}$$

Typically, experimental contact angles of different liquids with known γ_1^d on a dispersive solid surface ($\gamma_s = \gamma_s^d$) are employed to determine the surface tension of a solid.

Owens–Wendt–Kaelble

Fowkes' concept was extended by Owens and Wendt [37] to cases where both dispersion and hydrogen bonding forces may operate. The surface tension composes of two components such that:

$$\gamma = \gamma^{d} + \gamma^{h} \tag{2.18}$$

where γ^{h} denotes the component of surface tension due to both hydrogen bonding and dipole–dipole interactions. They postulated:

$$\gamma_{sl} = \gamma_{s} + \gamma_{l} - 2\sqrt{\gamma_{s}^{d}\gamma_{l}^{d}} - 2\sqrt{\gamma_{s}^{h}\gamma_{l}^{h}} \tag{2.19}$$

Combining this equation with Young's Equation 2.12 yields:

$$\gamma_{l}\left(1 + \cos\theta_{Y}\right) = 2\sqrt{\gamma_{s}^{d}\gamma_{l}^{d}} + 2\sqrt{\gamma_{s}^{h}\gamma_{l}^{h}} \tag{2.20}$$

Around the same time, Kaelble [38] published a very similar equation in terms of dispersion and polar forces. Thus, Equation 2.19 is often called the Owens–Wendt–Kaelble equation.

Equation 2.20 contains two unknowns: γ_{s}^{d} and γ_{s}^{h}. They can be determined by measuring the contact angle of at least two different liquids on one and the same solid surface and then solving the two simultaneous equations.

Lifshitz–van der Waals/acid–base (van Oss)

The Lifshitz–van der Waals/acid–base (van Oss) approach [39,40] is a generalization of the Fowkes' approach, by considering perceived acid–base interactions at the interface. van Oss et al. divided the surface tension into different perceived components (i.e., the so-called Lifshitz–van der Waals (LW), acid (+), and base (−) components) such that the total surface tension is given by:

$$\gamma_{i} = \gamma_{i}^{LW} + 2\sqrt{\gamma_{i}^{+}\gamma_{i}^{-}} \tag{2.21}$$

where i denotes either the solid or liquid phase. The interfacial tension was postulated both of solid–liquid and liquid–liquid systems as:

$$\gamma_{12} = \gamma_{1} + \gamma_{2} - 2\sqrt{\gamma_{1}^{LW}\gamma_{2}^{LW}} - 2\sqrt{\gamma_{1}^{+}\gamma_{2}^{-}} - 2\sqrt{\gamma_{1}^{-}\gamma_{2}^{+}} \tag{2.22}$$

For solid–liquid systems, combining Equation 2.22 with Young's equation yields:

$$\gamma_{l}\left(1 + \cos\theta_{Y}\right) = 2\sqrt{\gamma_{l}^{LW}\gamma_{s}^{LW}} + 2\sqrt{\gamma_{l}^{+}\gamma_{s}^{-}} + 2\sqrt{\gamma_{l}^{-}\gamma_{s}^{+}} \tag{2.23}$$

Equation 2.23 is used to determine the solid surface tension components (γ_{s}^{LW}, γ_{s}^{+}, and γ_{s}^{-}) from contact angles, using three simultaneous equations by inserting the properties of the test liquids.

Remarks

It must be noted that amorphous carbon is not a specific material, but a group of materials with a wide range of atomic bonding structures and properties depending on the deposition method. There are a number of "names" for this material. They include diamond-like carbon (DLC) and amorphous diamond (aD). In this chapter, "amorphous carbon" will be used as a general term for this group of materials. For ease of discussion, abbreviations will be used for specific classes as such:

Unhydrogenated amorphous carbon:	a-C
Hydrogenated amorphous carbon:	a-C:H
Unhydrogenated amorphous carbon with dopant:	a-C(X), where "*X*" is the dopant
Hydrogenated amorphous carbon with dopant:	a-C:H(X), where "*X*" is the dopant
Tetrahedral amorphous carbon:	ta-C

Tetrahedral amorphous carbon does not usually contain hydrogen. But if there are such cases, "ta-C:H" will be used.

Hemocompatibility

The major clinical issue in the use of blood's contacting artificial materials is blood compatibility. When biomaterials come into contact with internal body tissue, blood coagulation (i.e., thrombosis) may take place. The interaction of a biomaterial surface with blood stimulates platelet activation, coagulation, and thrombus formation. The reactions of the body to a blood-contacting surface crucially depend on the surface, especially the chemical situation present at the surface, the surface texture, the local flow conditions, and other such factors [41]. It is generally known that the increase in platelet adhesion, activation, and aggregation on the surface exposed to blood precede the formation of a thrombus. A high ratio of the proteins albumin/fibrinogen adsorbed on the surface prior to cell or platelet attachment can be correlated with a low number of adhering platelets and therefore a lower tendency of thrombus formation. Hence, a better inhibition of platelet and fibrinogen adhesion and enhancement of albumin adhesion on the surface are basic prerequisites for blood compatibility.

There are a number of regimes to characterize hemocompatibility. One of the most common methodologies is the use of platelet-rich plasma assay. Before we go into the topic, it is best we have some idea regarding the method. Below is one example.

Platelet-rich plasma preparation and assay. Four hundred and fifty milliliters of human whole blood from a drug-free donor was drawn and mixed with trisodium citrate. The ratio of blood to trisodium citrate was 9 to 1. To prepare the platelet-rich plasma (PRP), the blood was centrifuged at 3200 rpm for 10 min to separate the blood corpuscles. The plasma was extracted and centrifuged again at 3200 rpm for 15 min. Platelet clumps were obtained and allowed to redistribute back into the plasma, which was then 30 ml after draining away the excess. The platelet count in the PRP was determined by flow cytometry to be 1.6×10^6 cells/μL. The plasma was then held in a 37°C water bath for 30 min to allow the platelets to return to their original shape. After the cleaning (ultrasonic cleaning in acetone) and sterilization (4-h UV exposure) processes, the PRP was seeded onto the surfaces of the a-C(Si) coated substrates placed in a Petri dish. Incubation was carried out at 37°C in 5% CO_2 for 30 min. Afterward, the supernatant was discarded, and the samples were rinsed twice with Phosphate Buffered Saline (PBS) to remove the proteins and nonadherent platelets. The cells on the specimens were fixed with 2.5% gluteraldehyde for 30 min, followed by 1% osmium tetraoxide on ice for 45 min. After the fixation, the samples were washed and dehydrated in a graded ethanol series of 50%, 70%, 80%, 95%, and 100% (twice) for 10 min each. Critical point drying can be performed if desired.

A scanning electron microscope can be used to observe the platelets. The samples were coated with ~15 nm of gold to prevent surface charging. An average platelet count using the mean of six nonrepeating selected areas was conducted on each sample. Results were expressed as counts/unit area and standard error. The statistical analysis used was one-way analysis of variance (ANOVA) on an average of three replicates to compare data between different periods of culture, and Student's *t*-test was carried out to compare the culture data between coatings on each count. Statistical significance was considered at $p < 0.05$. The morphological shape changes were categorized according to Goodman et al. [42] and are illustrated in Table 2.1. There are five types of platelet morphologies. Inactivated platelets of Type I are ~2 μm in diameter and do not have a pseudopod. With increasing activation, the platelets develop pseudopodial extensions, which eventually

TABLE 2.1

Five Types of Platelet Morphologies in Relation to Their Activation Level Upon Adhesion to Foreign Surfaces

Type		Morphology Description
I		Round and discoid—No pseudopodia
II		Dendritic—Early pseudopodial with no flattening
III		Spread-dentritic—Intermediate pseudopodia with one or more pseudopodia flattened, no hyaloplasm between pseudopodia
IV		Spreading—Late pseudopodial with hyaloplasm spreading
V		Fully spread—Hyaloplasm fully spread with no distinct pseudopodia

become hyaloplasm at the highest state of activation (Type V). The platelets then can have a size up to ~5 µm.

Hydrogenated and Unhydrogenated Amorphous Carbon

Using PRP prepared from whole human blood and a parallel plate flow chamber, Krishnan et al. [43] showed that platelet adhesion is reduced on a-C compared to a titanium surface. Also, using radioscintigraphy, they showed that the adherence of platelets to the material is determined by the shear rates at which the materials are exposed to the PRP.

An in vitro experiment conducted by Jones et al. [44,45] showed that a-C:H surface expressed a lower area coverage of platelets when compared to titanium, titanium nitride (TiN), and titanium carbide (TiC). Water contact angle measurement of the films shows that the a-C:H is more hydrophobic as compared to the other films. Platelet activation, clotting of platelets, and thrombus formation were observed on titanium containing surfaces, but no such reactions took place on a-C:H surfaces.

A higher ratio of albumin/fibrinogen adsorption was observed on the a-C surfaces than on titanium, titanium nitride (TiN), and titanium carbide (TiC), indicating the ability of a-C to prevent thrombus formation [45]. Cui and Li [46] also showed the similar result when comparing a-C with carbon nitride (CN) and polymethylmethacrylate (PMMA) with a-C having a higher albumin/fibrinogen ratio. The albumin/fibrinogen ratios from the two research groups are summarized in Figure 2.9.

Gutensohn et al. [47] analyzed the intensity of the platelet activation antigens CD62p and CD63. In their in vitro experiment, they showed that a-C coating of AISI316L stainless steel coronary artery stents resulted in a decrease of the CD62p and CD63 antigens, indicating low platelet activation on a-C and, therefore, a low tendency for thrombus formation. Additionally, they showed that metal ion release from the stainless steel stents, which may negatively influence the hemocompatibility of a surface, could be suppressed by the a-C coating.

Platelet adhesion is found to be influenced by the sp^3/sp^2 ratio [48–52]. Recently, plasma immersion ion implantation (PIII) has been used to provide non–line-of-sight deposition of a-C:H films on large-sized substrates and on complicated-shaped substrates at room temperature. This technique is thus potentially useful for real medical devices with irregular geometries. Chen et al. [48] investigated the properties and blood compatibility of a-C:H

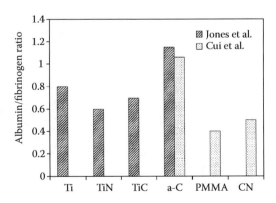

FIGURE 2.9
Albumin/fibrinogen ratios for different surfaces. (Data from Jones et al., *J. Biomed. Mater. Res.*, 52, 413, 2000; and Cui, F.Z., Li, D.J., *Surf. Coat. Technol.*, 131, 481, 2000. With permission.)

films fabricated on silicon substrates at room temperature using acetylene (C_2H_2) plasma immersion ion implantation-deposition (PIII-D). By changing the C_2H_2 to Ar ($F_{C_2H_2}/F_{Ar}$) flow ratios during deposition, they examined the effects of the reactive gas pressure and flow ratios on the characteristics and blood compatibility of the a-C:H films. The relationship between the sp^3 and sp^2 content ratio and adherent blood platelet quantity is specifically investigated.

Their FTIR data indicate that the a-C:H films are hydrogenated, but the atomic hydrogen in the films is free and not bonded to carbon. Rutherford backscattering spectrometry shows that the C concentration is uniform with depth in the a-C:H films. The Raman D band to G band intensity ratio is consistent with the platelet quantity. Both exhibit an initial increase and subsequent decrease with increasing $F_{C_2H_2}/F_{Ar}$ flow ratios. The blood compatibility of the amorphous carbon films is influenced by the ratio of sp^3 to sp^2, not by the absolute sp^3 or sp^2 content. The hemocompatibility becomes worse at larger sp^3 to sp^2 ratio. Their study suggests that a-C:H films with the proper sp^3/sp^2 ratio and good blood compatibility can be fabricated using C_2H_2 PIII-D. From Figure 2.10, the platelet count is lower when the intensity ratio of D band to G band (Raman spectroscopy) is lower (equivalent to higher sp^3/sp^2 ratio).

Yang et al. [49,52] also showed a similar phenomenon when they changed the D band to G band intensity ratio by changing the bias voltage (Figure 2.11). The surface energies are evaluated by solving the combined work of adhesion and van Oss equations. Platelet adhesion experiments were conducted to evaluate the surface thrombogenicity of the films and to examine the interaction between blood and the materials in vitro.

Platelet activation on the surface of a material can be assessed by their degree of spreading and changing shape [45]. Thus, platelets are strongly activated by films deposited at

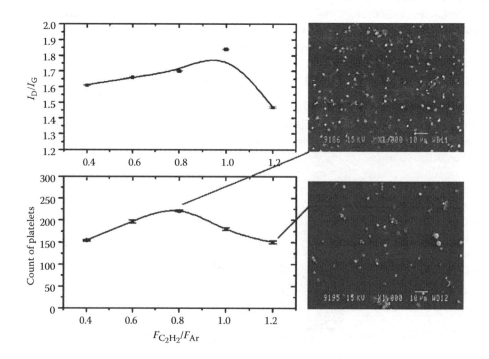

FIGURE 2.10
Effects of $F_{C_2H_2}/F_{Ar}$ flow ratios on intensity ratio of D band to G band and platelet counts. (Reprinted with permission from Chen et al., *Surf. Coat. Technol.*, 156, 289, 2002.)

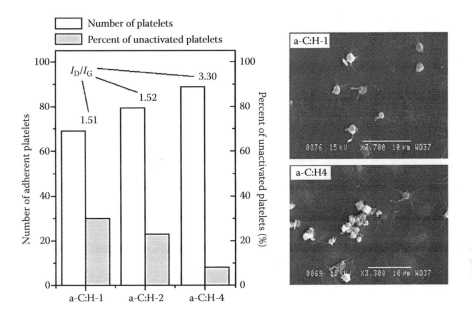

FIGURE 2.11

Quantity of platelets adhered on surface of a-C:H films synthesized at different bias voltages (15 min incubation in PRP). (Reprinted with permission from Yang et al., *Biomaterials*, 24, 2821, 2003.)

higher bias voltage compared to those at lower bias voltage. The platelet attachment and morphology studies suggest that the adhesion behavior is related to the surface energy of the film. From Figure 2.12, the higher the bias voltage (lower the sp^3/sp^2 ratio), the lower the value of the polar component of the surface energy and, accordingly, the higher the activation of adherent platelets.

Li and Gu [51] also found that the sp^3 fraction and surface energy of the film affects the adhering platelets. They coated a-C:H on polymethylmethacrylate (PMMA) using IBAD with different CH^{n+} beam bombarding energies. They investigated the effects of the bombarding energy on the chemical states and several sensitive cell attachments of the coatings by means of extensive spectroscopic experiments and cultured cells in vitro. Compared with the control sample (uncoated PMMA), a-C:H coatings show a lower platelet attachment. The highest 800 eV CH^{n+} beam bombardment during the film synthesis resulted in a more obvious decrease in the number of the platelets adhering to the surface of a-C:H coating. Analysis by XPS and Raman spectroscopy revealed an increase in sp^3 fraction within the 800 eV coating. A simple contact angle measurement using water showed the film to be more hydrophobic. In other words, the film had a lower surface energy that inhibited the adhesion of platelets. However, one should note that the surface energy's relation with cell adhesion is complex, and the study did not include comprehensive analysis of the films' surface characteristics.

Logothetidis et al. [53] studied the hemocompatibility of unhydrogenated, hydrogenated amorphous carbon and ta-C films based on the surface adsorption of the two proteins human serum albumin (HSA) and fibrinogen (Fib); both are contained in human plasma. The main characterization technique applied was Spectroscopic Ellipsometry (SE). From the analysis of the SE data, using the appropriate modeling, the HSA/Fib surface concentration ratio was derived. The higher the HSA/Fib ratio, the more hemocompatible the coating. By using the SE technique, it is possible to determine the optical functions of thin

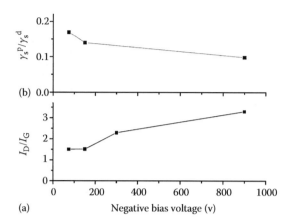

FIGURE 2.12
Effects of bias voltage on: (a) intensity ratio of D band to G band and (b) ratio of polar/dispersive components of surface energy. (Reprinted with permission from Yang et al., *Biomaterials*, 24, 2821, 2003.)

layers, such as the protein layers [54,55], that are formed after dipping the carbon-based surfaces into the protein solutions and drying them afterward. The sp^3 content was found to control the hemocompatibility of the a-C films. That is, the HSA/Fib ratio increases with the sp^3 fraction. Remarkable enhancement in the HSA/Fib ratio was observed for the a-C:H films grown with floating biased substrates and with 10 at.% H$_2$ concentration in plasma. The lowest HSA/Fib ratio was deduced for the ultrathin ta-C film examined in this work. This can be justified either by the surface properties of this type of film and/or its thickness, which is the lowest among the examined films.

A follow-up study by Logothetidis [56] with additional platelet morphology studies by AFM on hydrogenated a-C was carried out. On biased a-C:H films, platelets become aggregated and develop pseudopodia, as derived by AFM measurements, while on floating a-C:H thin films, platelets are round without pseudopodia. These morphological changes indicate platelets activation and the beginning of thrombus formation on biased films. The ratio HSA/Fib has a smaller value on biased a-C:H thin films compared with floating films, when protein adsorption is studied by SE. Therefore, hemocompatibility evaluation through both protein adsorption and platelet adhesion, by both techniques, verifies that the floating films are more hemocompatible than the biased ones. Protein adsorption mechanisms were also studied by SE and AFM. It was revealed that protein adsorption takes place very quickly. The fibrinogen adsorption rate is slower on the floating a-C:H film. Conformation of the proteins' changes during adsorption even after the equilibrium was observed. Based on the AFM measurements, a possible model of protein adsorption is suggested: protein molecules initially form islands and then coalesce until they fully cover the film's surface. The characteristics of the FIB molecule were preserved on the biased a-C:H film, even after a long incubation time (~70 min). Modification of FIB's conformation and interactions between molecules were also observed.

In another work by Karagkiozaki et al. [57], a study of platelets' response to a-C:H by the implementation of AFM enhanced by IR SE method was made in order to provide a more detailed description of nanoscale mechanisms of bio and non-bio interactions. The nondestructive FTIRSE technique was used for investigation of the vibrational properties of the bonding structure of the adsorbed platelets that preserve their viability, providing evidence about the platelets' adhesion onto a-C:H surfaces, paving the way for its utilization in the real-time study of cellular interactions with surfaces. The correlation between nanotopography, structural characteristics, and wettability of carbon-based thin films and their thrombogenicity was verified, whereas the different deposition conditions of RF reactive magnetron sputtering led to different structural and surface properties of the carbon thin films. The AFM study of a-C:H thin films concerning platelets aggregation (refer to Figure 2.13) shows that the films grown without ion bombardment during deposition with 5% H_2 in plasma exhibit less thrombogenicity compared to the biased ones grown with ion bombardment, attributing partially to their higher surface roughness and surface chemistry properties (e.g., lower contact angle and higher surface free energy). Lousinian

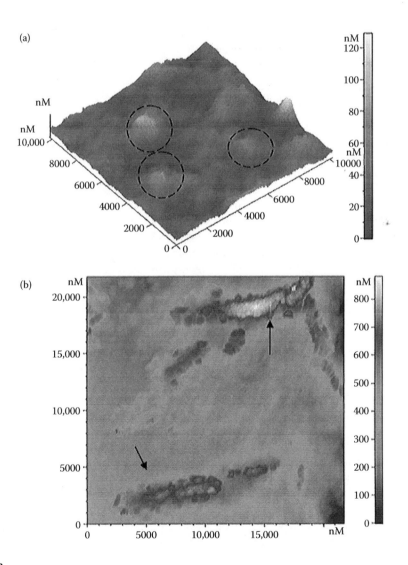

FIGURE 2.13
AFM topography image of (a) platelets on a-C:H (biased) after 1 h incubation. Circles show activated "egg-like" type platelets; (b) platelets on a-C:H (biased) after 2 h incubation. Arrows indicate platelet aggregation and formation of clusters. (Reprinted with permission from Karagkiozaki et al., *Mater. Sci. Eng. B*, 152, 16, 2008.)

et al. [58,59] also show better hemocompatibility of a-C:H deposited at a floating condition by studying the HSA/Fib ratio on the films.

The hemocompatibility of ta-C and low temperature isotropic pyrolytic carbon (LTI carbon) (a material used clinically used for artificial heart valves) was compared [60]. By evaluating the hemolysis ratio (measuring absorbencies of samples immersed in different diluted blood solutions) and observing the platelet morphology, their results indicate ta-C's having a better anticoagulation property than LTI carbon. The hemolysis ratio of ta-C film is much lower compared to LTI carbon, and there are significantly much lower platelet adhesion, aggregation, and activated platelets as well. In order to understand the observed hemocompatibility results, the surface energy of the films was evaluated to analyze surface adsorption of HSA and Fib. However, it was found that the ta-C films are identical to LTI carbon with respect to protein adsorption. It is reported that the formation of thrombus on the biomaterial surface is correlated with charge transferring from the inactive state of the protein (e.g., fibrinogen) to the material surface [61]. During this process, fibrinogen is oxidized and transforms to fibrin monomer, which then cross-links to give an irreversible thrombus. Fibrinogen has an electronic structure similar to a semiconductor with a band gap of 1.8 eV [62]. The effective work function of the ta-C films is approximately 1.0 eV, and LTI carbon's is a graphitic material with an effective work function of approximately 5.5 eV [60]. Therefore, the charge transferring from the inactive state of fibrinogen to the ta-C films is much more difficult than that to the surface of LTI carbon. Consequently, the platelet adhesion, which is related to fibrinogen adsorption and decomposing processes, is prevented, resulting in improved anticoagulation property.

Nurdin et al. [63] also show that amorphous carbon coating prolonged the clotting time and tended to suppress the platelet and complement convertase activation. Fedel et al. [64] conducted an extensive study on several commercially available amorphous carbon coated substrates. They showed that a low platelet activation and aggregation degree on the carbon-coated surfaces generally related to a low fibrinogen/albumin adsorption ratio. It was proposed that human serum albumin rapidly adsorbs on and strongly binds to the coated surfaces, causing amorphous carbon surface passivation and preventing high adsorption of fibrinogen and other platelet adhesive proteins.

Effects of Doping

Ong et al. [65] studied the effect of silicon incorporation on the hemocompatibility of magnetron sputter deposited amorphous carbon films. The number of adhered platelets and the fraction of inactivated platelets are presented in Figure 2.14. From a t-test, there is no significant difference between the count on a-C(Si7.4at.%) and a-C, while the rest are significantly different (having a p value smaller than 0.05, especially a-C(Si37.6at.%) with $p < 0.001$). In addition, the result from ANOVA shows that Si concentration in a-C indeed influenced the number of adhering platelets. The results clearly show a decrease in the number of adhering platelets as well as in the fraction of activated platelets as the Si concentration in the film is increased. The decrement is comparable to Raman spectroscopy results (refer to Figure 2.15), suggesting the increasing Si concentration and sp^3/sp^2 ratio improve the hemocompatibility of the film. However, the evolution of the surface properties of these films is not directly related to the platelet count. There is a decrease in the total surface energy until the Si concentration of 16.6 at.%. The decrease in the platelet count with decreasing total surface energy in the low Si concentration region is also shown by Okpalugo et al. [66] on hydrogenated a-C films. The results of films with higher Si concentration cannot be compared, as there is currently no hemocompatibility study done on

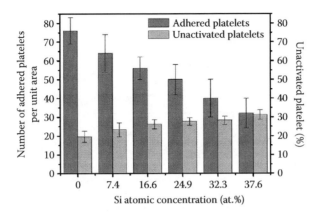

FIGURE 2.14
Number of adherent platelets and percentage of inactivated platelets with increasing Si concentration. Values are mean of six replicates, while error bars denote standard error. ANOVA was conducted, and effect of Si concentration on number of adherent platelet was significant, $F_{(5,30)} = 23.05$, $p = 1.89 \times 10^{-9}$.

such a-C films, whether hydrogenated or not. In this case, there is an increase in the surface energy when Si concentration is increased further, and it is attributed to the increase in the polar component (as shown in Figure 2.16).

The amount of adhered platelets and activation on the film surfaces is inversely proportional to the ratio of albumin to fibrinogen adhesion on the surfaces [45,46]. This is because the adhesion of albumin (a water-soluble protein in the blood plasma) on the film can prevent the adhesion of platelets. Fibrinogen is a protein that can enhance the adhesion and activation of platelets, and hence a thrombus when it is converted into fibrin by the action of the enzyme thrombin. The surface tensions of both albumin and fibrinogen are found to be similar at 65 mN/m [67], and the polar component of fibrinogen is higher than that of albumin: 40.3 mN/m as compared to 33.6 mN/m. The Lifshitz–van der Waals/acid–base approach allows a more in-depth analysis of the polar component. The polar component can further be differentiated into base (electron donor) and acid (electron

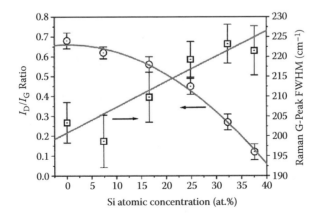

FIGURE 2.15
Raman D to G peaks intensity ratios with increasing Si concentration. (Reprinted with permission from Ong et al., *Biomaterials*, 28, 4033, 2007.)

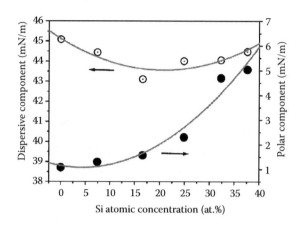

FIGURE 2.16
Dispersive and polar components of surface energy with increasing Si concentration. Polar component increases due to an increase in surface O concentration. Both Si–O and C–O bonds are polar in nature, thus increasing O promotes increment of polar component. Dispersive component is related to density of film. (Reprinted with permission from Ong et al., *Biomaterials*, 28, 4033, 2007.)

acceptor) components, and as Table 2.2 shows, the base components for all the films are very much larger than the acid component, indicating the polar component of the surfaces is predominantly negatively charged. This is beneficial toward hemocompatibility as the platelets and proteins tend to have a net negative zeta potential of –8 to –13 mV [68]. In other words, there will not be any preferential adsorption of any of the proteins and platelets due to electrostatic interaction. Computing the relative contribution of the respective surface energy components finds that the polar-to-dispersive ratio increases as the Si concentration is increased (see Figure 2.17). Therefore, the repulsion between the film surface and proteins should increase as the Si concentration increases. Albumin is also repelled, but the effect should be less intense than with fibrinogen due to its lower polar component. Furthermore, the dispersive component of all the films is relatively much larger than the polar component. Therefore, reflecting the interaction is predominantly based on dispersive forces. Since albumin has a higher dispersive component, it should have a more stable interaction with the film surfaces.

The phenomenon can be justified in Figure 2.14, where the amount of activated platelets decreases as the Si concentration is increased. The discouragement of fibrinogen adsorption is also evidential from the evolution of platelet morphology. As shown in Figure 2.18, the platelets on a-C film are mainly Type III–V, while mainly Types I–III for platelets on a-C(Si37.6at.%) film. (The platelet activation level is presented in Table 2.1.) This shows that the doping of Si not only reduces the number of adherent platelets, it can also deter their activation. Although the undoped a-C film causes a higher state of platelet activation, there is no evidence of any aggregation. Unlike the coated Si wafer, the bare Si surface (not chemically

TABLE 2.2

Base (–) and Acid (+) Contribution to Polar Component of a-C(Si) Films with Increasing Si Concentration

Si at.%	0	7.4	16.6	24.9	32.3	37.6
γ – (mN/m)	26.45	13.28	10.85	19.96	23.65	21.28
γ + (mN/m)	0.01	0.03	0.06	0.07	0.23	0.30

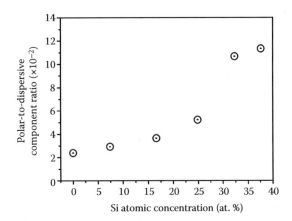

FIGURE 2.17
Polar-to-dispersive ratio with increasing Si concentration. Ratio increase is mainly due to increase in polar component. Since there is a higher surface O concentration when Si concentration is increased, polar bonds such as Si–O and C–O also increase, thereby causing increment of polar component of surface energy.

treated; there will be a presence of a native oxide layer) not only had a higher number of adherent platelets and activation, but there were also numerous aggregation sites. This marks the initial stage of thrombus formation. Okpalugo et al. [66,69] also observed silicon incorporation's improving the hemocompatibility of hydrogenated amorphous carbon films.

Hasebe et al. [70] investigated the hemocompatibility and biocompatibility of fluorinated a-C:H as surface coating for blood contacting devices in vitro and in vivo. Fluorinated a-C:H was compared to undoped a-C:H and medical grade SUS316L stainless steel (also used as substrate for the a-C:H coatings). The in vitro hemocompatibility was evaluated using a whole blood emersion and rotation model. After immersing rod specimens in the tubing and rotating at 37°C, blood was collected for in vitro assessment. Platelet counting was performed using an automated cell counter and markers of mechanically induced platelet activation [beta-thromboglobulin (beta-TG)], activated coagulation [thrombin–antithrombin three complex (TAT)], and acute inflammatory reaction (complement C3a) were assayed. Thrombogenicity of materials is predominantly associated with activated platelets. The group's quantitative measurements demonstrated that platelet loss was lower in the a-C:H and a-C:H(F) groups than in the SUS group, which suggests the adhesion of a smaller number of platelets on a-C:H and a-C:H(F) coated materials. Beta-TG, a platelet-specific alpha-granule protein marker reflecting platelet activation, was also lower in the a-C:H and a-C:H(F) groups than in the SUS group. TAT complex, a molecular marker of coagulation activity, was significantly lower in the a-C:H(F) group than in the SUS and a-C:H groups. These observations suggest that a-C:H(F) coatings have better anti-thrombogenic characteristics than SUS and a-C:H coatings. They have also reported quantitative and morphological studies on platelet adhesion to a-C:H films or a-C:H(F) coated silicon (Si) and bare Si substrates incubated in platelet-rich plasma [71]. In that study, it was found that a-C:H(F) coating reduced the number of platelets and also inhibited platelet activation on the film surface with statistically significant by SEM observation (refer to Figure 2.19). In the water contact angle test, a-C:H and a-C:H(F) have more hydrophobic surfaces than SUS, with a-C:H(F) having the most hydrophobic surface. This suggests that the wettability of a biomaterial surface *partially* determines its blood compatibility. The a-C:H(F) films showed higher levels of C–F bonds than C–H bonds. The stable bonding of

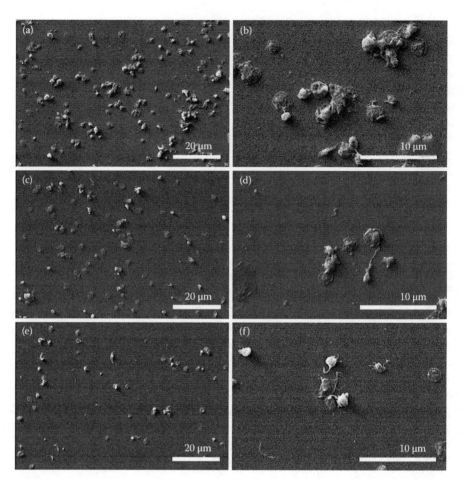

FIGURE 2.18
SEM micrographs of adherent platelets on: (a and b) uncoated Si wafer, (c and d) undoped a-C film, (e and f) a-C(Si37.6at.%) film. Number of adherent blood platelets decreases when Si concentration is increased. Platelet activation type for a-C is mainly Type III–V, while for a-C(Si37.6at.%) is mainly Type I–III. Numerous platelet aggregation sites are found on bare wafer, which marks the initial stage of thrombus formation.

carbon and fluorine atoms in a-C:H(F) films lowers the surface energy, which could result in the reduced adsorption of proteins. Results from the protein adsorption study show that a-C:H(F) film exhibited the highest albumin/fibrinogen ratio, which may be related to the low number of adhering platelets and, therefore, a low tendency to induce thrombus formation [72].

In the in vivo study, they assessed the systemic hematologic response and histocompatibility of a-C:H(F) coated disks and uncoated SUS316L disks in a rat implant model. As acute inflammatory markers, they evaluated the concentrations of TNF-alpha, IL-1beta, and C3a in rat serum or plasma. In both the SUS and a-C:H(F) groups, they found no detectable levels of these markers, which suggests that these materials do not induce an acute systemic inflammatory response. Taken together, the results from these studies suggest a favorable in vitro antithrombogenicity and an acceptable in vivo biocompatibility of a-C:H(F) coated materials.

(a)   (b)   (c)

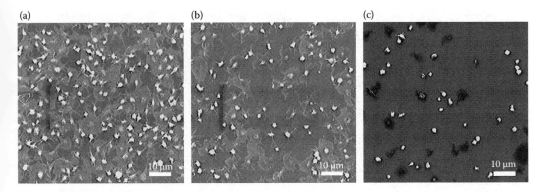

FIGURE 2.19
Morphology of adherent platelets on (a) Si, (b) a-C:H, and (c) a-C:H(F) surfaces observed using SEM. (Reprinted with permission from Saito et al., *Diamond Rel. Mater.*, 14, 1116, 2005.)

Liu et al. [73] evaluated the hemocompatibility of Ti alloys with and without phosphorus incorporated tetrahedral amorphous carbon (ta-C(P)) films. (These films may be hydrogenated as PH_3 was used as the precursor gas.) Platelet spreading and morphology are numerically estimated using the size and circularity indexes of platelets [74]. Low-phosphorus ta-C(P) film (<6at.% P) with the lowest indexes exhibits the slightest adhesion, spreading, and activation of platelets. However, a high content of phosphorus (~8 at.%) increases the fraction of sp^2-hybridized carbon atoms in ta-C(P) film and the ordering of structure, leading to a loss in blood compatibility (refer to Figure 2.20). They suggest the graphitized structure decreases the proportion of the polar component in surface energy, thus making the activation of platelets on the surface stronger.

In another study [75], they varied the deposition bias voltage of ta-C(P) (presumably <8at.% P) and found that all ta-C(P) films exhibit more hydrophilic surfaces than undoped ta-C film. Platelet adhesion tests show that ta-C(P) films with less spreading area and circularity index of platelets represent lower adhesion and activation of platelets in terms of the higher polar-dispersive ratio (as reviewed by the determined surface energy).

Kwok et al. [76] also observed a drastic increase in the polar component of the surface energy (which is also increased) of their phosphorus-doped a-C:H deposited by a plasma immersion ion implantation and deposition system as compared to undoped a-C:H. It is highly possible that this is due to the various PO_x and CP_xO_x species near the surface of the film. Platelet adhesion and activation are suppressed on the a-C:H(P) sample compared to the undoped a-C:H film. Their results suggest that one of the reasons for the good hemocompatibility is that the a-C:H(P) coating significantly minimizes the interactions with plasma protein, giving rise to slight changes in the conformation of adsorbed plasma proteins and preferentially adsorbed albumin.

Effects of Post-Deposition Treatment

Zhang et al. [77] studied the effect of post-deposition annealing temperature on the hemocompatibility of silicon-incorporated amorphous carbon. The number of adhered platelets and the fraction of inactivated platelets are presented in Figure 2.21 as a function of the annealing temperature. The number of adherent platelets increased when the annealing temperature was increased. Although this may be viewed as a degradation of blood

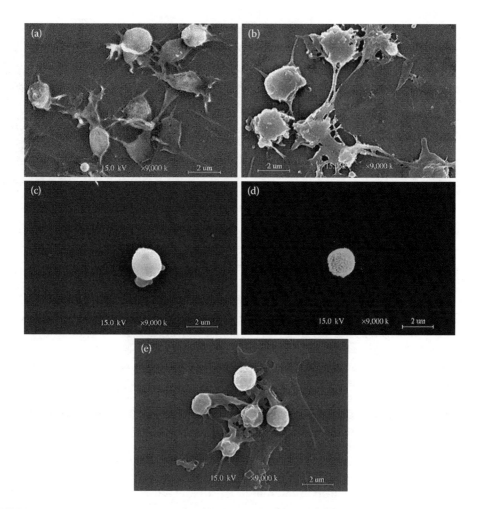

FIGURE 2.20
Morphology of adherent platelets on (a) Ti alloy, (b) ta-C, (c) ta-C(P2.9at.%), (d) ta-C(P5.8at.%), and (e) ta-C(P8.1at.%) surfaces. (Reprinted with permission from Liu et al., *Mater. Sci. Eng. C*, 28, 1408, 2008.)

compatibility of the films, only the platelets with a higher state of activation contributed significantly to the formation of thrombus.

Figure 2.22 presents the micrographs of the platelet morphologies adhering to the film surface. Type V platelets are present on all a-C(Si) films annealed at different temperatures, but there are a fraction of Type 1–3 platelets when the film is annealed at higher temperatures. From Figures 2.21 and 2.22, the fraction of activated platelets decreases with increasing annealing temperature.

Besides the surface chemistry, the surface morphology is another factor influencing the wetting behavior and blood compatibility of a solid-state material. The surface morphology can impart conformation changes to the protein, hence rendering it inactive [78]. Although there is an increase in the surface roughness when the annealing temperature is increased, the maximum attained average roughness value at 600°C is about 0.76 nm (R_{rms}). This roughness value is still too low to affect the wetting and, thus, the surface energy (i.e., ≪100 nm [79]). Even though the total surface area has increased, at such a low roughness

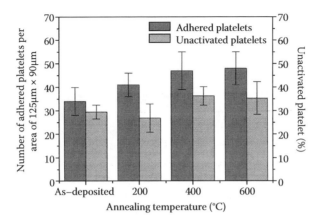

FIGURE 2.21
Number of adherent platelets and percentage of inactivated platelets on a-C(Si37.6at.%) film annealed at different temperatures. Values are mean of six replicates, while error bars denote standard error. ANOVA was conducted, and effect of annealing temperature on number of adherent platelet was significant, $F_{(3,20)} = 6.435$, $p = 0.003$. (Reprinted with permission from Zhang et al., *Thin Solid Films*, 515, 66, 2006.)

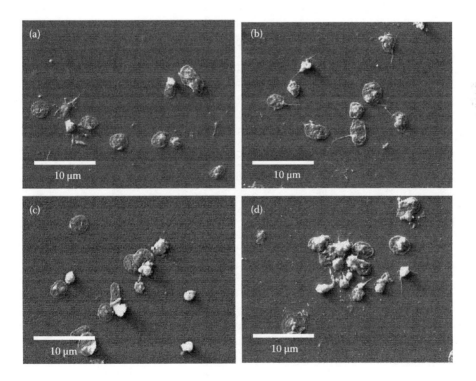

FIGURE 2.22
SEM micrographs of adherent platelets on a-C(Si) films of 37.6at.%Si: (a) as-deposited, (b) annealed at 200°C, (c) annealed at 400°C, and (d) annealed at 600°C. Type V platelets can be found on all sample surfaces, but Type I–III platelets seem to have a slight increase when annealing temperature is increased. Although platelet activation level is a little lower on sample annealed at 600°C, there seems to be an increase in aggregation sites. (Reprinted with permission from Zhang et al., *Thin Solid Films*, 515, 66, 2006.)

TABLE 2.3

Base (–) and Acid (+) Contributions to Polar Component of a-C(Si37.6at.%) with Increasing Annealing Temperatures

	As-deposited	200°C	400°C	600°C
$\gamma -$ (mN/m)	21.3	20.5	17.7	14.9
$\gamma +$ (mN/m)	0.30	0.32	0.36	0.08

Source: Zhang et al., *Thin Solid Films*, 515, 66, 2006. With permission.

value, no significant influence is expected for the adsorption of platelets since the platelets' size is about 2 μm. Proteins have a similar size of a few nanometers. For instance, albumin globule has a triangular shape of about 8 nm on the sides and 3 nm in thickness [80]. Therefore, the roughness (R_{rms} ~0.76 nm), though low, might have a certain effect on the adsorption of the proteins through mechanical interlocking. The changes in the number of adherent platelets and activation fraction are not likely to be affected by the changes in the internal bonding structure of the films as the films are thermally stable up to 600°C.

Table 2.3 shows that the base components for all the films are again much larger than the acid components, indicating that the polar component of the surface is predominantly negatively charged. Therefore, as discussed earlier, there will not be any preferential adsorption of any of the proteins and platelets due to electrostatic interaction if the polar component is increased. However, computing the relative contribution of the respective surface energy component reveals that the polar-to-dispersive ratio decreased as the annealing temperature was increased (see Figure 2.23). Therefore, the repulsion between the film surface and proteins decreases as the annealing temperature increases. The adsorption of both albumin and fibrinogen will now increase, with a slightly stronger effect on fibrinogen since it has a higher polar component. The result is a higher count of adherent platelets on the a-C(Si) annealed at higher temperatures. On the other hand, since the dispersive component of the films is much larger than the polar component, the interaction is predominantly based on dispersive forces. Since albumin has a higher dispersive component, it

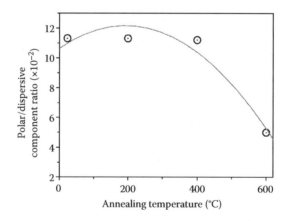

FIGURE 2.23
Ratio of polar to dispersive surface energy component on a-C(Si37.6at.%) film annealed at different temperatures. Ratio decrease at high annealing temperatures is mainly due to decrease in polar component. Since there is a decrease in surface and subsurface O level after thermal treatment, polar bonds such as Si–O and C–O also decrease, thereby causing decrement of the polar component of surface energy. (Reprinted with permission from Zhang et al., *Thin Solid Films*, 515, 66, 2006.)

will have a more stable interaction with the film surfaces, thus contributing to the decrease fraction of activated platelets.

Another study conducted by Okpalugo et al. [66,69] on hydrogenated silicon-incorpo-rated amorphous carbon also showed that thermal annealing can have a detrimental effect on the hemocompatibility of the films, but only at higher temperatures (~600°C and above). The results of the platelets aggregation study on a-C:H and a-C:H(Si) films for platelet incu-bation indicated an increase in the level of platelet aggregation at two extremes: when the films had a higher electrical resistivity and when graphitization had occurred in the films (see Figure 2.24). Silicon-doped films with lower electrical resistivity than the undoped films showed a much lower level of platelet aggregation. This trend is consistent with the report of Bruck on pyrolytic polymers [81,82]. Bruck observed clotting times six to nine times longer than those observed with nonconducting polymers and also observed little or no platelet aggregation on electroconducting polymers, when compared to nonconducting control samples. In the investigation by Okpalugo et al., thermal annealing of a-C:H below 400°C leads to lower levels of platelet aggregation similar to that observed in a-C:H(Si). This is attributed to the increased electronic conduction before graphitization at the lower annealing temperature for a-C:H. Zhang et al. [83] also observed more platelet adhesion and activation when annealing hydrogenated ta-C at 300°C and above.

The hemocompatibility of plasma-treated, silicon-incorporated hydrogenated amorphous carbon films was investigated by Roy et al. [84]. a-C:H(Si) films with a Si concentration of 2 at.% were prepared using a capacitively coupled radio frequency plasma assisted chemical vapor deposition method. The a-C:H(Si) films were then treated with O_2, CF_4, or N_2 glow discharge for surface modification. The aPTT determines the ability of blood to coagulate through the intrinsic coagulation mechanism. It measures the clotting time from the activa-tion of factor XII through to the formation of fibrin clot [86]. The aPTT also governs how a biomaterial affects the coagulation time. The enzymatic activities that lead to clot for-mation are measured through aPTT measurement. In Figure 2.25, the aPTT of untreated a-C:H(Si) film is compared with those of the plasma-treated films for an incubation time of 60 min. It is evident that the O_2 plasma–treated a-C:H(Si) films had a higher aPTT. This indicates that the O_2 plasma–treated a-C:H(Si) films have a tendency to retard the intrin-sic coagulation activities of blood compared with the other samples, which is consistent with the protein adsorption behavior. Similar behavior was observed with N_2 plasma–treated a-C:H(Si) films. In contrast, CF_4 plasma treatment did not induce a notable change in aPTT when compared with untreated a-C:H(Si) film. The N_2 and O_2 plasma–treated

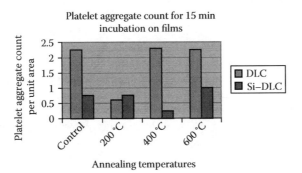

FIGURE 2.24
Platelet aggregate count on a-C:H and a-C:H:Si(7.6at.%) samples. (Reprinted with permission from Okpalugo et al., *Biomaterials*, 25, 239, 2004.)

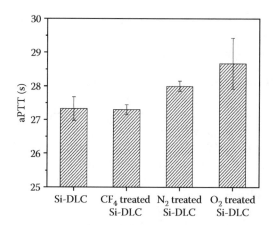

FIGURE 2.25
aPTTs of as deposited and O_2-plasma treated a-C:H(Si) films. (Reprinted with permission from Roy et al., *Acta Biomater.*, 5, 249, 2009.)

a-C:H(Si) films were also found to have considerably reduced platelet adhesion compared with untreated and CF_4 plasma–treated a-C:H(Si) films. The plasma treatment revealed an intimate relationship between the polar component of the surface energy and its hemocompatibility. All in vitro characterizations (e.g., protein absorption behavior, activated partial thromboplastin time measurement, and platelet adhesion behavior) showed improved hemocompatibility of the N_2- or O_2 plasma–treated surfaces where the polar component of the surface energy was significantly increased. Si–O or Si–N surface bonds played an important role in improving hemocompatibility. These results support the importance of a negatively charged polar component of the surface in inhibiting fibrinogen adsorption and platelet adhesion.

Cytocompatibility

Cytocompatibility studies of a-C films have been performed in vitro by exposing the coated materials to a variety of environments simulating the body ambience. In this section, the various cells relating to various physiological environment and function will be discussed. In vivo evaluation on a-C films will also be touched on.

Before we move on, we should at least have the basic concept of cell culturing, since most of the studies carried out require cells to be cultured and then analyzed. Below is one example, but do note the method is not limited to the one discussed here.

Cell culturing. The study of cellular behavior on biomaterials surface in vitro is an important aspect in determining the biocompatibility of the material. The healthy growth/proliferation and morphology of the biological cells on the material surface is an important prerequisite for compatibility.

Two types of cell lines were used in this study: African green monkey kidney fibroblast COS7; and human osteosarcoma MG63. Both cell lines were obtained from the American Type Culture Collection (ATCC, Rockwell, MD). Cells were cultured at 37°C in a humidified 5% CO_2 atmosphere. The standard medium used for culturing COS7 was Dulbecco's modified Eagle's medium (DMEM, ATCC) supplemented by 10% fetal calf serum (FCS, ATCC) and 1% penicillin (ATCC), while for MG63 Eagle's minimum essential medium (EMEM, ATCC) was used, also supplemented by 10% fetal calf serum (FCS, ATCC) and 1% penicillin (ATCC). For cell assay, the a-C samples were diced into 10×10 mm segments and exposed to UV for 4 h. After which, the samples are placed in a 24-well culture dish, and both cell lines were seeded at a density of 4×10^4 cells/ml and cultured up to 6 days. After each culture period (1, 3, and 6 days), the samples were rinsed twice with phosphate buffered saline solution, then the cells were detached using trypsin/ETDA. The detached cells were stained with trypan blue, and the living cells were counted using a hemacytometer (Becton Dickinson, Germany). The statistics of the cellular tests were conducted using one-way ANOVA on an average of three replicates to compare data between different periods of culture. Student's t-test was carried out to compare the culture data between coatings from each count. Statistical significance was considered at $p < 0.05$.

Endothelials

Endothelial cells, although not "blood cells," have functions that may relate directly to platelet interactions and blood compatibility. At the microvascular level, where most cellular–biomaterial interactions occur, these cells play key roles in the blood intravascular inner wall linings to keep the blood flowing without clotting. The inner endothelial lining of the endothelium is nature's blood compatible surface, and the performance of any biomaterial designed to be hemocompatible must be compared with that of the endothelium [86]. Under normal circumstances, platelets do not interact with the endothelial cells, that is, platelet adhesion to the blood vessel wall and the formation of platelet aggregates do not normally take place except when required for hemostasis. Hence the surface of endothelial cells does not promote platelet attachment [86]. The formation of platelet aggregates in close proximity to the endothelium is also rendered difficult by prostacyclin (PGI2), a powerful inhibitor of platelet aggregation secreted by the endothelial cells [87]. An increased platelets aggregation/adhesion on a material could be associated with increased potential of a material to induce clotting, while increased endothelial material adhesion could be associated with an increased potential of a material not to induce clotting, and vice versa. The functions of platelets and endothelial cells can therefore be said to be "opposing" but complementary in nature, and thus investigation of the interactions between both endothelial cells and platelets with a particular biomaterial can provide valuable insight [88].

In the previous section, we discussed hemocompatibility by addressing issues relating to blood platelet adhesion and activation. In this section, we will focus on tissue and blood compatibility of amorphous carbon films using endothelial cell cultures.

In most, if not all endothelial cell culture experiments, human microvascular endothelial cells (HMEC) are used. In a work by Okpalugo et al. [69], undoped and silicon-doped hydrogenated amorphous carbon films were annealed at various temperatures up to 600°C, and the attachment of HMEC was counted (refer to Figure 2.26a). For undoped films, without annealing the HMEC attachment is similar to that of the uncoated silicon control wafer. However, with increasing anneal temperature, cell attachment increases up to a maximum at 300°C and falls thereafter. For two values of Si doping, ~5% and ~7.6%, a high and approximately constant value of cell attachment occurs, irrespective of annealing temperature. In Figure 2.26b, the HMEC cell attachment is seen to rise with silicon doping between 0.36% Si and 5% Si and then "saturate" thereafter. The contact potential difference (CPD) between the Si-doped films and a reference (brass) probe, of known work function, falls in almost inverse relationship to HMEC attachment. The CPD change indicates either

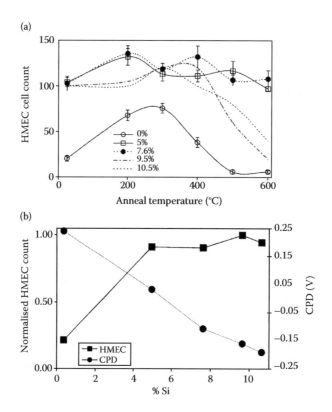

FIGURE 2.26
(a) Attachment of HMEC (after 6 h) as a function of anneal temperatures and silicon content; (b) contact potential difference (CPD) variation with silicon content compared with HMEC count (normalized). (Reprinted with permission from Okpalugo et al., *Diamond Rel. Mater.*, 13, 1088, 2004.)

a reduction in the a-C:H(Si) work function, due to an increased sp^3 fraction or a change in the density of surface charge [89].

HMEC attachment on a-C:H is lower than a-C:H(Si) and peaks at 300°C, beyond the onset of graphitization (as reviewed by an increasing I_D/I_G ratio of Raman spectroscopy), whereas attachment seems constant up to 600°C on a-C:H(Si). Without silicon, it appears that an optimal film structure exists at approximately 200–300°C, which promotes HMEC. It may be that loss of hydrogen is required for optimal attachment surfaces, but that continued hydrogen loss and the consequent conversion to sp^2 bonding has a negative effect. The polar nature of the surface is clearly modified with the introduction of silicon. Contact angle measurements show a change in surface structure from polar to dispersive and an increase in hydrophobicity. It may be that in a-C:H(Si), the nature of the surface remains sufficiently hydrophobic even as the sp^2/sp^3 ratio increases at high anneal temperatures.

In hydrogenated amorphous carbon films subjected to post-deposition nitrogen doping, Okpalugo et al. [90] found that the introduction of nitrogen atoms/molecules to the a-C:H structures leads to an atomic structural change favorable to the attachment of human microvascular endothelial cells. In this study a "sweep plate" was employed to attract charged ions, so these are excluded from the doping species (samples named SN). Nitrogen doping therefore involved either atomic species (named SN) or a mixture of nitrogen atoms and ions (named N), via post deposition exposure to the flux for up to 2.5 h.

The water contact angle increased with a-C:H coating when compared with an uncoated sample. However, the contact angle value for the N-doped film is slightly lower than that of a-C:H, whereas the values for the doping where the sweep plates (to remove ions) were employed is higher. The number of adherent cells seems to be highest for the doped films (where the sweep plates were employed), followed by the doped films, including the ionic species, then a-C:H (undoped films), and finally, uncoated samples (silicon wafer substrates). Typical SEM imaging of the adherent cells on the film surfaces are shown in Figure 2.27. Figure 2.27a, b shows the endothelial cell attachment to bare (uncoated) silicon wafer–substrate and a-C:H coated silicon wafer–substrate, respectively. The worst bioresponse (lowest number of cell attachments) occurs on the bare substrate (see Figure 2.27a),

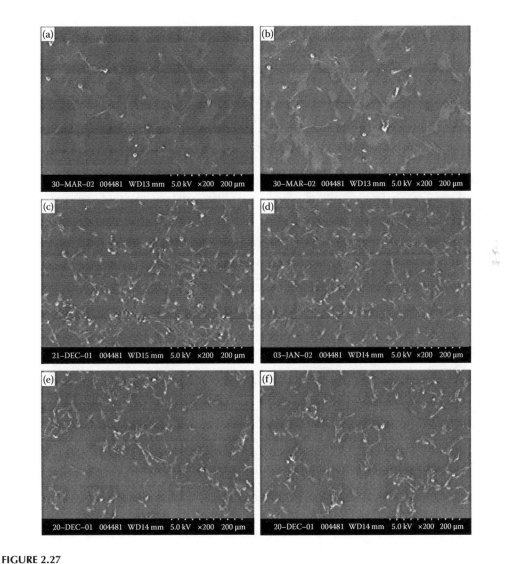

FIGURE 2.27
SEM micrographs of endothelial cells attached to a-C:H:N thin films, 3200: (a) uncoated substrate, (b) a-C:H coated substrate, (c) sample "SN1" (1 h exposure to nitrogen with use of sweep plates to exclude ions), (d) sample "SN2.5," sweep plate for 2.5 h, (e) "N1" (1 h, no sweep plate used), and (f) "N2.5" (2.5 h, no sweep plate used). (Reprinted with permission from Okpalugo et al., *J. Biomed. Mater. Res. B*, 85B, 188, 2008.)

followed by a-C:H coatings (see Figure 2.27b), and the best response is seen on the nitrogen doped counterparts. However, it can be seen from the SEM images that there are better endothelial cell adhesion and attachment on the SN films (Figure 2.27c, d) compared to N films (Figure 2.27e, f).

The results show that the trend in the endothelial behavior (attachment) seems not to be directly related to the degree of hydrophobicity alone. These preliminary results seem to suggest that hydrophobic films, with additional properties like increased atomic networks and decreased graphitic clusters as well as semiconductivity [91], may be favorable to human microvascular endothelial cellular attachment. It seems that the films obtained with the use of sweep plates (to remove ions, (i.e., atomic nitrogen doping)) encouraged more endothelial growth and proliferation compared to its counterpart. This is thought to be due to some changes in the films' microstructure and chemical bonding as revealed by XPS and SIMS techniques; whereas a better endothelial cell adhesion on all nitrogen doped species in comparison with the undoped samples is thought to be due to changes in electronic states and increased conductivity of N-doped a-C:H compared to insulating undoped a-C:H. The increased adhesion of endothelial cells on the atomic nitrogen and nitrogen-doped films could also be associated with the emergence of a suitable surface chemistry and surface energy resulting from nitrogen atom substitution in the carbon matrix.

These post-deposition a-C:H(N) films were compared to in situ deposition Si-doped a-C:H films in terms of HMEC attachment [92]. As shown in Figure 2.28, the a-C:H(Si) films have the highest number of attached HMEC. They also have the highest water contact angle and lowest I_D/I_G ratio. In this study, the lower Raman I_D/I_G ratios are associated with increased sp^3/sp^2 ratio, increased H concentration, increased photoluminescence intensity, and a higher endothelial cellular adhesion in the a-C:H(Si) films, but not necessarily with the a-C:H(N) films, where either a slight increase or decrease in the I_D/I_G ratios, photoluminescence intensity, and sp^3/sp^2 ratio improved endothelial attachment. These results seem to suggest that more hydrophobic films, with the properties of decreased compressive stress, increased atomic networks, decreased graphitic clusters, and semiconductivity, may be favorable to human microvascular endothelial cellular attachment.

The viability of various cells can be investigated by means of MTT (Tetrazolium) assay developed by Mosmann [93]. MTT (Tetrazolium) assay is a colorimetric assay that measures the reduction of 3-(4,5-dimethylthiazol-2-yl)-2,5-diphenyl tetrazolium bromide (MTT)

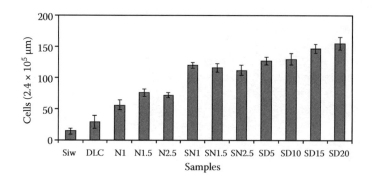

FIGURE 2.28
HMEC attachment per $2.4 \times 10^5 \, \mu m^2$ of a-C:H (DLC) and a-C:H(Si) (SD5–20, 5–20 sccm of TMS flow) thin films compared to a-C:H(N) (doped with N-neutrals) thin films. (Reprinted with permission from Okpalugo et al., *J. Biomed. Mater. Res. B*, 78B, 222, 2006.)

by the mitochondrial succinate dehydrogenase present in most cells. Thus, MTT assay is a semiquantitative colorimetric assay for mammalian cell survival and proliferation. According to Mosmann, the assay detects living, but not dead cells, and the signal generated is dependent on the degree of activation of the cells. However, according to Page et al. [94] nonviable cells could reduce the tetrazolium salt. The main advantages of the assay are rapidity and precision and a lack of radioisotope, thus requiring no washing steps [93]. In an MTT assay conducted on HMEC seeded on a-C:H and a-C:H(Si) films reviews no significant difference between coated and uncoated control samples (96-well tissue culture polystyrene) [95]. This shows that the coatings are not cytotoxic to the cells and could be said to be closely compatible when compared to the tissue culturing material.

Macrophages

Macrophages are white blood cells within tissues, produced by the division of monocytes. It is a suitable cell for in vitro biocompatibility testing, as it plays a major role in inflammation and the response to foreign bodies. Macrophages are known to produce a number of inflammatory mediators, which have an effect on the surrounding tissue [96]. They play a vital role in the development of atherosclerosis as well as in-stent restenosis. A minor population of macrophages can proliferate in the atherosclerotic lesions themselves, particularly in the early stage. Activated macrophages can accumulate cholesterol esters in the cytoplasm, which leads to foam cell formation in lesion development [97]. It is therefore desirable for a biomaterial material to have minimum macrophage adhesion and those that adhere should be viable.

Thomson et al. [98] studied the inflammatory potential of a-C coated tissue culture plates on a-C coating by measuring the levels of the lysosomal enzyme N-acetyl-D-glucosaminidase in the culture medium following the exposure of macrophages to a-C coatings. Since lysosomal enzymes are released from macrophages during inflammation, an increased enzyme level in the medium means that an inflammatory reaction has been elicited. They found no significant difference between the enzyme levels from a-C coatings and those from the control tissue culture plate. This shows that a-C does not induce inflammatory reactions in the cells any more than the tissue culture plate. Allen et al. [99] have also studied the effects of a-C–coated polystyrene plates on macrophages. The results showed that macrophages grew well on a-C–coated plates. Scanning electron microscopic examinations confirmed the normal behavior of cells and no evidence of extensive cell death, therefore showing no cytotoxicity was caused by the a-C coating. Lactate dehydrogenase (LDH), an enzyme released at cell death, has been used as a measure of cell viability [99], LDH assays carried out provided a measure of cell viability and have shown no evidence of overt cytotoxicity for a-C:H films [100]. No difference in LDH release between the a-C:H (with a-Si:H bonding layer) and control specimens has been observed. Furthermore, the absence of abnormal cellular morphology has been demonstrated by optical microscopy. Li and Gu [101] observed a decrease in the number of adhering macrophages when the sp^3 fraction and hydrophobicity were higher.

Increasing surface roughness and surface energy can lead to an enhancement of macrophage viability, and the higher the hydrogen content for a-C:H films, the lower the macrophage attachment [102]. The a-C:H films significantly suppressed attachment of viable macrophages, compared to the uncoated surface (Si), indicating possible lower inflammatory responses. This finding is in agreement with a previous report by Ball et al. [103], where J744 macrophages, cultured on ta-C surfaces, showed reduced hydrogen peroxide production compared to thermanox, stainless steel, and polyurethane-coated stainless steel. Therefore, hydrogen content may be an important factor for influencing the biological response of amorphous carbon surfaces. Macrophage cells spread well on all a-C:H film surfaces, and the surface results indicated the nontoxic nature of the surfaces on the cells (refer to Figure 2.29).

Fibroblasts

Fibroblast is a type of cell that synthesizes the extracellular matrix and collagen, the structural fibers, and ground substance of connective tissue, and it plays a critical role in wound healing. In growing individuals, fibroblasts are dividing and synthesizing ground substance. Fibroblasts can give rise to other cells, such as bone cells, fat cells, and smooth muscle cells. It is therefore widely used in cytocompatibility tests. A biomaterial should

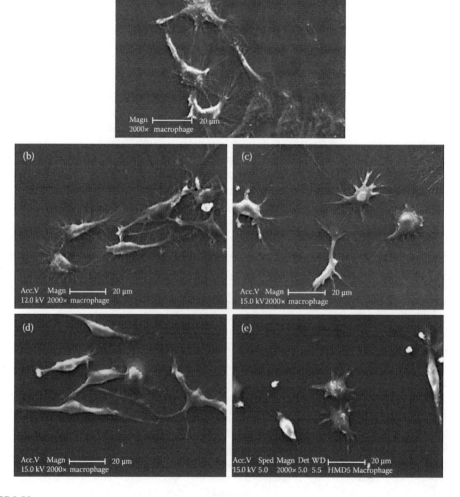

FIGURE 2.29
SEM micrographs of macrophage morphology: (a) Si, (b) ta-C, (c) a-C:H(C_2H_2), (d) a-C:H(CH_4), and (e) thermanox. (Reprinted with permission from Ma et al., *Biomaterials*, 28, 1620, 2007.)

be able to sustain healthy attachment, adhesion, spreading, proliferation, and growth of fibroblast.

The results of Allen et al. [99] have shown that there are no statistically significant differences between fibroblast grown on control polystyrene plate and those grown on a-C:H coating. Morphological examination showed no evidence of cellular damage to the fibroblasts. In vitro tests using maurine fibroblasts showed that a-C:H deposited on a titanium alloy has a low level of cytotoxicity and acts as a diffusion barrier between the titanium alloy and the fibroblasts [104]. These tests with maurine fibroblasts (different cell lines) also demonstrated good adhesion and spreading of the cells on the films' surface and no evidence of overt cytotoxicity [99–101,105]. Functional evaluation of viable cells (maurine L929 fibroblast cells) was done by assessing the metabolic activity via MTT assay of the cells after the contact of the cells with material extract [106]. Most of the cells were metabolically active, as they were able to convert MTT into formazan crystals by active mitochondrial enzymes. Ethidium bromide and acridine orange staining of adhered fibroblast cells on a-C:H-coated and uncoated Ti showed the intact nature of cell membrane.

In the study on cytotoxicity of silicon-doped unhydrogenated amorphous carbon using African green monkey kidney fibroblast COS7, Ong et al. [107] show that the cells proliferate better on a-C films with higher Si concentration (see Figure 2.30).

Raman spectroscopy results show a decrease in C sp^2-hybridized bondings with the incorporation of Si. But it does not translate to a more hydrophobic surface due to the polar Si–O and C–O bonds on the surface. The films become more hydrophilic with a higher polar/dispersive surface energy component ratio when Si concentration is increased. The COS7 adhere, spread, and proliferate well on a-C and a-C(Si) films. The more hydrophilic film a-C(Si37.6at.%) seems to be more conducive for cellular growth when the count is highest at the end of the incubation period.

Figure 2.31 shows the living cells' morphology on a-C(Si37.6at.%). The long and fine cytoplasmic extensions in multiple directions show that there is excellent adhesion of the cells to the film. The cells also exhibit long lamellipodes, indicating active cell migration leading to homogeneous colonization.

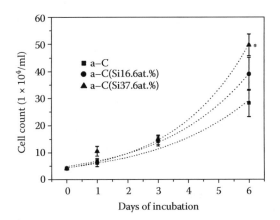

FIGURE 2.30

Cell attachment number of COS7 fibroblast cells. Values are mean of three replicates, while error bars denote standard error. ANOVA shows that cell type proliferated on a-C and a-C(Si) with $p < 0.001$. *Significant difference between COS7 count on a-C(Si37.6at.%) and a-C (*$p < 0.001$). (Reprinted with permission from Ong et al., *Thin Solid Films*, 516, 5152, 2008.)

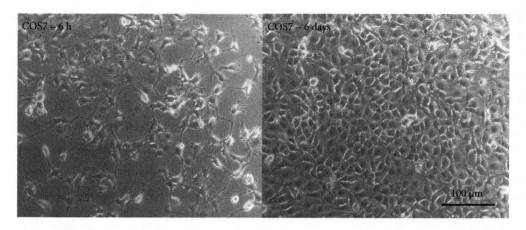

FIGURE 2.31
Optical micrographs of COS7 on a-C(Si37.6at.%). Cells exhibit long lamellipodes indicating active cell migration. Long and fine cytoplasmic extensions indicate that there is good adhesion of cells to film, and thus good initial attachment. On sixth day of culture, complete colonization of cell line is observed. (Reprinted with permission from Ong et al., *Thin Solid Films*, 516, 5152, 2008.)

Cell adhesion and spreading are influenced by the physicochemical characteristics of the underlying solid surface. The substrate surface free energy can affect the cell spreading. Poor spreading on hydrophobic surface and good spreading on hydrophilic surface can be observed in both the absence and presence of preadsorbed serum proteins [108]. Therefore, the substrate characteristics extend through the adsorbed proteins and affect cell adhesion and spreading. Cells can reach the underlying substrate by pseudopodia protruding through the preadsorbed protein layer, cells can consume preadsorbed proteins to make direct contact, and/or the substrate characteristics are reflected in the composition and conformation of adsorbed proteins, thus presenting different molecular groups to adhering and spreading cells. All proteins have NH_2 and COOH groups at their ends. The NH_2 tends to be positively charged and the COOH groups negatively charged [109]. a-C(Si) includes C–O and Si–O bonds at the surface that are polarized due to the difference in electronegativity between each element. Thus, the proteins can electrostatically bond with the film's surface. Since a-C(Si37.6at.%) has the highest polar component of the surface energy, it has better affinity with the proteins and in turn attracts more cells to adhere, spread, and proliferate.

L929 fibroblast adhesion is also improved when nitrogen is doped into hydrogenated amorphous carbon [110,111]. The cell adhesion percentages to silica substrates and a-C:H without nitrogen doping were about 28% and 67%, respectively. The cell adhesion percentage increased with increasing N concentration, and the best cell adhesion percentage was about 85%. The Raman I_D/I_G ratio is found to be increasing with increasing N concentration, that is, sp^3 fraction is decreasing. As can be expected, the film becomes more hydrophilic when N concentration is increased. It is considered that NH bonds and CN single and triple bonds exist at the surface in a-C:H(N). It is suggested that the surface of a-C:H(N) electrostatically bonds with protein molecules because a-C:H(N) polarizes at the surface due to the difference in electronegativity between carbon and nitrogen, and that a hydrogen bond is formed between electrically negative oxygen or nitrogen and NH_2 or NH groups. It is considered that the number of proteins attached on the material's surface increased with increasing the nitrogen concentration, and the cell adhesion percentage was enhanced.

Osteoblasts

Osteoblasts are mononucleate cells responsible for the formation of bone; in essence, osteoblasts are sophisticated fibroblasts that express all genes that fibroblasts express, with the addition of the genes for bone sialoprotein and osteocalcin. Osteoblasts produce osteoid, which is composed mainly of Type I collagen. Osteoblasts are also responsible for mineralization of the osteoid matrix. Bone mass is maintained by a balance between the activity of osteoblasts that form bone and other cells called osteoclasts (large multinucleate cells that differentiate from macrophages) that resorb bone. Osteoblast cells tend to decrease as individuals become older, thus decreasing the natural renovation of the bone tissue. One of the most promising applications of a-C is in the surface modification of artificial hip joint replacements. Therefore, a number of studies on the effects of these coatings on osteoblasts and osteoblast-like cells have been done.

The results of Allen et al. [99] indicated no statistical differences between osteoblasts grown on control polystyrene plates and those grown on a-C:H coatings. Scanning electron microscopy showed that the cells adhered well to the a-C coatings and produced extensive filopodia. Two osteoblast cell lines (MG-63 and SaOS-2) attached to and proliferated on both the uncoated and a-C:H–coated polystyrene substrates [112]. Analysis of culture medium and cell lysates showed that the cells maintained an osteoblastic phenotype on the a-C:H coating, with expression of alkaline phosphatase, osteocalcin, and type I collagen. Expression of each of the three markers was similar on uncoated and a-C:H–coated polystyrene. Because the tissue culture grade polystyrene that was used in these experiments is known to be biocompatible, one can conclude that the a-C:H coating is also biocompatible in vitro.

The results of Du et al. [113] showed that osteoblasts could migrate out of bone fragments and could attach, spread, and proliferate on the a-C coating in an attempt to colonize the entire substrate surface. But the situation was different with uncoated silicon. The osteoblasts were able to attach on the wafers, but were unable to follow this attachment with spreading. The osteoblasts showed a normal pattern of adhesion and spreading on a-C:H coated titanium [106]. There was no evidence of cytoplasmic vacuolization, membrane damage, or extensive cell death. The cells adhered well and produced extensive filopodia. The cells have not undergone any toxic reaction and showed proliferative capacity. Neighboring cells maintained cell–cell contact through multiple extensions. With proliferation and spreading, cells formed a continuous sheet. LDH assays carried out have also shown no evidence of overt cytotoxicity for a-C:H films [100].

Rodil et al. [114] and Olivares et al. [115] showed that the degree of osteoblasts adhesion measured at 24 h attained higher value for a-C when compared to titanium and bare stainless steel (see Figure 2.32). In vitro, osteoblasts cells grow and spread in the presence of culture medium, but to promote mineralization it is necessary to add β-glycerphosphate, dexamethasone, and ascorbic acid [116,117]. Biomineralization was studied by observing the samples in the scanning electron microscope [115]. The capacity of mineralization of the osteoblasts cells was not impeded by the a-C film. Moreover, Ca/P composition ratios of the mineralized areas were between 1.5 and 2.3, similar to human bone ratios.

Interactions between Saos-2 osteoblast-like cells were studied on microtextured ta-C, ta-C hybrid films (doped with Ti and PDMS; i.e., ta-C(Ti), and ta-C(PDMS), respectively) [118]. The results show that ta-C has the lowest contact angle (hence the highest surface

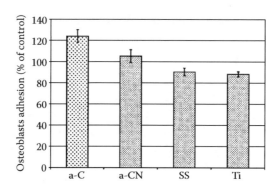

FIGURE 2.32
Adhesion of osteoblasts on the a-C, a-CN, Ti, and bare stainless steel substrates after 24 h. (Reprinted with permission from Olivares et al., *Surf. Coat. Technol.*, 177–178, 758, 2004.)

energy) and highest polar component of the surface energy among the three films. It also has the highest number of adhering cells on its surface (see Figure 2.33). It is once again shown that the adhesion of biological cells can be affected by modifying the contact angle and surface energy parameter. Pure ta-C with favorable physicochemical properties seemed to be most suitable for Saos-2 adhesion.

An evaluation on MC3T3-E1 osteoblast-like cells' response to a-C:H was done [119]. The a-C:H and deuterated a-C:H films were deposited by PECVD, and three types of precursor gas were applied for deposition: pure methane (CH_4), pure deuterated methane (CD_4), and their half/half mixture. All surface treatments were performed under two different self-bias voltages (V_{sb}): −400 and −600 V. The a-C:H films deposited under the V_{sb} of −600 V in pure methane (600CH4) or in pure deuterated methane (600CD4) offered a significantly higher cell proliferation rate as compared to silicon substrate. SEM observations confirmed that the optimal cell adhesion behavior, among all the treated surfaces, occurred on the surface of the 600CH4 and 600CD4 groups, which showed increased amounts of filopodia

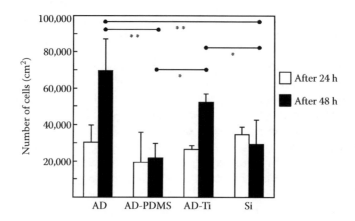

FIGURE 2.33
Cell proliferation for different coatings and silicon. Number of viable cells was determined at 24 and 48 h using MTT assay and a standard curve normalized to number of osteoblast-like cells. *Significant difference $p < 0.05$, **Significant difference $p < 0.01$. Error bars indicate standard deviations. (Reprinted with permission from Myllymaa et al., *Diamond Rel. Mater.*, 18, 1294, 2009.)

and microvilli to enhance cell–environment exchange. The results show that the films deposited at −600 V have a higher sp^2/sp^3 fraction, and 600CD4 has the highest polar component of the surface energy. The actin labeling with FITC–phalloidin reveals the cytoskeletal organization in Figure 2.34.

The attachment and proliferation of MG63 osteoblast-like cells were studied on Si-incorporated unhydrogenated a-C [107] and Si- and SiO_x-incorporated hydrogenated a-C [120]. Although substantial differences exist in surface and bulk compositions between these films (a-C:H, a-C:H(Si) and a-C:H(SiO_x)), osteoblast adhesion did not show trends in cell numbers, cell areas, or cell morphologies that can be attributed to either the Si/SiO_x content of the film or to the surface chemical structure of the films after a 3-day

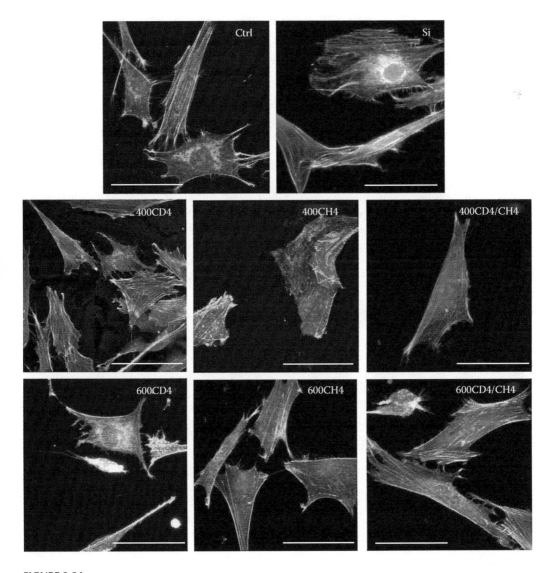

FIGURE 2.34
Cytoskeleton assessment MC3T3-E1 osteoblasts after a 3-day culture. All coatings induce a similar intensity and organization of actin stress fibers. (Reprinted with permission from Chai et al., *Acta Biomater.*, 4, 1369, 2008.)

culture [120]. The surface energy of a-C:H(SiO$_x$) films decreased with increasing Si content, whereas only small variations in surface energy were observed for a-C:H(Si) films as a function of Si content. The differences in surface chemistry between a-C:H, a-C:H(Si), and a-C:H(SiO$_x$) appear to have an undetectable impact on cell attachment.

The number of cells on a-C(Si) too shows no significant difference with counts on undoped a-C, but cell count is evidently higher on a-C(Si) on the sixth day of culture (see Figure 2.35) [107]. In this study though, the surface energy increases with Si concentration. The polar/dispersive component of the surface energy also exhibits an increasing trend. As mentioned earlier, a higher polar component can induce a surface to have better affinity with the proteins, and in turn attracts more cells to adhere, spread, and proliferate. Figure 2.36 shows the living cells' morphology on a-C(Si37.6 at.%). The long and fine cytoplasmic extension in multiple directions is evident of excellent adhesion of the cells to the film. The cells also exhibit long lamellipodes, indicating active cell migration leading to homogeneous colonization.

Other Cells

Bovine retinal pericytes. The survival and proliferation of bovine retinal pericytes (BRP) isolated from the eye were studied on a-C:H and a-C:H(Si)-coated tissue culture polystyrene (TCPS) [95]. Pericytes are associated with vasculature and appear to be present in most tissues. They are generally considered to be restricted to the microvessels (arterioles, venules, and capillaries where there are no smooth muscles) [121]. Pericytes are thought to contribute to endothelial cell proliferation via selective inhibition of endothelial cell growth. Thus, the understanding of these thin films' cytotoxicity to retinal pericytes is relevant to biomaterial application in the eye compartment, as well as the surrounding tissues of the vasculature. The a-C:H and a-C:H(Si) films seem not to be toxic to the BRP. Based on MTT assay results of the pericytes, it seems that these cells are more slightly activated in the a-C:H and a-C:H(Si) coated wells compared to uncoated TCPS conventionally used for cell culture.

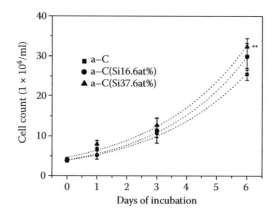

FIGURE 2.35
Cell attachment number of MG63 osteoblast cells. Values are mean of three replicates, while error bars denote standard error. ANOVA shows that cell type proliferated on a-C and a-C(Si) with $p < 0.001$. **Significant difference between MG63 count on a-C(Si37.6at.%) and a-C (**$p < 0.05$). (Reprinted with permission from Ong et al., *Thin Solid Films*, 516, 5152, 2008.)

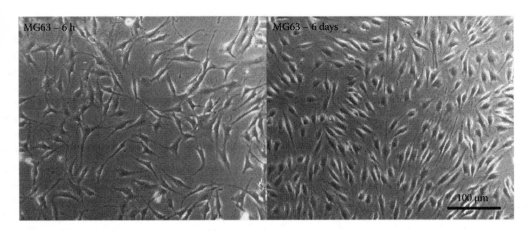

FIGURE 2.36
Optical micrographs of MG63 on a-C(Si37.6at.%). On sixth day of culturing, complete colonization of cell line is observed. (Reprinted with permission from Ong et al., *Thin Solid Films*, 516, 5152, 2008.)

Glial cell. Glial cells, commonly called neuroglia, are non-neuronal cells that maintain homeostasis, form myelin, and provide support and protection for the brain's neurons. The main functions of glial cells are to surround neurons and hold them in place, to supply nutrients and oxygen to neurons, to insulate one neuron from another, and to destroy pathogens and remove dead neurons. The glial cells' cytotoxicity was studied by culturing T98G human glioblastoma cell line on a-C:H [105]. The percent viability values for glial cells cultured on a-C:H coated substrates were calculated from experimental data that was collected using a commercial cytotoxicity assay kit. The results indicated that cell viability was not significantly different ($p < 0.05$) from positive control values (cells cultured on tissue culture plastic, $98 \pm 5\%$ viability). T98-G cell adhesion and spreading were robust on a-C:H, and the adhesion, spreading, and function were in comparison to normal culture conditions on tissue culture plastic. As such, a-C:H coatings were considered not toxic for cultured glial cells and fibroblasts.

Epithelial colorectal adenocarcinoma cell. Cell adhesion and viability studies were performed using Caco-2 human epithelial colorectal adenocarcinoma cell line on an "unconventional" a-C:H(PTFE) hybrid film [122]. These cells exhibit many characteristics of the human intestinal epithelium and are sensitive to cytotoxic effects. Thus, they are suitable for cytotoxicity studies of new biomaterials. Using this cell line and qualitative SEM and quantitative fluorescence microscopy experiments, a-C:H(PTFE) was shown to be biocompatible and noncytotoxic. Caco-2 cells adhered to its surface in the short-term 12 h experiments and spread and proliferated to cell monolayers in the longer-term 72 h experiments. In particular, the quantitative MTT test showed that there were no statistical differences between the coatings measured using the number and viability of the Caco-2 cells as indicators. It is interesting to note that the Teflon containing a-C:H has a high water contact angle of ~109°, which is around the value for bulk PTFE.

Bone marrow cells. Many implant materials are relatively inert in bulk form, but particles of these materials may cause adverse cellular reactions in surrounding bone, leading to a reduction of implant lifetime [123–126]. The biological response involves the accumulation and activation of inflammatory cells and subsequent bone resorption [127,128]. The rat bone marrow cell (RBMC) culture model composed of heterogeneous cell populations, which can advance along multiple differentiation pathways, one of which gives rise to the osteoblast lineage [129]. In addition, cells from the monocyte lineage can give rise to osteo-clastic, bone resorbing cells [130]. Osteoclasts have been shown to be phagocytose particles and to remain bone resorbing cells at the same time [131,132]. RBMC culture is suitable to investigate the effects of particle exposure on the formation and consequent function of osteoblastic and osteoclastic cells.

The cellular response of RBMC on a-C:H(Ti) coatings [133] and a-C:H(Ti) film fragments [134] were investigated. Increased proliferation and reduced osteoclast-like cell activity could be obtained on the a-C:H(Ti) coatings, while these reactions were not seen on pure a-C:H films or on glass control samples [133]. The results on the film particles showed that plain a-C:H and a-C:H(Ti) particles were inert. Both kinds of particles did not significantly stimulate the osteoclast-related enzyme tartrate-resistant acid phosphatase [134].

Neuronal cells. The potential for a-C to be used as biomaterials for the central nervous system was investigated [135]. The growth and survival of the N2a maurine neuroblastoma cell line and primary cortal neurons on a-C, surface-oxidized a-C and phosphorus-doped a-C films were studied. The results conclusively show that a-C is not cytotoxic to neurons or neural-like (N2a) cells. Cell adhesion and growth of neurons is greatly enhanced by either surface oxidation of the a-C or incorporation of phosphorus within the a-C matrix (up to 20 at.%). It is perhaps interesting to note that a-C(P) has the lowest water contact angle, followed by surface-oxidized a-C and then a-C. In this case, the adhesion and growth are better on surfaces with higher surface energy (hydrophilic). Furthermore, the different surface properties of a-C(P)/a-C can be exploited to generate spatially directed neuron growth via patterned deposition of these materials.

Endocrine cells. Cells release transmitters in discrete packets, a process called *quantal exo-cytosis*, as intracellular vesicles fuse with the cell membrane and release their contents. Electrochemical measurement of transmitter or hormone release from individual cells on microchips has applications both in basic science and drug screening. The ability of candidate electrode materials to promote the attachment of two hormone-secreting cell types (bovine adrenal chromaffin cell and insulin-secreting INS-1 cell line) was investigated [136]. From the result, nitrogen-doped a-C is better than several other commonly used electrochemical electrode materials for promoting cell attachment of endocrine cells. This is probably due to the optimal surface energy of a-C(N) as compared to the other candidates.

In Vivo Studies

An in vivo test performed by inserting 12-mm-long, 4-mm-diameter stainless steel cylin-ders coated with a-C:H into the cortical bone and muscular tissue of sheep [104]. Several implants were evaluated after 4 weeks and others after 12 weeks. It was found that the a-C:H coatings had no macroscopic adverse effects on the bone or muscle tissue. In another in vivo study, a-C:H coated cobalt–chromium (CoCr) cylinders were implanted in intra-muscular locations in rats and in transcortical sites in sheep (Figure 2.37). The specimens were retrieved 90 days after surgery, and their histological analysis showed that the a-C:H-coated specimens were tolerated well in both body sites [112].

The in vivo tissue response of a-C:H-coated titanium was investigated [137]. The mate-rials were implanted in the paravertebral muscles along both sides of the spine of New Zealand rabbits. Preparation of materials, methods used, and evaluation of the tissue response conformed to ASTM F981-93 (1999) standards. The parameters studied included evidence of necrosis, presence of inflammatory cells, fatty infiltration, calcification, and edema. Tissue-cell reaction studied on the samples explanted after 1, 3, 6, and 12 months

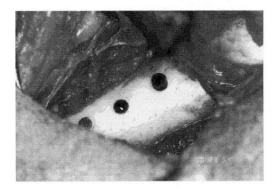

FIGURE 2.37
Transcortical implants in lateral femoral cortex of sheep. One (silver) uncoated CoCr alloy and two (black) a-C:H coated implants are shown in this intraoperative photograph. (Reprinted with permission from Allen et al., *J. Biomed. Mater. Res. B*, 58, 319, 2001.)

indicated that a-C:H followed the set pattern of response to an inert biocompatible material. At the end of 6 months, a-C:H/titanium implants were encapsulated by a 5- to 20-μm-thick layer of fibrous tissue, which reduced in thickness to 5–10 μm by 1 year. The surrounding muscle appeared to be normal. There was also no evidence of delamination of the coating or release of a-C:H particles into the surrounding tissue.

Tetrahedral amorphous carbon films (ta-C) coated Si die were implanted into male SV129 mice for in vivo tissue response [138]. The ta-C films were produced by pulsed laser deposition to be rich in either three- or four-fold (i.e., sp^2- or sp^3-bonded C) content. Tissue reaction to these materials over a period of 6 months was assessed following subcutaneous implantation of ta-C-coated silicon die. The reaction to ta-C particles injected near the sciatic nerve was studied as well. These particles were used as a simple analog to small, free-floating ta-C devices that might be used in vivo and as a well-characterized system to study tissue reaction to possible μm scale debris from a ta-C coated device.

The ta-C–coated die implants were easily removed with surrounding tissues and then processed for histologic evaluation of the tissue response at 4, 15, 23, and 56 days, and at 6 months after implantation. A typical ta-C–coated die is shown in Figure 2.38. This

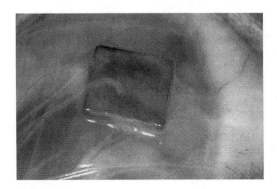

FIGURE 2.38
ta-C coated Si die in situ at the time of dissection. Implant dimensions are $5 \times 5 \times 0.5$ mm^3. (Reprinted with permission from LaVan et al., *Biomaterials*, 26, 465, 2005.)

sample had been in vivo for 6 months. There was no gross tissue reaction aside from the thin capsule that had formed around the implant. Specifically, there was no purulence or other evidence of inflammation, and surrounding tissues appeared intact. However, in vivo fragmentation seems to occur more readily on ta-C riched in three-fold bonding (more graphitic). There has been one report in the literature of damage to diamond-like carbon films [139] and another of increased inflammation reported in an in vivo study of diamond-like nanocomposite-coated stents [140]. Another report suggested that a-C films can have porosity, depending on the deposition conditions [141] that may have made them more susceptible to fragmentation. Those reports, along with the results presented by LaVan et al. [138] strongly suggest that amorphous carbon films with a higher four-fold bonding character (more diamond-like) are more resistant to in vivo fragmentation, and those films with more three-fold character (more graphitic) may be susceptible to in vivo fragmentation.

The tissue responses on ta-C particles were evaluated at 4-day, 8-week, and 6-month intervals. After 6 months of implantation, the group with 30 μm particles showed a foreign body giant cell reaction with mild fibrosis associated with the particles. In the 10 and 3 μm particle sizes, there was a foreign body giant cell reaction with fibrosis ranging from none to minimal. There was no evidence of acute inflammation, granulation tissue formation, or myocyte damage or histologic changes within the nerves, even when the particles were adjacent to these structures.

Antibacterial Behavior

Besides the ability of the implant surface to allow adhesion and proliferation of protective host cells, it is also desirable to develop implant coatings that are repellent to bacteria to minimize the colonization of the implant surface with circulating planktonic bacteria. Bacterial adhesion and colonization are followed by production of bacterial extracellular polymeric matrix and the development of a biofilm that protects bacteria against host defense, such as leukocytes, immunoglobulins, and complement as well as against antibiotics. These are often the major reasons for implant-related infections and failure. *Staphylococci* cause the majority of the nosocomial implant-related infections initiated by adhesion of planktonic bacteria to the implant surface.

The antibacterial behavior on polyethylene terephthalate (PET) coated with a thin layer of hydrogenated amorphous carbon (a-C:H) was investigated [142]. The capacities of *Staphylococcus aureus* and *Staphylococcus epidermidis* to adhere onto PET are quantitatively determined by plate counting and gamma-ray counting of ^{125}I radiolabeled bacteria in vitro. The results indicate that the adhesion of the two kinds of bacteria to PET is suppressed by a-C:H. From Figure 2.39, the adhesion efficiency of *S. epidermidis* on the coated surface is only about 14% of that of the untreated PET surface, and that of *S. aureus* is about 35% of that of the virgin surface. The electrokinetic potentials of the bacterial cells and substrates are determined by zeta potential measurement. All the substrates and the bacterial strain have negative zeta potentials. This means that bacterial adhesion is not mediated by electrostatic interactions. The surface energy components of the various substrates and bacteria are calculated later to obtain the interfacial free energies of adhesion of *S. aureus* and *S. epidermidis* onto various substrates. It is found that bacterial adhesion is energetically unfavorable on the a-C:H deposited on PET.

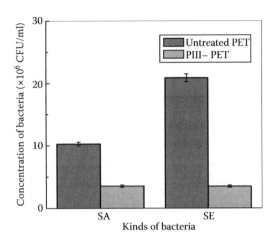

FIGURE 2.39
Number of bacteria adhering to untreated and a-C:H coated PET surfaces after incubation of 15 h. (Reprinted with permission from Wang et al., *Biomaterials*, 25, 3163, 2004.)

The number of adhered *S. aureus* and *S. epidermidis* on a-C:H(PTFE) hybrid film, which has the largest water contact angle (hydrophobic), is lowest when compared to a-C:H, titanium, and silicon [143]. The staphylococcal adhesion to the coatings is evaluated morphometrically from acridine orange-stained specimens. The bacterial adhesion is diminished at the same time when the noncytotoxic and cytocompatible properties for human cells were maintained (as discussed in Section 2.3.5). As such, a-C:H(PTFE) could be used to fight implant-related infections as it diminishes bacterial adhesion without affecting the capability of the surface to bind host cells.

Coating of stainless steel with ta-C reduced or almost eliminated adhesion and biofilm growth of *S. epidermidis*, *Deinococcus geothermalis*, *Meiothermus silvanus*, and *Pseudoxanthomonas taiwanensis* (*Psx. taiwanensis*) [144]. The latter three species are known to be pertinent biofilm formers in the wet-end of paper machines. It appears as if coating of the acid-proof steel coated with a ta-C prevented or reduced the formation of the appendages bridging the cells to each other or to the substrate. Field emission scanning electron microscopic analysis showed that *S. epidermidis*, *D. geothermalis*, and *M. silvanus* grew on stainless steel using threadlike organelles for adhesion and biofilm formation. *Psx. taiwanensis* adhered to the same surfaces by a mechanism involving cell ghosts on which the biofilm of live cells grew. *S. epidermidis* (a gram-positive coccus) and *Psx. taiwanensis* (a gram-negative gamma-proteobacterium) were effectively repelled by ta-C. The coating also has a similar effect on *D. geothermalis* and *M. Silvanus*, though not as significantly. The ta-C coating also reduced the accumulation of *S. epidermidis* biofilm on steel more efficiently than fluoropolymer coating, as reported by Katsikogianni et al. [145]. Besides hydrophobicity, the surface topology is also found to be affecting the microbe adhesion. High and positive surface skew (i.e., low film porosity) and high surface kurtosis (i.e., quantized height distribution) seem to decrease the attraction of the bacteria.

Titanium dioxide (TiO_2) in the anatase crystalline form is a strong bactericidal agent when exposed to near-UV light. The bactericidal activity of a-C:H films containing TiO_2 nanoparticles was investigated [146]. The films were grown on 316L stainless steel substrates from a dispersion of TiO_2 in hexane using PECVD. The antibacterial tests were

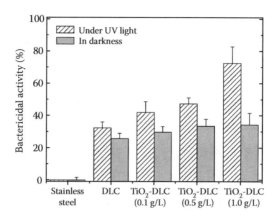

FIGURE 2.40
Antibacterial activity of the stainless steel-coated and uncoated with a-C:H and a-C:H(TiO₂) films in different TiO₂ concentrations. (Reprinted with permission from Marciano et al., *J. Coll. Interf. Sci.*, 340, 87, 2009.)

performed against *Escherichia coli,* and the results were compared to the bacterial adhesion force to the studied surfaces. As TiO₂ content increased, I_D/I_G ratio, hydrogen content, and roughness also increased. The films became more hydrophilic, with higher surface free energy, and the interfacial energy of bacteria adhesion decreased. Experimental results show that TiO₂ increased the a-C:H bactericidal activity (see Figures 2.40 and 2.41). Pure a-C:H films were thermodynamically unfavorable to bacterial adhesion. But the chemical interaction between the *E. coli* and the studied films can be increased for the films with higher TiO₂ concentration. As TiO₂ bactericidal activity starts its action by oxidative damage to the bacteria wall, a decrease in the interfacial energy of bacteria adhesion causes an increase in the chemical interaction between *E. coli* and the films, which is an additional factor for the increasing bactericidal activity. Another study of *E. coli* on silver-doped a-C:H also showed an increase in bactericidal activity [147].

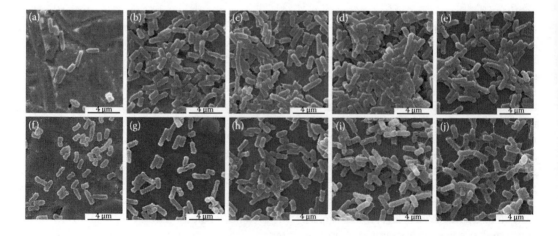

FIGURE 2.41
SEM images of *E. coli* in direct contact with (a) stainless steel, (b) a-C:H, (c) 0.1 g/L a-C:H(TiO₂), (d) 0.5 g/L a-C:H(TiO₂), and (e) 1.0 g/L a-C:H(TiO₂) films in darkness; and (f) stainless steel, (g) a-C:H, (h) 0.1 g/L a-C:H(TiO₂), (i) 0.5 g/L a-C:H(TiO₂), and (j) 1.0 g/L a-C:H(TiO₂) films under UV light. (Reprinted with permission from Marciano et al., *J. Coll. Interf. Sci.*, 340, 87, 2009.)

Besides the studies of undoped and doped a-C and a-C:H, polymer-, nanoparticle-incorporated a-C:H, another interesting study is on plasma-modified a-C:H [148]. The a-C:H treated with oxygen plasma exhibits superhydrophilicity with a contact angle of ~ 0°. Although there is a drastic change to the film surface energy, the level of bactericidal activity of *S. aureus, E. coli, Pseudomonas aeruginosa,* and *Salmonella typhimurium* is not affected significantly.

Biomedical Applications

Biocompatible implants allow the human body to reestablish biological and mechanical functions and thus increase the quality of life. Depending on the biomedical application, the implant has to withstand dynamic mechanical loads while performing a desirable long-term biological interaction with surrounding biological tissue. Bulk properties of the implant are mainly responsible for the load-bearing capabilities, whereas the interaction with the surrounding tissue is governed by the implant's surface. The surface influences the interaction and adsorption of different proteins, which, in turn, control the cell adhesion and behavior. However, the overall reaction of the body on an implant is a system property that includes many different aspects, such as surface chemistry and texture, implant movement, biodegradation, and surgical aspects. The highly corrosive environment and the low tolerance of the body to some dissolution products restrict the materials to be used for implants. As we already know from the previous sections, amorphous carbon is bio- and hemocompatible. Furthermore, the material can prevent the detrimental effects caused by the released metal ions from conventional metallic implants. Therefore, there is a growing interest in modifying implants' surface with amorphous carbon. In addition, amorphous carbon, due to its amorphous nature, is able to incorporate a certain amount of additional elements and even compounds into its matrix and still maintain its amorphous state. By this technique, several properties, including tribological properties, electrical conductivity, surface energy, and biological reactions of cells in contact with the surface, can be altered to suit specific applications. There are mainly two fields of biological applications of amorphous carbon: the application of amorphous carbon in blood-contacting implants, such as heart valves and stents, and the use of amorphous carbon to reduce wear in load-bearing joint implants. Amorphous carbon-coated heart valves and stents are already commercially available. But the situation for amorphous carbon-coated load-bearing implants is contradicting.

There are extensive reviews on amorphous carbon coatings for biological and biomedical applications [149–156]. In this section, some of the applications will be discussed. Some of these are readily available commercial coatings, while others are still under development.

Orthopedic Implants

Total hip replacement is one of the most challenging types of human implants from the materials science's point of view. The techniques developed for improving the hip implants can naturally be applied to other articulated or immovable implants. Since the human body is at the same time both a very hostile and sensitive environment for foreign objects, the lifespan of a hip implant is limited. The practical lifetime of the current artificial total hip replacements can be as low as 5–15 years because mechanical wear and stress, corrosion, and tissue reactions lead either to a mechanical failure or to aseptic loosening of the implant. The main problem with the prosthetic joints lies in its wear and corrosion during long-term use. The debris formed as a consequence of this wear results in tissue inflammation, osteolysis, and finally loosening of the implants [157–162]. When two material surfaces slide against each other and are in relative motion, the material with lower hardness is worn out. The material will also come in contact with human body fluids. Therefore, in prosthetic joints, the coating material should be hard and inert enough to prevent wear out and corrosion. The coating material should also have good adhesion on the substrate, especially in human body fluid. Besides amorphous carbon's biocompatibility, its excellent tribological properties [163–166] have made it a potential material to reduce the wear rate and corrosion in the physiological environment.

There are experiments using hip simulators to determine friction and wear of amorphous carbon-coated hip joint balls sliding against ultra high molecular weight polyethylene (UHMWPE) or of metal–metal joints with both sides coated with amorphous carbon. Tetrahedral amorphous carbon (ta-C) coated metal hip joint balls tested in 1 wt.% NaCl water by pin-on-disk and in a hip joint simulator reduce the wear of the UHMWPE cup by a factor of 10–100 [150,167]. In the case of a metal–metal joint with both sides coated, the wear could be reduced by a factor of 10^5. Additionally, the corrosion rate is significantly lowered when the coated substrate is exposed to a saline solution equivalent to body fluids in 37°C for 2 years [150]. Stainless steel femoral head is coated with a-C:H and the wear of the UHMWPE cups in a hip joint simulator using distilled water after six million cycles is determined [168]. The result is a decrease of wear by a factor of six. Tested in a knee wear simulator using distilled water as a lubricant, a decrease of a factor of five in wear of the UHMWPE by coating the cobalt chromium counter face with a-C:H can be obtained [169]. A comparative tribological test using ball-on-disk and pin-on-disk configuration, but in dry conditions, to investigate the wear of different materials used in hip joint prostheses against UHMWPE was conducted [170]. The wear rate of stainless steel, titanium, alumina, zirconium oxide, a-C:H coated stainless steel, and a-C:H coated titanium were compared. The results revealed the superiority of the a-C:H coatings. In a more recent tribological study using pin-on-disk in simulated body fluid, it was found that coating both surfaces of UHMWPE and Co–Cr–Mo implants by ta-C film enhanced the lifetime of the implant to a considerable extent [171,172].

The wear of UHMWPE acetabular cups against CoCr, alumina, and a-C:H coated CoCr with a biaxial hip wear simulator using diluted calf serum as the lubricant was studied [173]. It was found that there is no significant difference in the wear of UHMWPE for all three pairs of tested cups. The same result is obtained from another independent study [174]. The corrosion resistance and hardness of an orthopedic material like Co–Cr–Mo alloy can be significantly increased by ta-C coatings [175]. However, the wear resistance of the ta-C coated Co–Cr–Mo against UHMWPE measured by a pin-on-disk method in air, deionized water, and simulated body fluid did not show any significant improvement over Co–Cr–Mo/UHMWPE sliding pairs. Another pin-on-disk study on the tribological performance of UHMWPE against untreated, a-C coated by unbalanced magnetron sputtering of graphite, nitrogen-implanted, thermal oxygen-treated, and oxygen diffusion-treated Ti_6Al_4V alloy in distilled water environment was carried out [176]. There is improvement in tribological behavior with all the surface engineering techniques, but the thermal oxygen-treated Ti_6Al_4V alloy showed significantly less wear than the a-C coating.

Even though some studies reveal amorphous carbon film as a promising material to reduce the wear of UHMWPE, the effect of the amorphous carbon coating on artificial joints is still in debate. These conflicting findings may be the result of several issues. The liquid lubricant used in a tribological test has a crucial influence on the friction and wear values obtained as well as on the type of wear particles produced [177–179]. It was suggested that when bovine serum or synovial fluid was used as a lubricant, the different proteins, especially phospholipids, adsorbed on the surfaces strongly influence the tribological behavior in the joints [177,178]. Also, the surface texture has a decisive influence on the wear behavior of a joint. It was shown that even single scratches are capable of increasing the wear rate of UHMWPE by a factor of 30–70 [180]. To summarize, it can be stated that wear tests on load-bearing implants should be made in an adequate implant joint simulator. As a lubricant, a supply of synovial fluid (or any other fluid containing an adequate distribution of proteins) has to be maintained to compensate for the proteins decomposed due to high pressure between contact spots of the bearing [181]. Additionally, the surface texture of the areas involved in the tribological process must be characterized carefully.

There are also reports of failure of amorphous carbon coating in orthopedic implants. In 2001, the company Implant Design AG sold knee joints under the trade name Diamond Rota Gliding with the sliding area of the femur component coated with diamond-like nanocomposite (DLN), which was sliding against UHMWPE. Within a short time, some of the approximately 190 implanted joints showed increased wear and partial coating delamination and had to be replaced.

Coronary Stent

A coronary stent is a man-made tube that is inserted into a coronary artery to help open the artery so that blood can flow through it. The main purpose is to treat coronary heart disease as part of the procedure called percutaneous coronary intervention. Similar stents can also be used in noncoronary vessels. Such implantation is increasing day by day throughout the world. However, the application is largely limited by restenosis, occlusion, and stent-associated thrombosis. For implants in direct contact with blood, a key issue is the ability of the implant surface to prevent thrombus formation. The reactions of the body to a blood-contacting implant crucially depends on the surface of the implant, especially the chemical situation present at the surface, the surface texture, the local flow conditions, and other factors. It is generally known that increased platelet adhesion, activation, and aggregation on implant surfaces exposed to blood precede the formation of a thrombus. A high ratio of the proteins albumin/fibrinogen, adsorbed on a implant surface prior to cell or platelet attachment, can be correlated with a low number of adhering platelets and therefore with a low tendency of thrombus formation. As discussed in the earlier section, amorphous carbon coatings show promising results in being a hemocompatible material. Some of the findings even show the material may have the ability to suppress thrombus formation similar to or even better than glassy carbon, a material widely used for heart valves.

It has been observed that all metals corrode to some degree following implantation [182]. Release of metals like Ni, Cr, Mo, and Mn has been confirmed from uncoated stents in contact with human plasma for 4 days [183]. But no such metal release was observed for a-C–coated stents by the plasma-induced deposition technique. The a-C coating also reduced platelet activation and thrombogenicity to a significant extent. Some comparative studies were made on ta-C–coated, polyurethane-coated, and uncoated stainless steel vascular stents by observing their responses to macrophages [184]. It was noted that the spreading of macrophages and inflammatory activity was less on ta-C coating than that of polyurethane-coated and uncoated stents. In 2004, a successful implantation of nitinol (nickel–titanium shape memory alloy) stents coated with a-C:H was made for endovascular treatment of superficial femoral artery occlusive disease [185]. Primary results of this investigation showed a 100% patency rate 12 months after intervention. However, another clinical test in the year 2004 reported that a-C:H coating does not provide significant improvements over uncoated stainless steel stents [186]. A random study of the hemocompatibility of a-C:H coated stainless steel stents was made by comparing them with uncoated stents during the treatment of coronary artery disease in 347 patients. After 6 months' implantation, it was observed that the binary restenosis is 31.8% for a-C:H coated stents and 35.9% for stainless steel stents, while the major adverse cardiac effect is 30.5% for a-C:H coated stainless steel stents and 32.7% for uncoated ones.

Some of the amorphous carbon coatings have been incorporated into commercial stents or related products. The Cardio Carbon Company Limited has two amorphous carbon-coated titanium implants: Angelini Lamina-flo™ (mechanical heart valve) and Angelini Valvuloplasty™ ring that is used for heart valve repairs. Plasmachem of Germany produces a stent coated with 50 nm of amorphous carbon, marketed under the trade name BioDiamond Stent™. They use a plasma-induced cold deposition technique to coat amorphous carbon on stainless steel 316L stents. The company PHYTIS sells amorphous carbon-coated stents on which they report a reduced rate of restenosis due to the amorphous carbon coating and that target revascularization has been necessary in only 3.27% of the lesions treated. Another company, Sorin Biomedica of Italy, produces heart valves and stents (Carbonstent™) which are coated by approximately 0.5 μm thick Carbofilm™. This coating is produced by PVD from a carbon target, and the company states that Carbofilm™ has a turbostratic structure equivalent to that of pyrolytic carbon. In one clinical study, 165 Carbonstents™ were used in 129 coronary lesions of 110 patients [187]. At the 1-month follow-up, there were no sign of stent thrombosis or any other major adverse cardiac events. In another clinical study, the Carbonstent™ was implanted in 112 patients with 132 de novo lesions [188]. The 6-month angiographic follow-up was obtained in 108 patients (96%) (127 lesions); the angiographic restenosis rate was a low 11%.

Other Biomedical Applications

An amorphous carbon coated centrifugal ventricular blood pump device (made by SunMedical Technology Research Corporation, Nagano, Japan) was implanted in calves. Without any postoperative anticoagulation, only minor evidence of thrombosis was found on the amorphous carbon coated surfaces after explantation [189].

Hydrogenated amorphous carbon coatings have been investigated for oral implants [190–193]. It was observed that the RF-PECVD deposited a-C:H layers showed significant biointegration and resistance to saliva and other oral cavity elements [190]. Ion beam plated a-C:H films on orthodontic nitinol arch wires reduce the Ni ions release to a great extent [191–193]. The growth rate of Sa3 squamous carcinoma cells is also higher on coated wires [193].

There were studies on coating guide wires with amorphous carbon, and investigations of the films' lubrication, stability, and hemocompatible properties were addressed [194–196]. It was observed that a-C:H coated guide wires exhibited a lower coefficient of friction, better adhesion with stainless steel, higher hardness, and better hemocompatibility than other coatings, such as PTFE [195]. Si and F have been incorporated in a-C:H film to improve adhesion with the substrate and stability during guide wire windings. Use of an a-Si:H interlayer has increased the substrate adhesion significantly, while Si doping in FCVA deposited ta-C was reported to reduce film cracking [194]. Lubrication properties of stainless steel guide wires coated with a-C:H and a-C:H(F) was studied [196]. It was noted that a-C:H and a-C:H(F) improved smoothness, uniformity, and reduced polishing scars. Both films were found to improve the lubrication behavior by 30% when compared to uncoated guide wires. Fluorine incorporation in a-C:H also significantly reduced the thrombogenicity.

Some studies were done on the coating of contact lenses by carbon films to improve their ophthalmological applications [197,198]. Ion-assisted deposited a-C:H on contact lenses was found to adhere well to the lens materials, enhance stability, provide UV protection, and strengthen the lens life significantly [197]. The coating also minimized antibacterial activity and inflammatory processes and improved the chemical resistance to the sterilization and storage solution of contact lenses. Hydrogenated a-C coatings on contact lenses increased the refractive index, thereby reducing the thickness of contact lens [198]. The coatings of thickness in the range 20–200 nm have good transmission in the visible region, but minimize UV transmission by about 40–50%. Contact lens casings coated with a-C:H also showed significant surface integrity on exposure to saline solution, prevented the formation of microbial contamination, and proved to be a safe custodian of the contact lenses.

Summary

Amorphous carbon, renowned for its superior mechanical properties, is currently in the spotlight once again for its potential to be utilized in biomedical applications. Numerous studies in vitro, in vivo, and clinical have been done to prove the values of this material. However, there are multitudes of conflicting issues regarding its biological properties. As such, this class of "biomaterial" is complicated to characterize. Even so, some films are already utilized in commercial products.

The results on blood compatibility are very promising. The material is able to reduce blood platelet adhesion and activation to prevent thrombosis. In general, the property can be improved further if the material has a higher sp^3 to sp^2 fraction, becoming more hydrophobic. But studies have also shown hydrophobicity is not alone in determining the hemocompatibility. Surface energetics can affect the adhesion of proteins and hence the amount of adherent platelets. A surface is favorable when it can attract more albumin than fibrinogen. Results have also confirmed that material surface properties can be moderated by doping and surface treatment. There are already a couple of commercial biomedical implants utilizing this material in blood contacting applications (e.g., stents and heart valves).

Amorphous carbon has also proven to be noncytotoxic to a vast number of living biological cells, including the three cells (macrophages, fibroblasts, and osteoblasts) found in periprosthetic tissues and endothelial (found in blood intravascular inner wall linings). Doping and surface treatment have also helped to improve the material–cell interactions. Both hydrophobic and hydrophilic films have been proven to increase cellular proliferation and activity. Again, the surface energetics govern these interactions in addition to wettability. A number of experiments done on animal models have also shown minimal or no adverse effects.

The latest interesting studies are on the antibacterial properties of amorphous carbon. A number of bacteria have been used for these studies, and most results have shown reduced microbe adhesion and activity on the material. A hydrophobic surface is preferred, but hydrophilic surfaces have also been proven not to affect the antibacterial property. Besides surface energetics and its interaction with proteins and microbes, surface topography can play an important role as well. Generally, an ultrasmooth and ultralow porosity film is desired. Doping with known antibacteria elements can drastically improve bactericidal activity. This is one good example of the amorphous nature of the material where tuning and moderation is flexible.

There are already a number of application-specific studies. Coronary stents and other vascular stents have received great attention. Commercial products incorporating proprietary amorphous carbon coatings have been available for many years. Another promising application is orthopedic implants, where the biocompatibility and mechanical properties, such as high hardness and low friction, come together to reduce wear and failure. However, results have been contradicting. The conflicting results may be caused by different regimes used in the tests and simulation of actual physiological conditions. Human inner space is a harsh and unforgiving environment with a condition difficult to replicate in vitro.

Although much attention has been received and many studies have been done, the actual numbers of commercially available products that are useful in improving human life still only number a handful. Even so, these are good indicators of the potential amorphous carbons have. More work with good results, especially clinically, needs to be achieved before the material can be widely recognized and live up to its potential for widespread use.

References

[1] S. Aisenberg, R. Chabot: Ion-beam deposition of thin films of diamond-like carbon. *J. Appl. Phys.* 42 (1971) 2953.

[2] G. Galli, R.A. Martin, R. Car, M. Parrinello: Structural and electronic properties of amorphous carbon. *Phys. Rev. Lett.* 62 (1989) 555.

[3] N.A. Marks, D.R. McKenzie, B.A. Pailthorpe, M. Parrinello: Microscopic structure of tetrahedral amorphous carbon. *Phys. Rev. Lett.* 76 (1996) 768.

[4] Y. Lifshitz, S.R. Kasi, J.W. Rabalais: Subplantation model for film growth from hyperthermal species: Application to diamond. *Phys. Rev. Lett.* 62 (1989) 1290.

[5] Y. Lifshitz, S.R. Kasi, J.W. Rabalais, W. Eckstein: Subplantation model for film growth from hyperthermal species. *Phys. Rev. B* 41 (1990) 10468.

[6] W. Moller: Modeling of the sp^3/sp^2 ratio in ion beam and plasma-deposited carbon films. *Appl. Phys. Lett.* 59 (1991) 2391.

[7] H.J. Steffen, S. Marton, J.W. Rabalais: Displacement energy threshold for Ne^+ irradiation of graphite. *Phys. Rev. Lett.* 68 (1992) 1726.

[8] J. Koike, D.M. Parkin, T.E. Mitchell: Displacement threshold energy for type IIa diamond. *Appl. Phys. Lett.* 60 (1992) 1450.

[9] D.R. McKenzie, D. Muller, B.A. Pailthorpe: Compressive-stress-induced formation of thin-film tetrahedral amorphous carbon. *Phys. Rev. Lett.* 67 (1991) 773.

[10] J. Robertson: Deposition mechanisms for promoting sp^3 bonding in diamond-like carbon. *Diamond Rel. Mater.* 2 (1993) 984.

[11] J. Robertson: The deposition mechanism of diamond-like a-C and a-C:H. *Diamond Rel. Mater.* 3 (1994) 361.

[12] S. Uhlmann, T. Frauenheim, Y. Lifshitz: Molecular-dynamics study of the fundamental processes involved in subplantation of diamondlike carbon. *Phys. Rev. Lett.* 81 (1998) 641.

[13] H.P. Kaukonen, R.M. Nieminen: Atomic-scale modeling of the ion-beam-induced growth of amorphous carbon. *Phys. Rev. B* 61 (2000) 2806.

[14] K. Kohary, S. Kugler: Growth of amorphous carbon: Low-energy molecular dynamics simulation of atomic bombardment. *Phys. Rev. B* 63 (2001) 193404.

[15] J. Robertson: Diamond-like amorphous carbon. *Mater. Sci. Eng. R* 37 (2002) 129.

[16] H. Hofsäss, H. Feldermann, R. Merk, M. Sebastian, C. Ronning: Cylindrical spike model for the formation of diamondlike thin films by ion deposition. *Appl. Phys. A* 66 (1998) 153.

[17] J.P. Hirvonen, J. Koskinen, M. Kaukonen, R. Nieminen: Dynamic relaxation of the elastic properties of hard carbon films. *J. Appl. Phys.* 81 (1997) 7248.

[18] P.J. Fallon, V.S. Veerasamy, C.A. Davis, J. Robertson, G.A.J. Amaratunga, W.I. Milne, J. Koskinen: Properties of filtered-ion-beam-deposited diamondlike carbon as a function of ion energy. *Phys. Rev. B* 48 (1993) 4777.

[19] T. Diaz de la Rubia, R.S. Averback, R. Benedek, W.E. King: Role of thermal spikes in energetic displacement cascades. *Phys. Rev. Lett.* 59 (1987) 1930.

[20] H. Hsieh, T. Diaz de la Rubia, R.S. Averback, R. Benedek: Effect of temperature on the dynamics of energetic displacement cascades: A molecular dynamics study. *Phys. Rev. B* 40 (1989) 9986.

[21] M. Chhowalla, J. Robertson, C.W. Chen, S.R.P. Silva, G.A.J. Amaratunga: Influence of ion energy and substrate temperature on the optical and electronic properties of tetrahedral amorphous carbon (*ta*-C) films. *J. Appl. Phys.* 81 (1997) 139.

[22] Y. Lifshitz: Diamond-like carbon—present status. *Diamond Rel. Mater.* 8 (1999) 1659.

[23] J. Koskinen, J.P. Hirvonen, J. Keranen: Effect of deposition temperature and growth rate on the bond structure of hydrogen free carbon films. *J. Appl. Phys.* 84 (1998) 648.

[24] J. Filik, P.W. May, S.R.J. Pearce, R.K. Wild, K.R. Hallam: XPS and laser Raman analysis of hydrogenated amorphous carbon films. *Diamond Rel. Mater.* 12 (2003) 974.

[25] J. Diaz, G. Paolicelli, S. Ferrer, F. Comin: Direct evaluation of the sp^3 content in diamond-like-carbon films by XPS. *Phys. Rev. B* 54 (1996) 8064.

[26] P. Merel, M. Tabbal, M. Chaker, S. Moisa, J. Margot: Structural properties and surface morphology of laser-deposited amorphous carbon and carbon nitride films. *Appl. Surf. Sci.* 136 (1998) 105.

[27] E. Riedo, F. Comin, J. Chevrier, F. Schmithusen, S. Decossas, M. Sancroth, *Surf. Coat. Tech.* 125 (2000) 124.

[28] F. Tuinstra, J.L. Koenig: Raman spectrum of graphite. *J. Chem. Phys.* 53 (1970) 1126.

[29] A.A. Ogwu, R.W. Lamberton, S. Morley, P. Maguire, J. McLaughlin: Characterisation of thermally annealed diamond like carbon (DLC) and silicon modified DLC films by Raman spectroscopy. *Physica B* 269 (1999) 335.

[30] A.C. Ferrari, J. Robertson: Interpretation of Raman spectra of disordered and amorphous carbon. *Phys. Rev. B* 61 (2000) 14095.

[31] F. Li, J.S. Lannin: Radial distribution function of amorphous carbon. *Phys. Rev. Lett.* 65 (1990) 1905.

[32] F. Li, J.S. Lannin: Disorder induced Raman scattering of nanocrystalline carbon. *Appl. Phys. Lett.* 61 (1992) 2116.

[33] S. Prawer, K.W. Nugent, Y. Lifshitz, G.D. Lempert, E. Grossman, J. Kulik, I. Avigal, R. Kalish: Systematic variation of the Raman spectra of DLC films as a function of sp^2:sp^3 composition. *Diamond Rel. Mater.* 5 (1996) 433.

[34] S. Zhang, L. Li, A. Kumar (Eds.), *Materials Characterization Techniques.* CRC Press Taylor & Francis Group, Boca Raton (2008).

[35] T. Young: An essay on the cohesion of fluids. *Philos. Trans. R. Soc. London* 95 (1805) 65.

[36] F.M. Fowkes: Attractive forces at interfaces. *Ind. Eng. Chem.* 56 (1964) 40.

[37] D.K. Owens, R.C. Wendt: Estimation of the surface energy of polymers. *J. Appl. Polym. Sci.* 13 (1969) 1741.

[38] D.H. Kaelble: Dispersion-polar surface tension properties of organic solids. *J. Adhesion* 2 (1970) 66.

[39] C.J. van Oss, M.K. Chaudhury, R.J. Good: Interfacial Lifshitz-van der Waals and polar interactions in macroscopic systems. *Chem. Rev.* 88 (1988) 927.

[40] R.J. Good, C.J. van Oss: The modern theory of contact angles and the hydrogen bond components of surface energies, in: M. Schrader, G. Loeb (Eds.), *Modern Approaches to Wettability: Theory and Applications*. Plenum Press, New York (1992) 1–27.

[41] R. Hauert: A review of modified DLC coatings for biological applications. *Diamond Rel. Mater.* 12 (2003) 583.

[42] S.L. Goodman, T.G. Grasel, S.L. Cooper, R.M. Albrecht: Platelet shape change and cytoskeletal reorganization on polyurethaneureas. *J Biomed Mater Res* 23 (1989) 105.

[43] L.K. Krishnan, N. Varghese, C.V. Muraleedharan, G.S. Bhuvaneshwar, F. Derangere, Y. Sampeur, R. Suryanarayanan: Quantitation of platelet adhesion to Ti and DLC-coated Ti *in vitro* using 125I-labeled platelets. *Biomolecular Eng.* 19 (2002) 251.

[44] M.I. Jones, I.R. McColl, D.M. Grant, K.G. Parker, T.L. Parker: Haemocompatibility of DLC and TiC-TiN interlayers on titanium. *Diamond Rel. Mater.* 8 (1999) 457.

[45] M.I. Jones, I.R. McColl, D.M. Grant, K.G. Parker, T.L. Parker: Protein adsorption and platelet attachment and activation, on TiN, TiC, and DLC coatings on titanium for cardiovascular applications. *J. Biomed. Mater. Res.* 52 (2000) 413.

[46] F.Z. Cui, D.J. Li: A review of investigations on biocompatibility of diamond-like carbon and carbon nitride films. *Surf. Coat. Technol.* 131 (2000) 481.

[47] K. Gutensohn, C. Beythien, J. Bau, T. Grewe, R. Koester, K. Padmanaban, P. Kuehnl: *In vitro* analyses of diamond-like carbon coated stents: Reduction of metal ion release, platelet activation, and thrombogenicity. *Thrombosis Res.* 99 (2000) 577.

[48] J.Y. Chen, L.P. Wang, K.Y. Fu, N. Huang, Y. Leng, Y.X. Leng, P. Yang, J. Wang, G.J. Wan, H. Sun, X.B. Tian, P.K. Chu: Blood compatibility and sp^3/sp^2 contents of diamond-like carbon (DLC) synthesized by plasma immersion ion implantation-deposition. *Surf. Coat. Technol.* 156 (2002) 289.

[49] P. Yang, N. Huang, Y.X. Leng, J.Y. Chen, R.K.Y. Fu, S.C.H. Kwok, Y. Leng P.K. Chu: Activation of platelets adhered on amorphous hydrogenated carbon (a-C:H) films synthesized by plasma immersion ion implantation-deposition (PIII-D). *Biomaterials* 24 (2003) 2821.

[50] Y.X. Leng, J.Y. Chen, P. Yang, H. Sun, G.J. Wan N. Huang: Mechanical properties and platelet adhesion behavior of diamond-like carbon films synthesized by pulsed vacuum arc plasma deposition. *Surf. Sci.* 531 (2003) 177.

[51] D.J. Li, H.Q. Gu: Cell attachment on diamond-like carbon coating. *Bull. Mater. Sci.* 25 (2002) 7.

[52] P. Yang, S.C.H. Kwok, P.K. Chu, Y.X.Leng, J.Y. Chen, J. Wang, N. Huang: Haemocompatibility of hydrogenated amorphous carbon (a-C:H) films synthesized by plasma immersion ion implantation-deposition. *Nucl. Instrum. Methods Phys. Rev. B* 206 (2003) 721.

[53] S. Logothetidis, M. Gioti, S. Lousinian, S. Fotiadou: Haemocompatibility studies on carbon-based thin films by ellipsometry. *Thin Solid Films* 482 (2005) 126.

[54] H. Arwin: Ellipsometry on thin organic layers of biological interest: Characterization and applications. *Thin Solid Films* 377–378 (2000) 48.

[55] H. Wormeester, E.S. Kooij, A. Mege, S. Rekveld, B. Poelsema: Ellipsometric characterisation of heterogeneous 2D layers. *Thin Solid Films* 455–456 (2004) 323.

[56] S. Logothetidis: Haemocompatibility of carbon based thin films. *Diamond Rel. Mater.* 16 (2007) 1847.

[57] V. Karagkiozaki, S. Logothetidis, A. Laskarakis, G. Giannoglou, S. Lousinian: AFM study of the thrombogenicity of carbon-based coatings for cardiovascular applications. *Mater. Sci. Eng. B* 152 (2008) 16.

[58] S. Lousinian, S. Logothetidis, A. Laskarakis, M. Gioti: Haemocompatibility of amorphous hydrogenated cardbon thin films, optical properties and adsorption mechanisms of blood plasma proteins. *Biomol. Eng.* 24 (2007) 107.

[59] S. Lousinian. N. Kalfagiannis, S. Logothetidis: Albumin and fibrinogen adsorption on boron nitride and carbon-based thin films. *Mater. Sci. Eng. B* 152 (2008) 12.

[60] L.J. Yu, X. Wang, X.H Wang, X.H Liu: Haemocompatibility of tetrahedral amorphous carbon films. *Surf. Coat. Technol.* 128–129 (2000) 484.

[61] P. Baurschmidt, M. Schaldach: Alloplastic materials for heart-valve prostheses. *Med. Biol. Eng. Comput.* 18 (1980) 496.

[62] A. Wisbey, P.J. Gregson, L.M. Peter, M. Tuke: Effect of surface-treatment on the dissolution of titanium-based implant materials. *Biomaterials* 12 (1991) 470.

[63] N. Nurdin, P. Francois, Y. Mugnier, J. Krumeich, M. Moret, B.-O. Aronsson, P. Descouts: Haemocompatibility evaluation of DLC- and SiC-coated surfaces. *Eur. Cells Mater.* 5 (2003) 17.

[64] M. Fedel, A. Motta, D. Maniglio, C. Migliaresi: Surface properties and blood compatibility of commercially available diamond-like carbon coatings for cardiovascular devices. *J. Biomed. Mater. Res. B* 90B (2009) 338.

[65] S.E. Ong, S. Zhang, H. Du, H.C. Too, K.N. Aung: Influence of silicon concentration on the haemocompatibility of amorphous carbon. *Biomaterials* 28 (2007) 4033.

[66] T.I.T. Okpalugo, A.A. Ogwu, P.D. Maguire, J.A.D. McLaughlin: Platelet adhesion on silicon modified hydrogenated amorphous carbon films. *Biomaterials* 25 (2004) 239.

[67] S. Agathopoulos, P. Nikolopoulos: Wettability and interfacial interactions in bioceramic–body–liquid systems. *J. Biomed. Mater. Res.* 29 (1995) 421.

[68] P.N. Sawyer, J.W. Pate: Bioelectric phenomena as an etiological factor in intravascular thrombosis. *Surgery* 34 (1953) 491.

[69] T.I.T. Okpalugo, A.A. Ogwu, P.D. Maguire, J.A.D. McLaughlin, D.G. Hirst: In-vitro blood compatibility of a-C:H:Si and a-C:H thin films. *Diamond Rel. Mater.* 13 (2004) 1088.

[70] T. Hasebe, A. Shimada, T. Suzuki, Y. Matsuoka, T. Saito, S. Yohena, A. Kamijo, N. Shiraga, M. Higuchi, K. Kimura, H. Yoshimura, S. Kuribayashi: Fluorinated diamond-like carbon as antithrombogenic coating for blood-contacting devices. *J. Biomed. Mater. Res. A* 76A (2006) 86.

[71] T. Saito, T. Hasebe, S. Yohena, Y. Matsuoka, A. Kamijo, K. Takahahi, T. Suzuki: Antithrombogenicity of fluorinated diamond-like carbon films. *Diamond Rel. Mater.* 14 (2005) 1116.

[72] T. Hasebe, S. Yohena, A. Kamijo, Y. Okazaki, A. Hotta, K. Takahashi, T. Suzuki: Fluorine doping into diamond-like carbon coatings inhibits protein adsorption and platelet attachment and activation. *J. Biomed. Mater. Res. A* 83A (2007) 1192.

[73] A.P. Liu, J.C. Han, J.Q. Zhu, S.H. Meng, X.D. He: Evaluation on corrosion behavior and haemocompatibility of phosphorus incorporated tetrahedral amorphous carbon films. *Mater. Sci. Eng. C* 28 (2008) 1408.

[74] K. Park, F.W. Mao, H. Park: Morphological characterization of surface-induced platelet activation. *Biomaterials* 11 (1990) 24.

[75] A.P. Liu, J.Q. Zhu, M. Liu, Z.F. Dai, X. Han, J.C. Han: Platelet adhesion on phosphorus-incorporated tetrahedral amorphous carbon films. *Appl. Surf. Sci.* 255 (2008) 279.

[76] S.C.H. Kwok, J. Wang, P.K. Chu: Surface energy, wettability and blood compatibility of phosphorus doped diamond-like carbon films. *Diamond Rel. Mater.* 14 (2005) 78.

[77] S. Zhang, H. Du, S.E. Ong, K.N. Aung, H.C. Too, X. Miao: Bonding structure and haemocompatibility of silicon-incorporated amorphous carbon. *Thin Solid Films* 515 (2006) 66.

[78] B. Muller, R. Michel, S.M.D. Paul, R. Hofer, D. Heger, D. Grutzmacher: Impact of nanometer-scale roughness on contact-angle hysteresis and globulin adsorption. *J. Vac. Sci. Technol. B* 19 (2001) 1715.

[79] X. Zhang, S. Yu, Z. He, Y. Miao: Wetting of rough surfaces. *Surf. Rev. Lett.* 11 (2004) 7.

[80] X.M. He, D.C. Carter: Atomic structure and chemistry of human serum albumin. *Nature* 358 (1992) 209.

[81] S.D. Bruck: Intrinsic semiconduction, electronic conduction of polymers and blood compatibility. *Nature* 243 (1973) 416.

[82] S.D. Bruck: The role of electrical conduction of macromolecules in certain biomedical problems. *Polymer* 16 (1975) 25.

[83] L. Zhang, M. Chen, Z.Y. Li, D.H. Chen, S.R. Pan: Effect of annealing on structure and haemocompatibility of tetrahedral amorphous hydrogenated carbon films. *Mater. Lett.* 62 (2008) 1040.

[84] R.K. Roy, H.W. Choi, J.W. Yi, M.W. Moon, K.R. Lee, D.K. Han, J.H. Shin, A. Kamijo, T. Hasebe: Hemocompatibility of surface-modified, silicon incorporated diamond-like carbon films. *Acta Biomater.* 5 (2009) 249.

[85] F. Khan, L.M. Synder, L. Pechet: The laboratory of coagulation. A review of present laboratory techniques. *J. Thromb.Thrombolysis* 5 (1998) 83.

[86] J.L. Gordan in: J.P. Cazenave, J.A. Davies, M.D. Kazatchkine, W.G. van Aken (Eds), *Blood–Surface Interactions: Biological Principles Underlying Haemocompatibility with Artificial Materials.* Elsevier Science Publishers (Biomedical Division) (1986) 5.

[87] S. Moncada, J.R. Vane in: H.L. Nossel, H.J. Vogel (Eds), *Pathobiology of Endothelial Cells.* Academic Press, New York (1982) 253–285.

[88] T.I.T. Okpalugo, A.A. Ogwu, P.D. Maguire, J.A.D. McLaughlin, D.G. Hirst: In-vitro blood compatibility of a-C:H:Si and a-C:H thin films. *Diamond Rel. Mater.* 13 (2004) 1088.

[89] P.D. Maguire, D.P. Magill, A.A. Ogwu, J.A. McLaughlin: The insulating properties of a-C:H on silicon and metal substrates. *Diamond Rel. Mater.* 10 (2001) 216.

[90] T.I.T. Okpalugo, A.A. Ogwu, A.C. Okpalugo, R.W. McCullough, W. Ahmed: The human microvascular endothelial cells *in vitro* interaction atomic-nitrogen-doped diamond-like carbon thin films. *J. Biomed. Mater. Res. B* 85B (2008) 188.

[91] T.I.T. Okpalugo, A.A. Ogwu, P.D. Maguire, J.A.D. McLaughlin: Platelet adhesion on silicon modified hydrogenated amorphous carbon films. *Biomaterials* 25 (2004) 239.

[92] T.I.T. Okpalugo, H. Murphy, A.A. Ogwu, G. Abbas, S.C. Ray, P.D. Maguire, J. McLaughlin, R.W. McCullough: Human microvascular endothelial cellular interaction with atomic N-doped DLC compared with Si-doped DLC thin films. *J. Biomed. Mater. Res. B* 78B (2006) 222.

[93] T. Mosmann: Rapid colorimetric assay for cellular growth and survival: application to proliferation and cytotoxicity assays. *J. Immunol. Methods* 65 (1983) 55.

[94] M. Page, N. Bejaoui, B. Cinq-Mars, P. Lemieux: Optimization of the tetrazolium-based colorimetric assay for the measurement of cell number and cytotoxicity. *Int. J. Immunopharmacol.* 10 (1988) 785.

[95] T.I.T. Okpalugo, E. McKenna, A.C. Magee, J. McLaughlin, N.M.D. Brown: The MTT assays of bovine retinal pericytes and human microvascular endothelial cells on DLC and Si-DLC-coated TCPS. *J. Biomed. Mater. Res. A* 71A (2004) 201.

[96] J.M. Anderson, K.M. Miller: Biomaterial biocompatibility and the macrophage. *Biomaterials* 5 (1984) 5.

[97] K. Takahashi, M. Takeya, N. Sakashita: Multifunctional roles of macrophages in the development and progression of atherosclerosis in humans and experimental animals. *Med. Electron. Microsc.* 35 (2002) 179.

[98] L.A. Thomson, F.C. Law, N. Rushton, J. Franks: Biocompatibility of diamond-like carbon coating. *Biomaterials* 12 (1991) 37.

[99] M. Allen, F. Law, N. Rushton: The effects of diamond-like carbon coatings on macrophages, fibroblasts and osteoblast-like cells *in vitro*. *Clin. Mater.* 17 (1994) 1.

[100] R. Butter, M. Allen, L. Chandra, A.H. Lettington, N. Rushton: In vitro studies of DLC coatings with silicon intermediate layer. *Diamond Rel. Mater.* 4 (1995) 857.

[101] D.J. Li, H.Q. Gu: Cell attachment on diamond-like carbon coating. *Bull. Mater. Sci.* 25 (2002) 7.

[102] W.J. Ma, A.J. Ruys, R.S. Mason, P.J. Martin, A. Bendavid, Z. Liu, M. Ionescu, H. Zreiqat: DLC coatings: Effects on physical and chemical properties on biological response. *Biomaterials* 28 (2007) 1620.

[103] M. Ball, A. O'Brien, F. Dolan, G. Abbas, J.A. McLaughlin: Macrophage responses to vascular stent coatings. *J. Biomed. Mater. Res. B* 70A (2004) 380.

[104] D.P. Dowling, P.V. Kola, K. Donnelly, T.C. Kelly, K. Brumitt, L. Lloyd, R. Eloy, M. Therin, N. Weill: Evaluation of diamond-like carbon-coated orthopaedic implants. *Diamond Rel. Mater.* 6 (1997) 390.

[105] A. Singh, G. Ehteshami, S. Massia, J.P. He, R.G. Storer, G. Raupp: Glial cell and fibroblast cytotoxicity study on plasma-deposited diamond-like carbon coatings. *Biomaterials* 24 (2003) 5083.

[106] T.V. Kumari, P.R. Anil Kumar, C.V. Muraleeharan, G.S. Bhuvaneshwar, Y. Sampeur, F. Derangere, R. Suryanarayanan: *In vitro* cytotoxicity studies of diamond like carbon coarings on titanium. *Bio-Med. Mater. Eng.* 12 (2002) 329.

[107] S.E. Ong, S. Zhang, H. Du, Y.S. Wang, L.L. Ma: In-vitro cellular behavior on amorphous carbon containing silicon. *Thin Solid Films* 516 (2008) 5152.

[108] B.D. Ratner, A.S. Hoffman, F.J. Schoen, J.E. Lemons (Eds.), *Biomaterial Science*. Academic Press, New York (1996).

[109] S. Takashima, S. Takamoto, S. Hayakawa, A. Osaka: Blood compatibility and protein adsorption characteristics of sol–gel derived titania. *Bioceramics* 13 (2000) 889.

[110] T. Yokota, T. Terai, T. Kobayashi, M. Iwaki: Cell adhesion to nitrogen-doped DLCs fabricated by plasma-based ion implantation and deposition method. *Nucl. Instrum. Methods Phys. Res. B* 242 (206) 48.

[111] T. Yokota, T. Terai, T. Kobayashi, T. Meguro, M. Iwaki: Cell adhesion to nitrogen-doped DLCs fabricated by plasma-based ion implantation and deposition method using toluene gas. *Surf. Coat. Technol.* 201 (2007) 8048.

[112] M. Allen, B. Myer, N. Rushton: *In vitro* and *in vivo* investigations into the biocompatibility of diamond-like carbon (DLC) coatings for orthopedic applications. *J. Biomed. Mater. Res. B* 58 (2001) 319.

[113] C. Du, X.W. Su, F.Z. Cui, X.D. Zhu: Morphological behaviour of osteoblasts on diamond-like carbon coating and amorphous C–N film in organ culture. *Biomaterials* 19 (1998) 651.

[114] S.E. Rodil, R. Olivares, H. Arzate, S. Muhl: Properties of carbon films and their biocompatibility using in-vitro tests. *Diamond Rel. Mater.* 12 (2003) 931.

[115] R. Olivares, S.E. Rodil, H. Arzate: *In vitro* studies of the biomineralization in amorphous carbon films. *Surf. Coat. Technol.* 177–178 (2004) 758.

[116] M.J. Coelho, M.H. Fernandes: Human bone cell cultures in biocompatibility testing. Part II: effect of ascorbic acid, β-glycerophosphate and dexamethasone on osteoblastic differentiation. *Biomaterials* 21 (2000) 1095.

[117] C.H. Chung, E.E. Golub, E. Forbes, T. Tokuoka, I.M. Shapiro: Mechanism of action of β-glycerophosphate on bone cell mineralization. *Calcif. Tissue Int.* 51 (1992) 305.

[118] K. Myllymaa, S. Myllymaa, H. Korhonen, M.J. Lammi, V. Tiitu, R. Lappalainen: Interactions between Saos-2 cells and microtextured amorphous diamond or amorphous diamond hybrid coated surfaces with different wettability properties. *Diamond Rel. Mater.* 18 (2009) 1294.

[119] F. Chai, N. Mathis, N. Blanchemain, C. Meunier, H.F. Hildebrand: Osteoblast interaction with DLC-coated Si substrates. *Acta Biomater.* 4 (2008) 1369.

[120] L.K. Randeniya, A. Bendavid, P.J. Martin, Md.S. Amin, E.W. Preston, F.S. Magdon Ismail, S. Coe: Incorporation of Si and SiO_x into diamond-like carbon films: Impact on surface properties and osteoblast adhesion. *Acta Biomater.* 5 (2009) 1791.

[121] W.E. Thomas: Brain macrophages: On the role of pericytes and perivascular cells. *Brain Res. Rev.* 31 (1999) 42.

[122] T.J. Kinnari, A. Soininen, J. Esteban, N. Zamora, E. Alakoski, V.P. Kouri, R. Lappalainen, Y.T. Konttinen, E. Gomez-Barrena, V.M. Tiainen: Adhesion of staphylococcal and Caco-2 cells on diamond-like carbon polymer hybrid coating. *J. Biomed. Mater. Res. A* 86A (2007) 760.

[123] H.G. Willert, M. Semlitsch: Reactions of the articular capsule to wear products of artificial joint prostheses. *J. Biomed. Mater. Res.* 11 (1977) 157.

[124] H.J. Agins, N.W. Alcock, M. Bansal, E.A. Salvati, P.D. Wilson, P.M. Pellicci, P.G. Bullough: Metallic wear in failed titanium-alloy total hip replacements. A histological and quantitative analysis. *J. Bone Jt. Surg. Am.* 70 (1988) 347.

[125] E.J. Evans: Cell damage in vitro following direct contact with fine particles of titanium, titanium alloy and cobalt–chrome–molybdenium alloy. *Biomaterials* 15 (1994) 713.

[126] W.H. Harris: Osteolysis and particle disease in hip replacement—a review. *Acta Orthop. Scand.* 65 (1994) 113.

[127] T. Thornhill, R. Ozuna, S. Shortkroff, K. Keller, C. Sledge, M. Spector: Biochemical and histological evaluation of the synovial-like tissue around failed (loose) total joint replacement prostheses in human subjects and a canine model. *Biomaterials* 11 (1990) 69.

[128] A. Shanbhag, J. Jacobs, J. Black, J. Galante, T. Glant: Human monocyte response to particulate biomaterials generated in vivo and in vitro. *J. Orthop. Res.* 13 (1995) 792.

[129] D.J. Prockop: Marrow stromal cells as stem cells for nonhematopoietic tissues. *Science* 276 (1997) 71.

[130] J.M. Quinn, A. Sabokhar, N.A. Athanasou: Cells of mononuclear phagocyte series differentiate into osteoclastic lacunar bone resorbing cells. *J. Pathol.* 179 (1996) 106.

[131] W. Wang, D. Fergusson, J.M. Quinn, A. Simpson, N.A. Athanasou: Osteoclasts are capable of particle phagocytosis and bone resorption. *J. Pathol.* 182 (1997) 92.

[132] A. Sabokhar, R. Pandey, J.M. Quinn, N.A. Athanasou: Osteoclastic differentiation by mononuclear phagocytes containing biomaterial particles. *Arch Orthop. Trauma Surg.* 117 (1998) 136.

[133] A. Schroeder, F. Gilbert, A. Bruinink, R. Hauert, J. Mayer, E. Wintermantel: Titanium containing amorphous hydrogenated carbon films (a-C:H/Ti): surface analysis and evaluation of cellular reactions using bone marrow cell cultures in vitro. *Biomaterials* 21 (2000) 449.

[134] A. Bruinink, A. Schroeder, F. Gilbert, R. Hauert: In vitro studies on the effect of delaminated a-C:H film fragments on bone marrow cell cultures. *Biomaterials* 26 (2005) 3487.

[135] S. Kelly, E.M. Regan, J.B. Uney, A.D. Dick, J.P. McGeehan, Bristol Biochip Group, E.J. Mayer, F. Claeyssens: Patterned growth of neuronal cells on modified diamond-like carbon. *Biomaterials* 29 (2008) 2573.

[136] A. Sen, S. Barizuddin, M. Hossain, L. Polo-Parasa, K.D. Gillis, S. Gangopadhyay: Preferential cell attachment to nitrogen-doped diamond-like carbon (DLC:N) for the measurement of quantal exocytosis. *Biomaterials* 30 (2009) 1604.

[137] M. Mohanty, T.V. Anilkumar, P.V. Mohanan, C.V. Muraleedharan, G.S. Bhuvasneshwar, F. Derangere, Y. Sampeur, R. Suryanarayanan: Long term tissue response to titanium coated with diamond like carbon. *Biomol. Eng.* 19 (2002) 125.

[138] D.A. LaVan, R.F. Tadera, T.A. Friedmann, J.P. Sullivan, R. Langer, D.S. Kohane: In vivo evaluation of tetrahedral amorphous carbon. *Biomaterials* 26 (2005) 465.

[139] M. Allen, R. Butter, L. Chandra, A. Lettington, N. Rushton: Toxicity of particulate silicon carbide for macrophages, fibroblasts and osteoblast-like cells in vitro. *Biomed. Mater. Eng.* 5 (1995) 151.

[140] I. De Scheerder, M. Szilard, H. Yanming, X.B. Ping, E. Verbeken, D. Neerinck, E. Demeyere, W. Coppens, F. Van de Werf: Evaluation of the biocompatibility of two new diamond-like stent coatings (Dylyn) in porcine coronary stent model. *J. Invas. Cardiol.* 12 (2000) 389.

[141] J. Koskinen, U. Ehrnsten, A. Mahiout, R. Lahtinen, J.P. Hirvonen, S.P. Hannula: Porosity of thin diamond-like carbon films deposited by arc discharged method. *Surf. Coat. Technol.* 62 (1993) 356.

[142] J. Wang, N. Huang, P. Yang, Y.X. Leng, H. Sun, Z.Y. Liu, P.K. Chu: The effects of amorphous carbon films deposited on polyethylene terephthalate on bacterial adhesion. *Biomaterials* 25 (2004) 3163.

[143] T.J. Kinnari, A. Soininen, J. Esteban, N. Zamora, E. Alakoski, V.P. Kouri, R. Lappalainen, Y.T. Konttinen, E. Gomez-Barrena, V.M. Tiainen: Adhesion of staphylococcal and Caco-2 cells on diamond-like carbon polymer hybrid coating. *J. Biomed. Mater. Res. A* 86A (2007) 760.

[144] M. Rauli, M. Jarn, J. Ahola, J. Peltonen, J.B. Rosenholm, S. Tervakangas, J. Kolehmainen, T. Ruokolainen, P. Narko, M. Salkinoja-Salonen: Microbe repelling coated stainless steel analysed by field emission scanning electron microscopy and physiochemical methods. *J. Ind. Microbiol. Biotechnol.* 35 (2008) 751.

[145] M. Katsikogianni, I. Spiliopoulou, D.P. Dowling, Y.F. Missirlis: Adhesion of slime producing *Staphylococcus epidermidis* strains to PVC and diamond-like carbon/silver/fluorinated coatings. *J. Mater. Sci. Mater. Med.* 17 (2006) 679.

[146] F.R. Marciano, D.A. Lima-Oliveira, N.S. Da-Silva, A.V. Diniz, E.J. Corat, V.J. Trava-Airoldi: Antibacterial activity of DLC films containing TiO$_2$ nanoparticles. *J. Coll. Interf. Sci.* 340 (2009) 87.

[147] F.R. Marciano, L.F. Bonetti, L.V. Santos, N.S. Da-Silva, E.J. Corat, V.J. Trava-Airoldi: Antibacterial activity on DLC and Ag-DLC films produced by PECVD. *Diamond Rel. Mater.* 18 (2009) 1010.

[148] F.R. Marciano, L.F. Bonetti, N.S. Da-Silva, E.J. Corat, V.J. Trava-Airoldi: Wettability and antibacterial activity of modified diamond-like carbon films. *Appl. Surf. Sci.* 255 (2009) 8377.

[149] F.Z. Cui, D.J. Li: A review of investigation on biocompatibility of diamond-like carbon and carbon nitride films. *Surf. Coat. Technol.* 131 (2000) 481.

[150] V.M. Tiainen: Amorphous carbon as a bio-mechanical coating—mechanical properties and biological applications. *Diamond Rel. Mater.* 10 (2001) 153.

[151] R. Hauert: A review of modified DLC coatings for biological applications. *Diamond Rel. Mater.* 12 (2003) 583.

[152] R. Hauert, U. Muller: An overview on tailored tribological and biological behavior of diamond-like carbon. *Diamond Rel. Mater.* 12 (2003) 171.

[153] A. Grill: Diamond-like carbon coatings as biocompatible materials—an overview. *Diamond Rel. Mater.* 12 (2003) 166.

[154] G. Dearnaley, J.H. Arps: Biomedical applications of diamond-like carbon (DLC) coatings: A review. *Surf. Coat. Technol.* 200 (2005) 2518.

[155] R.J. Narayan: Nanostructured diamondlike carbon thin films for medical applications. *Mater. Sci. Eng. C* 25 (2005) 405.

[156] R.K. Roy, K.R. Lee: Biomedical applications of diamond-like carbon coatings: A review. *J. Biomed. Mater. Res. B* 83B (2007) 72.

[157] H. Malchau, P. Herberts, L. Ahnfelt: Prognosis of total hip replacement in Sweden. Follow-up of 96,675 operations performed 1978–1990. *Acta Orthop. Scand.* 64 (1993) 497.

[158] H.C. Amstutz, P. Campbell, N. Kossovsky, I. Clarke: Mechanism and clinical significance of wear debris-induced osteolysis. *Clin. Orthop. Rel. Res.* 276 (1992) 7.

[159] D. Nordstrom, S. Santavirta, A. Gristina, Y.T. Konttinen: Immune-inflammatory response in the totally replaced hip: A review of biocompatibility aspects. *Eur. J. Med.* 2 (1993) 296.

[160] M. Lind, R.L. Smith, M.C.D. Tindale, Y.T. Konttinen, S. Santavirta, S.B. Goodman: Implants for joint replacement and the host's immune response. *EOS-Riv Immunol.* 18 (1998) 15.

[161] W.H. Harris: The problem is osteolysis. *Clin. Orthop. Rel. Res.* 311 (1995) 46.

[162] R. Lappalainen, A. Anttila, H. Heinonen: Diamond coated total hip replacements. *Clin. Orthop. Rel. Res.* 352 (1998) 118.

[163] A. Grill: Tribology of diamond-like carbon and related materials: An update review. *Surf. Coat. Technol.* 94–95 (1997) 507.

[164] A. Grill: Diamond-like carbon: State of the art. *Diamond Rel. Mater.* 8 (1999) 428.

[165] B. Donnet: Recent progress on the tribology of doped diamond-like and carbon alloy coatings: A review. *Surf. Coat. Technol.* 100–101 (1998) 180.

[166] A. Gangopadhyay: Mechanical and tribological properties of amorphous carbon films. *Tribol. Lett.* 5 (1998) 25.

[167] R. Lappalainen, H. Heinonen, A. Anttila, S. Santavirta: Some relevant issues related to the use of amorphous diamond coatings for medical applications. *Diamond Rel. Mater.* 7 (1998) 482.

[168] D.P. Dowling, P.V. Kola, K. Donnelly, T.C. Kelly, K. Brumitt, L. Lloyd, R. Eloy, M. Therin, N. Weill: Evaluation of diamond-like carbon-coated orthopaedic implants. *Diamond Rel. Mater.* 6 (1997) 390.

[169] J.I. Onate, M. Comin, I. Braceras, A. Garcia, J.L. Viviente, M. Brizuela, N. Garagorri, J.L. Peris, J.I. Alara: Wear reduction effect on ultra-high-molecular-weight polyethylene by application of hard coatings and ion implantation on cobalt chromium alloy, as measured in a knee wear simulation machine. *Surf. Coat. Technol.* 142–144 (2001) 1056.

[170] F. Platon, P. Fournier, S. Rouxel: Trobological behaviour of DLC coatings compared to different materials used in hip joint prostheses. *Wear* 250 (2001) 227.

[171] D. Sheeja, B.K. Tay, L.N. Nung: Feasibility of diamond-like carbon coatings for orthopaedic applications. *Diamond Rel. Mater.* 13 (2004) 184.

[172] D. Sheeja, B.K. Tay, L.N. Nung: Tribological characterization of surface modified UHMWPE against DLC-coated Co–Cr–Mo. *Surf. Coat. Technol.* 190 (2005) 231.

[173] V. Saikko, T. Ahlroos, O. Calonius, J. Keranen: Wear simulation of total hip prostheses with polyethylene against CoCr, Alumina and diamond-like carbon. *Biomaterials* 22 (2001) 1507.

[174] S. Affatato, M. Frigo, A. Toni: An in vitro investigation of diamond-like carbon as femoral head coating. *J. Biomed. Mater. Res. B* 53 (2000) 221.

[175] E. Sheeja, B.K. Tay, S.P. Lau, L.N. Nung: Tribological characterization of diamond-like carbon coatings on Co–Cr–Mo alloy for orthopaedic applications. *Surf. Coat. Technol.* 146–147 (2001) 410.

[176] H. Dong, W. Shi, T. Bell: Potential of improving tribological performance of UHMWPE by engineering the Ti_6Al_4V counterfaces. *Wear* 225–229 (1999) 146.

[177] S.C. Scholes, A. Unsworth, A.A.J. Goldsmith: A frictional study of total joint replacements. *Phys. Med. Biol.* 45 (2000) 3721.

[178] V. Saikko, T. Ahlroos: Phospholipids as boundary lubricants in wear tests of prosthetic joint materials. *Wear* 207 (1997) 86.

[179] T. Ahlroos, V. Saikko: Wear of prosthetic joint materials in various lubricants. *Wear* 211 (1997) 113.

[180] J. Fisher, P. Firkins, E.A. Reeves, J.L. Hailey, G.H. Isaac: Influence of scratches to metallic counterfaces on the wear of ultra-high molecular weight polyethylene. *Proc. Inst. Mech. Eng. Part H, J. Eng. Med.* 209 (1995) 263.

[181] M.A. Wimmer, J. Loos, R. Nassutt, M. Heitkemper, A. Fischer: The acting wear mechanisms on metal-on-metal hip joint bearings: In vitro results. *Wear* 250–251 (2001) 129.

[182] A. Fergusson, P. Laing, E. Hodge: Ionization of metal implants in living tissues. *J. Bone Jt. Surg. A* 42 (1960) 77.

[183] K. Gutensohn, C. Beythien, J. Bau, T. Grewe, R. Koester, K. Padmanaban, P. Kuehnl: *In vitro* analyses of diamond-like carbon coated stents: Reduction of metal ion release, platelet activation, and thrombogenicity. *Thromb. Res.* 99 (2000) 577.

[184] M. Ball, A. O'Brien, F. Dolan, G. Abbas, J.A. McLaughlin: Macrophage responses to vascular stent coatings. *J. Biomed. Mater. Res. A* 70 (2004) 380.

[185] O. Schaefer, C. Lohrmann, J. Winterer, E. Kotter, M. Langer: Endovascular treatment of superficial femoral artery occlusive disease with stents coated with diamond-like carbon. *Clin. Radiol.* 59 (2004) 1128.

[186] F. Airoldi, A. Colombo, D. Tavano, G. Stankovic, S. Klugmann, V. Paolillo, E. Bonizzoni, C. Briguori, M. Carlino, M. Montorfano, F. Liistro, A. Castelli, A. Ferrari, F. Sgura, C. Di Mario: Comparison of diamond like carbon coated stents versus uncoated stainless steel stents in coronary artery disease. *Am. J. Cardiol.* 93 (2004) 474.

[187] A.L. Bartorelli, D. Trabattoni, P. Montorsi, F. Fabbiocchi, S. Galli, P. Ravagnani, S. Galli, P. Ravagnani, L. Grancini, S. Cozzi, A. Loaldi: Aspirin alone antiplatelet regimen after intracoronary placement of the Carbostent™: The Antares study. *Catheter. Cardiovasc. Interv.* 55 (2002) 150.

[188] D. Antoniucci, A. Bartorelli, R. Valenti, P. Montorsi, G.M. Santoro, F. Fabbiocchi, L. Bolognese, A. Loaldi, M. Trapani, D. Trabattoni, G. Moschi, S. Galli: Clinical and angiographic outcome after coronary arterial stenting with the carbonstent. *Am. J. Cardiol.* 85 (2000) 821.

[189] K. Yamazaki, P. Litwak, O. Tagusari, T. Mori, K. Kono, M. Kameneva, M. Watach, L. Gordon, M. Miyagishima, J. Tomioka, M. Umezu, E. Outa, J.F. Antaki, R.L. Kormos, H. Koyanagi, B.P. Griffith: An implantable centrifugal blood pump with recirculating purge system (Coll-Seal System). *Artif. Organs* 22 (1998) 466.

[190] A. Olborska, M. Swider, R. Wolowiec, P. Niedzielski, A. Rylski, S. Mitura: Amorphous carbon—Biomaterial for implant coatings. *Diamond Rel. Mater.* 3 (1994) 899.

[191] S. Kobayashi, Y. Ohgoe, K. Ozeki, K. Sato, T. Sumiya, K.K. Hirakuri, H. Aoki: Diamond-like carbon coatings on orthodontic archwires. *Diamond Rel. Mater.* 14 (2005) 1094.

[192] Y. Ohgoe, S. Kobayashi, K. Ozeki, H. Aoki, H. Nakamori, K.K. Hirakuri, O. Miyashita: Reduction effect of nickel ion release on diamond-like carbon film coated onto an orthodontic archwire. *Thin Solid Films* 497 (2006) 218.

[193] S. Kobayashi, Y. Ohgoe, K. Ozeki, K. Hirakuri, H. Aoki: Dissolution effect and cytotoxicity of diamond-like carbon coatings on orthodontic archwires. *J. Mater. Sci.: Mater. Med.* 18 (2007) 2263.

[194] P.D. Maguire, J.A. McLaughlin, T.I.T. Okpalugo, P. Lemoine, P. Papakonstantinou, E.T. McAdams, M. Needham, A.A. Ogwu, M. Ball, G.A. Abbas: Mechanical stability, corrosion performance and bioresponse of amorphous diamond-like carbon for medical stents and guidewires. *Diamond Rel. Mater.* 14 (2005) 1277.

[195] J.A. McLaughlin, B. Meenan, P. Maguire, N. Jamieson: Properties of diamond like carbon thin film coatings on stainless steel medical guidewires. *Diamond Rel. Mater.* 5 (1996) 486.

[196] T. Hasebe, Y. Matsuoka, H. Kodama, T. Saito, S. Yohena, A. Kamijo, N. Shiraga, M. Higuchi, S. Kuribayashi, K. Takahashi, T. Suzuki: Lubrication performance of diamond-like carbon and fluorinated diamond-like carbon coatings for intravascular guidewires. *Diamond Rel. Mater.* 15 (2006) 129.

[197] V.V. Sleptsov, V.M. Elinson, N.V. Simakina, A.N. Laymin, I.V. Tsygankov, A.A. Kivaev, A.D. Musina: Ophthalmological application of contact lenses modified by means of ion-assisted carbon films. *Diamond Rel. Mater.* 5 (1996) 483.

[198] V.M. Elinson, V.V. Sleptsov, A.N. Laymin, V.V. Potravsav, L.N. Kostuchenko, A.D. Moussina: Barrier properties of carbon films deposited on polymer-based devices in aggressive environments. *Diamond Rel. Mater.* 8 (1999) 2103.

3

Biomedical Applications of Carbon-Based Materials

Subbiah Alwarappan, Shree R. Singh, and Ashok Kumar

CONTENTS

Introduction 111
Methods of Synthesis of Various Carbon-Based Materials 112
    Pyrolytic Graphite 112
    Highly Oriented PG 113
    Glassy Carbon 114
    Carbon Fibers 114
    Carbon Black 114
    Carbon Film 115
    Diamond-Like Carbon 115
    Carbon Nanotubes 115
    Fullerenes 116
    Graphene 116
Biomedical Applications of Carbon-Based Materials 117
    Biomedical Utility of CNTs 117
        CNTs for Therapeutic Applications 117
        CNTs and Their Related Cellular Uptake 118
        CNTs for Drug Delivery 119
    Biomedical Utility of Diamond 120
        Diamond for Orthopedic Applications 121
        Diamond for Cardiovascular Applications 121
        DLC-Coated Guide Wires 122
        Other Biomedical Applications of Diamond 122
    Biomedical Applications of Fullerenes 123
        Functionalized Fullerenes as Drug Delivery Agents 123
        Suppression of Reactive Oxygen Species by Functionalized Fullerenes ... 124
        Functionalized Fullerenes as MRI Contrast Agents 125
        Other Important Applications of Functionalized Fullerenes 127
Acknowledgment 127
References 127

Introduction

Carbon materials possess excellent mechanical, tribological, and biological properties, and as a result, carbon-based materials find applications in biomedical devices including cardiovascular, orthopedic, and dental applications [1–3]. Pyrolytic graphite (PG) and other

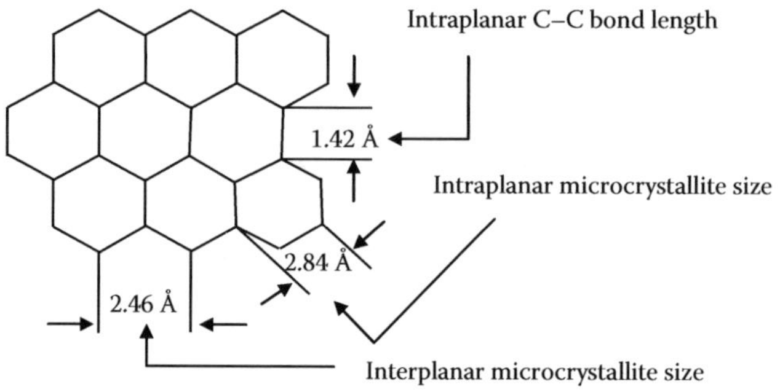

FIGURE 3.1
Schematic representation of crystallographic dimensions of sp^2 carbon.

forms of carbon coatings such as carbon nanotubes (CNTs), fullerenes, and diamond-like carbon (DLC) in its pure, hydrogenated, and doped forms [4, 5] have raised much interest as potential wear-resistant coatings for biomedical applications because of their attractive properties such as high hardness, high chemical inertness, and low-friction coefficient [6, 7]. Furthermore, carbon is widely used as a common electrode material in a great deal of electrochemical detection of biologically significant species. Usually, carbon materials are characterized by properties such as wide potential window, low background current, fast electron transfer rate, and stability. In electroanalytical chemistry, the carbon materials used are all sp^2 hybridized, as these sp^2 hybridized carbons are highly reactive and prone to required surface modification with ease. All these foretold carbon materials have identical C–C bonding but different bulk properties as a result of orientation and size of carbon crystallites. Carbon material possesses structural variables such as the intraplanar carbon–carbon bond distance, intraplanar carbon crystallite size (L_a), interplanar microcrystallite size (L_c), and the interplanar spacing as shown in Figure 3.1. Of these, the intraplanar C–C bond distance is estimated to be 1.42 Å [8]. L_a of the carbon crystallite is defined as the average size of the graphitic crystallite, and it can vary between 2 and 10^5 Å. The intraplanar size can be measured using x-ray diffraction technique [8]. A perfect single crystal of graphite has a larger L_a value. On the other hand, L_c is the distance perpendicular to the plane of the graphite sheet, which is usually 2.46 Å, and it can be increased by heating the carbon materials above 2000°C. Neutron scattering can also be used to measure the intraplanar spacing. For single crystal graphite, the intraplanar spacing value is 3.354 Å [9, 10], and for less ordered sp^2 carbon material, the intraplanar spacing value is 3.6 Å. Synthesis of various carbon materials such as PG, carbon fiber (CF), DLC, CNTs, fullerenes, and graphene is briefly described below.

Methods of Synthesis of Various Carbon-Based Materials

Pyrolytic Graphite

PG is highly ordered and anisotropic. It has been known since 1880, but its suitability for making electrode was only evident in the past 30 years. Miller and Zittel [11] were the first to identify PG as a suitable material for constructing an indicator electrode. The crystalline structure of PG closely approximates that of the ideal graphite crystal. The preparation, properties, and structure of PG have been described in detail by Walker [12]. PG can be obtained by the pyrolysis of gaseous hydrocarbons. PG materials usually consist of poly(aromatic rings) with sp²-hybridized carbon atoms. These aromatic planar rings are stacked together by π–π interaction of the electronic network [13]. A schematic representation of the layered structure of graphite is shown in Figure 3.2. The planar layer (i.e., the *ab* plane) formed by the aromatic ring system is usually termed as *basal plane*, whereas the planes perpendicular to the graphitic layer are the *bc* and *ac* planes and are called *edge planes*. Edge planes are usually active compared with the basal plane. The reactivity of the edge plane is due to the presence of various reactive groups such as carboxylic acid, ketonic, and hydroxyl groups [14]. Electron transport through *c*-axis accounts for the conductivity of PG. PG electrodes used in voltammetric studies can be prepared by cutting small rods (diameter 4 mm, length 10 mm) from a block of graphite [11]. The graphitic block must be positioned in such a way that it is cut exactly perpendicular to the *ab* plane [13]. The resulting small piece of graphitic rod [15] is then cemented in to long glass tubing with epoxy cement. The PG rod is mounted in such a way that only the *ab* planes are exposed. Care must be taken to avoid the occurrence of air pockets between the air tube and the PG rod. This is usually achieved by initially coating the inside of the glass tube with epoxy cement followed by coating the rod with epoxy and finally sliding the rod carefully into the tube. During this event, the rear end of the graphitic rod will be coated with epoxy that prevents the electrical contact to the graphitic rod. In certain cases, depending on the application, the end of the PG electrode can be polished using a silicon carbide paper. Various other forms of PG such as vapor-deposited PG and wax-impregnated PG have also emerged, and their preparation and properties have been described in detail [15–18].

Highly Oriented PG

Highly oriented PG (HOPG) is manufactured by the process of annealing PG under high compression force [19]. It is otherwise known as stress-annealed PG. The material has

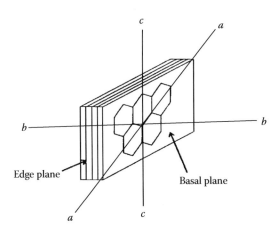

FIGURE 3.2
Schematic representation of the layered structure of pyrolytic graphite.

perfect orientation along the axis perpendicular to the planes of graphite. The structure of HOPG is well defined than PG, and its surface has a mirror-like finish. Several forms of HOPG have been developed [19–22].

Glassy Carbon

The possibility of using glassy carbon (GC) as an electrode material was pioneered by Zittel and Miller [23]. Unlike PG, which is anisotropic, GC has an isotropic structure. GC is highly resistant to chemical attack and electrically conductive. In addition, GC is impermeable to liquids and gases. GC can be prepared in several ways. Of all the methods reported, the simplest one is reported by McBride and Evans [24]. In this method, a GC rod of 3-mm diameter is sealed inside a 5-mm-long glass tubing with epoxy cement. A few millimeters of carbon are then exposed from the end of the glass rod and polished with emery paper, followed by alumina, until a mirror finish is obtained. In another method, GC can be obtained by the heat treatment of polymers of phenol or formaldehyde or by the heat treatment of poly(acrylonitrile). Upon heating the polymers at temperatures above 3000°C under pressure, atoms such as hydrogen, oxygen, and nitrogen are released from the polymeric chain, leaving behind the extended, conjugated, and interwoven sp^2 carbon structure, and this accounts for the hardness of GC. However, the original polymeric backbone remains unaltered, and it prevents the formation of extended graphitic domains. GC electrodes are reactive, and the functional groups present provide an opportunity for modifying the electrode surface [148] to detect targeted biological and biomedical applications.

Carbon Fibers

CFs are known for their high tensile strength and light weight. The diameter of the CFs varies between 0.1 and 100 µm. CFs can be obtained in many ways. However, most of the CFs used in these ways is made either by the heat treatment procedures that are used in the preparation of GC or by the catalytic chemical vapor deposition (CVD) technique. In the usual heat treatment method, the polymers are heated up to 3000°C. The molten polymer is then woven or extruded to obtain CFs. Methods involving heat treatment above 3000°C usually result in the formation of fibers that possess a high tensile strength [8]. At such a high temperature, carbon graphitizes and aligns its axis alongside the axis of the fiber, which accounts for a high Young's modulus [25–27]. The microstructure of CFs varies according to the method. Catalytic dehydrogenation of hydrocarbons on metals such as Fe and Ni forms the basis of catalytic CVD [8]. The fibers resulting in this manner possess onion type of structures and are stronger but shorter in length than the fibers obtained from polymers.

Carbon Black

Carbon black (CB) is not widely used in any applications. However, there are quite a few methods to synthesize CB. In all the methods, the basic principle involves thermal decomposition of hydrocarbons [8, 13]. The particles of the CB vary in its size from 300 to 5000 Å [13]. CB is a collection of many smaller microcrystallites. The surface area of the CB is on the order of 5000 m^2 g^{-1}. Unlike graphite, CB has a disordered structure that accounts for its lower conductivity and lower mechanical strength.

Carbon Film

Carbon film electrodes are generally prepared from conducting or semiconducting materials deposited either chemically or in vacuo on an appropriate substrate such as a glass slide [8]. The carbon films thus obtained can also be referred to as hard carbon. Film electrodes were developed for use in spectroelectrochemical studies where a beam of light is passed through an optically transparent film [8]. Besides this, the planarity of films deposited on an optically flat glass substrate makes them suitable for optical reflection spectroscopy. Unlike GC, carbon film is not hard and it has a density lower than that of graphite. In contrast to PG, carbon film possesses up to 10% sp^3-hybridized carbon atom. Carbon film with improved hardness can be obtained by the plasma deposition from CH_4 or CH_4/H_2 atmosphere [8]. Carbon films resulted from plasma method has enhanced hydrogen content. The presence of hydrogen in the carbon film was reported to result in improved hardness and lower density than nonhydrogenated carbon films.

Diamond-Like Carbon

In recent years, DLC has emerged as a potential material because of its high hardness, low frictional coefficient, high wear and corrosion resistance, chemical inertness, high electrical resistivity, infrared transparency, high refractive index, and excellent smoothness. Although it is called "diamond-like," DLC is in fact not like crystalline diamond and also not as hard and is virtually amorphous. Hydrogen is frequently present in amounts up to 40%, at occupying regions of low electron density in the matrix. Its presence strongly influences the mechanical and tribological behavior of DLC coatings. In addition, the microstructure of DLC allows the incorporation of other species such as nitrogen, silicon, tungsten, silver, and sulfur. DLC comprises a family of such materials, the properties of which can be tailored far more readily than those of diamond. Furthermore, DLC film comprises a mixture of sp^2 and sp^3 carbon bonds and is deposited by using high-energy carbon species. DLC films can be synthesized by a variety of techniques such as ion beam deposition [28], radio frequency plasma–enhanced CVD [28], filtered cathodic vacuum arc [29], ion plating [30], plasma immersion ion implantation and deposition [31], magnetron sputtering [32], ion beam sputtering [33], pulsed laser deposition [34], and mass-selected ion beam deposition [35]. The hydrogen content in DLC films varies up to 40%. Because of its amorphous structure, DLC films can be easily doped and alloyed with different elements. This leads to a wide range of properties depending on its sp^3, sp^2, and hydrogen content together with element incorporation.

Carbon Nanotubes

Since the discovery of CNTs, it has revolutionized the biomedical research as they can show superior performance because of their impressive structural, mechanical, and electronic properties such as small size and mass, high strength, higher electrical, and thermal conductivity [36–38]. They are hexagonal networks of carbon atoms possessing a diameter of about 1 nm and 1–100 nm in length and can essentially be thought of as a layer of graphite rolled up into a cylinder [39]. Furthermore, CNTs are of two types: single-walled nanotubes (SWNTs) and multiwalled nanotubes, and they differ in the arrangement of their graphene cylinders. SWNTs have only one single layer of graphene cylinders, whereas multiwalled nanotubes have several layers (approximately 50), as shown in Figure 3.3a [40]. Furthermore, the films of synthesized CNTs can be aligned or random in nature [36].

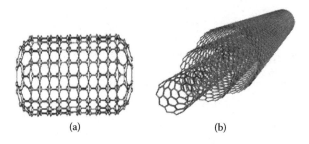

(a)   (b)

FIGURE 3.3
Structure of (a) SWCNTs and (b) MWCNTs. (Reproduced with permission from Wang, J., *Electroanalysis*, 17, 7–14, 2005.)

Sketches of aligned and random CNTs are shown in Figure 3.3b. Usually, CNTs were synthesized by the following three techniques, and they are (1) the carbon arc-discharge technique [41–45], (2) the laser-ablation technique [46–48], and (3) the CVD technique [49–51]. Of these, the arc-discharge technique results in high quality of single-walled CNTs (SWCNTs) and multiwalled CNTs (MWCNTs). Furthermore, during the growth process, MWCNTs do not require a catalyst, whereas the SWCNTs require a catalyst for its growth. Although CNTs look promising, they are also plagued with certain limitations, which prohibit their use on a large scale.

Fullerenes

Fullerenes, since their discovery in 1985, have captured the imagination of scientists because of their unique physical and chemical properties. Buckminsterfullerene (C_{60}) is considered a truncated icosahedron containing 60 carbon atoms with C5–C5 single bonds forming pentagons and C5–C6 double bonds forming hexagons [52]. The diameter of a C_{60} fullerene molecule is 0.7 nm, and it is an important member of the nanomaterials family. However, their poor solubility in aqueous solvents coupled with a tendency to form aggregates in aqueous solutions makes it an unattractive candidate in biological applications [53–55]. To overcome this problem, researchers functionalized fullerenes by various chemical and supramolecular approaches [56–58]. Some of the functionalized fullerenes have excellent solubility in polar solvents and easily overcome the hurdles posed by C_{60}. Usually, fullerenes are synthesized by vaporizing graphite by resistive heating under carefully defined condition and isolating the product of the resulting soot by chromatographic technique [59, 60]. On the other hand, fullerenes can also be obtained by the combustion of simple hydrocarbons in fuel-rich flames [61]. Isolable quantities of fullerenes are also resulted by chemical synthesis [62].

Graphene

Graphene is the name given to a two-dimensional crystalline form of carbon invented by Geim and Novoselov in 2004 [63]. Graphene can be further envisaged as a flat monolayer of carbon atoms firmly packed into a honeycomb-like crystalline lattice in a two-dimensional fashion [63, 64]. Graphene is considered a basic building block for graphitic materials of all other dimensionalities [65]. For instance, graphene can be wrapped up into zero-dimensional fullerenes, rolled into one-dimensional nanotubes, or stacked into three-dimensional graphite. Electrons in graphene were found to obey a linear dispersion relation; since they behave like massless relativistic particles, they form the base for all of graphene's peculiar electronic property. These electrons move ballistically in the graphene layer without scattering, with mobility exceeding 15,000 m^2 V^{-1} s^{-1} at room temperature. Graphene can be synthesized via chemical reduction of exfoliated graphitic oxide (GO) as described by Stankovich et al. [65]. GO can be produced by any of the oxidative treatments of graphite reported by Brodie [66], Hummers and Offeman [67], and Staudenmaier [68]. According to Wang et al. [69], few-layered substrate-free graphene can also be synthesized by the CVD of methane over cobalt supported on magnesium oxide at 1000°C in a gas flow of argon. Approximately 50 mg of few-layered graphene can be obtained under the experimental conditions set up by Wang et al. [69].

Biomedical Applications of Carbon-Based Materials

Biomedical Utility of CNTs

CNTs possess important characteristics such as high aspect ratio, ultralight weight, high mechanical strength, high electrical conductivity, high thermal conductivity, metallic or semimetallic behavior, and high surface area. The combination of all these characteristics makes CNTs an appropriate and unique material that holds potential for diverse applications [70–75]. To date, there has been an increasing interest among biomedical scientists in exploring all of the foretold properties that CNTs possess for nanobiotechnology applications. For instance, at present, CNTs are considered a suitable substrate for the growth of cells for tissue regeneration, as delivery systems for a variety of diagnostic or therapeutic agents, or as vectors for gene transfection [75]. Here we describe a few potential biomedical applications of CNTs that has been well established

CNTs for Therapeutic Applications

Initially, the application of CNTs as a template for targeting bioactive peptides to the immune system was studied in detail by Guiseppi-Elie et al. [76]. These peptide-modified CNTs bioconstructs were found to mimic the appropriate secondary structure for recognition by specific monoclonal and polyclonal antibodies. After this, the immunogenic features of peptide-based CNTs conjugates were subsequently assessed in vivo. Immunization of mice with peptide–CNTs conjugates provided high antibody responses than the free peptide upon comparison. Moreover, the antibodies displayed virus-neutralizing ability. The use of CNTs as a potential and novel vaccine delivery tools was further confirmed by studying the interaction with complement factors [77]. Surfactant proteins A and D are collectin proteins that are secreted by airway epithelial cells present in the lung, and they play an important role in first-line defense against infection within the lung. Furthermore, the interaction between CNTs and proteins contained in lung surfactant by using sodium dodecyl sulfate–polyacrylamide gel electrophoresis was demonstrated by Salvador-Morales et al. [78] (by using a novel technique known as affinity chromatography based on CNTs—Sepharose matrix and electron microscopy data), which showed that surfactant proteins selectively bind to CNTs. The study of CNTs mediated oligonucleotide transport inside living cells is another important research area. Liu and coworkers demonstrated [79] the possibility of using SWNTs as nonviral molecular transporters for the delivery of short interfering RNA (siRNA) into human T cells and primary cells. Furthermore, in their study, they found out that the delivery ability and RNA interference efficiency of CNTs exceed many more folds than those of several existing nonviral transfection agents, including four formulations of liposomes. It was suggested that CNTs could be used as generic molecular transporters for various types of biologically important cells, from cancer cells to T cells and primary cells, with superior silencing effects over conventional liposome-based nonviral agents.

In addition, the possibility of using CNTs as a culture substrate for neural cells was demonstrated by Hu et al. [80]. In this study, the authors grew freshly isolated rat hippocampal neuron cells onto chemically modified MWCNTs and illustrated that they could control the outgrowth and branching pattern of neuronal processes by manipulating the charge of MWCNTs. Furthermore, Gheith et al. [81] demonstrated the unique properties of biomodified SWCNTs as a biocompatible platform for potential neuroprosthetic implants. In this in vitro study, the behavior, viability, and differentiation of NG108-15 neuroblastoma cells grown in the presence of these biomodified CNTs constructs were assessed over time. More specifically, the authors demonstrated the biocompatibility of SWCNTs obtained by layer by layer and evidenced that cells grown on this film were able to preserve their important phenotype characteristics such as neurite outgrowth. Subsequently, Gheith et al. [82] exploited the electrical conductivity of these SWNT culture substrates and demonstrated that layer-by-layer SWCNTs films can be utilized to stimulate the neurophysiological activity of NG108-15 cells. All these examples clearly demonstrated the potential applications of CNTs in future therapeutic applications.

CNTs and Their Related Cellular Uptake

It is a well-known fact that biologically modified CNTs can be easily labeled with a fluorescent tag, internally injected, and monitored or tracked in the nucleus or in the cytoplasm using epifluorescence or confocal microscopy. The ability of functionalized CNTs to be taken up by a wide range of cells was first demonstrated by Kostas et al. [70]. Furthermore, it could traffic through different intercellular barriers. In this study, the intracellular trafficking of individual or small bundles of biomodified CNTs occurred, and the transportation of CNTs toward the perinuclear region was observed within a few hours after initial contact with the cells, even under endocytosis-inhibiting conditions. Other mechanisms (such as phagocytosis)—depending on cell type, size of CNTs, and extent of bundling—may also be contributing to or triggered by the ability of biomodified CNTs to penetrate the plasma membrane and therefore be directly involved in the intracellular trafficking of the biomodified CNTs. Based on the foretold behavior, it could be concluded that functionalized CNTs possess a capacity to be taken up by mammalian and prokaryotic cells and to intracellularly traffic through the different cellular barriers by energy-independent mechanisms. The cylindrical shape and high aspect ratio of CNTs possibly allow their penetration through the plasma membrane similar to a "nanosyringe." The mechanism of uptake of this type of biomodified CNTs appears to be passive and independent of endocytosis [83]. Incubation with cells in the presence of endocytosis inhibitors will not influence the cell penetration ability of biomodified CNTs. While demonstrating the cellular uptake, Kam and Dai [84] and Kam et al. [85] demonstrated that short SWCNTs with various functionalizations are capable of transporting proteins and oligonucleotides into living cells, and the cellular-uptake mechanism is an energy-dependent endocytosis. The detailed endocytosis pathway for short, well-dispersed SWNT conjugates is mainly through clathrin-coated pits rather than caveolae or lipid rafts. Biological systems are well known to be highly transparent to near-infrared (NIR) light. Jones et al. [98] reported that the strong optical absorbance of SWCNTs in this NIR spectral window, an intrinsic property of SWCNTs, could be used for optical stimulation of nanotubes inside living cells to afford multifunctional CNTs biological transporters. Their result demonstrated that if SWCNTs could be selectively internalized into cancer cells with specific tumor markers, NIR radiation of the CNTs in vitro can selectively activate or trigger cell death without destroying the normal cells, which would develop SWCNTs functionalization schemes with specific ligands for the identification and targeting the tumorous cells. The ability of the functionalized SWCNTs to conjugate with CNTs was exploited by Shao et al. [86]. According to them, functionalization of CNTs together with the combination of optical properties of these CNTs antibodies is capable of concomitantly targeting and destroying malignant breast cancer cells in vitro with the aid of photodynamic therapy. The strength of this method is that the SWCNTs constructs incorporated in the cytoplasm are able to absorb a certain amount of energy in NIR, which is sufficient to provoke cell death. Furthermore, control cells cultured in the presence of nonspecific antibody–SWCNTs complexes revealed a viability of more than 80%. It is noteworthy that this innovative approach of multicomponent targeting of cell surface receptors followed by subsequent NIR dosing of cancer cells using SWCNTs will set the scene for future investigations. Based on these in vitro results, everything is available from the technical perspective to successfully translate this molecular nanotargeting system toward related animal models and further toward the direction of long-term clinical applications.

CNTs for Drug Delivery

To maximize the efficacy of a drug, the choice of the delivery system is of fundamental importance. Conventional drug administration techniques often fails due to various factors such as low drug solubility, poor stability in biological environment, poor distribution among the cells, lack of selectivity, and damage of healthy tissues. Often, drug delivery systems are aimed and designed to minimize or avoid the drug degradation, to increase its bioavailability, to target it to specific cells, and to reduce the amount of drug needed, decreasing toxicity and harmful side effects. CNTs possess an enormous aspect ratio (ratio between the length and the diameter) compared with classical drug delivery systems such as liposomes or polymer-based carriers and are becoming a promising alternative in this field, and they have been successfully demonstrated for their ability to penetrate into cells. CNTs can be functionalized with antibiotics to deliver them into the cells. More specifically, CNTs were used in the administration of amphotericin B. AmB is a potential antifungal agent for the treatment of chronic fungal infections, but highly toxic for mammalian cells [87] due to the formation of aggregates, which reduce the solubility in water [88]. CNTs were also used as drug delivery systems concerns cancer therapy. Furthermore, Yinghuai et al. [89] studied the utility of CNTs as boron delivery agents for their use in boron neutron capture therapy. Substituted carborane cages were attached to the walls of SWCNTs via nitrene cycloaddition followed by subsequent treatment with sodium hydroxide, obtaining water-soluble carborane-appended SWCNTs. Boron tissue distribution studies indicated that there exists enhanced boron uptake and retention of the carborane nanotubes in tumor tissue compared with blood, lung, liver, or spleen. Although the mechanism of the accumulation of carborane nanotubes in tumor is not yet clear, these results are promising for the future use of CNTs as boron delivery vehicles in boron neutron capture therapy treatment of cancer.

Moreover, Liu et al. [79] had shown that the delivery of siRNA molecules is capable of suppressing the expression of the cell surface receptors CD4 and coreceptors CXCR4 in human T cells and peripheral blood mononuclear cells by CNTs. Because both cell-surface receptors are necessary for HIV binding and infection of T cells, the authors have suggested that siRNA-CNTs conjugates can potentially be used for the treatment of HIV. Furthermore, they observed that conjugates of CNTs covalently linked by disulfide bonds to siRNA had greatly improved the silencing in T cells compared with Lipofectamine 2000 and other liposome-based formulations. Furthermore, Zhang et al. [90] developed CNTs as siRNA delivery systems further, as they used ammonium-functionalized CNTs to mediate the delivery of *TERT*siRNA into tumor cells (human and murine) and silence the *TERT* gene, which is vital for the development and growth of tumors. They observed that treatment of different tumor cells with the *TERT*siRNA-CNTs complexes led to the suppression of the cell growth. These in vitro studies were extended to in vivo studies in the same report. The activity of *TERT*siRNA-CNTs was verified after intratumoral injections in mice-bearing Lewis lung carcinoma tumors or HeLa cell xenografts. Tumor growth was inhibited after treatment with *TERT*siRNA-CNTs complexes, and average tumor weight was significantly reduced when compared with that of tumors from untreated animals. In conclusion, CNTs can offer a promising new technology for the development of advanced cancer treatment applications. However, more experimental work in this direction is vital to further explore and to carefully define the opportunities and limitations of CNTs as delivery systems for nucleic acids using in vivo models.

Biomedical Utility of Diamond

Diamond or DLC exhibits several important properties such as superior mechanical, tribological properties with corrosion resistance, biocompatibility, and hemocompatibility. The biocompatibility of DLC was investigated in the beginning of the 1990s by cell culture methods followed by observing the corresponding biotolerance after implantation in laboratory animals [91–93]. After this, DLC were then used for studies in human fibroblast and human osteoblast-like cells for several days [94, 95]. In addition, DLC coatings also showed promising results as a hemocompatible material [96–98]. Furthermore, several studies have been performed to test the possibility of using DLC as a biocompatible material [99–101]. These investigations indicated that DLC has the potential to serve as an alternative to the existing materials for biomedical applications. The medical implants for orthopedic and cardiovascular applications are subject to drastic external forces during the implants lifetime in the body environment, which may sometimes leads to delamination and spallation of the coatings. To overcome this problem, several attempts were made to incorporate certain elements into the surfaces of biomaterials or use an interlayer that improves its adhesive properties, corrosive resistance, and biocompatibility. To attain superior biocompatible properties adapted for a specific biological function, DLC films have been successfully doped and alloyed with elements such as Si, P, Ti, N, F, Cu [102–106] and compounds such as CaO [35]. As a result, DLC has emerged as a promising material for numerous biomedical applications. DLC films with various atomic bond structures and compositions are routinely utilized in orthopedic, cardiovascular, and dental applications. Cells grew on DLC coating without any inflammation or cytotoxicity. DLC coatings in orthopedic applications minimize wear, corrosion, and debris formation. Furthermore, DLC coating minimizes thrombogenicity by decreasing the platelet adhesion and activation [107].

Diamond for Orthopedic Applications

Whenever the surface of two materials slide against each other and are in relative motion, the material having lower hardness will be worn out. If they are implanted inside the organ, under such conditions, the worn-out material or debris will come in contact with human body fluids and cause tissue inflammation, osteolysis, and finally loosening of the implants. As a result, the coating materials used in prosthetic joints should be hard and inert to prevent the wear out and corrosion. Furthermore, the coating material should also have good adhesion on the substrate (more specifically on the human body fluid). There have been several attempts made to understand the wear and corrosion of biomaterials in artificial joint fluids such as bovine serum, saline water, or phospholipids [108, 109]. DLC coatings have been explored over the past 10 years to overcome this issue, with some highly encouraging results. The goal is to demonstrate that DLC has lower wear than what occurs against metals and ceramics such as alumina or zirconia and have attracted interest regarding its use as a biomaterial in orthopedic applications because of its inertness, corrosion and wear resistance, high hardness, low frictional coefficient, and biocompatibility. Results over the past 5 years have indicated that DLC holds excellent potential to be used as a biomaterial in total joint replacements. However, the findings, although all good, have been variable, and it is interesting to arrive at an explanation for this in terms of coating roughness and test procedure. Saikko et al. [109] compared femoral heads of CoCr, alumina, and CoCr coated with DLC prepared by a remote plasma discharge in acetylene. Tests were done in bovine serum, with no additives, in an anatomical hip wear simulator operating at 1 Hz. The wear of ultra-high-molecular-weight polyethylene (UHMWPE) over 3 million cycles was found to be similar for each type of head. Next, Sheeja et al. [110] tested Co–Cr alloy disks coated with DLC and compared them with uncoated Co–Cr against UHMWPE pins in a simulated body fluid. The wear rates were identical, but it was found that the corrosion rate for the coated alloy was reduced by a factor of about 10,000. In another work, Sheeja et al. [111] explored the benefits of treating both the Co–Cr alloy and the UHMWPE with DLC and found a significant decrease in the wear rates of both sliding surfaces. From these observations, it is evident that when the polymer is coated alone, its wear rate is reduced, but there was found to be severe wear of the Co–Cr. Xu and Pruitt [112] examined DLC coatings on Ti–6Al–4V alloy against UHMWPE in pin-on-disk tests in water. Onate et al. [113] used a knee wear simulation machine to compare Co–Cr, alumina, and Co–Cr coated with DLC from acetylene. In this case, there was a substantial improvement over the uncoated alloy, by a factor of 4% and 40% less wear than against alumina. A hip joint simulator was used by Gutensohn et al. [114] to compare DLC coatings on stainless steel, Ti–6A–4V and Co–Cr–Mo alloy, by the filtered cathodic arc method, with a chromium bond coat. With ultrasmooth coatings with a roughness of 7 nm, the wear rate of UHMWPE was reduced by factors of 30 to 600 times compared with the uncoated metal.

Diamond for Cardiovascular Applications

Conventionally, heart valves are made from LTI carbon, and despite its utmost care during the manufacture, always there exists a very small but finite risk of failure due to fracture initiated at an undetected surface or subsurface flaw. Therefore, there has been considerable interest in replacing this brittle material with an alternate metal coated with hard carbon, which is nonthrombogenic. Work by Butter et al. [94] suggested the use of NiCr18 stainless steel coated by a non–line-of-sight method with carbon as a replacement. It has been reported that a silicon-containing DLC may be a better coating for cardiovascular purposes, but

Butter et al. [94] comment that in tests, it showed no difference from the controls. However, the works published indicated that DLC is a promising biomaterial for heart valve applications, and it is known that much research work is under progress on this topic. Furthermore, DLC-coated stents can be permanently inserted into an artery that will assist to open the artery through which the blood can flow through it. Cardiovascular implantation of stents is becoming famous and rapidly used worldwide, although it has several shortcomings such as restenosis and occlusion. Moreover, arterial stents can induce platelet activation and may initiate thrombosis by shear forces on the flow and by platelet adhesion to the metal. Alanazi et al. [115] evaluated in vitro the performance of stents coated with DLC. Growth arrays using smooth muscle cells and endothelial cells evidenced that DLC did not affect proliferation rates and no cytotoxic effects were observed. Flow cytometric analyses showed no significant changes in mean channel fluorescence intensity for the structural antigens CD41a and CD42b. On the other hand, contrast expression of the activation-dependent antigens CD62p and CD63 increased significantly in uncoated compared with DLC-coated stents. Release of metal ions into the bloodstream is a matter of concern, and Alanazi et al. [115] used atomic adsorption spectrometry to detect a significant release of nickel and chromium ions into human plasma over 4 days from uncoated stents. Similar results were obtained by inductively coupled plasma mass spectrometry analysis, and in this case, the release of metal ions from DLC coated stents was "virtually undetectable." From these observations, the authors concluded that the coating of intracoronary stents with DLC may contribute to a reduction in thrombogenicity and consecutively in the incidence of acute occlusion and restenosis in vivo. Furthermore, in vitro tests were performed by coating the catheters with a mixture of Ag and DLC, and the results confirmed the efficacy of this coating for local freedom from bacterial infection. DLC coatings on segmented polyurethane were tested for blood compatibility by McLaughlin et al. [116], and it was shown that they could be superior to an excellent nonthrombogenic polymer, 2-hydroxyethyl methacrylate, during the experiments performed in a parallel flow chamber. Finally, the authors concluded that greater attention should be paid to DLC for use in the medical field.

DLC-Coated Guide Wires

Guide wires are often used to introduce stents, catheters and other medical devices inside the human body. In practice, a good guide wire should possess high flexibility, low coefficient of friction, inertness, and biocompatibility. In the past decade, it is customary to use stainless steel as a guide wire material. Stainless steel is often coated with polytetrafluoroethylene or silicon to improve the lubricity or to lower the friction. Nevertheless, these coatings have serious shortcomings such as poor adhesion and less stability with stainless steel causing the release of coated materials. In principle, the guide wires should not have any implant trauma or harm the wall of the vessels during its insertion alongside the path of the vessels. Furthermore, studies were also performed to coat guide wires with DLC, and their stability, lubrication, and hemocompatibility were evaluated [117, 118]. The results are supportive of the fact that DLC containing suitable elements is capable of being used as guide wires. However, care must be taken to negate its delamination and spallation during winding of the guide wires.

Other Biomedical Applications of Diamond

To minimize the problem of biofilm formation, Elinson et al. [119] applied a thin layer of DLC over soft contact lenses. Furthermore, from their experiments, they confirmed that microbial contamination of the contact lenses can be resolved by storing the contact lenses inside the DLC-coated cases. Work by Butter and Lettington [120] indicated that microneedles coated with DLC causes the least possible distortion during an ophthalmic surgery. Next, hydrogenated DLC coatings have been investigated for implants in oral cavity [121, 122]. It was observed that the CVD-deposited C–H layers over DLC showed significant biointegration and resistance to saliva and other oral cavity elements [122].

Biomedical Applications of Fullerenes

Functionalized fullerenes have been extensively used in major areas of biomedicine such as drug delivery, reactive oxygen species quenching (ROS), and as magnetic resonance imaging (MRI) contrast agent, and they are all discussed in detail below.

Functionalized Fullerenes as Drug Delivery Agents

Paclitaxel-embedded buckysomes (PEBs) are spherical nanostructures in the order of ~200 nm and composed of the amphiphilic fullerene embedding the anticancer drug paclitaxel inside its hydrophobic pockets [123]. Similar to Abraxane®, the US Food and Drug Administration–approved drug for treating diseases such as metastatic breast cancer, the water-soluble fullerene derivatives enable the uptake of paclitaxel negating nonaqueous solvents, which can cause patient discomfort and other unwanted side effects. However, work by Partha et al. [124] indicated that PEBs are capable of delivering even higher amounts of paclitaxel than those delivered via Abraxane. By delivering an increased amount of paclitaxel, it is expected that infusion times were shortened and results in higher tumor uptake leading to greater anticancer efficacy. Another advantage of fullerene-based delivery vectors is that their nanoscale dimensions favor passive targeting and enables them to accumulate at tumor sites by entering through leaky vasculature present in the endothelial cells of the tumor tissue. Moreover, the fullerene moiety can be easily functionalized to attach targeting agents that facilitate active targeting. PEBs also provide an easy route to attach targeting groups to their fullerene moieties. In PEBs, both liposomal and nanoparticle technologies are combined together to create nanostructures that serve as novel drug carriers. This is an innovative approach because it will improve circulation times in the blood, shields the anticancer drug against enzymatic degradation, and reduces uptake by the reticuloendothelial system. Furthermore, the size of the PEBs is designed to be less than 200 nm to avoid reticuloendothelial system uptake. The presence of dendritic groups outside the PEBs can also provide stealth function to reduce the clearance. Fullerenes are capable of producing an ideal lipophilic slow release system and provide three-dimensional scaffolding for covalent attachment of multiple drugs, which will be used to create single dose "drug cocktails." Zakharian et al. [125] designed a fullerene paclitaxel conjugate to slowly release the drug for aerosol liposome delivery of paclitaxel for lung cancer therapy [125]. The aggregate size range for this conjugate was in the order of 120 nm and the size did not vary with concentration. This conjugate was designed to release paclitaxel via enzymatic hydrolysis with a half-life of release of 80 min in bovine plasma. A dilauroylphosphatidylcholine-based liposome formulation of the conjugate was reported to have a half maximal inhibitory concentration value virtually identical to the half-maximal inhibitory concentration (IC_{50}) for a paclitaxel–dilauroylphosphatidylcholine formulation in human epithelial lung carcinoma A549 cells. They concluded that together with clinically relevant kinetics of hydrolysis and significant cytotoxicity in tissue culture, the fullerene–paclitaxel conjugate had potential for enhanced therapeutic efficacy of paclitaxel in vivo. Apart from delivering drug molecules, functionalized fullerenes have also been studied as transfection vectors to deliver exogenous DNA into cells and tested for their ability to mediate gene transfer [126–129], and it has possible benefits in gene therapy. Although the first-generation fullerene transfection vectors showed promise, they also exhibited high cytotoxicity. Sitharaman et al. [130] successfully demonstrated that a new class of water-soluble C_{60} derivatives prepared using Hirsch–Bingel method can uptake DNA and transport them across the cell and elicit gene expression. However, their study reported only two positively charged C_{60} derivatives, an octa-amino derivatized C_{60} and a dodeca-amino derivatized C_{60} vector, that exhibited efficient in vitro transfection. Aggregation behavior was expected to cause increased cytotoxicity of certain functionalized fullerenes. Therefore, it was suggested that future studies should address this discrepancy of aggregation in the presence of DNA before designing the derivative. Furthermore, they have suggested the possibility to develop analogous gadofullerene vectors for a combinatorial approach of diagnosis and therapy.

Suppression of Reactive Oxygen Species by Functionalized Fullerenes

Fullerenes are very famous as antioxidant following Krusic et al. [131] work evidencing the ability of fullerenes to scavenge ROS. Furthermore, care must be taken to retain the scavenging properties while functionalizing the fullerenes. Dugan and coworkers [132] published an article on carboxyfullerenes as neuroprotective agents and suggested that C_{60} derivatives might constitute antioxidant compounds useful in biological systems. Carboxyfullerene were found to be efficient against excitotoxic necrosis and provided protection against the two forms of neuronal apoptosis. This led to the idea that oxidative stress is a critical downstream mediator in disparate necrotic and apoptotic neuronal deaths. In addition, the study showed that amphiphilicity is a desirable feature in the functionalization to increase the intercalation into brain membranes, and neuroprotective efficacy. The article further demonstrated that C_{60} derivatives can function as neuroprotective drugs in vivo. In another study, Monti et al. [133] presented in vitro data demonstrating that carboxyfullerenes possesses an antioxidative property and is capable of suppressing iron induced lipid peroxidation. Furthermore, the in vivo study showed neuroprotection by carboxyfullerene against iron-induced degeneration of the nigrostriatal dopaminergic system. Also, they reported that the intranigral infusion of carboxyfullerene was found to be nontoxic to the nigrostriatal dopaminergic system of rats. After this, various research studies also confirmed the protective activity of carboxyfullerenes against oxidative stress and their ability as a free radical scavenger. Santos et al. [134] demonstrated that carboxyfullerene was capable of protecting quiescent human peripheral blood mononuclear cells from apoptosis by a mechanism that partially involves the mitochondrial membrane potential integrity, which is known to be associated with early stages of apoptosis. Furthermore, in their work, the authors concluded that these results were the first indication of target activity of buckminsterfullerenes on cells of the immune system and their mitochondria. Daroczi et al. [135] demonstrated that the antioxidant properties of the dendrofullerene (DF-1) would help to alleviate the toxicity from radiation exposure. Furthermore, they compared the effect of DF-1 with the US Food and Drug Administration–approved drug amifostine in vivo in a zebrafish (*Danio rerio*) model. The article reported that radiation exposure of zebrafish embryos produced extensive edema in the developing fish, and this effect was reversed by DF-1 treatment. To obtain a more detailed view of DF-1–mediated radioprotection, they have further evaluated the effects of this drug on organ-specific, radiation-induced damage. They assessed the effects of

DF-1 on a commonly observed phenotype that was apparent within 1 to 2 days after ionizing radiation exposure (~40 Gy) of zebrafish. This phenotype is described as "curly-up" or cup and was ascribed to defects in midline development of zebrafish embryos. Finally, the study concluded that throughout the dose range tested, DF-1 markedly reduced the incidence of cup. Depending on the ionizing radiation dose, it either reduced the severity or abolished the dorsal curvature altogether. It was significant to note that DF-1 did not cause any adverse effects on normal zebrafish morphology or viability in the concentration range tested (1–1000 μmol/L). DF-1 (100 μmol/L) was reported to markedly attenuate overall and organ-specific radiation-induced toxicity when given within 3 h before or up to 15 min after radiation exposure. However, DF-1 is not capable of protecting within 30 min after ionizing radiation. The degree of DF-1 radioprotection was comparable with amifostine (4 mmol/L). Moreover, the study evidenced that protection against radiation-associated toxicity using DF-1 in zebrafish embryos was associated with marked reduction of radiation-induced ROS. Finally, the authors concluded that DF-1 offered excellent antioxidant properties against radiation-induced damage. This study has implications in developing drugs for the military during radiation attacks. Yin et al. [136] reported that three different types of water-soluble fullerenes materials may intercept all the major physiologically relevant ROS. They used a carboxyfullerene derivative [$C_{60}(C(COOH)_2)_2$] and a fullerenol derivative [$C_{60}(OH)_{22}$] and C_{82}-derived gadofullerene. The study demonstrated that these functionalized fullerenes can protect cells against hydrogen peroxide–induced oxidative damage, stabilize the mitochondrial membrane potential, and reduce intracellular ROS production. Furthermore, in vitro studies using human lung adenocarcinoma cell line A549 and rat brain capillary endothelial cell line indicated that these functionalized fullerenes reduces hydrogen peroxide–induced cytotoxicity, free radical formation, and mitochondrial damage. This result indicates that the gadofullerene derivative protected against oxidative injury to cellular mitochondria better than the other two fullerene derivatives [136]. Their study represented the first report that different types of fullerene derivatives can scavenge all physiologically relevant ROS. The article concluded that the role of oxidative stress and damage in the etiology and progression of many diseases suggests that these fullerene derivatives may be valuable in vivo cytoprotective and therapeutic agents.

Functionalized Fullerenes as MRI Contrast Agents

Fullerenes that are capable of encapsulating metal atom inside the fullerene cage are called *endohedral metallofullerenes,* and they represent another class of functionalized fullerenes. Similar to a liposome, protecting its encapsulated drug, the fullerene cage in a metallofullerene protects the metal inside both against chemical or enzymatic activity within the body and the unwarranted release of the metal. The ability to design water-soluble derivatives of endohedral metallofullerenes has played a key role in utilizing these compounds for medicinal applications. In this context, gadolinium-encapsulated fullerenes have been proposed as contrast agents to enhance MRI quality [137–142]. Another important reason to use gadofullerenes as a contrast agent for MRI is to ensure that the metal atom is held within the cage for applications that might require longer residency times. Toth et al. [139] reported the nuclear magnetic relaxation profiles for two water-soluble functionalized fullerenes: $Gd@C_{60}(OH)_x$ and $Gd@C_{60}[C(COOH)_2]_{10}$ [139]. From their experimental results, they have concluded that the strong pH dependency of the proton relaxivities made these functionalized fullerenes great candidates for MRI contrast agents with a stimulus based on pH. After this, in another study, Sitharaman et al. [140] showed that the anionic gadofullerene {Gd@C$_{60}$[C(COOH)$_2$]$_{10}$} was an attractive candidate for ex vivo labeling and noninvasive in vivo tracking of any mammalian cell via MRI [140]. Furthermore, the experiments on cellular internalization experiments indicated that complete labeling of the anionic gadofullerene was achieved for marrow stromal cells within 2–8 h of incubation with further increase in uptake beyond the 8-h time point. In addition, the supernatant obtained from the pulse-chase experiments showed no detectable Gd content, whereas the cells showed similar Gd concentrations at all time points. Based on these findings, they indicated the gadofullerene did not leach after labeling and the labeling process is irreversible under these conditions. Moreover, the results also confirmed that the cellular labeling with this fullerene derivative is intracellular, and the magnetic labels are intercalated deep within the cell membrane. Furthermore, in vitro cell viability and toxicity assays revealed no cell damage as a result of this labeling process. T$_1$-weighted MRI phantoms from the study clearly demonstrated that the signal intensity of Gd@C$_{60}$[C(COOH)$_2$]$_{10}$ was about 300% greater than that of clinically used Gd-DTPA (Magnevist™) at 0.04 mM concentration of gadolinium. They have also concluded that at the same concentration of Gd, commercially available Gd-DTPA exhibited a little enhancement compared with plain distilled water. They mentioned that the high relaxivity of the gadofullerenes substantially reduced the T$_1$ of labeled cells, even at modest concentrations of gadolinium, and this difference in T$_1$ between labeled and unlabeled cells might allow for their direct discrimination with clinical MRI imagers at 1.5 T. According to the study, this is significant for detection of stem cells by MRI at resolutions that can potentially be achieved in vivo in animals and humans. Fatouros and colleagues [142] conducted studies on water-soluble Gd$_3$N endohedral metallofullerenes functionalized with poly(ethylene glycol) and multihydroxyl groups (Gd$_3$N@ C$_{80}$[DiPEG$_{5000}$(OH)$_x$]) and demonstrated that they offer great potential for serving as MRI contrast agents due to their T$_1$–T$_2$ relaxivity characteristics—approximately 40 times greater than conventional gadolinium-containing MRI contrast agents.

TABLE 3.1

List of Biomedical Applications of Functionalized Fullerenes

Name of the Functionalized Fullerenes	Application	Reference
Amphiphilic fullerene (Buckysomes, AF-1)	Drug delivery	Brettreich and Hirsch [147], Burghardt et al. [148], Partha et al. [123, 124]
Fullerene—paclitaxel	Cancer therapy	Zakharian et al. [125]
Fullerene polyamine (tetra amino fullerene)	Gene delivery and transfection	Isobe et al. [127–129]
Hydrophilic or cationic fullerenes	Photodynamic cancer therapy	Goel and Howard [62], Geim and Novoselov [63]
Carboxy fullerene and ascorbic acid fullerene	Antioxidant	Monti et al. [133], Santos et al. [134]
Cystine C$_{60}$ and β-alanine C$_{60}$	Hydrogen peroxide induced apoptosis protection	Hu et al. [149, 150]
Amino fullerene adducts	Non viral gene delivery	Sitharaman et al. [130]
Fullerene vesicle	Oxidative stress reduction	Maeda et al. [137]
Fullerenol	Free radical scavenger	Tsai et al. [151], Lai et al. [152]

Other Important Applications of Functionalized Fullerenes

Fullerenes, when functionalized using peptides and amino acids, were found to substantially activate enzymes involved in the oxidative deamination of biogenic amines [143]. The presence of the fullerene-substituted amino acid in a peptide was found to have a significant effect on the secondary structures and self-assembly properties of peptides as compared with the native peptide [144]. Work by Gonzalez and coworkers [145] reported that a fullerene-based material can be successfully targeted to a selected tissue. In addition, they designed a tissue vectored *bis*-phosphonate fullerene to target bone tissue and evaluated in vitro. The whole idea was that an amide *bis*-phosphonate addend, in conjunction with multiple hydroxyl groups, conferred a strong affinity towards the calcium phosphate mineral hydroxyapatite of bone. Furthermore, functionalized fullerenes are capable of effectively photoinactivating either or both pathogenic microbial cells and malignant cancer cells. Mroz and coworkers [146] described that this mechanism involves superoxide anion as well as singlet oxygen, and under the right conditions, fullerenes have possible benefits over clinically applied photosensitizers for mediating photodynamic therapy of certain diseases. Furthermore, Table 3.1 provides a list of references that have investigated functionalized fullerenes for various other potential biomedical applications.

Acknowledgment

The authors thank the National Science foundation (NSF) for their support: NSF Center for Nanobiotechnology Research Grant 0734232.

References

1. Cunningham AJ. *Introduction to Bioanalytical Sensors: Techniques in Analytical Chemistry*. New York, NY: Wiley & Sons, 1998.
2. Clark LC and Lyons C. Electrode systems for continuous monitoring in cardiovascular surgery. *Annals of the New York Academy of Sciences*, 102 (1962) 29–45.
3. Updike SJ and Hicks JP. The enzyme electrode. *Nature*, 214 (1967) 986–988.
4. Wehmeyer KR, Halsall HB, Heineman WR, Volle CP, and Chen IW. Competitive heterogeneous enzyme immunoassay for digoxin with electrochemical detection. *Analytical Chemistry*, 58 (1986) 135–139.
5. Zhang S, Wright G, and Yang Y. Materials and techniques for electrochemical biosensor design and construction. *Biosensors and Bioelectronics*, 15 (2000), 273–282.
6. Amine A, Mohammadi M, Bourais I, and Palleschi G. Enzyme inhibition-based biosensors for food safety and environmental monitoring. *Biosensors and Bioelectronics*, 21 (2006) 1405–1423.
7. De Luca S, Florescu M, Ghica ME, Lupu A, Palleschi G, Brett CMA, and Compagnone D. Carbon film electrodes for oxidase-based enzyme sensors in food analysis. *Talanta*, 68 (2005) 171–178.
8. McCreery RL. *Electroanalytical Chemistry*. New York, NY: Marcel Dekker, 1991.
9. Clark RA, Zerby SE, and Ewing AG. *Electroanalytical Chemistry*. New York, NY: Marcel Dekker, 1991.
10. Kinoshita K. *Carbon: Electrochemical and Physiochemical Properties*. New York, NY: Wiley & Sons, 1988.

11. Miller FJ and Zittel HE. Fabrication and use of pyrolytic graphite electrode for voltammetry in aqueous solutions. *Analytical Chemistry*, 35 (1963) 1866–1869.
12. Walker PL. Carbon—an old but new material. *Carbon*, 10 (1972) 369–372.
13. Dryhurst G and McAllister DL. *Carbon Electrodes*. New York, NY: Marcel Dekker, 1994.
14. Kissinger, PT and Heineman, WR. *Laboratory Techniques in Electroanalytical Chemistry*. New York: M. Dekker, Inc., 1984.
15. Panzer RE and Elving PJ. Behavior of carbon electrodes in aqueous and in non aqueous systems. *Journal of the Electrochemical Society*, 119 (1972) 864–874.
16. Eisner U and Mark HB. Film formation on pyrolytic graphite electrodes. *Journal of Electroanalytical Chemistry*, 9 (1970) 305–310.
17. Laitinen HA and Rhodes DR. The electrochemistry of V_2O_5 in LiCl–KCl eutectic melt. *Journal of the Electrochemical Society*, 109 (1962) 413–419.
18. Beilby AL, Brooks W, and Lawrence GL. Comparison of the pyrolytic carbon film electrode with the wax-impregnated graphite electrode. *Analytical Chemistry*, 36 (1964) 22–26.
19. Randin J and Yeager E. Differential capacitance study of stress-annealed pyrolytic graphite electrodes. *Journal of the Electrochemical Society*, 118 (1972) 711–714.
20. Kozlowska HA, Klinger J, and Conway BE. Computer simulation of the kinetic behaviour of surface reactions driven by a linear potential sweep—Part I. Model 1—electron reaction with a single adsorbed species. *Journal of Electroanalytical Chemistry*, 75 (1977) 45–60.
21. Tse DCS and Kuwana T. Electrocatalysis of dihydronicotinamide adenosine diphosphate with quinones and modified quinone electrodes *Analytical Chemistry*, 50 (1978) 1315–1318.
22. Evans JF, Kuwana T, Henne MT, and Royer GP. Electrocatalysis of solution species using modified electrodes. *Journal of Electroanalytical Chemistry*, 80 (1977) 409–416.
23. Zittel HE and Miller FJ. A glassy-carbon electrode for voltammetry. *Analytical Chemistry*, 37 (1965) 200–203.
24. McBride HD and Evans DH. Rapid voltammetric method for the estimation of tocopherols and antioxidants in oils and fats. *Analytical Chemistry*, 45 (1973) 446–449.
25. Van der Linden WE and Dieker JW. Glassy carbon as electrode material in electro-analytical chemistry. *Analytica Chimica Acta*, 119 (1980) 1–24.
26. Elliot CM and Murray RW. Chemically modified carbon electrodes. *Analytical Chemistry*, 48 (1976) 1247–1254.
27. Moore A. *Chemistry and Physics of Carbon*. New York, NY: Marcel Dekker, 1981.
28. Sanchez-Lopez JC, Donnet C, Fontaine J, Belin M, Grill A, Patel V, and Jahnes C. Diamond-like carbon prepared by high density plasma. *Diamond and Related Materials*, 9 (2000) 638–642.
29. Lee CS, Lee KR, Eun KY, Yoon KH, and Han JH. Structure and properties of Si incorporated tetrahedral amorphous carbon films prepared by hybrid filtered vacuum arc process. *Diamond and Related Materials*, 11 (2002) 198–203.
30. Zou YS, Wang W, Song GH, Du H, Gong J, Huang RF, and Wen LS. Influence of the gas atmosphere on the microstructure and mechanical properties of diamond-like carbon films by arc ion plating. *Materials Letters*, 58 (2004) 3271–3275.
31. Thorwarth G, Hammerl C, Kuhn M, Assmann W, Schey B, and Stritzker B. Investigation of DLC synthesized by plasma immersion ion implantation and deposition. *Surface Coatings Technology*, 193 (2005) 206–212.
32. Sanchez NA, Rincon C, Zambrano G, Galindo H, and Prieto P. Characterization of diamond-like carbon (DLC) thin films prepared by r.f. magnetron sputtering. *Thin Solid Films*, 373 (2000) 247–250.
33. He X, Li W, and Li H. Bonding structure and tribological properties of DLC films synthesized by dual ion beam sputtering. *Vacuum*, 45 (1994) 977–980.
34. Shim KS, Kim SM, Bae SH, Lee SY, Jung HS, and Park HH. Fabrication and characterization of diamond-like carbon thin films by pulsed laser deposition. *Applied Surface Science*, 154–155 (2000) 482–484.
35. Hofsass H, Binder H, Klumpp T, and Recknagel E. Doping and growth of diamond-like carbon films by ion beam deposition. *Diamond Related Materials* 3, (1994) 137–142.

36. Niraj S and Yeow JTW. Carbon nanotubes for biomedical applications. *IEEE Transactions on Nanobioscience*, 4 (2005) 180–195.
37. Ijima S. Helical microtubules of graphitic carbon. *Nature*, 354 (1991) 56–58.
38. Dresselhaus MS. Fullerenes: down the straight and narrow. *Nature*, 358 (1998) 195–196.
39. Dresselhaus MS, Dresselhaus G, and Eklund PC. *Science of Fullerenes and Carbon Nanotubes*. New York, NY: Academic Press, 1996.
40. Wang J. Carbon nanotube based electrochemical biosensors: a review. *Electroanalysis*, 17 (2005) 7–14.
41. Bethune DS, Kiang CH, De Vries MS, Gorman G, Savoy R, Vazquez J, and Beyers R. Cobalt-catalyzed growth of carbon nanotubes with single-atomic-layer walls. *Nature*, 363 (1993) 305–305.
42. Ijima S, Ajayan PM, and Ichihashi T. Growth model for carbon nanotubes. *Physical Review Letters*, 69 (1992) 3100–3103.
43. Ebbesen TW and Ajayan PM. Large scale synthesis of carbon nanotubes. *Nature*, 358 (1992) 220–221.
44. Bethune DS, Kiang CH, De Vries MS, Gorman G, Savoy R, Vazquez J, and Beyers R. Cobalt-catalyzed growth of carbon nanotubes with single-atomic-layer walls. *Nature*, 363 (1993) 605–607.
45. Iijima S and Ichihashi T. Single-shell carbon nanotubes of 1-nm diameter. *Nature*, 363 (1993) 603–605.
46. Takahashi S, Ikuno T, Oyama T, Honda SI, Katayama M, Hirao T, and Oura K. Synthesis and characterization of carbon nanotubes grown on carbon particles by using high vacuum laser ablation. *Journal of Vaccum Society of Japan*, 45 (2002) 609–612.
47. Vanderwal RL, Berger GM, and Ticich TM. Carbon nanotube synthesis in a flame using laser ablation for *in situ* catalyst generation. *Applied Physics A*, 77 (2003) 885–889.
48. Braidy N, El Khakani MA, and Botton GA Carbon nanotubular structures synthesis by means of ultraviolet laser ablation. *Journal of Materials Research*, 17 (2002) 2189–2192.
49. Chatterjee AK, Sharon M, Banerjee R, and Neumann-Spallart M. CVD synthesis of carbon nanotubes using a finely dispersed cobalt catalyst and their use in double layer electrochemical capacitors. *Electrochimica Acta*, 48 (2003) 3439–3446.
50. Park D, Kim YH, and Lee JK. Synthesis of carbon nanotubes on metallic substrates by a sequential combination of PECVD and thermal CVD. *Carbon*, 41 (2003) 1025–1029.
51. Chaisitsak S, Yamada A, and Konagai M. Hot filament enhanced CVD synthesis of carbon nanotubes by using a carbon filament. *Diamond and Related Materials*, 13 (2004) 438–444.
52. Kroto HW, Heath JR, O'Brien SC, Curl RF, and Smalley RE. C_{60}: buckminsterfullerene. *Nature*, 318 (1985) 162–163.
53. Sivaraman N, Dhamodaran R, Kaliappan I, Srinivassan TG, Rao PRV, and Mathews CK. Solubility of C60 in organic solvents. *Journal of Organic Chemistry*, 57 (1992) 6077–6079.
54. Ruoff RS, Tse DS, Malhotra R, and Lorents DC. Solubility of fullerene (C60) in a variety of solvents. *Journal of Physical Chemistry*, 97 (1993) 3379–3383.
55. Partha R and Conyers JL. Biomedical applications of functionalized fullerene-based nanomaterials. *International Journal of Nanomedicine*, 4 (2009) 261–275.
56. Wilson SR. *Biological Aspects of Fullerenes. Fullerenes: Chemistry, Physics and Technology*. New York, NY: John Wiley & Sons, 2000.
57. Da Ros T and Prato M. Medicinal chemistry with fullerenes and fullerene derivatives. *Chemical Communications*, 8 (1999) 663–669.
58. Jensen AW, Wilson SR, and Schuster DI. Biological applications of fullerenes—a review. *Bioorganic and Medicinal Chemistry*, 4 (1996) 767–779.
59. Kratschmer W, Lamb LD, Fostiropoulos K, and Huffman DR. Solid C_{60}: a new form of carbon. *Nature*, 347 (1990) 354–358.
60. Alekseyev NI and Dyuzhev GA. Fullerene formation in arc discharge. *Carbon*, 41 (2003) 1343–1348.
61. Howard, JB, McKinnon JT, Makarovsky Y, Lafleur AL, and Johnson ME. Fullerenes C_{60} and C_{70} in flames. *Nature*, 352 (1991) 139–141.

62. Goel A and Howard JB. Reaction rate coefficient of fullerene (C_{60}) consumption by soot. *Carbon,* 41 (2003) 1949–1954.

63. Geim AK and Novoselov KS. The rise of graphene. *Nature Materials,* 6 (2007) 183–191.

64. Alwarappan S, Erdem A, Liu C, and Li C-Z. Probing the electrochemical properties of graphene nanosheets for biosensing applications. *Journal of Physical Chemistry C,* 113 (2009) 8853–8857.

65. Stankovich S, Dikin DA, Piner RD, Kohlhass KA, Kleinhammes A, Jia Y, Wu Y, Nguyen S, and Ruoff RS. Synthesis of graphene-based nanosheets *via* chemical reduction of exfoliated graphite oxide. *Carbon,* 45 (2007) 1558–1565.

66. Brodie BC. Sur le poids atomique du graphite *Annals of Chemical Physics,* 59 (1860) 466–472.

67. Hummers W and Offeman R. Preparation of graphitic oxide. *Journal of American Chemical Society,* 80 (1958) 1339.

68. Staudenmaier L. Verfahren zur Darstellung der Graphitsäure Berichte *der deutschen* chemischen *Gesellschaft,* 31 (1898) 1481–1487.

69. Wang X, You H, Liu F, Li M, Li W, Li S, Li Q, Xu Y, Tian R, Yu Z, Xiang D, and Cheng J. Large scale synthesis of few-layered graphene using CVD. *Chemical Vapor Deposition,* 15 (2009) 53–56.

70. Kostas K, Lara L, Giorgia P, Wei W, Sébastien W, Jacqueline L, Sylvie G, Davide P, Jean-Paul B, Sylviane M, Maurizio P, and Alberto B. Cellular uptake of functionalized carbon nanotubes is independent of functional group and cell type. *Nature Nanotechnology,* 2 (2007) 108–113.

71. Bianco A, Hoebeke J, Godefroy S, Chaloin O, Pantarotto D, Briand JP, Muller S, Prato M, and Partidos C D. Cationic carbon nanotubes bind to CpG oligodeoxynucleotides and enhance their immunostimulatory properties. *Journal of American Chemical Society,* 127 (2005) 58–59.

72. Pastorin G, Wu W, Wieckowski S, Briand JP, Kostarelos K, Prato M, and Bianco A. Double functionalisation of carbon nanotubes for multimodal drug delivery. *Chemical Communications* 11 (2006) 1182–1184.

73. Chou A, Bocking T, Singh NK, and Gooding JJ. Demonstration of the importance of oxygenated species at the ends of carbon nanotubes for their favourable electrochemical properties. *Chemical Communications,* 7 (2005) 842–844.

74. Boussaad S, Tao NJ, Zhang R, Hopson T, and Nagahara LA. *In situ* detection of cytochrome c adsorption with single walled carbon nanotube device. *Chemical Communications,* 13 (2003) 1502–1503.

75. Chen X, Tam UC, Czlapinski JL, Lee GS, Rabuka D, Zettl A, and Bertozzi CR. Interfacing carbon nanotubes with living cells. *Journal of American Chemical Society,* 128 (2006) 6292–6293.

76. Guiseppi-Elie A, Lei CH, and Baughman RH. Direct electron transfer of glucose oxidase on carbon nanotubes. *Nanotechnology,* 13 (2002) 559–564.

77. Salvador-Morales C, Flahaut E, Sim E, Sloan J, Green MLH, and Sim RB. Complement activation and protein adsorption by carbon nanotubes. *Molecular Immunoogy,* 43 (2006) 193–201.

78. Salvador-Morales C, Townsend P, Flahaut E, Venien-Bryan C, Vlandas A, Green MLH, and Sim RB. Binding of pulmonary surfactant proteins to carbon nanotubes; potential for damage to lung immune defense mechanisms. *Carbon,* 45 (2007) 607–617.

79. Liu Z, Winters M, Holodniy M, and Dai HJ. siRNA delivery into human T cells and primary cells with carbon-nanotube transporters. *Angewandte Chemie International Edition,* 46 (2007) 2023–2027.

80. Hu H, Ni YC, Montana V, Haddon RC, and Parpura V. Chemically functionalized carbon nanotubes as substrates for neuronal growth. *Nano Letters,* 4 (2004) 507–511.

81. Gheith MK, Sinani VA, Wicksted JP, Matts RL, and Kotov NA. Single walled carbon nanotube polyelectrolyte multilayers and freestanding films as a biocompatible platform for neuroprosthetic implants. *Advanced Materials,* 17 (2005) 2663–2670.

82. Gheith MK, Pappas TC, Liopo AV, Sinani VA, Shim BS, Motamedi M, Wicksted JR, and Kotov NA. Stimulation of neural cells by lateral layer-by-layer films of single-walled currents in conductive carbon nanotubes. *Advanced Materials,* 18 (2006) 2975–2979.

83. Bianco A, Kostarelos K, and Prato M. Applications of carbon nanotubes in drug delivery. *Current Opinion in Chemical Biology,* 9 (2005) 674–679.

84. Kam NWS and Dai HJ. Carbon nanotubes as intracellular protein transporters: generality and biological functionality. *Journal of American Chemical Society*, 127 (2005) 6021–6026.

85. Kam NWS, Liu ZA, and Dai HJ. Carbon nanotubes as intracellular transporters for proteins and DNA: an investigation of the uptake mechanism and pathway. *Angewandte Chemie International Edition*, 45 (2006) 577–581.

86. Shao N, Lu SX,Wickstrom E, and Panchapakesan B. Integrated molecular targeting of IGF1R and HER2 surface receptors and destruction of breast cancer cells using single wall carbon nanotubes. *Nanotechnology*, 18 (2007) 315101.

87. Zotchev SB. Polyene macrolide antibiotics and their applications in human therapy. *Current Medicinal Chemistry*, 10 (2003) 211–223.

88. Szlinder-Richert J, Cybulska B, Grzybowska J, Bolard J, and Borowski E. Interaction of amphotericin B and its low toxic derivative, N-methyl-N-D-fructosyl amphotericin B methyl ester, with fungal, mammalian and bacterial cells measured by the energy transfer method. *Il Farmaco*, 59 (2004) 289–296.

89. Yinghuai Z, Peng AT, Carpenter K, Maguire JA, Hosmane NS, and Takagaki M. Substituted carborane-appended water-soluble single-wall carbon nanotubes: new approach to boron neutron capture therapy drug delivery. *Journal of American Chemical Society*, 127 (2005) 9875–9880.

90. Zhang ZH, Yang XY, Zhang Y, Zeng B, Wang ZJ, Zhu TH, Roden RBS, Chen YS, and Yang RC. Delivery of telomerase reverse transcriptase small interfering RNA in complex with positively charged single-walled carbon nanotubes suppresses tumor growth. *Clinical Cancer Research*, 12 (2006) 4933–4939.

91. Evans AC, Franks J, and Revell PJ. Diamond-like carbon applied to bioengineering materials. *Surface Coating Technology*, 47 (1991) 662–667.

92. Mitura E, Mitura S, Niedzielski P, Has Z, Wolowiec R, Jakubowski A, Szmidt J, Sokolowska A, Louda P, Marciniak J, and Koczy B. Diamond-like carbon coatings for biomedical applications. *Diamond and Related Materials*, 3 (1994) 896–898.

93. Thomson LA, Law FC, Rushton N, and Franks J. Biocompatibility of diamond-like carbon coating. *Biomaterials*, 12 (1991) 37–40.

94. Butter R, Allen M, Chandra L, Lettington AH, and Rushton N. In vitro studies of DLC coatings with silicon intermediate layer. *Diamond and Related Materials*, 4 (1995) 857–861.

95. Du C, Su XW, Cui FZ, and Zhu XD. Morphological behaviour of osteoblasts on diamond-like carbon coating and amorphous CN film in organ culture. *Biomaterials*, 19 (1998) 651–658.

96. Yu LJ, Wang X, Wang XH, and Liu XH. Haemocompatibility of tetrahedral amorphous carbon films. *Surface and Coatings Technology*, 128/129 (2000) 484–488.

97. Nurdin N, Francois P, Moret M, Unal K, Krumeich J, Aronsson BO, and Descounts P. Hemocompatible diamond-like carbon (DLC) surfaces. *European Cells and Materials Journal*, 5 (2003) 17–28.

98. Jones MI, McColl IR, Grant DM, Parker KG, and Parker TL. Haemocompatibility of DLC and TiC–TiN interlayers on titanium. *Diamond and Related Materials*, 8 (1999) 457–462.

99. Linder S, Pinkowski W, and Aepfelbacher M. Adhesion cytoskeletal architecture and activation status of primary human macrophages on a diamond-like carbon coated surface. *Biomaterials*, 23 (2002) 767–773.

100. Mohanty M, Anilkumar TV, Mohanan PV, Muraleedharan CV, Bhuvaneshwar GS, Derangere F, Sampeur Y, and Suryanarayanan R. Long term tissue response to titanium coated with diamond like carbon. *Biomolecular Engineering*, 19 (2002) 125–128.

101. Sheeja D, Tay BK, and Nung LN. Feasibility of diamond-like carbon coatings for orthopaedic applications. *Diamond and Related Materials*, 13 (2004) 184–190.

102. Kim HG, Ahn SH, Kim JG, Park SJ, and Lee KR. Electrochemical behavior of diamond-like carbon films for biomedical applications. *Thin Solid Films*, 475 (2005) 291–297.

103. Kwok SCH, Wang J, and Chu PK. Surface energy, wettability, and blood compatibility phosphorus doped diamond-like carbon films. *Diamond and Related Materials*, 14 (2005) 78–85.

104. Hauert R. A review of modified DLC coatings for biological applications. *Diamond and Related Materials*, 12 (2003) 583–589.

105. Dorner-Reisel A, Schurer C, Nischan C, Seidel O, and Muller E. Diamond-like carbon: alteration of the biological acceptance due to Ca–O incorporation. *Thin Solid Films*, 420–421 (2002) 263–268.

106. Grill A. Diamond-like carbon coatings as biocompatible materials—an overview. *Diamond and Related Materials*, 12 (2003) 166–170.

107. Roy RK and Lee K-R. Biomedical applications of diamond-like carbon coatings: a review. *Journal of Biomedical Materials Research Part B: Applied Biomaterials*, (2007) 72–84.

108. Saikko V and Ahlroos T. Phospholipids as boundary lubricants in wear tests of prosthetic joint materials. *Wear*, 207 (1997) 86–91.

109. Saikko V, Ahlroos T, Calonius O, and Keranen J. Wear simulation of total hip prostheses with polyethylene against CoCr, alumina and diamond-like carbon. *Biomaterials*, 22 (2001) 1507–1514.

110. Sheeja D, Tay BK, and Nung LN. Tribological characterization of surface modified UHMWPE against DLC-coated Co–Cr–Mo. *Surface and Coatings Technology*, 190 (2005) 231–237.

111. Sheeja D, Tay BK, Lau SP, and Nung LN. Tribological characterization of diamond-like carbon coatings on Co–Cr–Mo alloy for orthopaedic applications. *Surface and Coatings Technology*, 146/147 (2001) 410–416.

112. Xu T and Pruitt L. Diamond-like carbon coatings for orthopaedic applications: an evaluation of tribological performance. *Journal of Material Science: Materials in Medicine*, 10 (1999) 83–90.

113. Onate JI, Comin M, Braceras I, Garcia A, Viviente JL, Brizuela M, Garagorri N, Peris JL, and Alava JI. Wear reduction effect on ultra-high-molecular-weight polyethylene by application of hard coatings and ion implantation on cobalt chromium alloy as measured in a knee wear simulation machine *Surface and Coatings Technology*, 142–144 (2001) 1056–1062.

114. Gutensohn K, Beythien C, Bau J, Fenner T, Grewe P, Koester R, Padmanaban K, and Kuehnl P. In vitro analyses of diamond like carbon coated stents: reduction of metal ion release, platelet activation and thrombogenicity. *Thrombosis Research*, 99 (2000) 577–585.

115. Alanazi A, Nojiri C, Noguchi T, Kido T, Komatsu Y, Hirakuri K, Funakubo A, and Sakai K. Improved blood compatibility of DLC coated polymeric material. *ASAIO Journal*, 46 (2000) 440–443.

116. McLaughlin JA, Meenan B, Maguire P, and Jamieson N. Properties of diamond like carbon thin film coatings on stainless steel medical guidewires. *Diamond and Related Materials*, 5 (1996) 486–491.

117. Hasebe T, Matsuoka Y, Kodama H, Saito T, Yohena S, Kamijo A, Shiraga N, Higuchi M, Kuribayashi S, Takahashi K, and Suzuki T. Lubrication performance of diamond-like carbon and fluorinated diamond-like carbon coatings for intravascular guidewires. *Diamond Related Materials*, 15 (2006) 129–132.

118. Sleptsov VV, Elinson VM, Simakina NV, Laymin AN, Tsygankov IV, Kivaev AA, and Musina AD. Ophthalmological application of contact lenses modified by means of ion assisted carbon films. *Diamond and Related Materials*, 5 (1996) 483–485.

119. Elinson VM, Sleptsov VV, Laymin AN, Potraysay VV, Kostuychenko LN, and Moussina AD. Barrier properties of carbon films deposited on polymer-based devices in aggressive environments. *Diamond and Related Materials*, 8 (1999) 2103–2109.

120. Butter RS and Lettington AH. Diamond-like carbon for biomedical applications *Journal of Chemical Vapor Deposition*, 3 (1995) 182–192.

121. Olborska A, Swider M, Wolowiec R, Niedzielski P, Rylski A, and Mitura S. Diamond-like carbon coatings for biomedical applications. *Diamond and Related Materials*, 3 (1994) 899–901.

122. Kobayashi S, Ohgoe Y, Ozeki K, Sato K, Sumiya T, Hirakuri KK, and Aoki H. Diamond-like carbon coatings on orthodontic arch wires. *Diamond and Related Materials*, 14 (2005) 1094–1097.

123. Partha R, Mitchell LR, Lyon JL, Joshi PP, and Conyers JL. Buckysomes: fullerene-based nanocarriers for hydrophobic molecule delivery. *ACS Nano*, 2 (2008) 1950–1958.

124. Partha R, Lackey M, Hirsch A, Casscells SW, and Conyers JL. Self-assembly of amphiphilic C_{60} fullerene derivatives into nanoscale supramolecular structures. *Journal of Nanobiotechnology*, 5 (2007) 6.

125. Zakharian TY, Seryshev A, Sitharaman B, Gilbert BE, Knight V, and Wilson LJ. A fullerene–paclitaxel chemotherapeutic: synthesis, characterization, and study of biological activity in tissue culture. *Journal of American Chemical Society*, 127 (2005) 12508–12509.

126. Nakamura E, Isobe H, Tomita N, Sawamura M, Jinno S, and Okayama H. Functionalized fullerene as an artificial vector for transfection. *Angewadte Chimie International Edition*, 39 (2000) 4254–4257.

127. Isobe H, Tomita N, Jinno S, Okayama H, and Nakamura E. Synthesis and transfection capability of multi-functionalized fullerene polyamine. *Chemistry Letters*, 30 (2001) 1214–1215.

128. Isobe H, Nakanishi W, Tomita N, Jinno S, Okayama H, and Nakamura E. Nonviral gene delivery by tetraamino fullerene. *Molecular Pharmaceutics*, 3 (2006) 124–134.

129. Isobe H, Nakanishi W, Tomita N, Jinno S, Okayama H, and Nakamura E. Gene delivery by aminofullerenes: Structural requirements for efficient transfection. *Chemistry: An Asian Journal* 1 (2006) 167–175.

130. Sitharaman B, Zakharian TY, Saraf A, Misra P, Pan S, Pham QP, Mikos AG, Wilson AJ, and Engler DA. Water-soluble fullerene (C_{60}) derivatives as non-viral gene delivery vectors. *Molecular Pharmaceutics*, 5 (2008) 567–578.

131. Krusic PJ, Wasserman E, Keizer PN, Morton JR, and Preston KF. Radical reactions of C_{60}. *Science*, 254 (1991) 1183–1185.

132. Dugan LL, Turetsky DM, Du C, Lobner D, Wheeler M, Almli CR, Shen CKF, Luh TY, Choi DW, and Lin TS. Carboxyfullerenes as neuroprotective agents. *Proceedings of the National Academy of Sciences USA*, 94 (1997) 9434–9439. Erratum in: *Proceedings of the National Academy of Sciences USA*, 94 (1997) 12241.

133. Monti D, Moretti L, Salvioli S, Malroni ESW, Pellicciari R, Schettini G, Bisaglia M, Pincelli C, Fumelli C, Bonafe M, and Franceschi C. C_{60} carboxyfullerene exerts a protective activity against oxidative stress-induced apoptosis in human peripheral blood mononuclear cells. *Biochemical and Biophysical Research Communications*, 277 (2000) 711–717.

134. Santos SG, Santana JV, Maia Jr FF, Lemos V, and Freire VN. Adsorption of ascorbic acid on the C_{60} fullerene. *Journal of Physical Chemistry B*, 112 (2008) 14267–14272.

135. Daroczi B, Kari G, McAleer MF, Wolf JC, Rodeck U, and Dicker AP. *In vivo* radioprotection by the fullerene nanoparticle DF-1 as assessed in a zebrafish model. *Clinical Cancer Research*, 12 (2006) 7086–7091.

136. Yin JJ, Lao F, Fu PP, Wamer WG, Zhao Y, Wang PC, Qiu Y, Sun B, Xing G, Dong J, Liang XJ, and Chen C. The scavenging of reactive oxygen species and the potential for cell protection by functionalized fullerene materials. *Biomaterials*, 30 (2009) 611–621.

137. Maeda R, Noiri E, Isobe H, Homma T, Tanaka T, Negishi K, Doi K, Fujita T, and Nakamura E. A water-soluble fullerene vesicle alleviates angiotensin II-induced oxidative stress in human umbilical venous endothelial cells. *Hypertension Research*, 31 (2008) 141–151.

138. Bolskar RD, Benedetto AF, Husebo LO, Price RE, Jackson EF, Wallace S, Wilson LJ, and Alford JM. First soluble M@C_{60} derivatives provide enhanced access to metallofullerenes and permit *in vivo* evaluation of Gd@C_{60}[C(COOH)$_2$]$_{10}$ as a MRI contrast agent. *Journal of the American Chemical Society*, 125 (2003) 5471–5478.

139. Toth E, Bolskar RD, Borel A, Gonzalez G, Lothar H, Merbach AE, Sitharaman B, and Wilson LJ. Water-soluble gadofullerenes: toward high-relaxivity, pH-responsive MRI contrast agents. *Journal of the American Chemical Society*, 127 (2005) 799–805.

140. Sitharaman B, Tran LA, Pham QP, Bolskar RD, Muthupillai R, Flamm SD, Mikos AG, and Wilson LJ. Gadofullerenes as nanoscale magnetic labels for cellular MRI. *Contrast Media Molecular Imaging*, 2 (2007) 139–146.

141. Bolskar RD. Gadofullerene MRI contrast agents. *Nanomedicine*, 3 (2008) 201–213.

142. Fatouros PP, Corwin FD, Chen ZJ, Broaddus WC, Tatum JL, Kettenmann B, Ge Z, Gibson HW, Russ JL, Leonard AP, Duchamp JC, and Dorn HC. *In vitro* and *in vivo* imaging studies of a new endohedral metallofullerene nanoparticle. *Radiology*, 240 (2006) 756–764.

143. Bianco A, Da Ros T, Prato M, and Toniolo C. Fullerene-based amino acids and peptides. *Journal of Peptide Science*, 7 (2001) 208–219.

144. Yang J, Alemany LB, Driver J, Hartgerink JD, and Barron AR. Fullerene derivatized amino acids: synthesis, characterization, antioxidant properties, and solid-phase peptide synthesis. *Chemistry*, 13 (2007) 2530–2545.

145. Gonzalez KA, Wilson LJ, Wu W, and Nancollas GH. Synthesis and *in vitro* characterization of a tissue-selective fullerene: vectoring $C_{60}(OH)_{16}AMBP$ to mineralized bone. *Bioorganic and Medicinal Chemistry*, 10 (2002) 1991–1997.

146. Mroz P, Tegos GP, Gali H, Wharton T, Sarna T, and Hamblin MR. Photodynamic therapy with fullerenes. *Photochemical and Photobiological Sciences*, 6 (2007) 1139–1149.

147. Brettreich M and Hirsch A. A highly water-soluble dendro[60]fullerene. *Tetrahedron Letters*, 39 (1998) 2731–2734.

148. Burghardt S, Hirsch A, Schade B, Ludwig K, and Bottcher C. Switchable supramolecular organization of structurally defined micelles based on an amphiphilic fullerene. *Angewandte Chemie International Edition*, 44 (2005) 2976–2979.

149. Hu Z, Guan W, Wang W, Huang L, Xing H, and Zhu Z. Protective effect of a novel cystine C_{60} derivative on hydrogen peroxide-induced apoptosis in rat pheochromocytoma PC12 cells. *Chemico-Biological Interactions*, 167 (2007) 135–144.

150. Hu Z, Guan W, Wang W, Huang L, Xing H, and Zhu Z. Synthesis of beta-alanine C_{60} derivative and its protective effect on hydrogen peroxide-induced apoptosis in rat pheochromocytoma cells. *Cell Biology International*, 31 (2007) 798–804.

151. Tsai MC, Chen YH, and Chiang LY. Polyhydroxylated C_{60}, fullerenol, a novel free-radical trapper, prevented hydrogen peroxide and cumene hydroperoxide-elicited changes in rat hippocampus *in vitro*. *Journal of Pharmacy and Pharmacology*, 49 (1997) 438–445.

152. Lai HS, Chen WJ, and Chiang LY. Free radical scavenging activity of fullerenol on the ischemia–reperfusion intestine in dogs. *World Journal of Surgery*, 24 (2000) 450–454.

4

Impedance Spectroscopy on Carbon-Based Materials for Biological Application

Haitao Ye and Shi Su

CONTENTS

Introduction 135
Impedance Theory 136
    Impedance Principle 136
    Conductivity Models 140
    Equivalent Circuits 143
        Resistor and Capacitor in Parallel 144
        Double Resistor and Capacitor Parallel in Series 145
    Formulae for Capacitance 145
        One-Layer Model 146
        Cross-Section Two-Layer Model 148
        In-Plane Two-Layer Model 150
Impedance Spectroscopy on Diamond-Based Materials 150
    Boron-Doped Single-Crystalline Diamond 151
    Polycrystalline Diamond 155
    Nanocrystalline Diamond 160
Diamond-Based Materials Applications 165
    Biosensors 165
    Diamond Electrodes 170
    Ultraviolet Sensors 172
Non-Diamond-Based Materials for Biological Application 172
    Cells Detection 173
    DNA Hybridization Sensor Applications 174
    Enzyme Detection 175
    Catalysts 178
    Lithium-Ion Battery Applications 179
    Supercapacitance 181
    DLC Biomedical Coating Materials 182
References 185

Introduction

Impedance spectroscopy is a powerful technique to characterize the electrical properties of materials and their interfaces with electrically conducting electrodes. The technique may be used to investigate the dynamics of bound or mobile charges in bulk or interface regions of any kind of ionic solids, or liquid materials, semiconductors, mixed ionic–electronic materials, and insulators (dielectrics). The technique measures the impedance as a function of frequency automatically in the range of 0.1 Hz to 10 MHz and is easily interfaced to the computer.

The complex impedance measurements are capable of separating the various contributions such as bulk, grain boundary, and electrode, to total conductivity. Hence, this technique is able to extract the data that allow these phenomena to be isolated. Spectroscopic impedance studies on diamond films form the basis of this chapter; as such, the current status, models, and fundamental applications and interpretations related to this technique are crucial to the chapter. This chapter provides detailed background information based on both theoretical and empirical knowledge in this area.

Starting with general concepts of electrochemical impedance, the principle of this technique is presented. The utilization of this technique to characterize the grains and grain boundaries contribution are discussed in details. The equivalent electrical circuits are presented to compare with real materials systems. Next, formulae for the capacitance of one-layer and two-layer dielectrics models, with either in-plane or cross-section electrode configuration, are presented as references for the following chapters. Finally, from the microscopic point of view, different mechanisms on dielectric relaxation and polarization are summarized.

Case studies on impedance spectroscopy of diamond films have been presented including single-crystalline, polycrystalline, and nanocrystalline. The potential applications for both diamond-based materials and non–diamond-based materials have been reviewed.

Impedance Theory

Impedance Principle

Electrochemical impedance is the frequency-dependent complex-valued proportionality factor that is a ratio between the applied potential and current signal. For the sake of simplicity, the impedance plots for the resistor–capacitor (R–C) in parallel with a series resistor network (see Figure 4.1) will be considered in some detail. The reason for choosing this circuit is because many of the electrochemical systems encountered in practice are actually modeled using this network [1].

The terms "resistance" and "impedance" both imply an obstruction to current or electron flow. When dealing with a direct current (DC), only resistors provide this effect. However, for the case of an alternating current (AC), circuit elements such as capacitors and inductors can also influence the electron flow. These elements can affect not only the magnitude of an AC wave form but also its time-dependent characteristics or phase. In DC theory, where the frequency equals 0 Hz, a resistance is defined by the Ohm's law:

$$E = IR \tag{4.1}$$

where E is the applied potential, I is the resulting current, and R denotes resistance.

For an AC current, where the frequency exceeds zero, this is represented by

$$E = IZ$$

Ohm's law with frequency > 0 (4.2)

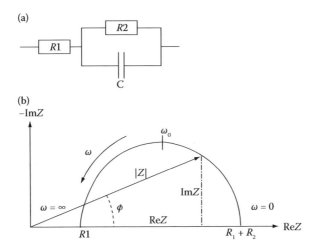

FIGURE 4.1
Equivalent circuit and AC impedance plots of an electrochemical cell with one time constant: equivalent circuit (a) and Cole–Cole plot in the complex plane (b), $\omega_0 = 1/(R_2C)$.

where E is the applied potential, I is the resulting current, and Z is impedance, the AC equivalent of resistance.

$$\text{High frequency: } Z'' \Rightarrow 0, Z' \Rightarrow R_1$$

$$\text{Low frequency: } Z'' \Rightarrow 0, Z' \Rightarrow R_1 + R_2$$

The mathematical contribution of the plot (Figure 4.1b) is based on a vector diagram, corresponding to a sine wave E and a sine wave I. This is because sine wave analysis is the most appropriate for electrochemical impedance studies to date. The current sine wave can be described by the following equation:

$$I = A \sin(\omega t + \phi) \tag{4.3}$$

$$\omega = 2\pi f \tag{4.4}$$

where A is the maximum amplitude, ω is the frequency in radians/s, f is the frequency in Hz, and ϕ is the phase shift in radians.

The impedance $Z(\omega)$ is a complex number that can be represented either in polar coordinates or in Cartesian coordinates:

$$Z(\omega) = |Z| e^{j\phi} \tag{4.5}$$

$$Z(\omega) = ReZ + j\,ImZ \tag{4.6}$$

where ReZ and ImZ are the real part and the imaginary part of the impedance, respectively. The relationships between these quantities are:

$$|Z|^2 = (\text{Re } Z)^2 + (\text{Im } Z)^2 \tag{4.7}$$

$$\phi = \text{Arc} \tan \frac{\text{Im } Z}{\text{Re } Z} \tag{4.8}$$

$$\text{Re } Z = |Z| \cos \phi \tag{4.9}$$

$$\text{Im } Z = |Z| \sin \phi \tag{4.10}$$

In Figure 4.1a, the equivalent circuit of an electrochemical interface is depicted; its impedance is:

$$Z(\omega) = \frac{E}{I} = R_1 + \frac{1}{\dfrac{1}{R_2} + jC\omega} = R_1 + \frac{R_2}{1 + \omega^2 C^2 R_2^2} - \frac{j\omega C R_2^2}{1 + \omega^2 C^2 R_2^2} \tag{4.11}$$

where E is the voltage, I is the current, R_1 and R_2 are the resistance values of the equivalent circuit, and C is the capacitance value of the equivalent circuit.

Furthermore,

$$|Z(\omega)| = \sqrt{\left(R_1 + \frac{R_2}{1 + \omega^2 C^2 R_2^2} \right)^2 + \left(\frac{\omega C^2 R_2^2}{1 + \omega^2 C^2 R_2^2} \right)^2} \tag{4.12}$$

When ω tends to zero, $|Z(\omega)|$ equals to $R_1 + R_2$. When ω tends to infinite, $|Z(\omega)|$ equals to R_1.

Note that the difference between the two limits is R_2. Therefore, the high-frequency intercept determines R_1 (the series resistance), whereas the low-frequency intercept yields the sum of $R_1 + R_2$. In simple terms, this means that at high frequencies, the capacitor conducts the current easily. Consequently, the impedance is solely due to the resistance R_1, whereas at low frequencies, the current flow via the capacitor is impeded. The current therefore flows through R_1 and R_2, and the impedance is given by the sum of the two resistors. At intermediate frequencies, the impedance takes a value somewhere between R_1 and $R_1 + R_2$ and thus has both real and imaginary components. This gives rise to the Cole–Cole plot semicircular shape, which corresponds to the equation as follows:

$$\left[Z' - \left(R_1 + \frac{R_2}{2} \right) \right]^2 + Z''^2 = \left(\frac{R_2}{2} \right)^2 \tag{4.13}$$

It has been shown that Equation 4.13 is analogous to the equation of a circle, with a radius of $\frac{R_2}{2}$ and a center at $(R_1 + \frac{R_2}{2}, 0)$. In all the materials studied, ω, R_1, and R_2 are greater than zero, thus resulting in a semicircle on the axis when plotted as function of frequency. $Z(\omega)$

is plotted in Figure 4.1b in terms of a Cole–Cole plot in the complex plane with the negative imaginary parts above the real axis, as is usually used in electrochemistry.

At the peak of the semicircle, the following condition is obtained:

$$\omega_{max} R_2 C = 1 \tag{4.14}$$

and hence

$$C = \frac{1}{2\pi f_{max} R_2} \tag{4.15}$$

where Equation 4.4 has been used. Knowing the value of R_2 and the frequency f_{max}, the value of the capacitance can be determined. It is possible to obtain all three parameters (R_1, R_2, and C) from the Cole–Cole plot as shown in Figure 4.1b, provided a sufficient frequency range is investigated.

The application of impedance spectroscopy to the characterization of polycrystalline materials started after Bauerle [2] showed that for zirconia with platinum electrodes, the individual polarizations of grain interiors, grain boundaries, and electrodes could be resolved in the admittance plane. He presented an equivalent circuit for his results, which have now proven to be typical of most solid electrolytes. In such a circuit, the individual elements correspond to grain interiors, grain boundaries, and electrodes connected in series. However, estimation of the circuit parameters was made complicated by Bauerle's choice of the admittance plane. Many subsequent researchers have therefore preferred to work in the impedance plane, that is, Cole–Cole plot, where a more direct relationship exists between the spectrum and the circuit [3,4]. The level of agreement between experiment and simulation is quite satisfactory for the grain interior and grain boundary arcs both in terms of shape and distribution of frequencies on the arcs, therefore supporting the view that equivalent circuits are a meaningful way of representing the data.

Measurement of the electrical conductivity for polycrystalline materials using impedance spectroscopy provides information related to the electrical behavior of the grain interiors, the grain boundary regions, and electrode. This is illustrated in Figure 4.2a, which contains the equivalent circuit for the electrical response of a polycrystalline material. The simple R–C parallel circuit in which three components are connected in series is often used to study the AC impedance behavior of materials. This circuit has a direct relationship to the complex impedance plot (Figure 4.2b) in which Z'', the imaginary part of the complex impedance, is plotted against Z', the real part, for a wide range of frequencies (typically 10^{-1}–10^7 Hz). The frequency increases as shown by the arrow in Figure 4.2b. The highest frequency is located at the origin. The resistances R_{gi}, R_{gb}, and R_e corresponding to the grain interior, grain boundary, and electrode, respectively, can be obtained from the intersections on the real axis of the corresponding semicircular arc. Comparing with the other two, R_e can normally be ignored except for the case of imperfect ohmic contacts which cause interfacial contact resistance. The capacitances C_{gi}, C_{gb}, and C_e corresponding to the grain interior, grain boundary, and electrode, respectively, can be obtained from Equation 4.15 [5].

The relationship between microstructural models and circuits shows its real merit when used to correlate the equivalent circuit parameters of a material with changes in the external conditions or the microstructure of the material. For example, in ceramics, where it is possible to resolve the resistances due to the grain interiors and the grain boundaries, it

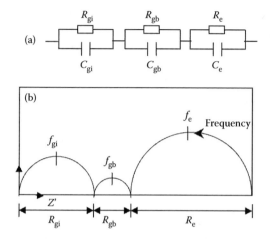

FIGURE 4.2

(a) An equivalent circuit representing a polycrystalline material. (b) An idealized complex impedance plot for a polycrystalline material showing contributions from the grain interiors (gi), grain boundaries (gb), and electrode interface (e). Note that $C_e \gg C_{gb} \gg C_{gi}$. (From Ye, H.T., PhD thesis, University College London, 2004. With permission.)

has facilitated the study of several important processes: sintering, grain growth, and solid-state precipitation. In diamond, it can facilitate the investigation of nucleation, growth, doping process, grain boundary deterioration, and nanocrystallization.

Conductivity Models

The impedance plots of polycrystalline materials can be related to their microstructure by means of physical models of the grain interior, grain boundary, and the electrode behavior. Three physical models used to describe the electronic materials are reviewed in details with their respective circuit equivalents [7].

The early model used to describe the properties of two-phase mixture is the series layer model. The model describes that the two phases are assumed to be stacked in layers parallel to the measuring electrodes, with total thickness of each phase made proportional to volume fractions X_1 and X_2. This model shows a linear mixing rule for the complex resistivity (ρ). The complex resistivity is the sum of the individual phase resistivity (ρ_1 and ρ_2):

$$\rho = X_1\rho_1 + X_2\rho_2 \tag{4.16}$$

In the parallel circuit model, the two phases are assumed to be stacked across the electrodes. For this model, the complex conductivity (σ) rather than resistivity follows a linear mixing rule:

$$\sigma = X_1\sigma_1 + X_2\sigma_2 \tag{4.17}$$

The widely used physical model is a more realistic one, which treats the microstructure as an array of cubic shaped grains with flat grain boundaries of finite thickness as shown in Figure 4.3 [8].

The volume fraction of grain boundaries is $3\delta/d$ (δ is grain boundary thickness and d is grain size) [7]. The current flow is assumed to be one-dimensional, and the current path

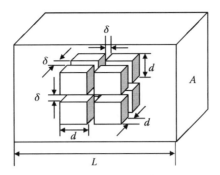

FIGURE 4.3
Brick layer model of idealized polycrystalline structure in which grains of dimensions d^3 are separated by grain boundaries of width δ. (From Maier, J., *Prog. Solid State Chem.*, 23, 171, 1995. With permission.)

at the corners of the grains is neglected. In this case, the two paths available to the current are either through the grains and across the grain boundary, or along grain boundaries, as depicted in Figure 4.3. Depending on the relative magnitudes of grain and grain boundary conductivity, one of the two paths may dominate. This model has been applied to many material systems, and according to this model, the bulk resistivity and the grain boundary resistivity may have different response [8].

In the brick layer model, the grain interior response will be displaced from the grain boundary response depending on the relaxation rate of charged species within each region. It is normal to compare the relaxation rates of different processes in terms of rate constant or relaxation time (τ); this can be defined as:

$$\tau = RC \tag{4.18}$$

In terms of grain interior rate constant, τ_{gi} can be expressed as follows:

$$R_{gi} = \frac{L}{A\sigma_{gi}} \tag{4.19}$$

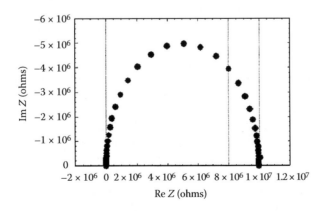

FIGURE 4.4
R–C in parallel. (From Ye, H.T., PhD thesis, University College London, 2004. With permission.)

$$C_{gi} = \frac{A\varepsilon_0\varepsilon_{gi}}{L} \tag{4.20}$$

and therefore

$$\tau_{gi} = \frac{\varepsilon_0\varepsilon_{gi}}{\sigma_{gi}} \tag{4.21}$$

where L is the sample length, A is the cross-sectional area, ε_0 is the permittivity of free space (8.854×10^{-12} F/m), and σ_{gi} and ε_{gi} are the electrical conductivity and relative dielectric constant of the grain interior, respectively.

The grain boundary relaxation time constant τ_{gb} can be expressed as follows [9]:

$$R_{gb} = \frac{L}{A\sigma_{sgb}}\frac{\delta}{d} \tag{4.22}$$

$$C_{gb} = \frac{A\varepsilon_0\varepsilon_{gb}}{L}\frac{d}{\delta} \tag{4.23}$$

and therefore

$$\tau_{gb} = \frac{\varepsilon_0\varepsilon_{gb}}{\sigma_{sgb}} \tag{4.24}$$

where d is the grain size, δ is the grain boundary width, and σ_{sgb} and ε_{gb} are the specific electrical conductivity and relative dielectric constant of the grain boundary, respectively. The resistance of the grain boundary is normally associated with the presence of a second phase or a constriction resistance, which can also result in a space charge region at the grain boundary. The capacitance of this region is thus associated with the polarization at the interface.

By applying the brick layer model and classic identification criteria comprehensively discussed in the literature [1,10–14], bulk (at high frequencies) and grain boundary (at low frequencies) contributions to the total materials' impedance were in each case distinguished.

This can be explained by the different relaxation rate of charged species within each region or the different R–C relaxation time of the elements. The defects, non-diamond phases, and impurities are believed to be accumulated preferentially within the grain boundaries than grain lattices [15]. The grain boundaries may induce dipole movements, which respond to an applied field with a delay [16]. Thus, the grain boundary contributions with a long relaxation time usually happen in the low frequencies and the grain bulk contributions with a short relaxation time in the high frequencies. In most cases, the sufficient difference in the capacitance of the R–C equivalent circuit rather than the resistance results in the two semicircles separated on the complex Cole–Cole plane [17].

The capacitance values of the grain boundary and grain interior are reported in the order of 10^{-9} and 10^{-12} F, respectively, for many polycrystalline material systems, for example, zirconia [7], bismuth titanate [18], ferroelectrics [19], and polycrystalline diamond [20].

One may ask why different materials show the similar capacitance values (10^{-9} F for grain boundaries and 10^{-12} F for the grain interiors) when analyzed in the Cole–Cole plot. The reason for this may be explained from the definition of the capacitance value itself as shown in Equations 4.20 and 4.23. The theoretical capacitance value associated with grain interiors has been defined in Equation 4.20. In practice, all the geometric parameters in this equation are not infinite to facilitate to carry out these experiments on a research laboratory basis. Thus, these geometric parameters normally have their expected magnitude order. L is the sample length within the order of millimeters (mm). A is the cross-sectional area within the order of 10 mm². ε_0 is the permittivity of free space (8.854×10^{-12} F/m). ε_{gi} is the relative dielectric constant of the grain interior of the sample. For high-purity diamond, the dielectric constant is reported to be about 5.7 [21]. Thus, formula 4.20 indicates that the grain interior capacitance from diamond is estimated about 0.5 pF.

The same A and L values can be applied to the grain boundary capacitance in Equation 4.23. In addition, the grain boundary–induced dipole polarization may cause the dielectric constant (ε_{gb}) to be slightly higher than that of grain bulk (ε_{gi}), but probably on the same magnitude order as grain bulk [15]. Furthermore, the grain size of a typical polycrystalline material is usually on the order of micrometers (μm), where the effective grain boundary width is expected to be on the order of nanometers (nm) [22]. Thus, the estimated grain boundary capacitance for a polycrystalline diamond is about 0.5 nF.

To gain further insight into these quantitative estimations, the ratio of the grain interior capacitance and grain boundary capacitance may be considered as follows:

$$\frac{C_{gi}}{C_{gb}} \approx \frac{\delta}{d} \tag{4.25}$$

Equation 4.25 indicates that the ratio of the grain capacitance and grain boundary capacitance is proportional to the ratio of the grain boundary width (δ) and grain size (d). In other words, the difference between the grain interior capacitance and grain boundary capacitance mainly originates from the geometric effect of the sample. This effect may be controlled by the following factors such as grain size, anisotropy, and porosity [1]. The typical geometric characteristic within a polycrystalline material leads to the grain boundary capacitance is normally two or three orders of magnitude higher than the grain interior capacitance.

The above discussion gives an explanation on the origin of the classic procedures and identification criteria for the grain boundary and grain bulk contributions in an ideal condition. In practice, it is difficult to calculate the theoretical capacitance of grain interior and grain boundaries for diamond. This is because the in-plane electrode measurement makes it unlikely to define the specific length and area of each sample. Cross-section electrode measurements make the geometric parameters solved easily, but most of impedance data cannot be detected across the samples due to extremely high resistance in diamond. Therefore, the conduction path identification criteria used in this chapter are emphasized on practical and empirical interpretations of materials based on the brick layer model discussed here.

Equivalent Circuits

This section presents impedance characterization on real electronic circuits made of resistors and capacitors rather than materials. Two types of circuits (R–C parallel and double

R–C parallel in series) have been studied. The impedance spectroscopy obtained from electronic circuits is analogous to that obtained from materials. Thus, impedance properties of materials can be represented by the relevant circuits, namely, equivalent circuits.

Resistor and Capacitor in Parallel

Figure 4.4 shows the impedance data for the circuit that has both a resistive and a capacitive component connected in parallel. The Cole–Cole plot is presented in a complex plane, where the negative values of the imaginary part (–ImZ) on the y-axis are versus the real part (ReZ) on the x-axis. Each data point corresponds to a different frequency. When represented in the Cole–Cole plot, the impedance spectra lead to a succession of semicircles. The resistor represents either ionic or electric conduction mechanism, whereas the capacitor represents the polarizability of the material.

The complex impedance Z^* measured by impedance spectroscopy can be expressed as a function of the resistance R and capacitance C, as follows:

$$Z^* = Z' - jZ'' \tag{4.26}$$

$$Z' = \frac{R}{1 + \omega^2 R^2 C^2} \tag{4.27}$$

$$Z'' = \frac{\omega R^2 C}{1 + \omega^2 R^2 C^2} \tag{4.28}$$

$$\left(Z' - \frac{R}{2}\right)^2 + Z''^2 = \left(\frac{R}{2}\right)^2 \tag{4.29}$$

Here, Z' and Z'' represent the real and imaginary parts of the impedance, respectively, and ω is the angular frequency. When plotted for different frequencies in a complex plane, Equation 4.29 takes the form of a semicircle. In this case, the second intercept of the semicircle with the real axis is the bulk resistance (R) of the sample. This equivalent circuit can be used to represent the properties of both single-crystalline diamond films and polycrystalline diamond films with one dominating conduction path. Table 4.1 compares the AC impedance for basic circuit elements, such as resistor (R), capacitor (C), and inductor (L). These are the basis of the AC electronic circuits.

TABLE 4.1

AC Impedances for Circuit Elements, Namely, Resistor (R), Capacitor (C), and Inductor (L)

Circuit Element	AC Impedance Equation
Resistor (R)	$z = R + 0j \quad j = \sqrt{-1}$
Capacitor (C)	$z = 0 - \dfrac{j}{\omega C} \quad \omega = 2\pi f$
Inductor (L)	$z = 0 + j\omega L \quad \omega = 2\pi f$

Double Resistor and Capacitor Parallel in Series

Figure 4.5 shows the impedance spectrum for the double resistor and capacitor parallel in series. The circuit has a direct relationship to the Cole–Cole plot. The highest frequency is located at the origin. The resistances R_1 and R_2 can be obtained from the diameters of the semicircles in this plot. Here the resistor R represents either an ionic or an electronic conduction mechanism, whereas the capacitor C represents the polarizability of the diamond. The symbols R_1, R_2, C_1, and C_2 have the same meaning as before for two-layer dielectrics.

The measured complex impedance Z^* can be expressed as a function of R_1, R_2, C_1, and C_2 in the following way:

$$Z^* = Z' - jZ'' \tag{4.30}$$

$$Z' = \frac{R_1}{1+\omega^2 R_1^2 C_1^2} + \frac{R_2}{1+\omega^2 R_2^2 C_2^2} \tag{4.31}$$

$$Z'' = \frac{\omega R_1^2 C_1}{1+\omega^2 R_1^2 C_1^2} + \frac{\omega R_2^2 C_2}{1+\omega^2 R_2^2 C_2^2} \tag{4.32}$$

where Z' and Z'' represent the real and imaginary portions of the impedance, respectively, and ω is the angular frequency. When plotted in a complex plane, Z'' versus Z' takes the form of two semicircles. In such a representation, a two-layer contribution is easily identified. Note that critical to the identification of each single resistor and capacitor in parallel is the simulated capacitance value for each semicircle. This model is well suited to simulate the resistance and capacitance associated with the grain boundary and grain interior.

Formulae for Capacitance

It is known that the electrical contribution from grains, grain boundaries, and/or electrodes for a certain polycrystalline material system can be extracted and separated. As

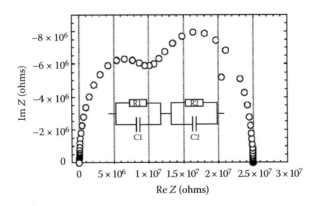

FIGURE 4.5
Double *R–C* parallel in series. (From Ye, H.T., PhD thesis, University College London, 2004. With permission.)

such the simulated capacitance value obtained in each Cole–Cole plot plays a crucial role in assigning the origin of each semicircle response. Therefore, understanding and calculating the dielectric parameters especially the capacitance value become essential. This section describes the formulae for the capacitance in both one-layer and two-layer dielectrics.

One-Layer Model

When a voltage is applied to a parallel-plate capacitor in vacuum, the capacitor will store charge. In the presence of a dielectric, an additional phenomenon happens within the dielectric, which allows the capacitor to store more charge.

For an empty plate capacitor, the capacitance in the electrostatic system is given by:

$$C_0 = \frac{\text{area}}{4\pi d} \tag{4.33}$$

where d is the distance between plates.

$$C = 4\pi\varepsilon_0 C_0 \tag{4.34}$$

Note that these formulae neglect the fringing of the field at the edges of the capacitor plates. When a capacitor is filled with a dielectric, its static capacitance is given by:

$$C = 4\pi\varepsilon_0\varepsilon_s C_0 \tag{4.35}$$

Here again, fringe fields have been neglected.

The capacitance under dynamic conditions may be expressed in terms of $\varepsilon^*(\omega)$.

The complex capacitance thus becomes:

$$C^*(\omega) = 4\pi\varepsilon_0 C_0\varepsilon^*(\omega) \tag{4.36}$$

Alternating current measurements give the impedance $Z^*(\omega)$ of the capacitor containing the dielectric, which is related to the complex capacitance by

$$Z^*(\omega) = \frac{1}{i\omega C^*(\omega)} \tag{4.37}$$

The impedance can be represented by an equivalent circuit. For a given frequency ω, an impedance can be represented by a large number of possible equivalent circuits, the simplest of which are the parallel and the series circuit.

Table 4.2 compares the characteristics of these circuits for a given ω. If the same dielectric is represented in one case by the parallel circuit and in the other case by the series circuit, then:

$$\tan\delta = \frac{1}{\omega C_p R_p} = \omega C_s R_s \tag{4.38}$$

TABLE 4.2

Characteristics of R–C Circuits in Series and in Parallel at a Given Frequency, Respectively

Circuit	R_s and C_s in Series	R_p and C_p in Parallel
$Z^*(\omega)$	$R_s - \dfrac{i}{\omega C_s}$	$\dfrac{R_p}{1 + i\omega C_p R_p}$
$\lvert Z(\omega) \rvert$	$\dfrac{1}{\omega C_s}\sqrt{1 + \omega^2 C_s^2 R_s^2}$	$\dfrac{R_p}{\sqrt{1 + \omega^2 C_p^2 R_p^2}}$
$C^*(\omega) = \dfrac{1}{i\omega Z^*(\omega)}$	$\dfrac{C_s}{1 + i\omega C_s R_s}$	$C_p - \dfrac{i}{\omega R_p}$
$\tan\delta$	$\omega C_s R_s$	$\dfrac{1}{\omega C_p R_p}$
τ	$C_s R_s$	$\dfrac{1}{\omega^2 C_p R_p}$

whereas the values of the equivalent series and parallel components are related by

$$\frac{C_p}{C_s} = \frac{1}{1 + \tan^2\delta} \tag{4.39}$$

and

$$\frac{R_p}{R_s} = \frac{1 + \tan^2\delta}{\tan^2\delta} \tag{4.40}$$

In the parallel representation, it is convenient to work with the resistivity of a material, which is measured as the resistance between electrodes applied to opposite faces of a cube of unit edge. A capacitor of these dimensions has, in the electrostatic system, a capacitance $C_0 = 1/4\pi$ cm, so that Equation 4.37 gives

$$\varepsilon^*(\omega) = \frac{1}{\varepsilon_0} C^*(\omega) \tag{4.41}$$

or, in the parallel representation,

$$\varepsilon^*(\omega) = \frac{1}{\varepsilon_0}\left(C_p(\omega) - \frac{i}{\omega R_p(\omega)} \right) = \frac{1}{\varepsilon_0}\left(C_p(\omega) - \frac{i}{\omega}\gamma(\omega) \right) \tag{4.42}$$

where $\gamma(\omega)$ is the conductivity, C_p is the capacitance, and $\varepsilon^*(\omega)$ is expressed in e.s.u.

Frequency dependence of permittivity (ε), conductivity (γ), resistivity (ρ), and dielectric loss ($\tan\delta$) in the one-layer dielectrics model is shown in Figure 4.6. From the position

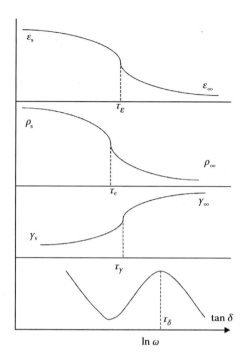

FIGURE 4.6
Examples of calculated curves give the dependence of permittivity (ε), conductivity (γ), resistivity (ρ), and dielectric loss (tan δ) on ln ω in the one-layer dielectrics model. (From Ye, H.T., PhD thesis, University College London, 2004. With permission.)

of the curves along the frequency axis, the relevant dielectric relaxation times may be derived.

Cross-Section Two-Layer Model

Apart from the simple R–C circuits described above, the most useful equivalent circuits are that of the two-layer model. Figure 4.7 shows the electrode configuration of cross-section measurements of the two-layer model. The two-layer model represents two layers of dielectric of thicknesses d_1 and d_2, static dielectric constants ε_1 and ε_2, and direct conductivities γ_1 and γ_2.

Volger [23] evaluates the frequency dependent behavior of this model in terms of the following formulae:

$$\varepsilon(\omega) = \frac{\varepsilon_s + \varepsilon_\infty \tau_\varepsilon^2 \omega^2}{1 + \tau_\varepsilon^2 \omega^2} \tag{4.43}$$

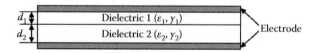

FIGURE 4.7
Electrode configuration of cross-section measurement of two-layer dielectrics model. (From Volger, J., *Prog. Semicond.*, 4, 209, 1960. With permission.)

$$\gamma'(\omega) = \frac{\gamma_s + \gamma_\infty \tau_\gamma^2 \omega^2}{1 + \tau_\gamma^2 \omega^2} \tag{4.44}$$

$$\rho''(\omega) = \frac{\rho_s + \rho_\infty \tau_\rho^2 \omega^2}{1 + \tau_\rho^2 \omega^2} \tag{4.45}$$

$$\tan\delta = \frac{\gamma_\infty}{\varepsilon_0 \omega \varepsilon_\infty} \frac{\left(\dfrac{\varepsilon_\infty \gamma_s}{\varepsilon_s \gamma_\infty}\right) + \tau_\delta^2 \omega^2}{1 + \tau_\delta^2 \omega^2} \tag{4.46}$$

with

$$\tau_\varepsilon = \tau_\gamma = \varepsilon_0 \frac{\varepsilon_s - \varepsilon_\infty}{\gamma_\infty - \gamma_s} = \varepsilon_0 \frac{\varepsilon_1 d_2 + \varepsilon_2 d_1}{\gamma_1 d_2 + \gamma_2 d_1} \tag{4.47}$$

$$\tau_\rho = \left(\frac{\gamma_\infty}{\gamma_s}\right)^{1/2} \cdot \tau_\varepsilon \tag{4.48}$$

$$\tau_\delta = \left(\frac{\varepsilon_\infty}{\varepsilon_s}\right)^{1/2} \cdot \tau_\varepsilon \tag{4.49}$$

$$\varepsilon_s = \frac{(d_1 + d_2)}{\left(\dfrac{d_1}{\gamma_1} + \dfrac{d_2}{\gamma_2}\right)^2} \cdot \left(\frac{d_1 \varepsilon_1}{\gamma_1^2} + \frac{d_2 \varepsilon_2}{\gamma_2^2}\right) \tag{4.50}$$

$$\varepsilon_\infty = \frac{d_1 + d_2}{\dfrac{d_1}{\varepsilon_1} + \dfrac{d_2}{\varepsilon_2}} \tag{4.51}$$

$$\gamma_s = \frac{d_1 + d_2}{\dfrac{d_1}{\gamma_1} + \dfrac{d_2}{\gamma_2}} \tag{4.52}$$

$$\gamma_\infty = \frac{(d_1 + d_2)}{\left(\dfrac{d_1}{\varepsilon_1} + \dfrac{d_2}{\varepsilon_2}\right)^2} \cdot \left(\frac{d_1 \gamma_1}{\varepsilon_1^2} + \frac{d_2 \gamma_2}{\varepsilon_2^2}\right) \tag{4.53}$$

Equations 4.50 through 4.53 give the static and high-frequency values for the composite dielectric, whereas the meaning of the three relaxation times is clearly shown.

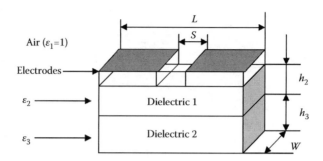

FIGURE 4.8
Electrode configuration of in-plane measurement of two-layer dielectrics model.

In-Plane Two-Layer Model

Figure 4.8 illustrates the electrode configuration of in-plane measurement of the two-layer dielectrics model. Formulae for the in-plane capacitance of the two-layer structure are shown below.

The total capacitance of the multilayer capacitor is calculated as the sum of partial capacitances

$$C = C_1 + C_2 + C_3 \tag{4.54}$$

where C_1, C_2, and C_3 are the capacitances of air, dielectric 1, and dielectric 2, respectively [24,25]. More complicated formulae corresponding to n parallel circuits have been given by Volger [23].

$$C_1 = w\varepsilon_0 \frac{2}{\pi} \ln\left(\frac{4L}{S}\right) \tag{4.55}$$

$$C_2 = \frac{w\varepsilon_0(\varepsilon_2 - \varepsilon_3)}{s/h2 + (4/\pi)\ln 2} \tag{4.56}$$

$$C_3 = w\varepsilon_0(\varepsilon_3 - 1)\frac{1}{\pi}\ln\left(16\frac{h2 + h3}{\pi s}\right) \tag{4.57}$$

Impedance Spectroscopy on Diamond-Based Materials

In this section, impedance measurements on a variety of diamond-based materials will be discussed, which include single-crystalline, polycrystalline, and nanocrystalline.

Boron-Doped Single-Crystalline Diamond

The most effective method of modifying electronic properties of a material is through intentional doping. Boron is known to promote the formation of acceptor states giving rise to p-type conductivity in the diamond films [26–29]. The investigation of boron impurities as a deep acceptor (0.37 eV ionization energy) has been extremely fruitful over the past 30 years. Collins et al. [30] determined the activation energy of the p-type behavior in type IIb diamond based on the model containing both acceptors and donors levels. They measured a mean value of 0.368 eV. Lightowlers et al. [31] utilized the *I–V* and *C–V* characteristic of a Au Schottky barrier to correlate quantitatively the active carriers in the diamond film to the boron concentration in the film. They concluded that the acceptors responsible were probably substitutional boron. Sandhu et al. [32] reported a sharp optical absorption at 2963 cm^{-1} (0.37 eV) in diamond films coimplanted by carbon and boron. Masood et al. [33] reported a simple method of boron doping using a solid boron source and the dopant activation energies in the range of 0.30–0.38 eV.

Malta et al. [34] compared the electronic transport properties in boron-doped homoepitaxial, polycrystalline and natural single-crystalline diamond using Hall-effect and resistivity measurements. They proposed that carrier trapping at grain boundaries result in charge build-up that impedes the motion of carriers from one crystallite to the next, thereby decreasing their mobility. If grain size and acceptor concentration are both sufficiently large, the grain boundaries will significantly degrade mobility but have a negligible effect on carrier concentration. The intragranular structural defects commonly exist as stacking faults, twins, and dislocations. They are not expected to dominate over the effect of grain boundaries; however, they may be still contributing to the degradation of mobility. Kalish et al. [35] concluded that graphitization along grain boundaries that one might have expected to happen due to boron implantation and following annealing does not seem to affect the electrical properties of the implantation-doped material. In the same year, Werner et al. [36] reported the charge transport in heavily B-doped polycrystalline diamond films. They found that the decrease in activation energy with increasing doping concentration can be explained in terms of impurity conduction. At sufficiently high doping concentrations, the impurity band merges with the valence band and metallic conduction occurs. Won et al. [37] reported that the crystalline quality and phase purity are much better for the boron-doped diamond (BDD) than for the undoped diamond through cathodoluminescence spectrum. Boron incorporation eliminates the exciton-related emission. Negative electron affinity has been observed in BDD using scanning filed emission spectroscopy by Wang et al. [38]. They described detailed spatial correlation between filed emission sites and diamond morphology, surface work function, and diamond quality. Sternschulte et al. [39] observed the bound exciton spectrum and demonstrated the presence of isolated boron on substitutional lattice sites which implies electrical acceptor activity.

Liu et al. [40] reported a very small electron affinity of about 0.025 eV and a work function of 5.165 eV for the BDD (100) surface from frequency dependence capacitance–voltage spectroscopy measurements. They measured the boron acceptor concentration of ~10^{17} cm^{-3} in diamond using capacitance spectroscopy. They argued that there might be several electronic processes in a material, each with its specific time constant; the time constant connected to the Schottky barrier may overlap with other time constants. It may not be possible to obtain doping concentration just from CV measurement at a single frequency, and complex impedance measurement and analysis are necessary. A year after, from the same group Liu et al. [41] reported the activation energy of 0.36 eV for BDD using the flat-band capacitance method. Jaeger et al. [42] calculated the internal electrostatic potential distribution and resistivity of BDD using a finite element analysis. They found the dominating conduction mechanism shifts from the valence-band conduction at intermediate temperature to the hopping conduction at low temperatures. Chen et al. [43] correlated the electron field emission properties of BDD with secondary ion mass spectroscopy and infrared absorption and concluded that the solubility limit of boron in diamond is $(B^{+3})_s = 5 \times 10^{21}$ cm^{-3}, and the largest boron concentration that can be incorporated as substitutional dopants is only one-tenth of the solubility limit, $(B^{+3})_d = 5 \times 10^{20}$ cm^{-3}. The diamond lattices are strongly strained when heavily doped. Krutko et al. [44] produced p-type polycrystalline diamond layers by rapid diffusion of boron. Gevrey et al. [45] used a contactless method to measure the conductivity of BDD films at microwave frequencies, which has an advantage to avoid parasitic resistance or grain boundaries, although the skin effect has to be considered. Lyman spectra in the infrared, electronic Raman scattering, and cathodoluminescence in the UV have revealed much of the complex electronic structure of this shallow acceptor. Nebel et al. [46] detected the long living excited states in BDD in the energy regime 3.2–3.5 eV.

To date, only boron has clearly demonstrated and established itself conclusively to be an active electrically active dopant, and a wide range of techniques have been applied to BDD to investigate their electrical activation energy and defect levels. However, less work has been found to characterize BDD films using AC impedance spectroscopy to the best of the author's knowledge. Narducci and Cuomo [47] investigated the boron diffusivity in diamond single crystals by impedance spectroscopy at a very early stage. They reported that diffusivity of boron in diamond at up to 800°C will not make the thermal drift of impurities a major path to device failure. However, their impedance measurement was only up to 10^5 Hz without temperature dependence; the results presented still did not give full understanding of responsible mechanism behind.

In this section, initial attention has been paid on boron-doped single-crystalline diamond films. Room-temperature DC current–voltage measurements between two symmetric electrodes across the surface of the diamond films were carried out. Voltage is set from –10 to 10 V. Direct current current–temperature measurements were investigated using Keithley 487 Picoammeter under rough vacuum from –185°C to 256°C. Voltage is set to 50 V as power supply. Impedance measurement of the films was determined using a Solartron 1260A electrochemical impedance spectroscopy (EIS) in the frequency range from 0.1 Hz to 10 MHz, and in the temperature range from –100°C to 300°C. The setup parameters are 0.05 V of AC amplitude, 1 s integration time, and no delay time.

Figure 4.9 shows room temperature DC current–voltage measurement on the surface of the diamond films in two electrode directions: (1) from up to down and (2) from left to right. Comparing the curves in both directions, Figure 4.9b measured from left electrode to right shows nearly a perfect ohmic contact, which has a symmetric and linear characteristic from the negative to positive voltage. It is easily estimated that the room temperature resistance is about 1.1 MΩ. To investigate the DC temperature effect in this electrode direction, the current–temperature (–185°C to 256°C) curves are shown in Figure 4.10. It is found that the current increases exponentially with the temperature increasing, which indicates thermally activated conduction process. Linear curve fitting shows the sample has activation energy of 0.36 eV. The result is consistent with most of the other people reported on BDD [29].

Simple DC electrical experiments have now been repeated to achieve the activation energy of BDD, 0.37 eV, which is already well known within diamond community for a number of years. For the first time, we applied impedance spectroscopy to the boron-doped single-crystalline diamond sample to compare the AC results with DC and to

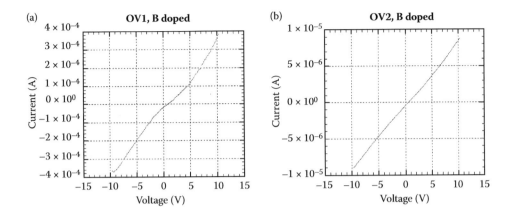

FIGURE 4.9
Room temperature current–voltage measurements between two symmetric electrodes across the surface of the diamond films. (From Ye, H., *Phys. Status Solidi A Appl. Res.*, 193, 462, 2002. With permission.)

prove if this technique is valid on this type of film. The Cole–Cole plots of boron-doped single-crystalline diamond films from 50°C to 300°C are shown in Figure 4.11a–c. Figure 4.11a presents the data measured at 50°C showing the presence of a single semicircular response, with some scatters at the low frequency impedance range (right end). Similar data are shown in Figure 4.11b for the temperature range from 125°C to 200°C. The diameter of the semicircles reduces dramatically with the temperature increasing: (a) 50°C and 100°C, (b) 125°C and 200°C, and (c) 225°C and 300°C.

It is found that each Cole–Cole plot shows only one depressed semicircle. The single semicircle indicates that only one primary mechanism exists for the electrical conduction within the diamond film at temperatures below 300°C. The depressed semicircles make their centers on a line below the real axis, which indicates the departure from the ideal Debye behavior [1]. The diameter of each semicircle indicates the electrical resistance of

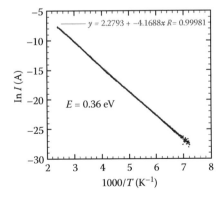

FIGURE 4.10
DC current–temperature measurement using TSC chamber from –185°C to 256°C. Voltage is set to 50 V as power supply. Linear curve fitting from –134°C to 147°C shows the sample has a DC activation energy of 0.36 eV. OV1 is from up to down, and OV2 is from left to the right as shown in Figure 4.9. (From Ye, H., *Phys. Status Solidi A Appl. Res.*, 193, 462, 2002. With permission.)

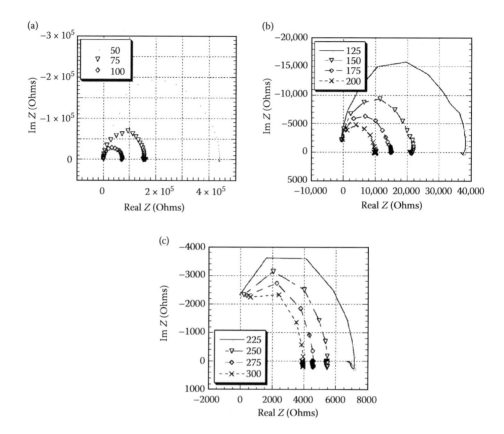

FIGURE 4.11

AC impedance measurements on boron-doped single-crystalline diamond films, from 0.1 Hz to 10 MHz, vacuum pressure: 0.05 mbar, AC amplitude: 0.1 V, from 50°C to 300°C. (From Ye, H., *Phys. Status Solidi A Appl. Res.*, 193, 462, 2002. With permission.)

diamond films. With the increase in temperature, the diameter decreases indicating the reduction of the resistance from 400 kΩ at 50°C to 5 kΩ at 300°C.

A central issue to be addressed is what portion of the equivalent circuit (see Figure 4.2) corresponds to the observed single semicircular response. This interpretation is centered to determine the dominance of impedance from grain interiors or grain boundaries or otherwise injection from the electrodes. For ionic conductors, electrode porosity and polarization must be considered for the general impedance analysis [2], whereas for diamond, different electrode configuration effects have been investigated, and the results show no significant variation in impedance spectroscopy due to its large resistance discrimination between diamond and electrode. Therefore, the impedance contribution from the electrodes could be ignored in diamond-based high-resistive materials.

Critical to the identification of the grain boundary and grain interior contribution is the simulated capacitance value for each semicircle. It has already been established in literature that the lower frequency dispersion corresponds to the grain boundaries and the higher frequency dispersion corresponds to the grain bulk interior if two semicircles appear, which normally have a capacitance value in the range of nF and pF, respectively [48–50].

The parallel resistance, capacitance, and relaxation frequency in each semicircle have been simulated using Zview software supplied by Solartron Inc. The detailed values are shown by M'peko et al. [14]. It is obvious that all the capacitance values is in the range of pF. This implies that the single semicircular response is from grain interiors, which is expected from a single-crystal diamond (SCD) where no grain boundaries are being involved. Huang et al. [51] reported a very interesting result that boron atoms are deseg-regated at grain boundaries and are uniformly distributed inside each diamond grain by using Auger and secondary ion mass spectroscopy (SIMS) techniques. Based on their observation, it was suggested that boron dopants make a significant contribution in the conduction path within grain interiors instead of grain boundaries either for polycrystal-line diamond films or single-crystalline.

The electrical resistance is plotted against temperature in an Arrhenius plot shown in Figure 4.12. Linear curve fitting shows that the sample has an activation energy of 0.37 eV, which is possibly the data at low carrier concentrations [28]. Comparing activation energy from AC impedance with the one from DC measurements (0.36 eV), we can summarize that they are consistent with each other.

Impedance spectroscopy on boron-doped single-crystalline diamond has proved to be an effective way to provide electrical information on a microscopic basis. Another advan-tage is its low amplitude of source voltage, which offers a nondestructive method to char-acterize the system. Thus, it could become an alternating approach to traditional electrical characterization techniques in many other semiconductor materials, correlating electrical with physical properties in both materials science and electronic engineering.

Polycrystalline Diamond

For many industrial applications such as cutting tools, optical components, and microelec-tronic devices, the control of film structure and morphology is of great importance. The crystallite size, orientation, and surface roughness have a profound effect on the mechani-cal, electrical, and optical properties of the films deposited. A few research papers on scan-ning electron microscopy (SEM) analysis of diamond films have related the morphological

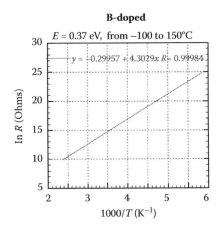

FIGURE 4.12
Temperature dependence of resistance from the impedance spectroscopy. (From Ye, H., *Phys. Status Solidi A Appl. Res.*, 193, 462, 2002. With permission.) Linear curve fitting from −100°C to 150°C shows that the sample has AC activation energy of 0.37 eV, which is consistent with the theoretical value published.

development to the deposition parameters. Moreover, the polycrystalline morphology has been related to Raman spectroscopy and x-ray diffraction measurements. An excellent review has been given by Zhu et al. [52]. A morphology field map has been presented [53] that depicts different zones of surface texture of diamond films as a function of methane concentration in hydrogen and substrate temperature. Tang et al. [54] reported that the film of best quality has very smooth crystalline facets free of second nucleation, and the full width at half maximum of the diamond Raman peak is 2.2 cm^{-1}, as narrow as that of IIa natural diamond. Larson and Girshick [55] concluded increasing substrate temperature causes the film morphology to shift from {100} toward {111} faceting. Although a number of different chemical vapor deposition (CVD) techniques have been developed to deposit diamond films, the study of the factors controlling the morphology, quality, and related properties of the deposited films is far from complete [56,57]. Among the multitude of diamond CVD processes that have been developed for about 20 years, the microwave plasma–enhanced CVD process (MPECVD), together with the hot-filament CVD method (HFCVD), has continued to be one of the most used diamond deposition processes. This section compares the impedance properties of polycrystalline films deposited using both MPECVD and HFCVD methods.

Free-standing diamond films grown by microwave plasma–enhanced CVD and hot-filament CVD were used to investigate the influence of the film quality on the impedance spectrum.

SEM photographs of investigated films are shown in Figure 4.13. MPECVD diamond film shows a well-faceted and polycrystalline morphology with (111) triangle crystal orientation dominating. However, HFCVD diamond shows a rather rougher surface than MPECVD with the merging surface of different crystal orientations. Rounded and layered morphology was also observed for HFCVD diamond. The corresponding Raman spectra are shown in Figure 4.14. MPECVD diamond has a sharp peak at 1331 cm^{-1}, which is characteristic of high-purity diamond and a tiny shoulder at about 1580 cm^{-1}, which is the signal of graphite phases embedded in this sample. The HFCVD film shows a typical diamond peak at 1331 cm^{-1} as well, but the intensity of this peak is much lower in the HFCVD diamond than in the MPECVD diamond. In addition, there is a broader shoulder

(a)   (b)

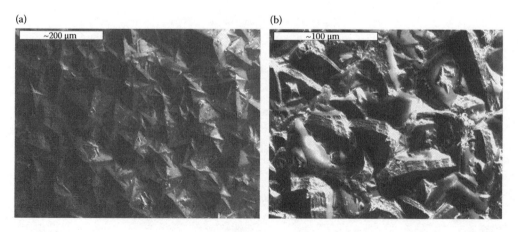

FIGURE 4.13
SEM photographs of MPECVD diamond film (a) and HFCVD diamond film (b). (From Ye, H.T., PhD thesis, University College London, 2004. With permission.)

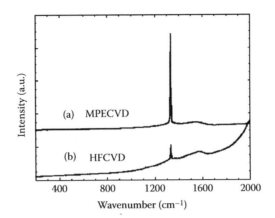

FIGURE 4.14
Raman spectroscopy of MPECVD (a) and HFCVD (b) diamond films. (From Ye, H.T., PhD thesis, University College London, 2005. With permission.)

at 1580 cm^{-1} that indicates that the HFCVD diamond has more graphite and non-diamond phases formed during the CVD process.

The Cole–Cole plots for MPECVD diamond films from 25°C to 400°C are shown in Figure 4.15. The Cole–Cole plot at room temperature shows the presence of a single semi-circular response, with some scatters in the data of the low frequency range. Similar data are shown for the other temperature ranges. The diameters of the semicircle response reduce dramatically with the temperature increase. At 400°C, the semicircular response is accompanied by a linear tail extended to low frequency. It is found that each Cole–Cole plot shows only one depressed semicircle. The single semicircle indicates that only one primary mechanism exists for the electrical conduction within the diamond film at temperatures below 300°C. The depressed semicircles make their centers on a line below the real axis, which indicates the departure from the ideal Debye behavior [1]. The diameter of each semicircle indicates the electrical resistance of diamond films. With increasing temperature, the diameter decreases indicating the reduction of the resistance from 62 MΩ at room temperature to 4 kΩ at 300°C. The Cole–Cole plot at 400°C shows a small semicircle and a long linear tail at low frequency. Such phenomena have been observed in other systems and have been attributed to the AC polarization of diamond/electrode interface at this high temperature [48].

The Cole–Cole plots for HFCVD diamond films from 25°C to 300°C are shown in Figure 4.16. The Cole–Cole plot at room temperature shows the presence of an arc, instead of a complete semicircle, with a linear trend at the low-frequency impedance range. Similar data are shown at other temperatures. The diameters of these arcs reduce dramatically with the temperature increase. It is difficult to derive the thermal activation energy for HFCVD diamond because there are no clear semicircles in their Cole–Cole plots. However, through the simulation of the each arc, it was found that the capacitance value for each arc is maintained at 0.7 pF, which indicates that the impedance spectrum is from the grain interior.

A central issue to be addressed is which portion of the equivalent circuit in Figure 4.2 corresponds to the observed single semicircular response. This interpretation is centered to determine the dominance of conduction from grain interiors or grain boundaries or otherwise injection from the electrodes. For ionic conductors, electrode porosity and polarization must be considered for the general impedance analysis [2], whereas for diamond, different electrode configuration effects have been investigated [48], and the results show

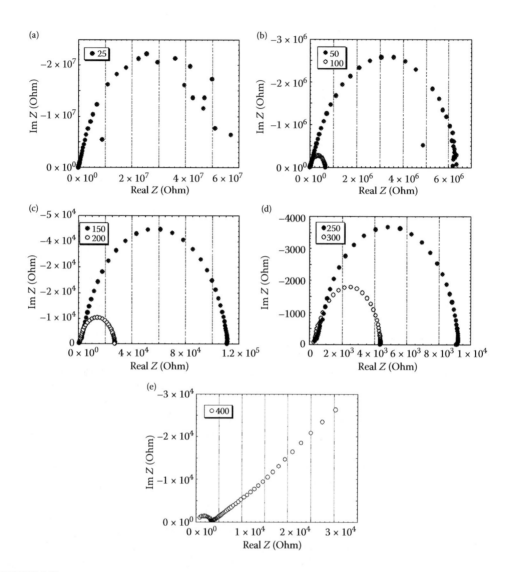

FIGURE 4.15

Cole–Cole plots of MPECVD diamond films at different temperatures: (a) 25°C, (b) 50°C and 100°C, (c) 150°C and 200°C, (d) 250 and 300°C, and (e) 400°C. (From Ye, H.T., PhD thesis, University College London, 2006. With permission.)

no significant variation in impedance spectroscopy because of its large resistance difference between diamond and electrode. Therefore, the impedance contribution from the electrodes could be ignored in diamond-based materials that are less conductive.

Critical to the identification of the grain boundary and grain interior contribution is the simulated capacitance value for each semicircle. Experimentally, the low-frequency dispersion corresponds to the grain boundaries and the higher-frequency dispersion corresponds to the grain bulk interior if two semicircles appear, which normally have capacitance values in a nF and pF range, respectively [59]. The resistance and capacitance values for each semicircle (in Figure 4.15) have been simulated using Zview software supplied by Solartron Inc. It is apparent that all the capacitance values are in the range of 0.2 nF.

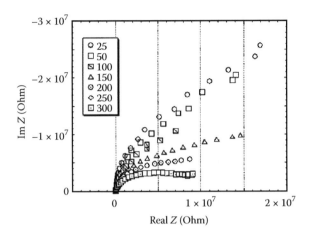

FIGURE 4.16
Cole–Cole plots of HFCVD diamond films at different temperatures. (From Ye, H.T., PhD thesis, University College London, 2007. With permission.)

This indicates that these single semicircular responses for MPECVD diamond films are attributed to grain boundaries. In Figure 4.17, the calculated resistance for the MPECVD diamond within the Cole–Cole plot, which persists over the whole temperature range investigated here, is presented in a logarithmic plot against reciprocal of temperature. A straight line is apparent, enabling a single electrical activation energy to be estimated from the slope of the curves. The activation energy is found to be about 0.51 eV, which is consistent with the results on deep-level transient spectroscopy [60].

HFCVD diamond is also called *thermal management grade diamond* or *low electronic grade diamond*. It contains more defects and non-diamond phases incorporated during the process of CVD. The growth speed for HFCVD diamond is 10 times faster than for MPECVD, and the quality within both grains and grain boundaries deteriorates [61]. In the HFCVD diamond, both grains and grain boundaries are thought to have contributions to the impedance value. Since the contribution from grains is much stronger

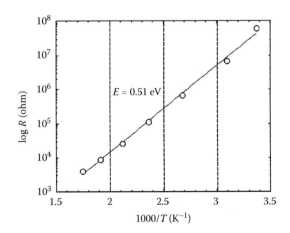

FIGURE 4.17
Temperature dependence of electrical resistance on MPECVD diamond films. (From Ye, H.T., PhD thesis, University College London, 2008. With permission.)

than that from grain boundaries, the effect from grain boundaries are negligible. In the MPECVD diamond, the grain boundary conduction is dominating because the high resistance associated with the high-purity diamond grain interiors prevents the current from flowing through the grains. In MPECVD diamond, the only possible way for the current to flow is through the grain boundaries, where graphite and non-diamond phases are embedded.

It can be seen that MPECVD and HFCVD diamond films have different dominating conduction paths within the material itself. This is due to the specific chemical reactions of different CVD processes. The HFCVD technique is the simplest commonly used CVD method for diamond synthesis. It was first described by Matsumoto et al. [62]. The thermal energy required for dissociation of molecular hydrogen into atomic hydrogen is supplied by a refractory metal filament (Ta and W) usually heated to about 1900–2000°C; at these temperatures, a dissociation efficiency of approximately 10% can achieved [63]. However, the filaments have a limited lifetime due to carburization of filament, and physical degradation of the filament usually contaminates the diamond film with metallic impurities. MPECVD technique is also the most commonly used method for activation of hydrogen, which was first reported by the National Institute for Research in Inorganic Materials in Japan [64]. Microwaves are introduced into a deposition chamber that is designed such that a standing wave is created producing a plasma ball just above the substrate; microwaves at 2.45 GHz are usually used. MPECVD produces some of the best-quality CVD diamond, with slower growth rates and larger area than that of HFCVD method. These two different growth techniques have resulted in the deposition of CVD diamond films with different quality as witnessed by SEM, Raman, and impedance spectroscopy. Both materials have led to widespread interest in the field of electronic device and electronic packaging application as potentially revolutionary materials.

Nanocrystalline Diamond

The emergence of CVD technique for the growth of thin film diamond has led to widespread interest in the use of this material for electronic applications. The focus of most growth studies to date has been in the production of high-quality, large-grain polycrystalline diamond, with the realization of single-crystalline material remaining a key aim of the diamond research community. Early reports on fine-grained nanocrystalline diamond received less attention, since they did not appear to fit with these aims [65]. However, this position has recently changed, with the properties of nanocrystalline films themselves being recognized as potentially useful for many applications in fields as diverse as electrochemical electrodes, tribology, cold cathodes, corrosion resistance, and conformal coatings on microelectromechanical systems (MEMS) devices [66–73].

A variety of deposition techniques and conditions have been used to grow the nanocrystalline diamond films. Among these are remote microwave plasma [74], microwave plasma [75], direct current arc [76], hot filament CVD [77], glow discharge radiofrequency (RF) [78], carbon sputtering [79], and electron–cyclotron resonance [80]. Erz et al. [74] grew 800-nm-thick films with 10% CH_4 in H_2, which were characterized by x-ray diffraction, Raman, and visible infrared spectroscopy. Konov et al. [80] and Nistor et al. [81] produced 0.2- to 1-µm-thick films from $CH_4/H_2/Ar$ mixtures that were characterized chiefly with XRD, Raman, and high-resolution transmission electron microscopy (TEM). The Ar ratio in the mixtures was kept at 50%. Grain sizes were found to be in the range 30–50 nm. TEM did not reveal amorphous carbon in significant quantities, but disordered sp^3- and sp^2-bonded amorphous carbon was detected, presumably located at grain boundaries. The diamond crystallites are highly defected with many twins and other planar defects. Khomich et al. [76] deposited 100- to 200-nm crystallites with the appearance of polycrystalline conglomerates. Lee et al. [75] prepared nanocrystalline films from CH_4/H_2 mixtures and concluded real-time spectroscopic ellipsometry to measure activation energies. Microhardness, electrical conductivity, and the effect of methane pressure on film growth rate were studied by Fedoseev et al. [77]. Films produced by Zarrabian et al. [79] from an electron cyclotron resonance (ECR) plasma were studied by TEM and electron energy loss spectroscopy (EELS) and found to consist of 4- to 30-nm crystallites embedded in diamond-like carbon (DLC). Magnetron sputtering of vitreous carbon produced films in which the nanocrystallites were embedded in an amorphous carbon matrix [78]. By adjusting the ratio of noble gas to hydrogen in the gas mixture, Gruen's group [82] has achieved a continuous transition from microcrystalline to nanocrystalline.

However, in essence, the technique allows an equivalent circuit representation of the material system under study to be proposed, and the experimental data determined to be compared with simulated data based on manipulation of the circuit parameters within the equivalent circuit. This chapter shows evidence for both grain boundaries and grain interior conduction within the silicon-supported nanocrystalline diamond films used here.

All films studied here were produced using a commercial supplied 2.45-GHz resonant standing wave cavity microwave plasma–enhanced CVD system. It has been already demonstrated that good quality, microcrystalline diamond films can be really produced on suitably treated Si substrates using $CH_4/H_2/O_2$ gas mixtures [83–86]. The introduction of Ar in place of the oxygen has been shown to lead to nanocrystalline film production [73,87]; this approach has been used here.

The films synthesized comprise randomly oriented fine grains 50–100 nm in size. The temperature dependence of the characteristic Cole–Cole plots measured for these diamond films is shown in Figure 4.18a–e. Figure 4.18a presents the data measured at 25°C and 100°C, respectively, showing the presence of a single semicircular response, with some scatter in the data in the low-frequency impedance range. Similar data are shown in Figure 4.18b for the temperatures of 150°C and 200°C. The diameter of the semicircular response is reduced dramatically with the increase in temperature. Beyond 250°C, shown in Figure 4.18c–e, the semicircular response is accompanied by an additional semicircle (or an arc) that extends to low frequencies.

In Figure 4.19, the calculated resistance for the higher-frequency semicircular response within the Cole–Cole plot, which persists over the whole temperature range investigated here, is presented in a logarithmic plot against reciprocal temperature. A straight line is apparent, enabling a single electrical activation energy to be estimated from the slope of the curves. Attention should be paid to the steep transition of the activation energy from 0.13 to 0.67 eV at 250°C, coincident with the emergence of the second semicircular response.

It has been found that each Cole–Cole plot below 250°C shows only one depressed semicircle, as indicated in Figure 4.18a and b. The single semicircle indicates that one primary mechanism exists for the polarization within the diamond film at these temperatures. The presence of the single semicircle in this frequency range corresponds to the electrical conduction from bulk grain interior. The diameter of each semicircle corresponds to the resistance for the particular contribution from the diamond grain interior at each temperature. As the temperature increases, the diameter of the semicircle decreases, indicating a reduction of the grain interior resistance. There appears to be no secondary semicircular response over the frequency range measured here for temperatures below 250°C; it can therefore be summarized that the electrical conduction within these diamond films is being dominated by the diamond grain interiors.

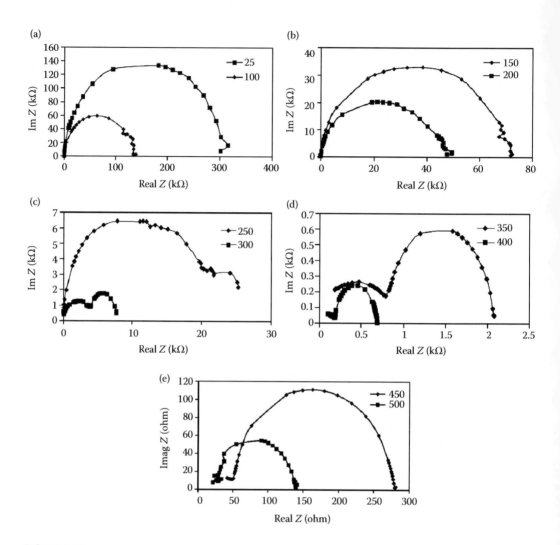

FIGURE 4.18
Temperature dependence of the Cole–Cole plots of the diamond films: (a) 25°C and 100°C, (b) 150°C and 200°C, (c) 250°C and 300°C, (d) 350°C and 400°C, and (e) 450°C and 500°C. (Ye, H., *J. Appl. Phys.*, 94, 7878, 2003. With permission.)

When the temperature is raised above 250°C, the dominant electrical conduction mechanism changes. It is found that a secondary semicircular response occurs in the low-frequency range. In this case, two distinct semicircular relaxations were observed in Figure 4.18c–e, although the high-frequency response is incomplete at higher temperatures and is replaced by an arc. It is now possible to identify the contributions from the grain interior and grain boundary resistances from the visible arcs or semicircles of the Cole–Cole plots [2]. The arc on the left (high frequency) is assigned to the electrical behavior within the grain interior, as discussed above, whereas the feature on the right (low frequency) is assigned to the grain boundaries. The high-frequency semicircular response (left) changes from a perfect semicircle into an imperfect arc and begins to disappear with increasing temperature. This is due to the frequency limitation of the equipment used here [88], which can measure only up to 1 MHz. The low-frequency semicircular response

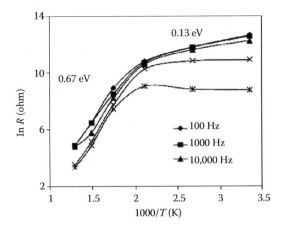

FIGURE 4.19
Temperature and frequency dependence of the bulk grain interior resistance obtained by fitting the impedance spectra. The activation energy is estimated from the slope as 0.13 eV below 250°C and 0.67 eV above 250°C, respectively. (From Ye, H., *J. Appl. Phys.*, 94, 7878, 2003. With permission.)

(right) becomes more complete and begins to dominate the spectra with increasing temperature. Comparing the diameters of the semicircles in each Cole–Cole plot, it is apparent that the ratio of the low-frequency to the high-frequency semicircle diameter increases with an increase in temperature. This indicates that impedance from grain boundaries becomes more significant at higher temperatures; that is, electrical conduction through grain boundaries dominates at temperatures above 250°C.

Theoretically, a double R–C parallel circuit model in series [2] could be used to simulate the electrical conduction of diamond films contributed from both grain interiors and grain boundaries. Each parallel R–C equivalent circuit model accurately fits each Cole–Cole semicircle. The fitting procedure used here is the same as the one described by Kleitz and Kennedy [89] and allows the determination of resistance and relaxation frequencies with a good precision. Here the resistor R represents ionic or electronic conduction mechanisms, whereas the capacitor C represents the polarizability of the diamond. The symbols R_{gi}, R_{gb}, C_{gi}, and C_{gb} are defined as before. The complex impedance Z^* measured by the RCL meter can be expressed as the following function of the R_{gi}, R_{gb}, C_{gi}, and C_{gb} of the specimen:

$$Z^* = Z' - j\, Z'' \tag{4.58}$$

$$Z' = \frac{R_{gi}}{1+\omega^2 R_{gi}^2 C_{gi}^2} + \frac{R_{gb}}{1+\omega^2 R_{gb}^2 C_{gb}^2} \tag{4.59}$$

$$Z'' = \frac{\omega R_{gi}^2 C_{gi}}{1+\omega^2 R_{gi}^2 C_{gi}^2} + \frac{\omega R_{gb}^2 C_{gb}}{1+\omega^2 R_{gb}^2 C_{gb}^2} \tag{4.60}$$

where Z' and Z'' represent the real and imaginary portions of the impedance, and ω is the angular frequency. When plotted in a complex plane, Z'' versus Z' takes the form of two semicircles. In this representation, the grain interior and grain boundary contributions are easily identified, and the electrical conduction paths of the bulk material can be studied separately from grain boundary interference; this task has been performed above.

As previously mentioned, the diameter of each semicircle indicates the resistance (R) contributed either from grain interiors or from grain boundaries. To understand the different semicircular response quantitatively, the resistance for the contribution from both grain interiors and grain boundaries was estimated and extracted as shown in Table 4.3. R_{gi}, R_{gb}, and R_{gi}/R_{gb} are the resistance from the grain interior, the resistance from grain boundaries, and the ratio between them. The first observation is that the resistance either from grain interiors or from grain boundaries decreases with increasing temperature. Particular attention should be paid to the marked decrease in diamond grain interior resistance (from 300 to 0.02 kΩ) with increasing temperature (from 25°C to 500°C). The resistance contributed from the grain boundaries is not measurable below 250°C, implying that it is relatively small. Comparison of the relative variation of both resistances shows that the resistance from grain boundaries made more dominant contribution with increasing temperature.

Recent studies of the temperature-dependent resistance of polycrystalline CVD diamond films have shown that the thermal activation energy can cover a wide range between 0.09 and 1.5 eV [90]. However, the grain interior and grain boundary resistances have not previously been identified and separated. In the field of CVD diamond, it is often difficult to make direct comparisons with a body of published work, since films grown in different laboratories can display significantly different properties. Jin et al. [90] have reported activation energy changes from 0.4 to 0.9 eV with increasing temperature. They suggested that the weakly temperature-dependent resistivity at lower temperature was due to leakage along the grain boundaries; however, no directly evidence was presented. The resistance they reported became nearly independent of frequency at the high temperature end, which is consistent with similar observations by Nath and Wilson [91].

A few reports exist that discuss different mechanisms to explain the electrical conduction properties of microcrystalline diamond films, rather than the nanocrystalline diamond films studied here [92–96]. Landstrass and Ravi [97] proposed that the conduction transition they observed with temperature was caused by the movement of hydrogen and other defects from electrically active deep levels to nonactive sites during annealing. Mori et al.

TABLE 4.3

Temperature Dependence of Grain Boundary Resistance (R_{gb}), Grain Interior Resistance (R_{gi}), and the Relative Resistance (R_{gb}/R_{gi}) between Them

T (°C)	R_{gi} (kΩ)	R_{gb} (kΩ)	R_{gb}/R_{gi}
25	300.00	–	–
100	133.00	–	–
150	71.00	–	–
200	50.00	–	–
250	28.00	–	–
275	14.00	5.20	0.37
300	5.60	3.68	0.66
350	1.00	1.32	1.32
375	0.50	0.80	1.60
400	0.22	0.54	2.45
425	0.11	0.35	3.18
450	0.05	0.24	4.80
500	0.02	0.12	6.00

Source: Ye, H. *J. Appl. Phys.*, 94, 7878, 2003. With permission.

[98] suggested the existence of a surface conductive layer combined with chemical absorption and oxidation. Werner et al. [99] and Huang et al. [100] have presented space charge–limited currents and the Poole–Frenkel mechanism as origin for the nonlinear increase of conduction with temperature. Frequency-independent and frequency-dependent band conduction and hopping conduction mechanisms have also been discussed [101]. Some studies have shown that a number of different defects are present within the grain boundaries, which influence the conduction and the mobility of the charge carriers [102,103].

It is worth noting that nanocrystalline material containing a high density of grain boundaries has a high surface area/volume ratio [104]. With external heating, the grain boundaries may undergo the deformation and distortion caused by the thermal expansion, thermal stress, and even oxidation. The total area of grain boundaries, where defects and non-diamond carbon phases are believed to be most densely accumulated, can increase enormously [75,105]. These impurities are not as thermally stable as diamond grains. Diamond crystals begin to oxidize in air at about 500°C and begin to graphitize under vacuum at about 800°C [106], whereas impurities at grain boundaries are thermally activated at lower temperatures (250°C), as observed. Therefore, oxidation, diffusion, and space charge transportation can easily take place. An alternative explanation involves the interfaces between the diamond and the electrode, and/or between the diamond and the silicon substrate. If the accumulation and trapping of charges at structural interface reaches a certain value, interfacial or boundary polarization will happen with increasing temperature and will subsequently cause a responding secondary relaxation in the impedance data.

As indicated above, the effect of current conduction through the silicon substrate is assumed to be absent. However, it is interesting to note that the change in activation energy found in the grain interior resistance to a value of 0.67 eV above 250°C is exactly the same as the activation energy found for the radio frequency losses due to thermal activation of intrinsic charge carriers in silicon (over the band gap) [107]. Therefore, another possible explanation would be that the contribution of silicon becomes significant over 250°C. Further investigations will look into the in situ observation of grain boundaries using high-resolution TEM with temperature control to provide more direct proof of the physical mechanisms suggested.

Diamond-Based Materials Applications

Recently, diamond is considered as a promising candidate for bioelectronics applications for its electronic [108–111] and chemical properties [109,112,113]. Successful applications of impedance spectroscopy have been reported for immunosensors [114,115], enzyme sensors [116–118], and DNA sensors [119–125]. In this chapter, the electrochemical equivalent circuit models and impedance spectroscopy experiments of different kinds of diamonds will be discussed.

Biosensors

DNA molecule detection is one of the basic applications in molecular diagnostics. Faradic and non-Faradic impedance spectroscopy have been applied for the studies of DNA hybridization by recording the impedance changes in DNA layers before and after hybridization. If a semiconductor is used as the signal transducer, a field effect could be induced by the binding of the negatively charged DNA, resulting in distinct changes in the interfacial impedance at certain measuring frequencies. In 2000, Takahashi et al. [126] investigated the chlorination/amination/carboxylation process on H-terminated diamond for persevering and analyzing DNA clip. In 2002, Yang et al. [127] modified the nanocrystalline diamond with alkenes and concluded that DNA bonding on diamond material would be much better than that on other substrates. Then, several methods including chemical reduction [128] and direct amination [129] on diamond with DNA [127], enzyme [130], and proteins [131] were investigated by using cyclic voltammetry and other electrochemistry methods. To understand the electrical response and the hybridization-induced changes, the impedance data were analyzed using equivalent circuit models with constant phase elements (CPEs). The electrochemical equivalent circuit of DNA-modified diamond film, which was given by Yang et al. [130] and Rao et al. [132], is shown in Figure 4.20.

In the equivalent circuit, R_s represents the ohmic resistance of the electrolyte solution. The paralleled resistor R_1 and capacitor C_{dl} reflect the properties of the molecular layer and the double layer. R_2 and CPE $(=A^{-1}(j\omega)^{-\alpha})$, where A and α are nonintegral, adjustable parameters, which describe the impedance of the space charge region of the BDD electrode.

From 2006 to 2007, Nebel et al. [133–135] applied the photochemistry technology to attach alkene modules on undoped diamond and electrochemical reduction of diazonium salts to form nitrophenyl-linker molecules on boron-doped CVD diamond [133,136,137]. Thiol-modified single-stranded probe DNA (ss-DNA) was bonded to diamond by hetero-bifunctional cross-linker. Then, such surfaces were exposed to fluorescence-labeled target ss-DNA to investigate hybridization on the DNA-FET (field-effect transistor) structure. CVD diamond growth process and photochemistry method were introduced in the article of Nebel et al. [138], and x-ray photoelectron spectroscopy, atomic force microscopy, fluorescence microscopy were utilized to characterize the surface with DNA. Figure 4.21 shows the EIS properties of DNA-modified nanodiamond films. The impedance shown on Nyquist plot was detected from ss-DNA exposure to 4-base mismatched DNA and after exposure to complementary DNA in pH 7.4 phosphate buffer containing 1 mM $Fe(CN_6)^{3-/4-}$. The Nyquist plot, indicated discriminating hybridization of matched and mismatched DNA. The author gave an interpretation of these results, which depended on several factors including variations of ss-DNA and double-strand DNA layers, applied external electric fields, as well as the effect of redox molecules such as $Fe(CN_6)^{3-/4-}$ on the dielectric and conductivity properties of DNA films on diamond.

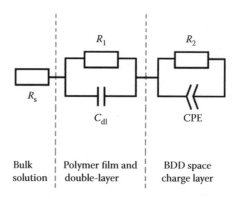

FIGURE 4.20
EIS equivalent circuit of DNA-modified diamond film.

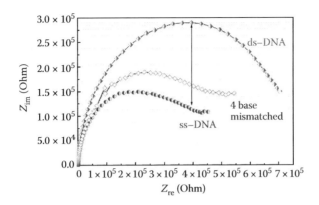

FIGURE 4.21
Nyquist plot of the nanodiamond films with 1 mM Fe(CN$_6$)$^{3-/4-}$ (From Nebel et al., *Br. J. Soc. Interface*, 4, 439, 2007. With permission.) [133].

A recent report on BDD verifies that material is qualified to be the next generation of DNA electrode, for its widely electrochemical potential window both in aqueous and non-aqueous media, relative low double-layer capacitance, as well as insensitivity to dissolved oxygen [139]. In 2005, Gu et al. [131] investigated polyaniline/polyacrylate (PANI/PAA)-modified BDD electrode in DNA hybridization applications. The BDD was fabricated on MWCVD with methanol and boron oxide mixture gas. Then, the PANI/PAA-modified BDD electrodes were dipped into a mixture of the NH$_2$-ssDNA (2 μM in 0.1 M Na$_3$PO$_4$ buffer) solution with 20 mg/mL of *N*-ethyl-*N'*-[3-(dimethylamino)-propyl], and the EIS Nyquist plot for the polymer-modified BDD and DNA-modified BDD was measured by the potentiostat at a given open-circuit voltage, from 100 kHz down to 0.1 Hz, with AC amplitude of 10 mV.

Figure 4.22a shows the Nyquist plot of probe-immobilized BDD electrodes measured at different potential (open-circuit potential vs. Ag/AgCl) in phosphate-buffered solution (pH 7.4). The characteristic potential dependence of the BDD electrode could be obtained at the high-frequency range ($f > 10$ kHz), which was a region dominated by the space charge region of diamond. After the immobilization of the probe DNA on the polymer-modified BDD electrode, the diameter derived from the Nyquist plot semicircle (in Figure 4.22b) increases significantly comparing with the naked BDD and the PANI/PAA-modified BDD.

Figure 4.23 shows the Nyquist plot of DNA-immobilized PANI/PAA-modified BDD electrode, before (solid squares) and after (solid triangles) exposure to fully complementary target, with one-base mismatch (hollow circles), after denature (hollow triangles) and renature (hollow squares) with the fully complementary target, measured at –1.0 V open-circuit potential vs. Ag/AgCl.

At the frequency range between 10 and 100 Hz, the impedance modulus decreased from 13 to 6 kΩ. The author explained that phenomenon was due to the effect of DNA hybridization, which reduced the electron-transfer resistance on the electrode, clearly manifested as a much smaller diameter of the semicircle in the Nyquist plot after DNA hybridization. The BDD electrodes/electrolyte interface was divided into three physical regions, the bulk electrolyte solution, the molecular layer (including the DNA and the polymer composite thin film), and its associated double layer, as well as the space-charge layer in the BDD electrode based on equivalent circuit elements [142]. The schematic equivalent circuit

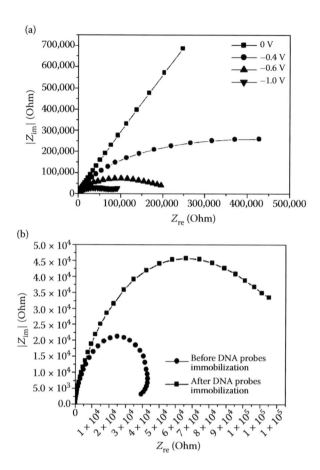

FIGURE 4.22
(a) Nyquist plot of DNA probes-immobilized PANI/PAA modified BDD measured at the different open-circuit potentials. (b) Nyquist plot of PANI/PAA-modified BDD before and after DNA probes immobilization, measured at –0.8 V open-circuit potential vs. Ag/AgCl. (From Gu et al., *J. Phys. Chem. B*, 109, 13611–13618, 2005. With permission.) [131]

model has been demonstrated by Yang et al. [143] for DNA-modified diamond. After fitting the data from the equivalent circuit, the capacitance C_{dl} of the polymer/double layer in the target-hybridized DNA reached the highest value of 42 µF comparing with the probe-immobilized BDD electrode before hybridization which was 1.59 µF. This meant that the presence of the double-stranded helix generates more charges on the electrolyte–electrode interface. The increase in capacitance and the decrease in polymer film resistance (R_1) indicated that the density of ionic charges increased at the interface after DNA hybridization. The author assumed that hybridization of DNA in the polymer scaffold decreased the impedance of the polymer significantly. Therefore, this process led to dramatic changes in R_1 and C_{dl} at the frequency range of 10–100 Hz.

Yang et al. [143] in 2007 investigated the property of the antibody–antigen–modified BDD surface. The diamond samples were all *p*-type BDD (deposition concentration: 10^{18} cm^{-3}), which grow on *p*-type Si (100) substrate by MWCVD method. EIS experiments were performed using human immunoglobulin G (human IgG, Sigma I4506) and human immunoglobulin M (human IgM, Sigma I8260) linked to surfaces, whereas binding experiments were performed using the complementary antibodies antihuman IgG (Fc specific, Sigma

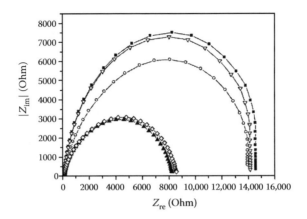

FIGURE 4.23
Nyquist plot of DNA PANI/PAA-modified BDD before and after hybridization. (From Gu et al., *J. Phys. Chem. B*, 109, 13611–13618, 2005. With permission.)

F9512) and antihuman IgM (m-chain specific, Sigma F5384). The Nyquist plot after covalent linking of antigen to surfaces is shown in Figure 4.24.

Figure 4.24 shows Nyquist plots of Z' and Z'' from 100 to 1.1 MHz, with 10-mV root-mean-square (rms) modulation for different kinds of antibody–antigen-modified diamond surfaces. After anti-IgG and anti-IgM modified, the Cole–Cole plot has only slightly changes in real component response (Z' changes from 110 to 112 Ω at 200 kHz). Then the impedance Z' (before and after exposure to anti-IgG) increased from 110 to 190 Ω at 200 kHz. The author also gave the electrochemistry equivalent circuit, which is shown in Figure 4.25.

To analyze the principle, an electrochemistry equivalent circuit model with discrete element has been established, as shown on Figure 4.25. The author separated the interface into three layers: (1) the space-charge layer of the semiconductors, (2) the tightly packed organic modification layers, and (3) the more diffuse ionic region and the biomolecular layer. In this model, R_{sc} and C_{sc} represented the space charge layer of the semiconducting substrates. R_{dl} and a CPE reflected the densely packed initial functionalization layer

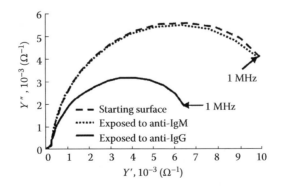

FIGURE 4.24
Nyquist plot measured on a diamond sample modified with IgG and exposed to anti-IgM and anti-IgG (From Yang, W., *Analyst*, 132, 296, 2007. With permission.) [143].

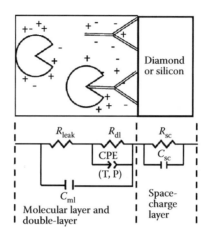

FIGURE 4.25
Equivalent circuit model representation of the IgG-modified semiconductor interfaces and used to fit the data on n-type and p-type silicon. (From Yang, W., *Analyst*, 132, 296, 2007. With permission.) [143]

and its ionic environment. R_{leak} and C_{ml} represented the properties of the biomolecular layer and its associated ionic charge distribution. The CPE component is a generalized capacitor with an impedance defined by $Z = 1/(T\omega)^P$, where T and P are adjustable parameters.

Diamond Electrodes

The BDD applications for surface electrochemistry pretreatment have been reported. For the chemical stability and surface reproducibility, BDD is an excellent candidate for contaminated water treatment. Different studies on BDD and diamond electrodes have been reported by Rao et al. [144], Terashima et al. [145], Yagi et al. [146], and Latto et al. [147]. To present differences after cathodic or anodic pretreatment of the diamond films, Suffredini et al. [148] utilized EIS measurement. A 0.62 cm × 1.0 cm BBD electrode that was deposited by HFCVD technique on a silicon wafer was used as a working electrode in EIS experiments. The gases in vapor deposition were methane, H_2, and trimethylboron, and the boron content was 4500–5000 ppm. The EIS experiments were carried on with 0.5 mol L^{-1} H_2SO_4 and 1×10^{-3} mol L^{-1} $K_4Fe(CN)_6$ or 0.5×10^{-3} mol L^{-1} ferrocene. Figure 4.26 shows the Nyquist plot obtained at 0.06 V after anodic and cathodic pretreatments.

Ferro and Battisti [149], as well as Becker and Jüttner [150], had previously reported the similar phenomenon in the Nyquist plot. Ferro and Battisti explained that the high-frequency element decreased, whereas the redox couple concentration increased. Becker and Jüttner presented that this element increased as the overpotential increased and explained that this unexpected increase was due to a partial blocking of the electrode surface. The resistance of the high-frequency element for the anodically treated BDD (Figure 4.27a) is quite similar to the previous reports for the same solution at an oxidized BDD. When the BDD surface undergoes the cathodic treatment, the resistance reduced, as it can be seen in Figure 4.27b. However, the factor is relatively smaller than the previous reports. The author assumed the cathodical BDD surface impedance decrease indicated that the

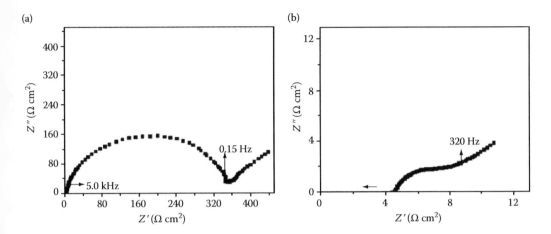

FIGURE 4.26
The Nyquist plots for the BDD electrode in $K_4Fe(CN)_6$ + H_2SO_4 aqueous solution after (a) anodic pretreatment at 3.0 V or (b) cathodic pretreatment at –3.0 V. Frequency intervals: 50 kHz to 30 MHz (a) and 50 kHz to 10 Hz (b). Measurements carried out at 0.60V. (From Suffredini, H.B., *Electrochim. Acta*, 49, 4021, 2004. With permission.) [148]

inner or the surface structure of the BDD material is obviously altered by this treatment and leads to faster electron transfers consequence.

Figure 4.27 presents Nyquist plots obtained at 0.37 V in a 0.5×10^{-3} mol L^{-1} ferrocene + 0.5 mol L^{-1} H_2SO_4 aqueous solution for the BDD electrode after anodic and cathodic pretreatments. The value of the high-frequency resistance element after the cathodic surface pretreatment is also significant but not as in the case of the $Fe(CN)_6^{4-/3-}$ couple. The EIS experiments demonstrate that a discontinuous passive layer or an internal transformation of the BDD will decrease the surface blocking, which is caused by the cathodic pretreatment.

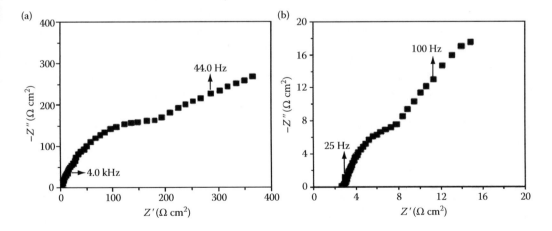

FIGURE 4.27
The Nyquist plots for the BDD electrode for a 0.5×10^{-3} mol L^{-1} ferrocene + 0.5 mol L^{-1} H_2SO_4 aqueous solution with measurements carried out at 0.37 V. (From Suffredini, H.B., *Electrochim. Acta*, 49, 4021, 2004. With permission.) [148]

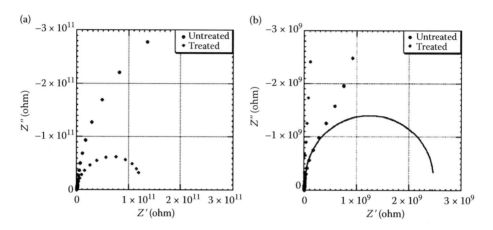

FIGURE 4.28
(a) Impedance spectroscopy of treated and untreated SCD samples. (b) High-frequency impedance data. The solid line is a mathematical fitting to the semicircular response of the untreated device. (From Bevilacqua, M., *Appl. Phys. Lett.*, 95, 243501, 2009. With permission.) [151]

Ultraviolet Sensors

Bevilacqua et al. [151] successfully fabricated diamond as a UV photodetector in 1995. Recently, their group invested SCD in this area and found that it represented an extreme sensitivity to deep UV light. The SCD, which had an rms value of 3.5 nm, was performed a passivation treatment in an environment full of methane at about 700°C for 15 min, and then annealed at a temperature of 400°C for 1 h. The frequency range of the impedance spectroscopy measurement was varied from 0.1 Hz up to 10 MHz. The Nyquist plot is shown in Figure 4.28.

The impedance spectroscopy is plotted by real component, Z' versus imaginary component Z'' for both treated and untreated SCD samples in Figure 4.28. The presence of impedance spectroscopy plot indicates that the equivalent circuit of the SCD sample is a resistance parallel with a capacitance (R–C parallel circuit). After using mathematical method fit on the data, the resistance/capacitance value after passivation treatment is simulated to be 8×10^{11} Ω/0.5 pF with untreated surface and 1×10^{11} Ω/3 pF, respectively. The high-frequency impedance is given in Figure 4.28b, and the solid semicircular line is a mathematical fitting, where R/C value is 4×10^9 Ω/0.3 pF. The author explained that the disorder materials on the surface of the SCD samples were removed, so a lower resistivity was conducted from the impedance spectroscopy measurement. After the passivation process, the external quantum efficiency was more comparably optimistic than other homoepitaxial films and it enhanced the UV photoconductive device performance.

Non-Diamond-Based Materials for Biological Application

Non-diamond carbon–related materials include multiwalled carbon nanotubes (MWCNTs), DLC, hydrogenated amorphous carbon (a-C:H), fullerene, and graphene. They have a wide range of applications in different fields, and EIS is also introduced as an assistance to find their performance in specific areas.

MWCNTs are the strongest and stiffest materials, which have been discovered in term of tensile, elastic modulus, inertness to react with other chemical material, as well as bio-compatibility. These characteristics endow CNTs a candidate for cells (Section 4.5.1), DNA (Section 4.5.2), and enzyme (Section 4.5.3) detection. Another critical property of CNTs is the surface/volume ratio and the ability to fabricate on other polymer and alloy as a catalyst (Section 4.5.4). Meanwhile, graphene, which has similar characters as CNTs, has been considered as a proper material in fabricating electrode in lithium ion batteries (Section 4.5.5) and supercapacitor (Section 4.5.6). The family of amorphous carbon-based films include a wide range of films having different properties, such as DLC films, which are very hard and, under certain environmental conditions, might have friction coefficients in the 10^{-2} range that makes them excellent candidates for coating (Section 4.5.7) the moving parts of orthopedic implants.

Cells Detection

The electrical conductivity and impedance of biological materials have been investigated over the past century using conventional electrodes [152]. Recently, with the advance of nanotechnology, nanoelectrodes based on electrochemistry method can offer advantages such as reduced double-layer capacitance, fast convergence to a steady-state signal, enhanced current density arising from increased mass transport at the working electrode interface, low detection limits, and improved signal-to-noise ratios. Electrochemical impedance has been utilized for human body measurement to cells detection. In 2007, Yun et al. [153] reported on nanoelectrode array embedded into a polydimethylsioxane channel to distinguish LNCaP (lymph node carcinoma of the prostate) prostate cancer cells. In this report, 8-mm-tall high-density MWCNTs arrays were synthesized by water-assisted CVD. The gold-coated MWCNTs were then fabricated on 5-mm-square $Fe/Al_2O_3/$ SiO_2/Si substrate, and the substrates were embedded into a polydimethylsioxane channel. Each tower (1×1 mm) of the patterned array contained about 50 million nanotubes. The nanotubes' average diameter was 20 nm, and the aspect ratio was 200,000. The surface area of each tower (average diameter: 20 nm and length: 8 mm MWCNTs) was 2500 mm². Electrochemical impedance characterization of nanotubes electrodes was measured under a fluidic channel with different solutions and LNCaP prostate cancer cells.

From the phase and magnitude plot, the phase angle is different between the HBSS and the LNCaP prostate cells, which is more capacitive with the increase in incubation time. In Figure 4.29, the Nyquist plot shows that the diameter of the semicircle at high-frequency increases obviously with incubation time. The EIS equivalent circuit was given by Randles model with a CPE. As the HBSS is only a one-layer capacitance, the equivalent circuit of LNCaP prostate cell was given by $[R_u(C_{cl}R_{cl})Z_{CPE}]$, where C_{cl} and R_{cl} are the cell capacitance and resistance. Extracted parameters were CPE = 0.134 μ S, α = 0.83, and R_u = 950 Ω. A higher value of α was indicative of the closeness of the CPE to an ideal capacitor (α = 1). The author assumed that the reason was because the LNCaP cells formed a tight contact and a cover to the electrodes, and then blocked the ion movement. Extracted parameters show that both C_{cl} and R_{cl} increased after incubation time increased. Since the solution resistance represents the bulk properties of the electrolyte solution and the LNCaP cells settled on the electrode's surface, solution resistance does not change much. On the other hand, the cell layer capacitance C_{cl} and cell layer resistance R_{cl} affect the interface property of the electrode–electrolyte due to insulating or coating the surface by LNCaP cells. The EIS results showed that the MWCNTs electrode could characterize different solutions, which suggested that its applications as a cell-based biosensor and gold functionalized nanotube

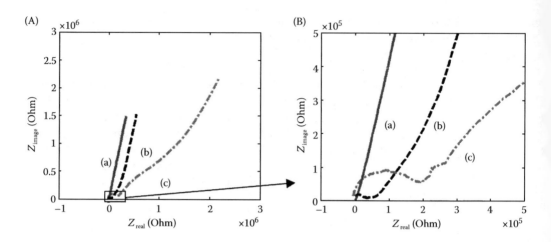

FIGURE 4.29
Electrochemical impedance measurement result (A) with magnified plot (B) with (a) HBSS and then HBSS with LNCaP with different incubation times: 5 min (b) and 2 h (c). (From Yun, Y.H., *Nanotechnology*, 18, 465505, 2007. With permission.) [153]

array electrodes would be useful for further bioconjugation such as antibodies and special receptors to detect specific cancer cells.

DNA Hybridization Sensor Applications

Electrochemistry DNA sensors provide a novel method of detecting selected DNA sequence and mutated genes that lead to human disease. Different approaches have been developed, such as direct and indirect electrochemistry of DNA, polymer-modified electrodes, amplification nanoparticles, and so on. In these years, EIS was used to characterize a DNA hybridization sensor to realize sensitive indicator-free detection of gene sequence. Hybridization reaction of DNA on the electrode surface causes the changing of R_{ct} value upon formation of duplex between probe and target DNA. The quantity if there is a negative charge on the surface of the electrode increases greatly because of the hybridization formation, and then impedes the electron transfer with the negative charge such as $[Fe(CN)_6]^{3-/4-}$ at the electrode surface is observed. Electrode modified with CNTs has been used for detecting important biomolecules [154,155]. Traditional method of DNA detection is based on radio-isotopic and fluorescent technology, which is not efficient and not compatible for routine and rapid medical analysis. The combination of conducting polypyrrole with CNTs was applied to detect oligonucleotides (a short fragment of DNA), since it enhanced the charge density, electrical conductivity, and electrocatalytic activity [156–158]. In 2010, Lien and Lam [159] developed MWCNT-doped polypyrrole DNA biosensors, and EIS plot was utilized to study the DNA hybridization. In the genome, promoter sequence has been found out as the CaMV 35S extracted from cauliflower mosaic virus. The EIS measurements were performed in the frequency range between 200 kHz and 100 MHz with 5-mV alternating voltage on DC potential. The electrochemical equivalent circuit is given by Randles mode (with lower CaMV 35S concentration) and Vorotyntsev's model (with higher CaMV 35S concentration) [160]. The fitting values extracted from the EIS plot were applied to explain "Signal-on" behavior, which represented the decreasing process of R_{ct} during hybridization. The signal-on effect indicates that DNA hybridization at the vicinity of the polymer–solution interface increases the switching speed of electronically conducting polymer. The

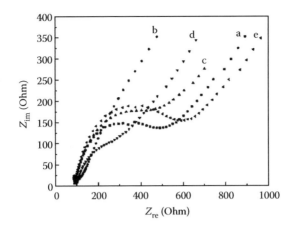

FIGURE 4.30
Nyquist plots obtained from bare electrode: MWCNT-modified electrode (a), ABA/MWCNT-modified electrode (b), AuNPs/PABA/MWCNT-modified electrode (c), and ssDNA/AuNPs/PABA/MWCNT-modified electrode (d). (e) The supporting electrolyte was 0.1 M phosphate-buffered solution (pH 7.0) containing 10.0 mM $K_4Fe(CN)_6$/ $K_3Fe(CN)_6$ (1: 1). (From Zhang et al., *Colloids Surf B: Biointerfaces*, 75, 179–185, 2010. With permission.) [161]

author gave the explanation that the electrostatic effect and the steric effect was due to the polyelectrolyte character of oligonucleotides strands; thus, the ionic transportation across the polymer–solution interface changed.

Zhang and Wang [161] fabricated a sensitive electrochemical DNA biosensor with aminobenzoic acid (ABA) electropolymerized on the surface of glassy carbon electrode (GCE) modified with MWCNTs. ABA was electropolymerized on the surface of GCE modified with MWCNTs, and then gold nanoparticles (AuNPs) were subsequently introduced to the surface of poly-ABA-MWCNTs by electrodeposition mode. Finally, the probe DNA was immobilized on the surface of AuNPs through Au–S bond. The EIS measurements were carried on with a frequency range between 1 and 10^5 Hz at the formal potential of +0.15 V, with the amplitude of 5 mV alternative voltage, and used 10 mM $K_3[Fe(CN)_6]/K_4[Fe(CN)_6]$ (1:1) mixture as a redox probe.

Figure 4.30 shows the Nyquist plot of the sensing electrode response at different stages in assembly process. When the MWCNTs were assembled on the GCE surface, the electron transfer resistance (R_{ct}) decreased greatly (curve b) compared with that of bare GCE (curve a) due to the promotion from the MWCNTs. When ABA was electropolymerized onto the surface of the MWCNTs/GCE, the R_{ct} value increased. After AuNPs was introduced, the R_{ct} decreased, and when probe DNA was immobilized on the electrode surface, R_{ct} obviously increased. The author explained that DNA was negatively charged and had electrostatic repulsion toward negatively charge $[Fe(CN)_6]^{3-/4-}$. The experimental results proved that different species had been immobilized on the surface of modified electrode from change in electron transfer resistance.

Enzyme Detection

Recently, nitrogen-doped carbon nanotubes (CNx-MWCNTs) are extremely attractive as important nanomaterials in biosensing applications. Because of the hydrophobic characteristics of CNTs surface, it is necessary to functionalize CNTs with polymers, guest molecules, or side wall substituents to improve the biocompatibility [162]. Compared with

CNTs, CNx-MWCNTs have larger surface-active, group-to-volume ratio, thermal stability, superb electrical and mechanical properties [163–165]. Several reports studied the electro-catalytic behavior of CNx-MWCNTs toward the glucose oxidase (GOx). Deng and Jian [166] investigated the direct electron transfer of GOx at CNx-MWCNT–modified electrode and its applications. CNx-MWCNTs suspension (3.5 µL) was dropped on the prepolished GCE surface and dried at room temperature. The EIS experiments were carried out with 0.1 M KCl solution containing 5 mM $K_3[Fe(CN)_6]/K_4[Fe(CN)_6]$. The frequency range is between 10^{-2} and 10^5 Hz, and the amplitude of the potential is 5 mV. The Nyquist plots are shown on Figure 4.31.

In Figure 4.31, the bare GCE shows an electron-transfer resistance of about 2800 Ω, which is larger than the CNx-MWCNT–modified GCE. It proves that the CNx-MWCNTs could act as a good electron–transfer interface. Then, when the GOx was coated on the bare electrode, the resistance increased significantly, which proved that the bulky GOx molecules blocked the electron exchange between the redox probe and electrode surface. After GOx was absorbed on CNx-MWCNT–modified GCE, the semicircle diameter in Nyquist plot was lower than CNx-GOx–modified GCE. The author explained that it could also accelerate the electron transfer between the electroactive sites embedded in enzyme and electrode.

The nucleotide sequence of the HIV-1 genome1 reveals that the HIV-1 virus encodes an aspartic protease (HIV-1 PR), an essential enzyme for virion assembly and maturation [167]. The enzyme will be inactivated because of mutation or chemical inhibition, leading to the production of immature, noninfectious viral particles [168]. The approach to assay HIV protease has been developed both in vitro and in vivo, including applying polyprotein or oligopeptide substrates, utilizing gel electrophoresis, as well as introducing high-performance liquid chromatography for ascertaining the presence of cleavage product [169–171]. These methods can only detect the inhibitor in the micromolar range, whereas only a nanomolar or lower range of such drugs can be used in HIV-1 therapy [172]. EIS is a quite efficient and highly sensitive electroanalytical method that can provide direct detection of immunospecies by measuring the change in impedance. Besides the convenience and operation simplicity, EIS provides a nondestructive method to characterize the electrical properties at biological interfaces [173,174]. Another application in HIV-1 PR detection

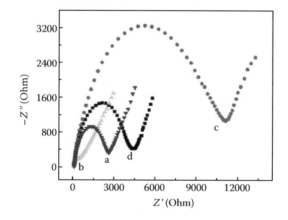

FIGURE 4.31
EIS of bare (a), CNx-MWCNTs (b), GOx (c), and GOx/CNx-MWCNTs (d) modified by GCEs in 0.1 M KCl solution. (From Deng, C., *Biosens. Bioelectron.*, 25, 373, 2009. With permission.) [161]

with gold-modified MWCNT was developed by Mahmoud and Luong [175]. Their works describe an ultrasensitive impedance procedure for detecting HIV-1 PR and screening its potent inhibitors using ferrocene (Fc)-pepstatin–modified surfaces. The gold electrode surface was treated with thiolated single-walled carbon nanotube/AuNP. The single-walled carbon nanotube samples (diameter: 1 nm; CNTs purity: >90 wt.%; length: 5–30 μm; specific surface area: 407 m^2/g; electrical conductivity: >10^{-2} S/cm) were supplied by Carbon Nanotechnology (Houston, TX). The HIV-1 PR recombinant was expressed in *Escherichia coli*. The human serum albumin and human male serum were obtained from Sigma (St. Louis, MO), and DTT (±threo-2,3-dihydroxy-1,4-butanedithiol) was obtained from Fluka. The other two HIV-1 drugs Kaltera and Telzir were obtained from Dr. Chris Tsoukas from the McGill University Health Center (Montreal, QC, Canada). The electrodes were then incubated in four different kinds of solutions with a fixed enzyme concentration (10 pM) and increasing concentrations of the desired inhibitor as the following ratios: HIV-1 PR/inhibitor: 1:0, 1:1, 1:10, and 1:100. Impedance measurement, using 1 mM $Fe(CN)_6^{3-/4-}$ as the redox probe, shows a typical Nyquist plot for the CNT/AuNP-modified gold electrode, as is shown in Figure 4.32.

The EIS equivalent circuit can be described as a Randles model: $[R_s(C_{dl}(R_{ct}W))]$, with mixed kinetic and diffusion control component. The binding event between a target analyte and its corresponding ligand will block the diffusion and, on the other hand, serves as a passage between the redox probe and the active area of the detecting electrode. Consequently, R_{ct} becomes increasingly high and can be used to monitor the binding event. Therefore, R_{ct} is the most directive and sensitive parameter that responds to changes on the electrode interface, as represented by the diameter of the semicircle in the Nyquist plot [176]. A considerable increase in R_{ct} was observed with the Fc-pepstatin/CNT/AuNP electrode compared with the CNT/AuNP-modified electrode (4814 vs. 19.6 Ω). Such behavior demonstrated that the electron transfer to the electrode was significantly reduced for the binding between Fc-pepstatin and CNTs. The subsequent HIV-1 PR binding (10 and 100 pM) to Fc-pepstatin caused an R_{ct} increase to 10,230 and 11,620 Ω, respectively. As expected, changes in R_s, C_{dl}, and W were insignificant compared with the change in R_{ct}. The modified circuit also

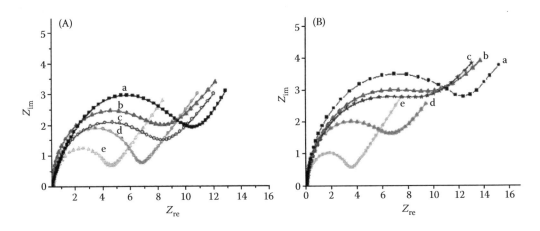

FIGURE 4.32
The Nyquist plot for the impedance in a pH 7.4 buffer with $Fe(CN)_6^{3-/4-}$ as the redox probe for the CNT/AuNP-modified gold electrode after incubation with 10 pM HIV-1 PR in the presence of saquinavir (A) and indinavir (B). HIV-1 PR/inhibitor ratios: (a) 1:0, (b) 1:1, (c) 1:10, (d) 1:100, and (e) 0:100. (From Mahmoud, K.A., Luong, J.H.T., *Anal. Chem.*, 80, 7056–7062, 2008. With permission.) [175]

provided an accurate fitting to the experimental data at both low and high frequency for the Fc-pepstatin/CNT/AuNP–modified electrode, as well as the subsequent binding event with HIV-1 PR (Figure 4.32b). The binding of HIV-1 PR (10 pM) to the Fc-pepstatin/CNT/AuNP–modified electrode led to an obvious change in R_{ct}. The Fc-pepstatin binding site became almost saturated, since further increase in the HIV-1 PR concentration beyond this level only effected a slight increase in R_{ct}. On the basis of this finding, the Fc-pepstatin/CNT/AuNP–modified electrode together with 10 pM HIV-1 PR was used as a starting point for testing the selected HIV-1 PR inhibitors. This result has demonstrated the possibility of using MWCNTs together with AuNPs and ferrocene-conjugate nanomaterials in impedance spectroscopy for detecting HIV-1 protease and subsequent evaluation of the enzyme inhibitors at picomolar levels.

Catalysts

The direct methanol fuel cell (DMFC) is commonly accepted as a potential material for energy-generating devices because of its simple structure, liquid fuel, and environmental cleanliness [177,178]. However, the electrochemistry performance of DMFCs is greatly hampered by the slowly oxidation rate of methanol. It is widely accepted that Pt surface poisoning by CO-like species produced during methanol oxidation is the critical reason for the low reaction rate. To solve this problem, Pt-based alloys (including PtRu and PtSn) [179,180] and Pt/metal oxide composites (including Pt/SnO_2 and Pt/RuO_2) [181–183] have been used to increase the activity and CO tolerance of the catalysts. Song and Xiao [184] utilized Pt, S, TiO_2, and CNT composite as a catalyst in DMFC. As is generally accepted that CO-like species can lead to Pt surface poisoning and reduce the rate of reaction, the author introduced the $Pt–S–TiO_2/CNT$ electrode to improve the catalytic activity and CO tolerance of Pt, as well as high electron and proton conductivities. The $S–TiO_2/CNTs$ were prepared by an improved sol–gel and ethylene glycol reduction methods. The content of sulfated TiO_2 in the $S–TiO_2/CNTs$ was 40 wt.%. The EIS studies were carried out in the solution containing 1.0 M CH_3OH and 1.0 M $HClO_4$, as is shown in Figure 4.33.

From the Nyquist plot, the diameter of right semicircle is a measurement of the charge transfer resistance, which is related to the reaction kinetics of charge transfer. The diameter of right semicircle of $Pt–S–TiO_2/CNTs$ is smaller than that of $Pt–TiO_2/CNTs$, indicating

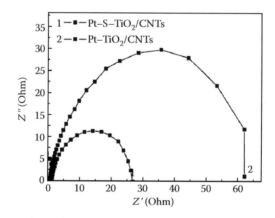

FIGURE 4.33
Electrochemistry Nyquist plot of impedance spectroscopy in 1 M CH_3OH and 1 M $HClO_4$ solution at 0.4 V (sample: $Pt–S–TiO_2/CNTs$ and $Pt–TiO_2/CNTs$). (From Song, H., *J. Power Sources*, 195, 1610. With permission.) [184]

that Pt–S–TiO$_2$/CNTs decrease the charge transfer resistance. Thus, it demonstrates an improvement about the kinetic of methanol oxidation of Pt–S–TiO$_2$/CNTs catalyst.

Lithium-Ion Battery Applications

Recently, rechargeable lithium batteries have become the main energy storage systems for a wide range of applications [185,186]. Arie and Chang [187] applied fullerene coating film on Si for rechargeable lithium batteries. For anode materials, rechargeable lithium batteries with graphite only give a limited capacity of about 372 mA h g^{-1}. Due to the theoretical capacity of silicon, it demonstrates a promising capacity to replace graphite material. Some approaches were utilized to modify the surface property of Si thin films to give it a better electrical contact and lower cell failure. Here, the author applied fullerene coating on Si thin films, which have a high specific capacity of 3000 mA h g^{-1} and a good retention for 40 cycles. The fullerene-coated silicon thin films have been synthesized by RF plasma–assisted deposition techniques. It is generally expected that fullerene films could serve as a buffer layer to reduce the effect of the volume expansion during the repeated cycling as well as to improve the Li-ion kinetic property at the interface of both the Si electrode and the electrolyte.

Figure 4.34 shows EIS plot of Si thin films and the first cycle after fullerene coating. The semicircle in the high-frequency range indicates the migration progress of Li ions on the surface of the electrode, whereas the semicircle in medium frequency range shows the charge transfer process at the interface between the electrode and the electrolyte. The impedance of Si thin film is larger than fullerene-coating film due to the continuous formation of the solid electrolyte interface (SEI) layer, which is unstable and makes the charge transfer process difficult. The higher value of surface film resistance (R_{f_1}) is caused by the direct contact with electrolyte, and certain percentage of the electrolyte decomposition occurs and then forms on the SEI layer. It is then followed by a high-charge transfer resistance (R_{ct_1}). For the fullerene-coating film, its impedance is much smaller than bare Si film, since it could provide a relatively more stable surface against the side reactions with the electrolyte. It demonstrates lower resistance both for the surface film resistance (R_{f_2}) and the charge transfer resistance (R_{ct_2}), so it provides a favorable path for Li ion transfer and suppresses the side reaction between the electrode–electrolyte interfaces.

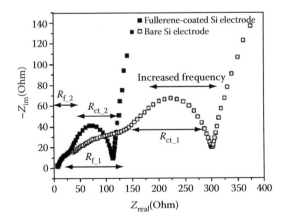

FIGURE 4.34
EIS plot of bare Si thin films and fullerene-coating Si thin films. (From Arie, A.A., *J. Solid State Electrochem.*, 14, 51. With permission.) [187]

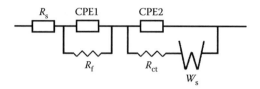

FIGURE 4.35
Electrochemistry equivalent circuit with Warburg component (Vorotyntsev's model) [160].

Another lithium-ion battery cathode material, $LiNi_{1/3}Co_{1/3}Mn_{1/3}O_2$, was reported by Ohzuku and Makimura [188] in 2001. To enhance the performance of cycling rate, Guo and Shi developed the carbon coating on $LiNi_{1/3}Co_{1/3}Mn_{1/3}O_2$ using polyvinyl alcohol (PVA) as a carbon source, because PVA could be pyrolyzed in air at low temperature conveniently [189]. Different amounts of PVA were added into the $LiNi_{1/3}Co_{1/3}Mn_{1/3}O_2$ with the ratio of 5:100, 10:100, 15:100, and 20:100, and then marked as PVA5, PVA10, PVA15, and PVA20, respectively.

Electrochemistry equivalent circuit is the same as shown in Figure 4.35. R_s denotes the ohmic resistance, whereas R_f and CPE1 represent the surface resistance and associated capacitance. R_{ct} is the charge transfer resistance, CPE2 is allocated with its interfacial capacitance, and W_s represents the Warburg component. The EIS plot is given in Figure 4.36a and b. We can conclude from the plot that the surface film resistance R_f is relatively small. It indicates that R_f has little effect on the performance of $LiNi_{1/3}Co_{1/3}Mn_{1/3}O_2$. In contrast, the charge transfer resistance (in the low-frequency region, as shown in Figure 4.36a) decreases remarkably when carbon content increases. To explain this phenomenon, the author suggests that the carbon on the surface makes the lithium ion transfer across the interface between the bulk of active material and the SEI film easier. Thus, the carbon coating is helpful for improving the electrochemical performance of $LiNi_{1/3}Co_{1/3}Mn_{1/3}O_2$ as well as cycle performance and rate capability. Kim and Chung [190] also investigated the

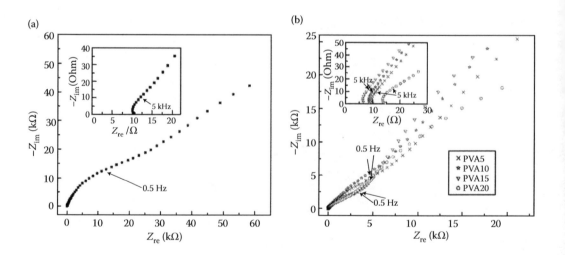

FIGURE 4.36
Electrochemistry impedance plot of the bare $LiNi_{1/3}Co_{1/3}Mn_{1/3}O_2$ (a) and with carbon coating (b) in the frequency range between 0.01 Hz and 100 kHz. The insert plots give the enlarged view of high-frequency domains. (From Kim, H.S., *Electrochim. Acta*, 54, 3606, 2009. With permission.) [190]

carbon coating applications on SnS_2 for lithium ion batteries applications. Similar conclusions were also given by EIS plots.

Supercapacitance

Supercapacitors are highly attractive energy storage devices for their exceptionally high-power and energy-density characteristics compared with conventional dielectric capacitors and to their long cycle life in the applications of batteries. Certain kinds of metal oxide, such as RuO_2, MnO_2, and NiO_2, have already been applied as a contribution for carbon-based supercapacitors [165,191]. Recently, graphene material has been considered for high mobility, chemical, and mechanical stability due to its unique structure of two-dimensional layer hexagonal lattice of carbon atoms [192]. Kalpana et al. [193] fabricated ZnO/carbon aerogel composite electrode with a specific high capacitance of 500 F/g. In 2009, Zhang and Pan [194] investigated graphene–ZnO composite film as an electrode for supercapacitor. The graphene was pasted on the indium tin oxide glass substrate. The graphene was fabricated by a modified Hummers method, and then ZnO was deposited by ultrasonic spray pyrolysis at a frequency of 1.65 MHz. The as-made graphene, pure ZnO film, and graphene–ZnO composite films were named ITO-G, ITO-ZnO, and ITO-G-ZnO, respectively, for EIS study. 1 M KCl solution was used as electrolyte, and the frequency range is from 10 kHZ to 10 MHz. Figure 4.37 shows the Nyquist plots of different electrodes.

In Figure 4.37, the high-frequency arc is ascribed to the double-layer capacitance (C_{dl}) in parallel with the charge transfer resistance (R_{ct}) at the contact interface between the electrode and the electrolyte solution. In the low frequency, the result is explained by the electrode surface inhomogeneity and the existence of CPE. The resistance R_{ct} values, which is calculated from the diameter of the high-frequency arc, are 17 and 3 Ω for ITO-G and ITO-G-ZnO, respectively. The electrochemical measurement shows that graphene–ZnO composite film enhances the capacitive properties more than pure graphene or ZnO electrode.

Guo et al. [195] used graphene nanosheets (GNSs) as anode material for lithium-ion batteries. The GNSs were prepared using artificial graphite (AG) as material by a rapid

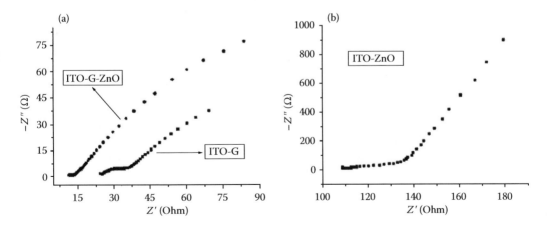

FIGURE 4.37
Nyquist plots for ITO-G-ZnO, ITO-G (a), and ITO-ZnO (b). (From Zhang, Y., *J. Electroanal. Chem. Interfacial Electrochem.*, 634, 68, 2009. With permission.) [194]

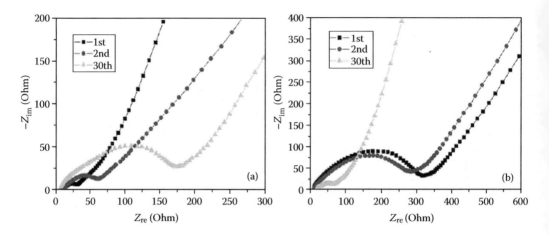

FIGURE 4.38
Nyquist plots of AG (a) and GNS (b). (From Guo et al., *Electrochem. Commun.*, 11, 1320, 2009. With permission.) [195]

heating process and were then ultrasonically treated. EIS of the electrodes was performed utilizing an electrochemical workstation (CHI 660B) with amplitude of 5.0 mV over the frequency range from 100 kHz to 0.01 Hz. From Figure 4.38, the high-frequency semicircle is corresponded to the formation of SEI film and/or contact resistance; the semicircle in the medium-frequency region is assigned to the charge transfer resistance on the electrode–electrolyte interface, and the inclined line at an approximate 45° angle to the real axis corresponds to the lithium diffusion process within carbon electrodes. In high-frequency areas, the diameter of the semicircle for GNSs electrode is decreased evidently after 30 cycles. The author explained that the presence of functional groups at the unorganized carbon sites results in more irreversible lithium inserting in the electrode with the growth of cycle number, which could lead to the increase in electrical conductivity of GNSs. The variation in impedance in the medium-frequency region is investigated by modeling AC spectra according to modified Randles equivalent circuit presented. On the contrary, for the AG electrode, the diameter of the semicircle increases with the cycle process, which is due to the SEI on the surface of AG electrode, and grows thicker with cycle process, implying that the electrochemical activity of GNSs is enhanced.

Lee and Sivakkumar [165] developed VGCF (vapor-grown carbon fiber)/$RuO_2 \cdot xH_2O$ nanocomposite for supercapacitor applications as well. $RuO_2 \cdot xH_2O$ has been proved to be one of the best candidates for supercapacitor material becaue of its specific capacitance and long cycle life. Analysis from Nyquist plot of the pristine $RuO_2 \cdot xH_2O$ electrode indicates that the diffusion of solvated ions within the pristine $RuO_2 \cdot xH_2O$ matrix is the rate-determining step in the charge–discharge process. Both the pristine $RuO_2 \cdot xH_2O$ and its composite electrodes prove stability and the capacitance retention over 10^4 cycles, at 90% and 97%, respectively.

DLC Biomedical Coating Materials

DLC thin films have excellent properties for biological and medical applications because of their excellent biocompatibility, chemical inertness, and superior mechanical properties. It is important for the surface properties of DLC thin films for these applications.

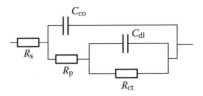

FIGURE 4.39
Basic electrochemical equivalent circuit of DLC as coating materials.

Several reports about DLC coating in biomedical implant application have been published. Nam et al. [196] studied DLC-Si coating stress effect in 0.89 wt.% NaCl-simulated body environment, and Turcio-Ortega et al. [197] investigated the corrosion behavior. For electrochemistry corrosion character, impedance plot is always used as a measurement for related coating resistance R_p in the electrolyte. The electrochemical equivalent circuit of DLC is introduced in Figure 4.39. Here, R_s is the electrolyte resistance corresponding to the geometrical configuration of the electrodes. R_{ct} and C_{dl} represent the charge transfer resistance and double-layer capacitance existing at the interface between the electrolyte and substrate, whereas R_p and C_{co} are the resistance and capacitance of the DLC coating related to the total effective coverage, material thickness, and other surface characteristics, respectively. This model can be applied in most of the DLC materials, with combining or simply changing some element parameters. In some previous reports, the resistance R_p can be replaced by R_{pf}, which represents the pore resistance on the sample surface [198]. A higher R_{ct} implies a slow corrosion rate and good anticorrosion property.

In several previous reports, C_{co} and C_{dl} can be expressed with another impedance Z_{cpe}, which is a CPE representing the deviation from the true capacitive behavior. The complex impedance is given by $Z_{cpe}=[C(j\omega)a]^{-1}$. The coefficient a is the deviation index related to surface roughness and inhomogeneity of the electrode. The whole equivalent circuit model is simplified (Figure 4.40) and widely applied in many DLC samples.

In 2002, Papakonstantinou et al. [199] applied this model on a-C:H with Si incorporation. After the Si content grew onto the substrate, the corrosion resistance increased 11.8 %. Kim et al. [200] studied DLC corrosion performance in simulated body fluid environment in 2005 (0.89% NaCl solution, pH 7.4 at 37°C) and concluded that Si incorporation in a-C:H could increase corrosion resistance R_p, as well as charge transfer resistance R_{ct}.

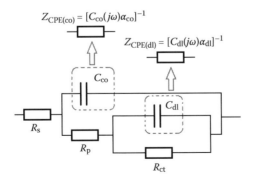

FIGURE 4.40
Combined electrochemical equivalent circuit of DLC.

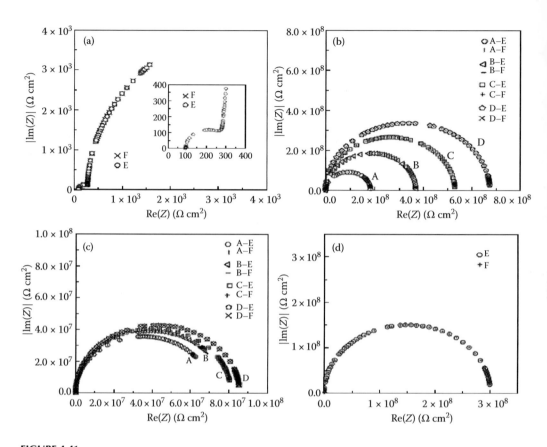

FIGURE 4.41
Cole–Cole (Nyquist) plots of EIS results: The frequency range is 10^4–10^{-3} Hz, and amplitude is 15 mV. The E curve gives out experimental data, and F curve presents fitting data. The b–d plots on DLC film samples deposited at different puttering powers: 500–650 W (b), 700–850 W (c), and 900 W (d). The double-layer capacitance on the DLC films is approximately 0.571–3.91 × 10^{-6} F cm^{-2}, which is smaller than that of some popular electrode materials and comparable with that of diamond. (From Zeng, A., *Thin Solid Films*, 426, 258, 2003. With permission.) [201]

In 1999, Zeng and Liu [201] carried out electrochemical measurements on DLC, which was deposited on AlTiC (70% Al_2O_3 + 30% TiC) substrate. The different DLC films with four types of thickness (2, 5, 10, and 100 nm) are deposited on silicon-coating AlTiC substrates by plasma-assisted ion beam technique. The C_2H_2 gas pressure is 0.1 mTorr with an inductively coupled radio frequency (13.56 MHz). Under the measurement, the resistance R_{ct} and R_p are relatively low (corresponding to 2-nm DLC thickness) and increase dramatically when the DLC layer becomes thicker (R_{ct} = 500 MΩ cm^2, R_p > 10^5 MΩ cm^2 at 100 nm). The author explained that the low-frequency coefficient, α, was decreased from 0.93 to 0.80 whereas coating thickness increased. The polarization plot demonstrates that the corrosion potential of DLC-coated sample is at least 90 mV$_{SCE}$ higher than the uncoated AlTiC substrate. In 2002, Zeng et al. [202] used magnetron sputtering method to form DLC conductive materials on silicon substrate. The DLC films were deposited with DC magnetron sputtering (500–900 W) using a graphite target of high purity (nominal purity, >99.995%) on highly conductive (1–6 × 10^{-3} Ω cm) silicon wafers (111). The potential measurement was carried on with respect to a saturated calomel reference electrode, and a platinum plate counter electrode was used. The Cole–Cole plot result is given by Figure 4.41. Pleskov et al. [203], in the same year, researched the electrochemical behavior of DLC on p-type silicon and glassy carbon substrate. From the electrochemical study, they proved that reasonable admixture of Pt (10% platinum in DLC) made the film suitable for fabrication as electrodes.

References

[1] J. R. Macdonald, *Impedance Spectroscopy: Theory, Experiments and Applications, 2nd Ed.*, Edited by Barsoukov, Wiley-Interscience 2005.

[2] J. E. Bauerle, Study of solid electrolyte polarization by a complex admittance method, *The J. Phys. Chem. Solids* 1969, 30, 2657.

[3] C. M. Armstrong and F. Bezanilla, Charge movement associated with the opening and closing of the activation gates of Na channels, *J. Gen. Physiol.* 1974, 63, 533–552.

[4] E. J. L. Schouler, M. Kleitz, E. Forest, E. Fernandez, and P. Fabry, Overpotential of H_2-H_2O, Ni/ YSZ electrodes in stream electrolyzers, *Proceeding of the International Conference on Fast Ionic Transport in Solids* 1981, 5, 559–562.

[5] L. L. Hench and J. K. West, The sol-gel process, *Chem. Rev.* 1990, 90, 33–72.

[6] H. T. Ye, PhD Thesis, University College London, 2004.

[7] N. Khan, PhD Thesis, University College London, 1990.

[8] H. L. Tuller, Ionic conduction in nanocrystalline materials, *Solid State Ionic* 2000, 131, 143.

[9] J. Maier, Ionic conduction in space charge regions, *Progress in Solid State Chemistry* 1995, 23, 171–263.

[10] T. V. Dijk and A. J. Burggraaf, Gain boundary effects on ionic conductivity in ceramic $Gd_xZr_{(1-x)}O_{(2-(x/2))}$ solid solutions, *Phys. Stat. Sol. A* 1981, 63, 229–240.

[11] M. J. Verkerk, B. J. Middelhuis, and A. J. Burggraat, Effect of grain boundaries on the conductivity of high-purity ZrO_2-Y_2O_3 ceramics, *Solid State Ionics* 1982, 6, 159–170.

[12] M. Gödickemeier, B. Michel, A. Orliukas, P. Bohac, K. Sasaki, and L. Gauckler, Effect of intergranular glass films on the electrical conductivity of 3Y-TZP, *J. Mater. Res.* 1994, 9, 1228.

[13] J. Fleig, The influence of non-ideal microstructure on the analysis of grain boundary impedances, *Solid State Ionics* 2000, 131, 117–127.

[14] J. C. M'Peko, D. L. Spavieri, and M. F. de Souza, In situ characterization of the grain-boundary electrical response of zirconia ceramics under uniaxial compressive stresses, *Appl. Phys. Lett.* 2002, 81, 2827.

[15] L.C. Nistor, J. V. Landury, V. G. Ralchnko, E. D. Obraztsova, and A. A. Smolin, Nanocrystalline diamond films: transmission electron microscopy and Raman spectroscopy characterization, *Diam. Rel. Mater.* 1997, 6, 159–168.

[16] V. V. Daniel, *Dielectric Relaxation*, Academic Press: London, 1967.

[17] I. M. Hodge, M. D. Ingram, and A. R. West, New method of analyzing the ac behavior of polycrystalline solid electrodes, *J. Electroanal. Chem.* 1975, 58, 429–432.

[18] A. Huanosta, O. A. Fregoso, and E. Amano, AC impedance analysis on crystalline layered and polycrystalline bismuth titanate, *J. Appl. Lett.* 1990, 69, 404.

[19] M. M. Kumar, and Z. G. Ye, Dielectric and electric properties of donor- and acceptor-doped ferroelectric $SrBi_2Ta_2O_9$, *J. Appl. Lett.* 2001, 90, 934.

[20] I. Garcia, J. S. Olías, F. A. Rueda, and A. J. Vázquez, Dielectric characterization of oxyacetylene flame-deposited diamond thin films, *Diam. Rel. Mater.* 1997, 6, 1210–1218.

[21] R. F. Davis, Deposition and characterization of diamond, silicon carbide and gallium nitride thin films, *J. Cryst. Growth.* 1994, 137, 161–169.

[22] M. Aoki, Y. M. Chiang, I. Kosacki, L. J. Lee, H. Tuller, and Y. Liu, Solute segregation and grain-boundary impedance in high-purity stabilized zirconia, *J. Am. Ceram. Soc.* 1996, 79, 1169–1180.

[23] J. Volger, *Progress in semiconductor (ed.)*, Edited by A. F. Gibson, New York: John Wiley, 1960.

[24] I. B. Vendik, O. G. Vendik, A. N. Deleniv, V. V. Kondratiev, M. N. Goubina, D. V. Kholodniak, Development of CAD tool for a design of microwave planar HTS filters, *IEEE Trans. Microwave. Theory Tech.* 2000, 48, 1247–1255.

[25] O. G. Vendik, S. P. Zubko, and M. A. Nikol'skiĭ, Modeling and calculation of the capacitance of a planar capacitor containing a ferroelectric thin film, *Tech. Phys.* 1999, 44, 349–355.

[26] J. Mott, D. Kuhman, M. Morgan, F. Jansen, K. Okumura, Y. M. LeGrice, and R. J. Nemanich, Boron doping of diamond thin film, *Appl. Phys. Lett.* 1989, 55, 1121.

[27] J. Mort, M. A. Machonkin, and K. Okumura, Infrared absorption in Boron-doped diamond thin films, *Appl. Phys. Lett.* 1991, 58, 1908.

[28] K. Miyata, K. Kumagai, K. Nishimura, and K. Kobashi, Morphology of heavily B-doped diamond films, *J. Mater. Res.* 1993, 8, 2847–2857.

[29] K. Liu, B. Zhang, M. Wan, J. H. Chu, C. Johnson, and S. Roth, Measurement of electron affinity in boron-doped diamond from capacitance spectroscopy, *Appl. Phys. Lett.* 1997, 70, 2891.

[30] A. T. Collins and A. W. S. Williams, The nature of the acceptor centre in semiconductor diamond, *J. Phys. C: Solid State Phys.* 1971, 4, 1789.

[31] E. C. Lightowler and A. T. Collins, Determination of boron in natural semiconducting diamond by prompt particle nuclear microanalysis and Schottky barrier differential-capacitance measurement, *J. Phys. D: Appl. Phys.* 1976, 9, 951.

[32] G. S. Sandhu, M. L. Swanson, and W. K. Chu, Doping of diamond by coimplantation of carbon and boron, *Appl. Phys. Lett.* 1989, 55, 1397–1399.

[33] A. Masood, M. Aslam, M. A. Tamor, and T. J. Potter, Synthesis and electrical characterization of boron-doped thin diamond films, *Appl. Phys. Lett.* 1992, 61, 1832.

[34] D. M. Malta, J. A. von Windheim, and B. A. Fox, Comparison of electronic transport in boron-doped homoepitaxial polycrystalline, and natural single-crystal diamond, *Appl. Phys. Lett.* 1993, 62, 2926-2928.

[35] R. Kalish, C. U. Saguy, B. Philosoph, V. Richter, and S. Prawer, Loss of electrical conductivity in boron-doped diamond due to ion-induced damage, *Appl. Phys. Lett.* 1997, 70, 999.

[36] M. Werner, O. Dorsch, H. U. Baerwind, E. Obermeier, L. Haase, W. Seifert, A. Ringhandt, C. Johnston, S. Romani, H. Bishop, and P. R. Chalker, Charge transport in heavily B-doped polycrystalline diamond films, *Appl. Phys. Lett.* 1994, 64, 595–597

[37] J. H. Won, A. Hatta, H. Yagyu, N. Jiang, Y. Mori, T. Ito, T. Sasaki, and A. Hiraki, Effect of boron doping on the crystal quality of chemical vapor deposited diamond films, *Appl. Phys. Lett.* 1996, 68, 2882.

[38] W. N. Wang, N. A. Fox, J. W. Steeds, S. R. Lin, and J. E. Butler, Negative electron affinity observed in boron-doped p-type diamond scanning field emission spectroscopy, *Appl. Phys. Lett.* 1996, 80, 6809–6812.

[39] H. Sternschulte, S. Wahl, K. Thonke, M. Dalmer, C. Ronning, and H. Hofsäss, Observation of boron bounded excitons in boron-implanted and annealed natural IIa diamond, *Appl. Phys. Lett.* 1997, 71, 2668.

[40] D. M. Gvozdić, Analysis of transfer function of metal-semiconductor-metal photodetector equivalent circuit, *Appl. Phys. Lett.* 1997, 70, 286.

[41] K. Liu, J. Chu, C. Johnston, and S. Roth, Measurement of electrical activation energy in boron doped diamond using the flatband capacitance method, *J. Appl. Phys.* 1998, 83, 4202–4205.

[42] M. D. Jaeger, S. Hyun, A. R. Day, M. F. Thorpe, B. Golding, Resistivity of boron-doped diamond microcrystals, *Appl. Phys. Lett.* 1998, 72, 2445–2447.

[43] Y. H. Chen, C. T. Hu, and I. N. Lin, Defect structure and electron field-emission properties of boron-doped diamond films, *Appl. Phys. Lett.* 1999, 75, 2857.

[44] O. B. Krutko, P. B. Kosel, R. L. C. Wu, S. J. Fries-Carr, S. Heidger, and J. Weimer, P-type polycrystalline diamond layers by rapid thermal diffusion of boron, *Appl. Phys. Lett.* 2000, 76, 849.

[45] F. Gevrey, A. Gire, D. Gaudiot, J. Theobald, E. Gheeraert, M. Bernard, and F. Torrealba-Anzola, Conductivity and photoconductivity in boron doped diamond films: microwave measurement, *J. Appl. Phys.* 2001, 90, 4251–4255.

[46] C. E. Nebel, E. Rohrer, and M. Stutzmann, Long living excited states in boron doped diamond, *J. Appl. Lett.* 2001, 89, 2237.

[47] D. Narducci and J. J. Cuomo, Boron diffusion in nonimplanted diamond single crystals measured by impedance spectroscopy, *J. Appl. Phys.* 1990, 68, 1184–1186.

[48] H. Ye, O. A. Williams, R. B. Jackman, R. Rudkin, and A. Atkinson, Electrical conduction in polycrystalline CVD diamond: Temperature dependent impedance measurement, *Phys. Status Solidi (A)* 2002, 193, 462–469.

[49] A. Huanosta, O. A. Fregoso, and E. Amano, AC impedance analysis on crystalline layered and polycrystalline bismuth titanate, *J. Appl. Lett.* 1990, 69, 404.

[50] H. Ye, O. Gaudin, R. B. Jackman, P. Muret and E. Gheeraet, DC current and AC impedance measurements on boron-doped single crystalline diamond films, *Phys. Status Solidi (A)* 2003, 199, 92–96.

[51] J. T. Huang, C. S. Hu, J. Hwang, H. Chang, and L. J. Lee, Desegregation of boron at the grain boundary of the *in situ* doped diamond films, *Appl. Phys. Lett.* 1995, 67, 2382.

[52] W. Zhu, B. R. Stoner, B. E. Williams, and J. T. Glass, Growth and characterization of diamond films on nondiamond substrate for electronics applications, *Proceeding of IEEE* 1991, 79, 621.

[53] W. Zhu, A. R. Badzian, and R. F. Messier, Morphological phenomena of CVD diamond (Part I), *Proc. SPIE Diamond Optics III* 1990, 1325, 187–201.

[54] C. J. Tang, A. J. Neves and A. J. S. Fernandes, Influence of nucleation density on film quality, growth rate and morphology of thick CVD diamond films, *Diam. Rel. Mater.* 2003, 12, 1488–1494.

[55] J. M. Larson, and S. L. Girshick, The effect of substrate temperature on the morphology of diamond films grown under acetylene-lean and acetylene-rich conditions, *Diam. Rel. Mater.* 2003 12, 1584–1593.

[56] W. A. Yarbrough and R. Messier, Current issue and problems in the chemical vapor deposition of diamond, *Science* 1990, 247, 688–696.

[57] W. Piekarczyk and W. A. Yarbrough, Application of thermodynamics to the examination of the diamond CVD process II. A model of diamond deposition process from hydrocarbon-hydrogen mixtures, *J. Cryst. Growth* 1991, 108, 583–597.

[58] R. Ramesham, Effect of annealing and hydrogen plasma treatment on the voltammetric and impedance behavior of the diamond electrode, *Thin Solid Films* 1998, 315, 222–228.

[59] H. Ye, R. B. Jackman, and P. Hing, Spectroscopic impedance study of nanocrystalline diamond films, *J. Appl. Phys.* 2003, 94, 7878.

[60] D. Troupis, PhD Thesis, University College London, 2004.

[61] O. A. Williams, R. B. Jackman, and C. E. Nebel, Hydrogenated black diamond: An electrical study, *Phys. Status Solidi (A)* 2002, 193, 577–584.

[62] S. Matsumoto, M. Hino, and T. Kobayashi, Synthesis of diamond films in a rf induction thermal plasma, *Appl. Phys. Lett.* 1987, 51, 737–739.

[63] S. Matsumoto, Y. Sato, M. Tsutsumi, and N. Setaka, Growth of diamond particles from methane-hydrogen gas, *J. Mater. Sci.* 1982, 17, 3106–3112.

[64] M. Kamo, Y. Sato, S. Matsumoto, and N. Setaka, Diamond synthesis from gas phase in microwave plasma, *J. Cryst. Growth* 1983, 62, 642–644.

[65] R. B. Jackman, J. Beckman, and J. S. Foord, The growth of nucleation layers for high-quality diamond CVD from an r.f plasma, *Diam. Rel. Mater.* 1995, 4, 735–739.

[66] R. B. Jackman, J. Beckman, and J. S. Foord, Diamond chemical vapor deposition from a capacitively coupled radio frequency plasma, *Appl. Phys. Lett.* 1995, 66, 1018.

[67] I. P. Hayward, Friction and wear properties of diamond and diamond coatings, *Surf. Coat. Tech.* 1991, 49, 554–559.

[68] S. Chandrasekhar and S. K. Prasad, Recent development in discotic liquid crystals, *Contemp. Phys.* 1999, 40, 237–245.

[69] G. M. Swain, A. B. Anderson, and J. C. Angus, Applications of diamond thin films in electrochemistry, *J. C. MRS Bulletin* 1998, 23, 56–60.

[70] S. Rotter, Applications of conformal CVD diamond films, *Israel J. Chem.* 1998, 38, 135–140.

[71] D. Zhou, D. M. Gruen, L. C. Qin, T. G. McCauley, and A. R. Krauss, Control of diamond film microstructure by Ar additions to CH_4/H_2 microwave plasma, *J. Appl. Phys.* 1998, 84, 1981.

[72] A. R. Krauss, O. Auciello, M. Q. Ding, D. M. Gruen, Y. Huang, V. V. Zhirnov, E. I. Givargizov, A. Breskin, R. Chenchen, E. Shefer, V. Konov, S. Pimenov, A. Karabutov, and N. Suetin, Electron field emission for ultracrystalline diamond films, *J. Appl. Lett.* 2001, 89, 2958.

[73] S. Jiao, A. Sumant, M. A. Kirk, D. M. Gruen, A. R. Krauss, and O. Auciello, Microstructure of ultrananocrystalline diamond films grown by microwave Ar-CH$_4$ plasma chemical vapor deposition with or without added H$_2$, *J. Appl. Lett.* 2001, 90, 118.

[74] R. Erz, W. Dötter, K. Jung, and H. Ehrhardt, Preparation of smooth and nanocrystalline diamond films, *Diam. Rel. Mater.* 1992, 2, 449–453.

[75] J. Lee, B. Hong, R. Messier, and R. W. Collins, Nucleation and bulk film growth kinetics of nanocrystalline diamond prepared by microwave plasma-enhanced chemical vapor deposition on silicon substrate, *Appl. Phys. Lett.* 1996, 69, 1716.

[76] A. V. Khomich, V. I. Polyakov, P. I. Perov, V. P. Varnin, I. G. Teremetskata, V. G. Balakirev, and E. D. Obraztsova, Surface chemical effects on the optical properties of thin nanocrystalline diamond films, *III-nitride, SiC and Diamond Materials for Electronics Devices, Proc. Symposium San Francisco* 1996, 723–728.

[77] D. V. Fedoseev, V. P. Varnin, and B. V. Deryagin, Synthesis of diamond in its thermodynamic metastability region, *Russ. Chem. Rev.* 1996, 70, 1594.

[78] S. N. Kundu, M. Basu, A. B. Maity, S. Chaudhuri, and A. K. Pal, Nanocrystalline diamond films deposited by high pressure sputtering of vitreous carbon, *Mater. Lett.* 1997, 31, 303–309.

[79] M. Zarrabian, N. Fourches-Coulon, G. Turban, C. Marhic, and M. Lancin, Observation of nanocrystalline diamond in diamondlike carbon films deposited at room temperature in electron cyclotron resonance plasma, *Appl. Phys. Lett.* 1997, 70, 2535–2537.

[80] V. I. Konov, A. A. Smolin, V. G. Ralchenko, S. M. Pimenov, E. D. Obraztsova, E. N. Loubnin, S. M. Metev, and G. Sepold, DC arc plasma deposition of smooth nanocrystalline diamond films, *Diam. Rel. Mater.* 1995, 4, 1073–1078.

[81] L. Nistor, J. Van Landuyt, V. G. Ralchenko, E. D Obratzova, K. G. Korotushenko, and A. A. Smolin, Structural studies of nanocrystalline diamond thin films, *Mater. Sci. Forum* 1997, 239–241, 115–118.

[82] D. M. Gruen, Nanocrystalline diamond films, *Annual Rev. Mater. Sci.* 1999, 29, 211–259.

[83] R. Spitzl, V. Ralko, and J. Engemann, Diamond deposition on porous silicon by plasma-assisted CVD, *Diam. Rel. Mater.* 2003, 3, 1256–1261.

[84] S. Jin, M. Fanciulli, T. D. Moustakas, and L. H. Robins, Electronic characterization of diamond films prepared by electron cyclotron resonance microwave plasma, *Diam. Rel. Mater.* 1994, 3, 878–882.

[85] D. V. Fedoseev, V. L. Bukhovets, Y. N. Tolmachev, I. G. Varshavskaya, and V. B. Kvaskov, Deposition and properties of polycluster diamond films, *Diam. Rel. Mater.* 2003, 2, 1327–1329.

[86] W. Zhu, G. P. Kochanski, L. Seibles, D. C. Jacobson, M. McCormack, and A. E. White, Electron field emission from ion-implanted diamond, *Appl. Phys. Lett.* 1995, 67, 1157.

[87] D. Zhou, T. G. McCauley, L. C. Qin, A. R. Krauss, and D. M. Gruen, Synthesis of nanocrystalline diamond thin films from an Ar-CH$_4$ microwave plasma, *J. Appl. Phys.* 1998, 83, 540.

[88] H. Ye, C. Q. Sun, H. Huang, and P. Hing, Single semicircular response of dielectric properties of diamond films, *Thin Solid Films* 2001, 381, 52–56.

[89] P. Vashishta, J. N. Mundy, and G. K. Shenoy, *Fast ion transport in solid: electrodes and electrolytes*, Elsevier North Holland, Inc., New York, NY, 1979.

[90] S. Jin, M. Fanciulli, T. D. Moustakas, and L. H. Robins, Electronic characterization of diamond films prepared by electron cyclotron resonance microwave plasma, *Diam. Rel. Mater.* 1994, 3, 878–882.

[91] S. Nath, and J. I. B. Wilson, Impedance measurement on CVD diamond, *Diam. Rel. Mater.* 1996, 5, 65–75.

[92] J. D. Hunn, N. R. Parikh, M. L. Swanson, and R. A. Zuhr, Conduction in ion-implanted single-crystal diamond, *Diam. Rel. Mater.* 1993, 2, 847–851.

[93] B. R. Stoner, S. R. Sahaida, J. P. Bade, P. Southworth, and P. J. Ellis, Highly oriented, texture diamond films on silicon via bias-enhanced nucleation and textured growth, *J. Mater. Res.* 1993, 8, 1334.

[94] J. G. Ran, C. Q. Zheng, J. Ren, and S. M. Hong, Properties and texture of B-doped diamond films as thermal sensor, *Diam. Rel. Mater.* 1993, 2, 793–796.

[95] T. Sugino, Y. Muto, K. Karasutani, J. Shirafuji, and K. Kobashi, Trap states elucidated by A.C conductance measurement in polycrystalline chemically vapour-deposited diamond films, *Diam. Rel. Mater.* 1993, 2, 803–807.

[96] K. Miyata, and D. L. Dreifus, Effect of annealing in air on electrical resistance of B-doped poly-crystalline diamond films, *Jpn. J. Appl. Phys.* 1994, 33, 4526–4533.

[97] M. I. Landstrass, and K. V. Ravi, Hydrogen passivation of electrically active defects in diamond, *Appl. Phys. Lett.* 1989, 55, 1391–1393.

[98] Y. Mori, Y. Show, M. Deguchi, H. Yagi, H. Yagyu, N. Eimori, T. Okada, A. Hatta, K. Nishimura, M. Kitabatake, T. Ito, T. Hirao, T. Izumi, T. Sasaki, and A. Hiraki, Characterization of surface conductive diamond layer grown by microwave plasma chemical vapor deposition, *Jpn. J. Appl. Phys.* 1993, 32, L987–L989.

[99] M. Werner, O. Dorsch, A. Hinze, E. Obermeier, R. E. Harper, C. Johnston, P. R. Chalker, and I. M. Buckley-Golder, Space-charge-limited current flow and trap density in undoped diamond films, *Diam. Rel. Mater.* 1993, 2, 825–828.

[100] B. Huang, and D. K. Reinhard, Electric field-dependent conductivity of polycrystalline dia-mond thin films, *Appl. Phys. Lett.* 1991, 59, 1494–1496.

[101] P. Extance, S. R. Elliott, and E. A. Davis, Frequency-dependent conductivity in sputtered amor-phous phosphorus thin film, *Phys. Rev. B* 1985, 32, 8184.

[102] D. M. Malta, J. A. Windheim, H. A. Wynands and B. A. Fox, Comparison of the electric prop-erties of simultaneously deposited homoepitaxial and polycrystalline diamond films, *J. Appl. Phys.* 1995, 77, 1536.

[103] B. Fiegl, R. Kuhnert, M. Ben-Chorin, and F. Koch, Evidence for grain boundary hopping trans-port in polycrystalline diamond films, *Appl. Phys. Lett.* 1994, 65, 371–371.

[104] J. Chen, S. Z. Deng, J. Chen, Z. X. Yu, and N. S. Xu, Graphitization of nanodiamond powder annealed in argon ambient, *Appl. Phys. Lett.* 1999, 74, 3651.

[105] H. Hirai, K. Kondo, M. Kim, and H. Koinuma, Transparent nanocrystalline diamond ceramics fabricated from C_{60} fullerene by shock compression, *Appl. Phys. Lett.* 1997, 71, 3016.

[106] C. Q. Sun, H. Xie, W. Zhang, H. Ye, and P. Hing, Preferential oxidation of diamond {111}, *J. Phys. D: Appl. Phys.* 2000, 33, 2196.

[107] R. Heidinger, and A. Kumlin, The impact of extrinsic conductivity on the mm-wave dielectric loss in high resistivity silicon, *16th Internat. Conf. on Infrared and Millimeter Waves, Lausanne, Aug. 26-30, Conf. Digest Lausanne: Ecole Polytechnique* 1576. 1991, 450–451.

[108] C. E. Nebel, and J. Ristein, *Thin Film Diamond: I 76*, 2003.

[109] C. E. Nebel, and J. Ristein, *Thin Film Diamond: I 77*, 2004.

[110] O. A. Williams, S. Curat, J. E. Gerbi, D. M. Gruen, and R. B. Jackman, *n*-type conductivity in ultrananocrystalline diamond films, *Appl. Phys. Lett.* 2004, 85, 1680.

[111] P. W. May, *Diamond thin films: a 21st-century material*, Philosophical Transactions of The Royal Society A: Mathematical Physical & Engineering Sciences 2000, 358, 473.

[112] J. C. Angus, Y. V. Pleskov, and S. C. Eaton, *Chapter 3 Electrochemistry of diamond*, Semiconductors and Semimetals 2004, 77, 97–119.

[113] A. Fujishima, Y. Einaga, and T. N. Rao, *Diamond Electrochemistry*, Elsevier, 2005.

[114] A. B. Kharitonov, L. Alfonta, E. Katz, and I. Willner, Probing of bioaffinity interactions at interface using impedance spectroscopy and Chronopotentiometry. *J. Electro. Chem.* 2000, 487, 133–141.

[115] L. Alfonta, E. Katz, and I. Willner, Sensing of acetylcholine by a tricomponent-enzyme layered electrode using faradic impedance spectroscopy, cyclic voltammetry, and microgravimetric quarts crystal microbalance transduction method, *Anal. BioChem.* 2000, 75, 927–935.

[116] L. Alfonta, A. Bardea, O. Khersonsky, E. Katz, and I. Willner, Chronopotentiometry and Faradic impedance spectroscopy as signal transduction methods for the biocatalytic precipitation of an insoluble product on electrode supports: Route for enzyme sensors, immunosensors and DNA sensors, *Biosens. Bioelectron.* 2001, 16, 675–687.

[117] A. Bardea, F. Patolsky, A. Dagan, and I. Willner, Sensing and amplification of oligonucleotride-DNA interactions by means of impedance spectroscopy: A route to a Tay-Sachs sensor, *Chem. Comm.* 1999, 21–22.

[118] F. Patolsky, A. Liochtenstein, and I. Willner, Electrochemical transduction of liposome-amplified DNA sensing, *Chem. Inter. Ed.* 2000, 39, 940.

[119] F. Patolsky, Y. Weizmann, and I. Willner, redox-active nucleic-acid replica for the amplified bioelectrocatalystic detection of viral DNA, *J. American Chem. Soc. Communication* 2002, 124, 770–772.

[120] M. Y. Vagin, A. A. Karyakin, and T. Hianik, Surfactant bilayers for the direct electrochemical detection of affinity interactions, *Biochem.* 2002, 56, 91–93.

[121] T. Y. Lee and Y. B. Shin, Direct DNA hybridization based on the oligonucleotide-functionalized conductive polymer, *Anal. Chem.* 2001, 73, 5629–5632.

[122] H. Cai, Y. Xu, P. G. He, and Y. Z. Fang, Indicator free DNA hybridization detection by impedance measurement based on the DNA-doped conducting polymer film formed on the carbon nanotube modified electrode, *Electroanalysis* 2003, 15, 1864.

[123] C. A. Marquette, I. Lawrence, C. Polychronakos, and M. F. Lawrence, Impedance based DNA chip for direct T_m measurement, *Talanta* 2002, 56, 763–768.

[124] C. Berggren, B. Bjarnason, and G. Johansson, Capacitive biosensors, *Electroanalysis* 2001, 13, 173.

[125] C. D. Feng, Y. D. Ming, P. J. Hesketh, S. M. Gendel, and J. R. Stetter, Confirmation of immobilizing IgG on different surfaces with AFM and impedance investigations of a Pt electrode during the immobilization, *Sensor. Actuat. B-Chem.* 1996, 36, 431.

[126] K. Takahashi, M. Tanga, O. Takai, and H. Okamura, DNA preservation using diamond chips, *Diam. Rel. Mater.* 2003, 12, 572–576.

[127] W. Yang, O. Auciello, J. E. Butler, W. Cai, J. A. Carlisle, J. E. Gerbi, D. M. Gruen, T. Knickerbocker, T. L. Lasseter, J. N. Russell, Jr, L. M. Smith, and R. J. Hamers, DNA-modified nanocrystalline diamond thin-films as stable, biologically active substrate, *Nat. Mater.* 2002, 1, 253–257.

[128] J. Wang, M. A. Firestone, O. Auciello, and J. A. Carlisle, Surface functionalization of ultrananocrystalline diamond films by electrochemical reduction of aryldiazonium salts, *Langmuir* 2004, 20, 11450–11456.

[129] G. J. Zhang, K. S. Song, Y. Nakamura, T. Ueno, T. Funatsu, I. Ohdomari, and H. Kawarada, DNA micropatterning polycrystalline diamond via one-step direct amination, *Langmuir* 2006, 22, 3728–3734.

[130] W. Yang, J. E. Bulter, J. N. Russell, Jr, and R. J. Hamers, Interfacial electrical properties of DNA-modified diamond thin films: Intrinsic response and hybridization-induced field effects, *Langmuir* 2004, 20, 6778–6787.

[131] Y. Gu, D. Chen, and X. Jiao, Synthesis and electrochemical properties of nanostructured $LiCoO_2$ fiber as cathode materials for lithium-ion batteries, *J. Phys. Chem.* 2005, 109, 17901–17906.

[132] T. N. Rao, I. Yagi, T. Miwa, D. A. Tryk, and A. Fujishima, Electrochemical oxidation of NADH at highly boron-doped diamond electrode, *Anal. Chem.* 1999, 71, 2506–2511.

[133] C. E. Nebel, D. Shin, B. Rezek, N. Tokuda, H. Uetsuka, and H. Watanabe, Diamond and biology, *J. R. Soc. Interface* 2007, 4, 439–461.

[134] C. E. Nebel, D. Shin, D. Takeuchi, T. Yamamoto, H. Watanabe, and T. Nakamura, Photochemical attachment of amine linker molecules on hydrogen terminated diamond, *Diam. Rel. Mater.* 2006, 15, 1107–1112.

[135] Alkene/diamond liquid/solid interface characterization using internal photoemission spectroscopy, *Langmuir* 2006, 22, 5645–5653.

[136] D. Shin, N. Tokuda, B. Rezek, and C. E. Nebel, Periodically arranged benzene-linker molecules on boron-doped single-crystalline diamond film for DNA sensing, *ElectroChem. Comm.* 2006, 8, 844–850.

[137] D. Shin, B. Rezek, N. Tokuda, D. Takeuchi, H. Watanabe, T. Nakamura, T. Yamamoto, and C. E. Nebel, Photo- and electrochemical bonding of DNA to single crystalline CVD diamond, *Phys. Status Solidi A* 2006, 203, 3245–3272.

[138] C. E. Nebel, B. Rezek, D. Shin, H. Uetsuka, and N. Yang, Diamond for bio-sensor applications, *J. Phys. D: Appl. Phys.* 2007, 40, 6443.

[139] G. M. Swain, and R. Ramesham, The electrochemical activity of boron-doped polycrystalline diamond thin film electrodes, *Anal. Chem.* 1993, 65, 345–351.

[140] H. B. Martin and W. M. Morrison, Jr, Application of a diamond thin film as a transparent electrode for *in situ* infrared spectroelectrochemistry, *ElectroChem. Solid-State Lett.* 1996, 143, L133.

[141] T. Yano, D. A. Tryk, K. Hashimoto, and A. Fujishima, Electrochemical behavior of highly conductive boron-doped diamond electrodes for oxygen reduction in alkaline solution, *J. ElectroChem. Soc.* 1998, 145, 1870–1876.

[142] S. Sano. K. Kato, and Y. Ikada, Introduction of functional groups onto the surface of polyethylene for protein immobilization, *Biomaterials* 1993, 14, 817–822.

[143] W. Yang, J. E. Bulter, J. N. Russell, Jr, and R. J. Hamers, Direct electrical detection of antigen-antibody binding on diamond and silicon substrate using electrical impedance spectroscopy, *Analyst* 2007, 132, 296–306.

[144] T. N. Rao, T. A. Ivandini, C. Terashima, B. V. Sarada, and A. Fujishima, application of bare and modified diamond electrodes in electroanalysis, *New Diam. Front. C. Tech.* 2003, 13, 79.

[145] C. Terashima, T. N. Rao, B. V. Sarada, D. A. Tryk, and A. Fujishima, electrochemical oxidation of chlorophenols at a boron-doped diamond electrode and their determination by high-performance liquid chromatograph with amperometric detection, *Anal. Chem.* 2002, 74, 895–902.

[146] I. Yagi, H. Nostu, T. Kondo, D. A. Tryk, and A. Fujishima, Electrochemical selectivity for redox systems at oxygen-terminated diamond electrodes, *J. ElectroAnal. Chem.* 1999, 473, 173–178.

[147] M. N. Latto, D. J. Riely, and P. W. May, Impedance studies of boron-doped CVD diamond electrodes, *Diam. Rel. Mater.* 2000, 9, 1181–1183.

[148] H. B. Suffredini, V. A. Pedrosa, L. Codognoto, S. A. S. Machado, R. C. Rocha-Filho, and L. A. Avaca, Enhanced electrochemical response of boron-doped diamond electrodes brought on by a cathodic surface pre-treatment, *Electro. Acta.* 2004, 49, 4021–4026.

[149] S. Ferro, and A. D. Battisti, Electron transfer reactions at conductive diamond electrodes, *Electro. Acta.* 2002, 47, 1641–1649.

[150] D. Becker, and K. Jüttner, Impedance measurements on boron-doped diamond electrodes at different doping levels, *New Diam. Front. C. Tech.* 2003, 13, 67.

[151] M. Bevilacqua, and R. B. Jackman, Extreme sensitivity displayed by single crystal diamond deep ultraviolet photoconductive devices, *Appl. Phys. Lett.* 2009, 95, 243–501.

[152] R. M. Wightman, Probing cellular chemistry in biological systems with microelectrodes, *Science* 2006, 311, 1570–1574.

[153] Y. Yun, Z. Dong, V. N. Shanov, and M. J. Schulz, Electrochemical impedance measurement of prostate cancer cell using carbon nanotube array in a microfluidic channel, *Nanotechnology* 2007, 18, 465–505.

[154] V. Raffa, G. Clofani, S. Nitodas, T. Karachalios, D. D'Alessandro, M. Masini, and A. Cuschieri, *Carbon* 2008, 46, 1600–1610.

[155] R. K. Gupta, and V. Saraf, Nanoelectronics: Tunneling current in DNA-single electron transistor, *Current Appl. Phys.* 2009, 9, S149–S152.

[156] T. Ahuja, I. A. Mir, D. Kumar, and Rajesh, Potentiometric urea biosensor based on BSA embedded surface modified polypyrrole film, *Sensor. Actuat. B-Chem.* 2008, 134, 140–145.

[157] E. Paleček, M. Fojta and F. Jelen, New approaches in the development of DNA sensors: Hybridization and electrochemical detection of DNA and RNA at two different surface, *Bioelectrochemical* 2002, 56, 85–90.

[158] E. Paleček, and M. Fojta, Magnetic beads as versatile tools for electrochemical DNA and protein biosensing, *Talanta* 2007, 74, 276–290.

[159] T. T. N. Lien, T. D. Lam, V. T. H. An, T. V. Hoang, D. T. Quang, D. Q. Khieu, T. Tsukahara, Y. H. Lee, and J. S. Kim, Multi-wall carbon nanotubes (MWCNTs)-doped polypyrrole DNA biosensor for label-free detection of genetically modified organisms by QCM and EIS, *Talanta* 2010, 80, 1164–1169.

[160] M. A. Vorotyntsev, C. Deslouis, M. M. Musiani, B. Tribollet, and K. Aoki, Transport across an electroactive polymer film in contact with media allowing both ionic and electronic interfacial exchange, *Electrochimical Acta.* 1999, 44, 2105–2115.

[161] Y. Zhang, J. Wang, and M. Xu, A sensitive DNA biosensor fabricated with gold nanoparticles/ploy(p-aminobenzoic acid)/carbon nanotubes modified electrode, *Col. Sur. B: Biointerfaces* 2010, 75, 179–185.

[162] M. Varcárcel, S. Cárdenas, and B. M. Simonet, Role of carbon nanotubes in analytical science, *Anal. Chem.* 2007, 79, 4788–4797.

[163] S. Maldonado, S. Morin, and K. J. Stevenson, Electrochemical oxidation of cathecholamines and catechols at carbon nanotubes electrodes, *Analyst* 2006, 131, 262–267.

[164] Y. Tang, B. L. Allen, D. R. Kauffman, and A. Star, Electrocatalytic activity of nitrogen-doped carbon nanotubes cups, *J. ACS. Communication* 2009, 131, 13200–13201.

[165] B. J. Lee, S. R. Sivakkumar, J. M. Ko, J. H. Kim, S. M. Jo, and D. Y. Kim, Carbon nanofibre/hydrous RuO2 nanocomposite electrodes for supercapacitors, *J. Power Sources* 2007, 168, 546–552.

[166] S. Deng, G. Jian, J. Lei, Z. Hu, and H. Ju, A glucose biosensor based on direct electrochemistry of glucose oxidase immobilized on nitrogen-doped carbon nanotubes, *Biosens. Bioelectron.* 2009, 25, 373–377.

[167] L. Ratner, W. Haseltine, R. Patarca, K. J. Livak, B. Starcich, S. F. Josephs, E. R. Doran, J. A. Rafalski, E. A. Whitehorn, K. Baumerster, L. Ivanoff, S. R. Petteway, Jr, M. L. Pearson, J. A. Lautenberger, T. S. Papas, J. Ghrayeb, N. T. Chang, R. C. Gallo, and F. Wong-Staal, Complete nucleotide sequence of AIDS virus, HTLV-III, *Nature* 1985, 313, 277–284.

[168] S. Seelmeier, H. Schmidt, V. Turk, and K. Von der Helm, Human immunodeficiency virus has an aspartic-type protease that can be inhibited by pepstatin A, *Proc. Natl. Acad. Sci. USA* 1988, 85, 6612–6616.

[169] A. Molla, S. Vasavanonda, G. Kumar, H. L. Sham, M. Johnson, B. Grabowski, J. F. Denissen, W. Kohlbrenner, J. J. Plattner, J. M. Leonard, D. W. Norbeck, and D. J. Kempf, Human serum attenuates the activity of protease inhibitors towards wild-type and mutant human immunodeficiency virus, *Virology* 1998, 250, 255–262.

[170] H. G. Kräusslich, R. H. Ingraham, M. T. Skoog, W. Wimmer, P. V. Pallari, and C. A. Carter, Activity of purified biosynthetic proteinase of human immunodeficiency virus on natural substrates and synthetic peptides, *Proc. Natl. Acad. Sci. USA* 1989, 86, 807.

[171] L. Gillim, G. L. Gusella, J. Vargas, Jr, D. Marras, M. E. Klotman, and A. Cara, Development of a novel screen for protease inhibitors, *Clin. Diagn. Lab Immunol.* 2001, 8, 437.

[172] K. Hu, J. Clément, L. Abrahamyan, K. Strebel, M. Bouvier, L. Kleiman, and A. J. Mouland, A human immunodeficiency virus type 1 prtease biosensor assay using bioluminescence resonance energy transfer, *J. Viro. Met.* 2005, 128, 93.

[173] Y. Shan, and L. Gao, Formation and characterization of multi-walled carbon nanotubes/Co_3O_4 nanocomposites for supercapacitors, *Mater. Chem. Phys.* 2007, 103, 206–210.

[174] G. Arabale, D. Wagh, M. Kulkarni, I. S. Mulla, S. P. Vernekar, K. Vijayamohanan, and A. M. Rao, Enhanced supercapacitance of multiwalled carbon nanotubes functionalized with ruthenium oxide, *Chem. Phys. Lett.* 2003, 376, 207–213.

[175] K. A. Mahmoud, and J. H. T. Luong, Impedance method for detecting HIV-1 protease and screening for its inhibitors using ferrocene-peptide conjugate/au nanotubes/single walled carbon nanotube modified electrode, *Anal. Chem.* 2008, 80, 7056–7062.

[176] J. Marciniszyn, Jr, J. A. Hartsuck, and J. Tang, Mode of inhibition of acid protease by pepstatin, *J. Bio. Chem.* 1976, 251, 7088–7094.

[177] T. Hyeon, S. S. Lee, J. Park, Y. Chung, and H. B. Na, Synthesis of highly crystalline and monodisperse maghemite nanocrystallites without a size-selection process, *J. Am. Chem. Soc.* 2001, 123, 12798–12801.

[178] A. Lam, D. P. Wilkinson, and J. Zhang, A novel single electrode supported direct methonal fuel cell, *ElectroChem. Comm.* 2009, 11, 1530–1534.

[179] A. Lan, and A. S. Mukasyan, Complex $SrRuO_3$-Pt and $LaRuO_3$-Pt catalyst for direct alchol fuel cell, *Industr. & Eng. Chem. Res.* 2008, 47, 8989.

[180] Z. Liu, L. Hong, M. P. Tham, T. H. Lim, and H. Jiang, Nanostructured Pt/C and Pd/C catalysts for direct formic acid fuel cells, *J. Power Sources* 2006, 161, 831–835.

[181] J. Choi, K. Park, I. Park, W. Nam, and Y. Sung, Methanol electro-oxidation and direct methanol fuel cell using Pt/Rh and Pt/Ru/Rh alloy catalysts, *Electrochimica Acta* 2004, 50, 787–790.

[182] S. Jayaraman, T. F. Jaramillo, S. Baeck, and E. W. McFarland, Synthesis and characterization of Pt-WO_3 as methanol oxidation catalysts for fuel cell, *J. Phys. Chem. B* 2005, 109, 22958–22966.

[183] L. P. R. Profeti, D. Profeti, and P. Olivi, Pt-RyO_2 electrodes prepared by thermal decomposition of polymeric precursors as catalysts for direct methanol fuel cell applications, *Inter. J. Hydrogen Energy* 2009, 34, 2747–2757.

[184] H. Song, P. Xiao, X. Qiu and W. Zhu, Design and preparation of highly active carbon nanotube-supported sulfated TiO_2 and platinum catalysts for methanol electrooxidation, *J. Power Sources* 2010, 195, 1610–1614.

[185] P. Poizot, S. Laruelle, S. Grugeon, L. Dupont, and J. Tarascon, Nano-sized transition-metal oxides as negative-electrode materials for lithium-ion batteries, *Lett. Nat.* 2000, 407, 496–499.

[186] Y. Nishi, Lithium ion secondary batteries; past 10 years and the future, *J. Power Sources* 2001, 100, 101–106.

[187] A. A. Arie, W. Chang, and J. K. Lee, Effect of fullerene coating on silicon thin film anodes for lithium rechargeable batteries, *J. Solid State Electr.* 2010, 14, 51.

[188] T. Ohzuku, and Y. Makimura, Layeres lithium insertion material of $LiCo_{1/3}Ni_{1/3}Mn_{1/3}O_2$ for lithium ion batteries, *Chem. Lett.* 2001, 30, 642–643.

[189] R. Guo, P. Shi, X. Cheng, and C. Du, Synthesis and characterization of carbon-coated $LiN_{1/3}Co_{1/3}Mn_{1/3}O_2$ cathode material prepared by polyvinyl alcohol pyrolysis route, *J. Alloys & Compounds* 2009, 473, 53–59.

[190] H. S. Kim, Y. H. Chung, S. H. Kang, and Y. Sung, Electrochemical behavior of carbon-coated SnS_2 for use as the anode in lithium-ion batteries, *Electrochimica Acta* 2009, 54, 3606–3610.

[191] Y. Zheng, M. Zhang, and P. Gao, Preparation and electrochemical properties of multiwalled carbon mamotubes-nikel oxide porous composite for supercapacitors, *Mater. Res. Bulletin* 2007, 42, 1740–1747.

[192] T. P. Gujar, V. R. Shinde, C. D. Lokhande, and S. Han, Electrosynthesis of Bi_2O_3 thin films and their use in electrochemical supercapacitors, *J. Power Sources* 2006, 161, 1479–1485.

[193] D. Kalpana, K. S. Omkumar, S. S. Kumar, and N. G. Renganathan, A novel high power symmetric ZnO/carbon aerogel composite electrode for electrochemical supercapacitors, *Electrochimica Acta* 2006, 52, 1309–1315.

[194] Y. Zhang, H. Li, L. Pan, T. Lu, and Z. Sun, Capacitive behavior of graphene-ZnO composite film for supercapacitors, *J. ElectroAnal. Chem.* 2009, 634, 68–71.

[195] P. Guo, H. Song, and X. Chen, Electrochemical performance of graphene nanosheets as anode materials for lithium-ion batteries, *ElectroChem. Comm.* 2009, 11, 1320–1324.

[196] N. D. Nam, S. H. Lee, J. W .Yi, and K. R. Lee, Effect of stress on the passivation of Si-DLC coating as sheet materials in simulated body environment, *Diam. Rel. Mater.* 2009, 18, 1145–1151.

[197] D. Turcio-Ortega, S. E. Rodil, and S. Muhl, Corrosion behavior of amorphous carbon deposite in 0.89% NaCl by electrochemical impedance spectroscopy, *Diam. Rel. Mater.* 2009, 18, 1360–1368.

[198] Mechanical stability, corrosion performance and bioresponse of amorphous diamond-like carbon for medical stents and guidewires, *Diam. Rel. Mater.* 2004, 14, 1277–1288.

[199] P. Papakonstantinou, J. F. Zhao, P. Lemoine, E. T. McAdams, and J. A. McLaughlin, The effects of Si incorporation on the electrochemical and nanomechanical properties of DLC thin films, *Diam. Rel. Mater.* 2002, 11, 1074–1080.

[200] H. Kim, S. Ahn, J. Kim, S. J. Park, and K. Lee, Corrosion performance of diamond-like carbon (DLC)-coated Ti alloy in the simulated body fluid environment, *Diam. Rel. Mater.* 2004, 14, 35–41.

[201] A. Zeng, E. Liu, S. Zhang, S. N. Tan, P. Hing, I. F. Annergren, and J. Gao, Impedance study on electrochemical characteristics of spttered DLC films, *Thin Solid Films* 2003, 426, 258–264.

[202] A. Zeng, E. Liu, I. F. Annergren, S. N. Tan, S. Zhang, P. Hing, and J. Gao, EIS capacitance diagnosis of nanoporosity effect on the corrosion protection of DLC films, *Diam. Rel. Mater.* 2002, 11, 160–168.

[203] Y .V. Pelskov, A. Y. Sakharova, M. D. Krotova, L. L. Bouilov, and B. V. Spitsyn, Photoelectrochemical properties of semiconductor diamond, *J. ElectroAnal. Chem.* 1987, 228, 19–27.

5

Control of Drug Release from Coatings: Theories and Methodologies

Lei Shang, Sam Zhang, Subbu S. Venkatraman, and Hejun Du

CONTENTS

Introduction 196
   Coating Technology in Release Rate Control 196
   Sustained Release Profile 197
   Pulsatile Release Profile...197
Release Rate Control Principles 199
   Diffusion..199
      Diffusivity Control Theory..202
   Porous Perspective..203
      Nonporous Perspective 210
      Partition/Solubility Oriented 215
      Equilibrium Condition of Partition..217
      Partition of Protein in Aqueous Two-Phase Systems 217
      Partition of Protein in Hydrogel Membrane 218
      Excess Function and Activity Coefficient (for Nonelectrolytes)...............219
      Polymer Solution 226
      Modeling of Charged Solute Partitioning in Hydrogel 230
   Erosion Controlled 235
      Degradation Kinetics 236
      Diffusion in a Degrading Coating..236
   Osmotic Pressure Controlled...237
Coating Materials and Techniques 238
   Coating Materials...238
      Collagen..238
      Gelatin..238
      Alginate..238
      Chitosan..239
      Cellulose and Its Derivatives 239
      Polyvinyl-Based Polymers 239
      Acrylate-Based Materials 239
      Polyethylene Glycol 240
      Polyesters...240
   Coating Techniques...240
      Fluid Bed..240

Compression Coating 241
Plasticizer Dry Coating..241
Hot–Melt..241
Supercritical Fluid Coating 242
Electrospinning...242
Precipitation Method 242
Drug Delivery Systems with Coating 243
Summary 249
References..249

Introduction

There are three phases that a drug has to undergo before it takes effect in the human body: pharmaceutical phase, pharmacokinetics phase, and pharmacodynamic phase. Pharmaceutical phase is the initial phase when the formulation breaks apart and the active ingredient dissolves. The pharmacokinetics phase concerns how the drug is affected by the physiological system. Pharmacodynamic phase is the one in which the drug reaches the targeted site and takes action. From the site of administration to the targeted site, various mechanisms, both biochemical and physical, take place in the human body. Drugs are selected or transformed or even destroyed and its therapeutic effects are limited [1]. The objective of drug delivery research is to neutralize the negative effects and to improve the efficacy of the medicine by bypassing those undesirable processes.

The demand for a delivery system becomes more urgent in recent years because new technologies and clearer biological insights have led to new classes of therapeutic agents. Typical examples are antibodies, gene-based drugs, antisense oligonucleotides, virus-like particles, recombinant proteins, and hormones. The potency and activity of these biotechnological agents are often thwarted by the wrong or improperly constructed delivery systems, because of the fact that these agents frequently have short half-lives, poor permeability in membranes, and serious toxicity when delivered systemically in large doses [1].

Drug delivery system design has been an integral part of drug development in the pharmaceutical industry. It provides the functions of protection, targeting, and release rate control. Protection of therapeutic agents can be realized by packing the drug in a carrier so that the direct contact between the drug and the physiological environment is avoided. If the packaging material is well selected, it could enable drug permeation across membranes and physiochemical barriers (such as the blood–brain barrier and skin). Surface modification of the packaging materials using highly specific recognition molecules could induce localized accumulation of the drug in a preferred site for action (targeting). Eventually, drug molecules have to be released from the package to take effect.

Coating Technology in Release Rate Control

Drug delivery system design is essentially a step of the formulation development in the overall drug development process. Coating technology has been used extensively in different formulations to address different issues: taste masking [2], protection [3], coloring, release rate control, and targeting. Among different applications of the coating technology in the drug delivery, this chapter focuses on release rate control by coating technology. The advantages of applying coating in release rate control are its flexibility to be used in the realization of both sustained and pulsatile drug release profiles.

Sustained Release Profile

One of the main objectives of drug delivery is to maintain the concentration of the drug sufficiently high at the site of action to exert the therapeutic effect, while ensuring that it is not too high to cause any detrimental side effects. The concentration range bound by these upper and lower limits of the drug concentration is also known as the therapeutic window. To maintain an essentially constant blood drug level within this therapeutic window over a period of time, Smith, Kline, and French designed and commercialized sustained drug delivery systems in the late 1940s. Sustained drug delivery is ideal for drugs that have a short half-life and a narrow therapeutic window (potent drugs). Sustained drug delivery is also a better option for the treatment of chronic diseases, which requires prolonged drug action time (e.g., cancer, high blood pressure). Therefore, toxicity and the inconvenience of the repeated dosage are greatly reduced. Depending on the nature of the disease and the medicine, the therapeutic window could be large or narrow. This imposes stringent requirements for drug delivery systems to provide a narrow therapeutic window and control release rate precisely. A rate-limiting coating on the drug carrier is commonly used to achieve a sustained release profile.

Pulsatile Release Profile

Most physiological systems work in a negative feedback manner, and only vary in a narrow range. A typical example is the blood glucose concentration. Glucose is a major energy source for human beings. It is taken from food and converted into glycogen in liver and muscles, where glycogen is also able to convert back to glucose, as shown in Scheme 1.

$$\text{Glucose} \underset{k_2}{\overset{k_1}{\rightleftharpoons}} \text{Glycogen} \qquad\qquad \text{Scheme 1}$$

At equilibrium, k_1 is equal to k_2, resulting in a constant blood glucose concentration of 70–100 mg/dL (3.9–6.1 mmol/L) for healthy people to guarantee that a sufficient amount of energy is supplied to the system.

In a simplified picture, if the glucose concentration goes higher than the normal level (after food), the body will send messengers (insulin) to the liver and the muscle to speed up the conversion of glucose to glycogen ($k_1 > k_2$), to reduce the glucose concentration, whereas if the blood glucose concentration is lower than the normal level (hungry), messengers will be absent; hence, the reverse reaction is dominating ($k_1 < k_2$), resulting in an increase in the glucose concentration.

Many physiological peptides and proteins, which act as messengers to maintain the equilibrium of the physiological system, are collectively known as hormones. They are released in the body in a pulsatile fashion on an as-needed basis as opposed to a continuous release. Diseases caused by functionality or secretion deficiency of this kind of proteins are often treated by the administration of the same kind of proteins obtained from other sources (animal or human recombinant proteins). A significant challenge in hormone delivery is to prepare delivery systems that release hormones in a non–zero-order fashion to better mimic physiological hormone release. Using pulsatile/controlled delivery systems function in an on–off manner to deliver protein or peptide drugs in response to internal or external stimuli is the ideal choice (Figure 5.1).

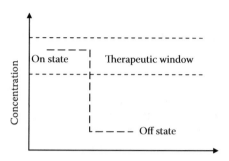

FIGURE 5.1
Pulsatile release profile.

Externally regulated pulsatile delivery systems may be considered open-loop systems (Figure 5.2a) and the internal or self-regulated systems may be considered closed-loop systems (Figure 5.2b). It is obvious that the closed-loop system is a more suitable choice because of its ability to be self-controlled. Overdose of hormone drugs such as insulin is highly undesirable because it leads to coma and death [4]. A good control over the release rate, especially at off-state, is thus the key issue in pulsatile/controlled delivery systems to minimize any leakage. To realize pulsatile drug delivery and to control its release rate at different states, a responsive material can be coated onto the conventional drug carrier.

This chapter is devoted to address four fundamental questions: (1) What mechanisms are used to control release by coating? (2) What materials are usually used for coating the drug delivery systems? (3) How are different release profiles achieved, and can their release rates by different types of coatings be controlled? (4) What techniques are used to realize different coatings in both large-scale production and research laboratories?

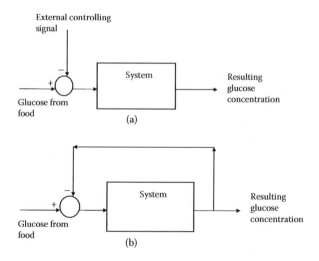

FIGURE 5.2
Open- and closed-loop control systems.

Release Rate Control Principles

Release rate control is eventually a control over the driving force for the drug release. Among different driving forces, diffusion, erosion, and osmotic pressure are the most commonly encountered ones in coated drug delivery systems.

Diffusion

The most commonly used driving force in drug delivery systems is probably diffusion. At device level, there are two basic configurations of diffusion-controlled systems: matrix based (tablets) and membrane based (capsules and tablets) (Figure 5.3). In matrix-based systems, also known as monolith systems, drug molecules are entrapped in a polymeric matrix, and its release rate is controlled by the diffusivity of the drug. On the other hand, in membrane-based systems, drugs are carried in a separate reservoir, and one or more surfaces of the reservoir are permeable to the drug. Drug molecules have to dissolve or partition into the membrane and then diffuse out from it.

Although it is more popular to use matrix-based systems for drug delivery, a lot of them require modifications to alter their release profiles. One of the most commonly used modifications is to coat the surface of the original matrix with another material. Such systems are more similar to membrane-based systems when their release mechanisms are concerned: the core serves the same function like the reservoir. Drug molecules have to dissolve into the coating/membrane first (partition step), diffuse along a concentration gradient in that layer, and then release to the surroundings. In other words, there are two factors governing the overall release rate of diffusion-controlled systems: diffusivity and partition coefficient.

The release mechanism of such a system is more complex compared with a simple matrix-based system for two reasons: (1) drug molecules diffuse in two different regions with different diffusivity, and (2) besides diffusion, there is an extra step governing the overall release rate, which is partition. The complication due to the partition step is because only drug molecules inside the membrane/coating could be released, but drug concentration in the membrane might not be equal to the drug concentration in the donor/matrix. This scenario is illustrated in Figure 5.4 where C_D and C_R are the donor and receptor drug concentration, respectively; C_A and C_B are the drug concentration in the membrane at two interfaces; and L is the membrane thickness. Under a perfect sink condition ($C_R(t) = 0$), it is reasonable to assume that $C_B = C_R$, but C_D is usually different from C_A, and the ratio between these two is called partition coefficient $\left(K_p = \dfrac{C_A}{C_D}\right)$.

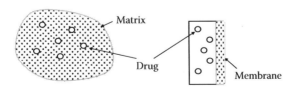

FIGURE 5.3
Matrix and membrane-based drug delivery systems.

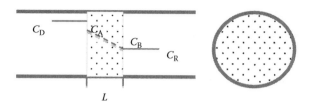

FIGURE 5.4
Illustration of diffusion process through membrane-based system (left) and coated microsphere (right).

In this situation, Fick's first law inside the membrane can be written as

$$\frac{ds}{dt} = -D\frac{dC}{dx} \tag{5.1}$$

where s is the mass per unit area.

Due to mass conservation, the amount of drug transported from region A to region B results in that the concentration in region A is reduced by $\frac{s}{V_A} A$, whereas the concentration in region B of the membrane is increased by $\frac{s}{V_B} A$. Therefore, at any instance, the concentration difference in the membrane is $V_A - \frac{V_B}{V_A} C_B - C_B$. V_A and V_B denote the volumes of regions A and B, respectively, and A denotes the effective area of the membrane. Therefore, the equation becomes

$$\frac{V_B}{A}\frac{dC_B}{dt} = -D\frac{C_A - C_B\dfrac{V_B}{V_A} - C_B}{L} \tag{5.2}$$

Under an infinite source condition, there is a constant source outside the system (membrane) to maintain C_A at a constant value at all times; and initial condition $C_B(0) = 0$, Equation 5.2 becomes

$$-\frac{\ln\left(C_A - C_B - C_B\dfrac{V_B}{V_A}\right)}{\left(1 + \dfrac{V_B}{V_A}\right)} = \frac{AD}{V_B L}t - \frac{\ln C_A}{\left(1 + \dfrac{V_B}{V_A}\right)} \tag{5.3}$$

Since A and B are interfacial regions, it can be inferred that $V_A = V_B$ as long as surface area of the membrane at both sides are equal; therefore, the above equation can be simplified to be

$$\ln\left(\frac{C_A - 2C_B}{C_A}\right) = -2\frac{AD}{V_B L}t \tag{5.4}$$

The model, derived in 1931 [5], assumes the donor chamber to be an infinite source for diffusion, and a linear concentration distribution inside the membrane (same assumption to derive equation).

The above derivation is based on membrane only. If we extend the domain of interest slightly to include a layer of water in both sides of the membrane, then the above equation becomes

$$\ln\left(\frac{C_D - 2C_B}{C_D}\right) = -2\frac{AD_{eff}}{V_B L}t \tag{5.5}$$

Where D_{eff} is the effective diffusion coefficient, taking into account of the transport from donor to the membrane. It is equal to

$$D_{eff} = K_p D \tag{5.6}$$

In practice, a finite period of time is needed to establish the equilibrium in the membrane. By non–steady-state analysis, under the condition such that concentrations at both sides of the membrane are constant and the initial concentration in the membrane is constant C_0 as well, then the concentration inside the membrane is given by

$$C(x,t) = C_A + (C_B - C_A)\frac{x}{L} + \frac{2}{\pi}\sum_{n=1}^{\infty}\frac{C_B\cos n\pi - C_A}{n}\sin\frac{n\pi x}{L}\exp(-D_n^2\pi^2 t/L^2)$$

$$= \frac{4C_0}{\pi}\sum_{m=0}^{\infty}\frac{1}{2m+1}\sin\frac{(2m+1)\pi x}{L}\exp\left\{-D(2m+1)^2\pi^2 t/l^2\right\} \tag{5.7}$$

If the exponential terms vanish as time goes to the infinity, the concentration gradient inside the membrane will be a straight line, which proves the assumption in the previous model is reasonable.

Total solute (Q, g/cm^2) passes through the membrane at time t is obtained by integrating flux with respect to time

$$Q_t = D(C_A - C_B)\frac{t}{L} + \frac{2L}{\pi^2}\sum_{n=1}^{\infty}\frac{C_A\cos n\pi - C_B}{n^2}\left\{1 - \exp\left(-\frac{D_n^2\pi^2 t}{L^2}\right)\right\}$$

$$+ \frac{4C_0 L}{\pi^2}\sum_{m=0}^{\infty}\frac{1}{(2m+1)^2}\left\{1 - \exp\left(-\frac{D(2m+1)^2\pi^2 t}{L^2}\right)\right\} \tag{5.8}$$

In most experimental setup $C_0 = C_B = 0$ (perfect sink condition), so that

$$\frac{Q_t}{LC_A} = \frac{Dt}{L^2} - \frac{1}{6} - \frac{2}{\pi^2}\sum_{n=1}^{\infty}\frac{(-1)^2}{n^2}\exp\left(-\frac{D_n^2\pi^2 t}{L^2}\right) \tag{5.9}$$

When the equilibrium is established (exponential term vanishes):

$$Q_t = \frac{DC_A}{L}\left(t - \frac{L^2}{6D}\right) \tag{5.10}$$

From the intercept of Q_t vs. t curve on t-axis, the effective diffusion coefficient could be obtained from the slope, whereas C_A could be calculated from the y-axis intersection.

Another form of solution under the same condition (constant donor concentration, constant diffusion coefficient, and perfect sink), flux ($g/(cm^2 \cdot t)$) at the donor side is given by

$$J(t) = -D\left(\frac{\partial C}{\partial x}\right)_{x=1} = 2C_A \sum_1^\infty \left(\frac{D}{\pi t}\right)^{\frac{1}{2}} \exp\left\{-(2m+1)^2 l^2/(4Dt)\right\} \tag{5.11}$$

By taking only the leading term, the flux at the donor side of the membrane is simplified to [6]

$$\ln(t^{0.5} J_t) = \ln\left\{2C_A\left(\frac{D}{\pi}\right)^{0.5}\right\} - \frac{L^2}{4Dt} \tag{5.12}$$

According to this equation, the effect of partition and diffusion in the membrane can be separately calculated.

Chen and Lee [7] ignored the partition effect and studied the drug distribution and release behavior for the case where the core and the coating have different drug diffusivity. Their theoretical study showed that the ratio between the diffusivity of the drug in the coating and the diffusivity in the core was a major factor that affects the release rate and the lag time (the time between onset of the experiment and the instance when drug can be detected in the medium): the higher the ratio, the higher the release rate and the shorter the lag time. This finding has been intuitively applied in numerous coating designs.

Diffusivity Control Theory

The diffusion coefficient is extremely important in diffusion because it measures the number of solute being transported through a unit cross-sectional area in a unit time, so it tells how fast a solute molecule could travel in a given system. Because diffusion is eventually a type of motion, any factors, that is, the interaction between solute molecules, the interaction between solute and solvent, and barriers to move and influence the mobility of a solute, would affect its diffusion coefficient. In drug delivery devices, where the drug (solute) is often released (through diffusion) from membrane or matrix, the release rate could be affected by all the factors that affect its diffusion coefficient. Control of the drug release rate is one of the essential issues in drug delivery; therefore, it is the control of the diffusion coefficient critical in the design of drug delivery devices. In this section, limiting factors of the diffusion coefficient and their mathematical models will be discussed.

The simplest case of diffusion in a solution is a binary system where solutes are nonelectrolytes, and the interaction between solutes is ignored (dilute solution). By considering the thermal energy as a force exerted onto the solute, and assuming solute molecules are sphere in shape (with radius a) and are much greater than solvent molecules, the well-known Stokes–Einstein equation would be derived [8]:

$$D = \frac{k_B T}{6\pi\mu a} \tag{5.13}$$

where k_B is Boltzmann's constant, 1.38054×10^{-23} J/K, and T is the absolute temperature. If the solute is not a sphere, yet its diffusion coefficient is known, the resulting radius is called hydrodynamic radius. Sometimes, the denominator of the above equation is also known as the frictional drag coefficient, denoted by f.

The diffusion system described by Stokes–Einstein equation considers only hydrodynamic interactions between the solute and the solvent. In drug delivery systems, the medium that drugs diffuse through is composed of not only the solvent but also other components (i.e., polymer chains), which contributes to dragging forces in diffusion. The effect of the membrane or the matrix on diffusion could be described from different perspectives: porous and nonporous. In the porous consideration, polymeric chains are thought to construct randomly oriented channels, which allow solvent and solute to flow through. In the nonporous consideration, solute molecules dissolve in the membrane and diffuse through it [9]. As more dragging forces exist, the diffusion coefficient through polymers is generally smaller than that in a pure solvent.

Porous Perspective

The simplest case of diffusion through pores is that all long-range interactions (i.e., electrostatic force, van der Waal force) are ignored but only considered restriction of pore walls on solute motion. Two main factors hindering diffusion in porous polymers should be considered: steric hindrance at the entrance to pores and the frictional resistance within the pores (Figure 5.5). It is reasonable to expect that the degree of hindrance depends on the relative size of the solute and the pore. If we assume cylindrical shape for the pores, it

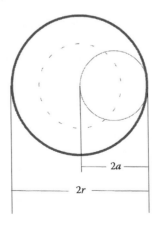

FIGURE 5.5
Hindrance effect.

is possible to describe the two hindering factors discussed above theoretically. Ferry [10] addressed the steric hindrance issue by only allowing molecules without striking the edge to enter the pore. Assuming the pore is cylindrical with inner diameter r, and the solvent molecule is so small that the system could be treated as a continuum, solutes of radius a could pass through the pore only if $r - a > 0$. Hence, the effective area of opening A_{eff} (the area inside the dashed line) is given by

$$A_{eff} = A_0 \left(1 - \frac{a}{r} \right)^2 \qquad (5.14)$$

where A_0 is the total cross-sectional area of the pore. With a given geometry of the pore, the effective opening is very sensitive to the shape of the solute. Although we limit our discussion on spherical solutes, even proteins classified as globular proteins are not necessarily sphere, bovine serum albumin (BSA) is an ellipsoid of axial ratio 3.4 [11]. Fifty percent reduction of the effective diffusion coefficient of BSA through a noncharged membrane was reported [12] as compared with the value predicted by taking BSA as a sphere; therefore, caution has to be taken when a hydrodynamic radius is used to predict the effective diffusion coefficient in a release medium.

The second factor, friction of the solute moving inside the pore, was correlated to the effective surface area by [13]

$$\frac{A_{eff}}{A_0} = 1 - 2.104 \left(\frac{a}{r} \right) + 2.09 \left(\frac{a}{r} \right)^3 - 0.95 \left(\frac{a}{r} \right)^5 \qquad (5.15)$$

The total effect due to steric hindrance and frictional resistance is given by the Renken equation [14]

$$\frac{A_{eff}}{A_0} = \left(1 - \frac{a}{r} \right)^2 \left[1 - 2.104 \left(\frac{a}{r} \right) + 2.09 \left(\frac{a}{r} \right)^3 - 0.95 \left(\frac{a}{r} \right)^5 \right] \qquad (5.16)$$

After we obtained the total effective area of pore opening, we need to relate it to the total surface area (A) to formulate the relationship between the effective diffusion coefficient (D_{eff}) and the diffusion coefficient in a pure solvent (D). To do so, the volume fraction of the void space, also known as porosity (ε) is introduced, such that

$$A_0 - A\varepsilon \qquad (5.17)$$

Another factor that needs to be considered is the distance traveled by the solute. In pore models, solute molecules are only transported through pores. However, the pore length and the distance that the solute travels are not necessarily equal to each other. To take this factor into account, tortuosity, which is defined as the ratio of the path length traveled by the solute d to the end distance L is introduced (Figure 5.6).

Since only the total surface area, the porosity, and the membrane thickness can be measured, the diffusion coefficient calculated from the Fick's first law is only an effective value (D_{eff})

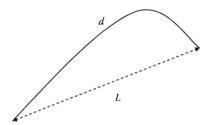

FIGURE 5.6
Definition of tortuosity.

$$\frac{m}{A \cdot t} = -D_{\text{eff}} \frac{\partial C}{L}$$ (5.18)

But in fact, solute has traveled a distance d, and the area for diffusion is only A_{eff}, so we should have

$$\frac{m}{A_{\text{eff}} \cdot t} = -D \frac{\partial C}{L \cdot \tau}$$ (5.19)

Therefore,

$$\frac{D_{\text{eff}}}{D} = \frac{A_{\text{eff}}}{A \cdot \tau}$$ (5.20)

Substituting Equation 5.17 into the above equation:

$$\frac{D_{\text{eff}}}{D} = \frac{A_{\text{eff}} \cdot \varepsilon}{A_0 \cdot \tau}$$ (5.21)

Therefore, the effective diffusion coefficient would be correlated to the diffusion coefficient in a pure solvent by the following equation

$$\frac{D_{\text{eff}}}{D} = \left(1 - \frac{a}{r}\right)^2 \left[1 - 2.104\left(\frac{a}{r}\right) + 2.09\left(\frac{a}{r}\right)^3 - 0.95\left(\frac{a}{r}\right)^5\right] \varepsilon / \tau$$ (5.22)

Due to the steric hindrance, the solute concentration in the membrane (mass of the solute in the membrane divided by volume of solution in the membrane) is smaller than the concentration outside. Therefore, the first term in Equation 5.22 is also known as partition coefficient (K_p). Similarly, the second term is known as the fraction reduction in diffusivity or hydrodynamic dragging factor (K_d). The above equation therefore could be written in a compact form:

$$D_{\text{eff}} = D \frac{\varepsilon K_d K_p}{\tau}$$ (5.23)

If the pore size is so small that the entrance of solvent molecules (radius: b) is hindered as well, partition coefficient would be written as [15]:

$$A_{\text{eff}} = A_0 \frac{\left(1 - \dfrac{a}{r}\right)^2}{\left(1 - \dfrac{b}{r}\right)^2} \tag{5.24}$$

A more rigorous and general derivation was reviewed by Deen [11]. Diffusion of the solute inside solvent-filled pore was described by Langevin equation for a sphere of mass m, radius a with velocity v (Figure 5.7) [16].

$$m\frac{dv}{dt} = -6\pi\mu av + F(t) \tag{5.25}$$

The first term on the right-hand side of the above equation is also known as Stokes force on the sphere in an unbounded fluid [17].

Substituting the expression for driving forces [18] to produce diffusion motion into the above equation by considering only the concentration difference, we have

$$m\frac{dv}{dt} = -6\pi\mu av - kT\frac{\partial \ln C}{\partial x} \tag{5.26}$$

At equilibrium, the diffusion motion force (second term of the right-hand side) is exactly balanced by the hydrodynamic force (first term of the right-hand side). A factor K is introduced to account the effect of the sidewall:

$$0 = -6\pi\mu aKv - kT\frac{\partial \ln C}{\partial x} \tag{5.27}$$

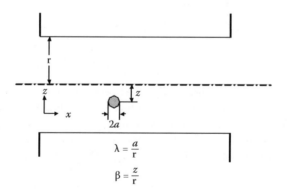

FIGURE 5.7
Solute in a pore.

By dimensional analysis, it is easy to show flux $J = vC$, and Equation 5.27 is rewritten as

$$J = -K^{-1}D\frac{\partial C}{\partial x} \tag{5.28}$$

So far, the analysis is on a single-solute molecule (Brownian motion). To understand the macroscopic diffusion behavior, we consider the average flux in the pore. The average flux averaged over the pore cross section is

$$\bar{J} = 2\int_0^{1-\lambda} J\beta\,d\beta \tag{5.29}$$

By combining Equations 5.28 and 5.29, the relationship between the flux and the concentration could be established:

$$\bar{J} = 2\int_0^{1-\lambda} -K^{-1}D\frac{\partial C}{\partial x}\beta\,d\beta \tag{5.30}$$

Now we need an expression for $\bar{C}$ so as to substitute C in Equation 5.30. The two-dimensional concentration distribution along the z direction was found to be a function of x, $g(x)$, and the long range interaction between solute and the pore wall, $E(\beta)$, which is

$$C = g(x)\exp\left[-\frac{E(\beta)}{kT}\right] \tag{5.31}$$

From Equations 5.30 and 5.31, a local flux equation is obtained:

$$\bar{J} = -K_d D\frac{\partial \bar{C}}{\partial z}$$

$$\text{where } K_d = \frac{\displaystyle\int_0^{1-\lambda} K^{-1}\exp\left(-\frac{E(\beta)}{kT}\right)\beta\,d\beta}{\displaystyle\int_0^{1-\lambda} \exp\left(-\frac{E(\beta)}{kT}\right)\beta\,d\beta} \tag{5.32}$$

To solve the above partial differential equation, we need two boundary conditions, which are concentrations at both ends of the pore C_0 and C_L. Because of the exponential distribution of concentration in the z direction, the average number of solutes enter/leave the pore $(\bar{C}_b)$ is less than the number of solutes available in the bulk (C_b) by a factor of K_p

$$K_p = \frac{\bar{C}_b}{C_b} = 2\int_0^{1-\lambda} \exp\left(-\frac{E}{kT}\right)\beta\,d\beta \tag{5.33}$$

Integrate Equation 5.33 over the total pore length L:

$$\bar{J} \cdot L = -K_p K_d D(C_L - C_0) \tag{5.34}$$

Comparing Equation 5.34 with Fick's first law, the flux equation obtained here is equivalent to Fick's first law when the concentration gradient is linear. It is worth noting that Equation 5.34 was derived based on a single straight pore, with number of pores per unit area and channel orientation in consideration, and ignore any long-range interaction ($E(\beta) = 0$). Equations 5.34 and 5.23 are in fact identical, and the coefficients in both equations share the same physical meaning.

To estimate the effective diffusion coefficient in porous membranes, an expression of K_d is required. Different hydrodynamic dragging factors have been presented by Deen [11]. An exact expression of the hydrodynamic dragging factor was given by Brenner and Gaydos [17]:

$$K_d = 1 + \frac{9}{8}\lambda \ln \lambda + 0.461\lambda + \frac{9}{4}\lambda^2 \ln \lambda + O(\lambda^2) \tag{5.35}$$

Equation 5.15 was proved to be a special case of Equation 5.35 when the average hydrodynamic dragging factor across the channel is assumed to be equal to the hydrodynamic dragging factor along the centerline (centerline approximation). The centerline approximation is a reasonable assumption because the viscosity of the solution is constant until a distance from the wall of one solvent molecule (water molecule size = 2 Å) [19]. The minimum distance of a solute to the pore side wall of the pore is defined by Bohor repulsion distance = 1.54 Å, which means the viscosity of the solvent in which a solute could be found is equal to the viscosity in the centerline. Hence, the most sensitive parameter to external potential energy is the partition coefficient (K_p).

At low solute concentration, the pore model presented above works well for neutral solutes without interacting with the membrane. However, in practice, the interaction between solute and membrane could be prominent, and more sophisticated models concerning the solute–membrane interaction ($E(\beta) \neq 0$) were recently summarized briefly by Ladero et al. [19]. van der Waals interaction between solute and pore wall was formulated by Hamker [20], and van der Waals interaction for different geometries were given by Tadmor [21]. Shao and Baltus [22] incorporated the van der Waals interaction energy with the pore model, such that

$$E(\beta) = \frac{A}{6}\left\{\frac{\lambda}{1-\beta-\lambda} + \frac{\lambda}{1-\beta-\lambda} + \ln\frac{1-\beta-\lambda}{1-\beta+\lambda}\right\} \tag{5.36}$$

where A is the Hamaker constant (J), which varies from case to case. The Hamaker constant A_{312} for the interaction between solutes 2 and 3 in medium 1 was given in terms of the interaction between molecules of the same type separated by vacuum (A_{11}, A_{22}, A_{33}) [23]:

$$A = A_{312} = \left(A_{33}^{0.5} - A_{11}^{0.5}\right)\left(A_{22}^{0.5} - A_{11}^{0.5}\right) \tag{5.37}$$

Hamaker constant ($A_{water-water} = 3.51 \times 10^{-20}$ J) of some commonly used solute and solvent could be found in literature [19, 22]. As a result of introduction of van der Waals interaction, when the solute is very close to the pore wall, the interaction energy is blooming up infinitely, which implies deposition of the solute on the pore wall. For nonabsorbing solutes, it is necessary to define a region in which van der Waals interaction is present (region I), and in the region that is very close to the pore wall, van der Waals interaction is absent (region II). Typically, the region I extend from centerline to $z = r - 0.05a$, so that partition coefficient is

$$K_p = \frac{\overline{C_b}}{C_b} = 2 \int_0^{1-1.05\lambda} \exp\left(-\frac{E(\beta)}{kT}\right)\beta\,d\beta + 2 \int_{1-1.05\lambda}^{1-\lambda} \beta\,d\beta \tag{5.38}$$

The effects of the electrostatic double-layer and the acid–base interaction between solute and pore wall have been added to the external potential function [24,25]. Experimental results [19] suggested that the model proposed by Bhattacharjee and Sharma [24] fitted for protein solution (BSA) the best. In the same report [19], an empirical correction of Hamaker constant dramatically improved the performance of Shao's model dramatically.

The last but not the least factor that controls diffusion coefficient of macromolecules through fine pores is the solute concentration. It has been reported that the partition coefficient was shown to increase with bulk solution concentration. This could be explained by the change in molecular size with concentration. For a dilute solution in a good solvent, coiled molecules expand; however, as the concentration increases, the repulsion force between solute molecules pushes the entangled molecule segments back. Therefore, the molecule becomes smaller. At high concentrations, the dimensions approach their unperturbed values [26]. However, literature results show the inverse for some flexible solutes, such as BSA [27] and polyethylene glycol (PEG) [28]. Pioneer work by Batchelorz [29], who eliminated the solution constraint, offers a concentration dependent expression of the diffusion coefficient.

$$D(\phi) = \frac{K(\phi)}{6\pi\mu a}\left(\frac{d\Pi}{dn}\right) \tag{5.39}$$

where ϕ is the volume fraction of the particles ($\phi = C\dfrac{NV}{MW}$), and n is the mean number density of the particles, $\dfrac{d\Pi}{dn}$ is the derivative of chemical potential per particle, which serves as the thermodynamic driving force for diffusion. $K(\phi)$ is the sedimentation coefficient. The first term of the above equation is in fact a concentration dependent friction dragging coefficient $f(\phi)$ similar to f in the Stokes–Einstein equation. For hard spheres in bulk solution, in which only two body interactions are considered, the effective diffusion coefficient is given:

$$\frac{D(\phi)}{D_0} = 1 + 1.45\phi + O(\phi^2) \tag{5.40}$$

D_0 is the diffusion coefficient at an infinite dilution. According to Equation 5.40, diffusion coefficient increases with increases in concentrations. In the case of BSA, coefficient of $O(\phi)$

is negative [30,31] when pH is close to its PI, suggesting a decrease in diffusion coefficient with increase in concentration.

The diffusion phenomenon discussed above can be described by Maxwell–Stefan theory. Maxwell–Stefan theory [32,33] is a generalized mathematical description of mass transportation, which is also applicable to multicomponent systems. Transport of mass could be divided according to driving forces: diffusive and convective transports. Diffusive transport is caused by electrochemical potential gradient, and convective transport is driven by the total force on the mixture as a whole. Microscopic force balance could be written similarly to the pore model, and an overall macroscopic relation between the solute velocity and the driving force could also be obtained. Because both describe the same physical phenomenon, parameters used in each of them could be related, and normalized diffusion coefficient could also be found.

Nonporous Perspective

In most polymeric membranes, no distinct pores could be identified; therefore, the application of Maxwell–Stefan theory is less accurate in determining effective diffusion coefficient across the membrane. The permeation through polymeric membrane could be more realistically described by a two-step process: solute dissolves in the membrane material and then diffuses through it down a concentration gradient. Two factors limit solute permeation, solubility, and diffusivity. Membranes made of porous substrate and filled by selective soluble polymer were successfully applied to organic liquid separation based on this two-step mechanism [34]. Models based on this description are therefore called solution-diffusion models. The fundamental assumption of solute-diffusion models is that chemical potentials of all components in the solution at both sides of the membrane are in equilibrium with the adjacent membrane surfaces [35]. For a passive diffusion where no chemical reaction is involved, this assumption is valid. Here, chemical potential is used because all the common driving forces of diffusion can be reduced to chemical potential gradient. The chemical potential of ith component is given by

$$u_i = u_i^0 + RT\ln(\gamma_i C_i) + v_i(p - p_{i,\text{sat}}) \tag{5.41}$$

μ_i^0 is the chemical potential of pure I at pressure $p_{i,\text{sat}}$, γ_i is the activity coefficient, v_i is the molar volume of ith component, and R is the ideal gas constant.

Because of the equilibrium between the solution and the membrane, the chemical potential of the bulk solution and the solution in the membrane is equal:

$$u_i^0 + RT\ln(\gamma_i C_i) + v_i(p - p_{i,\text{sat}}) = u_i^0 + RT\ln(\gamma_{i,\text{m}} C_{i,\text{m}}) + v_i(p - p_{i,\text{sat}}) \tag{5.42}$$

Therefore,

$$C_{\text{m}} = \frac{\gamma_i}{\gamma_{i,\text{m}}} C_i = K_{\text{p}} C_i \tag{5.43}$$

Substitute this relation into Fick's first law, where the effective diffusion coefficient is used:

$$J = \frac{DK_p}{L}(C_A - C_B) \tag{5.44}$$

D measures the diffusivity of the solute in the membrane. The activity coefficient measures the solute–solvent interaction, which will be discussed in more detail in the subsequent section. For the sake of discussion, in the following sections, the effective diffusion coefficient is defined as the product of the partition coefficient and the diffusivity of the solute, which accounts for the combined effect of partition (K_p) and diffusion (D) on the flux.

Free Volume

In the nonporous description of membrane, diffusion is a result of the random movement of molecules through the free volume in the membrane. Free volume is defined as the difference between the actual volume of the liquid and the minimum volume, which it would occupy, of its molecules, which were packed firmly in contact with each other [36]. It could also be interpreted as the volume difference between temperature T and absolute zero. Molecules in the liquid at temperature T are moving at the average thermal velocity but, most of the time, is confined to a cage bounded by their immediate neighbors. Fluctuation in molecular arrangement opens up a hole in the cage, which is big enough to permit a considerable displacement of the molecule contained in the cage. Net movement of the displaced molecule could result only if another molecule jumps into the hole before the displaced molecule returns to its original position. Diffusion occurs as a result of redistribution of the free volume within the liquid. This description of diffusion by Cohen and Turnbuli [37] was originally to describe self-diffusion of liquid with impurities (solute). Because another molecule has to fill the void left by the displaced molecule, the free volume (difference between the cage volume and volume of the molecule) has to be large enough to permit another molecule to jump in after displacement.

In a solvent–solute binary system, solute diffusion coefficient is therefore proportional to the probability of finding a free volume, which is greater than its own volume. The total probability of finding a hole of volume exceeding v^* is [37]

$$P(v^*) = \exp[-\kappa v^*/v_f] \tag{5.45}$$

where k is a factor to correct for overlap of free volume ($0.5 \leq \kappa \leq 1$ [38]), and v_f is the average free volume. κ is introduced because the total free volume is not the summation of individual free volume:

$$v_f = \frac{V_f}{N} = \frac{\kappa \sum_i N_i v_i}{\sum_i N_i} \tag{5.46}$$

Diffusion coefficient of solute in a liquid at infinite dilution is given by

$$D \propto a^* u \exp(-\gamma v^*/v_f) \tag{5.47}$$

a^* is the diameter of the cage or the rough diameter of the molecule [37].

By assuming immobile, impenetrable polymer chains suspended in a mobile solvent continuum, diffusion of solute may only proceed through the solvent phase permeating the whole membrane. The polymer molecules of the solvated membrane are forming a network immersed in the solvent and exhibiting a wide spectrum of holes. The solute can diffuse through the membrane if it finds a hole larger than the solute molecules. Average free volume in the membrane is contributed by solvent molecules and polymer chains:

$$v_f = (1 - \phi_p)V_{f,water} + \phi_p V_{f,polymer} \tag{5.48}$$

By assumption, the free volume contributed by polymer chains is not permeable to solutes; therefore,

$$v_f \cong (1 - \phi_p)V_{f,water} \tag{5.49}$$

where ϕ_p is the polymer volumetric fraction (distinguish it from solute volumetric ratio ϕ). Volume degree of swelling is

$$Q = \frac{1}{\phi_p} \tag{5.50}$$

Instead of volume, Yasuda et al. [39–41] considered the cross-sectional area of the free volume as the permeating criteria. The normalized diffusion coefficient (D/D_0) as a function of the probability of finding a hole larger than solute $P(\pi a^2)$:

$$\frac{D}{D_0} = P(\pi a^2)\exp\left[-B\left(\frac{\pi a^2}{V_{f,water}}\right)\left(\frac{\phi_p}{1-\phi_p}\right)\right] \tag{5.51}$$

where B is a constant of water and $V_{f,water}$ is the free volume of water.

For cross-linked systems, Peppas et al. [42] considered volume as a permeating parameter and expressed the normalized diffusion coefficient as a function of polymer volume ratio and solute size:

$$\frac{D}{D_0} = f(\overline{M_c})\exp\left(\frac{-v_{solute}}{V_{solvent}\left(\frac{1}{\phi_p}-1\right)}\right) \tag{5.52}$$

$\overline{M_c}$ is the number average molecular weight between cross-links, $f(\overline{M_c})$ is the probability function of finding a void big enough to allow diffusion, v_{solute} is the solute volume, and $v_{solvent}$ is the free volume of solvent. Molar weight between cross-links M_c and cross-linking density ρ_x is determined using [43]

$$\frac{1}{\overline{M_c}} = \frac{2}{\overline{M_n}} - \frac{(\overline{v}/\overline{V_1})[\ln(1-v_{2,s})+v_{2,s}+\chi v_{2,s}^2]}{v_{2,r}\left[\left(\dfrac{v_{2,s}}{v_{2,r}}\right)^{1/3} - \dfrac{1}{2}\left(\dfrac{v_{2,s}}{v_{2,r}}\right)\right]}$$

$$\rho_x = \frac{1}{\overline{v}\,\overline{M_c}}$$

$$v_{2,r} = \frac{m_p/\rho_p}{(m_{\text{membrane-air}} - m_{\text{membrane-hep}})/\rho_h} \tag{5.53}$$

$$v_{2,s} = \frac{m_p/\rho_p}{(m'_{\text{membrane-air}} - m'_{\text{membrane-hep}})/\rho_h}$$

$$N = 2\frac{\overline{M_c}}{M_r}$$

The volume of the polymer could be obtained by considering buoyancy. Conventionally, heptane and air were chosen as the weighting medium because heptane does not induce swelling. After synthesis, sample was weighed in air $m_{\text{membrane-air}}$ and in heptane $m_{\text{membrane-hep}}$; after swelling, sample was weighed in air $m'_{\text{membrane-air}}$ and heptanes $m'_{\text{membrane-hep}}$ again. Finally, sample was dried to a constant weight m_p. ρ_p and ρ_h are the density of polymer and heptane, respectively. $\overline{v}$ is the specific volume of the membrane (cm^3/g), $\overline{V_1}$ is the molar volume of water (volume per water molecule is 30 Å^3 [44]; therefore, $V_1 = 18$ cm^3/g), $\overline{M_n}$ is the number average molecular weight of the uncross-linked polymer [45], and M_r is the molecular weight of the repeating unit. N is the number of repeating units between two cross-links. χ is Flory thermodynamic interaction parameter, which varies between 0.49 and 0.51 for polyvinyl alcohol (PVA) [45]. For HEMA [48]:

$$\chi = 0.022 + 0.904v_{2,s} \tag{5.54}$$

The empirical relationship between glass transition temperature and $\overline{M_c}$ is also available [46].

$$\overline{M_c} = \frac{3.9 \times 10^4}{T_g - T_{g0}} \tag{5.55}$$

T_g is the glass transition temperature of the cross-linked polymer, and T_{g0} is the glass transition temperature of the uncross-linked polymer with the same chemical composition.

Instead of the number average molecular weight between cross-links, it is more physically sound to use a length scale in describing the structure of the polymer for diffusion, which is defined as the radius of gyration of a chain between cross-links or the mesh size of the polymer [47]. Mesh size is proportional to the end-to-end distance of polymer chain:

$$\overline{r_0^2} = Nl^2C_n \tag{5.56}$$

l is the C–C bond length 1.54 Å and C_n is the Flory characteristic ratio, or rigidity factor (6.95 for poly(methyl methacrylate) and poly(2-hydroxyethyl methacrylate [48], whereas 8.9 for poly(vinyl alcohol) [45] and 14.4 in case of a methacrylate chain).

Mesh size is

$$\xi = Q^{1/3}(\overline{r_0^2})^{1/2} \tag{5.57}$$

In a highly swollen hydrogel, diffusion coefficient can be calculated from [47]

$$D \cong \left(1 - \frac{a}{\xi}\right) \exp\left(-\frac{Y}{Q-1}\right) \tag{5.58}$$

Y is a structural parameter, near unity. For most polymers, $Y = 1$ is a good approximation [47]. In the case where mesh size is unknown, another form of Equation 5.58 was derived for a highly swollen hydrogel:

$$D \cong aQ^{-3/4} \exp\left(-\frac{Y}{Q-1}\right) \tag{5.59}$$

On the other perspective, the diffusion coefficient of solute depends on solvent content as following [49–51]:

$$D_2 = D_{2,s} \exp(-\beta(1 - C_1)) \tag{5.60}$$

where $D_{2,s}$ is the diffusion coefficient in the fully swollen polymer, β is a constant, and C_1 is the solute concentration normalized with respect to the equilibrium solvent content in the membrane. Clearly, cross-linking density affects mesh size, which further influences the diffusivity of the drug in the membrane.

Temperature Effect

The free volume of the polymer predicts that the diffusivity of the solute in the polymeric membrane is related to the solute size and the swelling behavior of the membrane; hence, the release rate of a given drug is controlled by swelling of the polymer. Recall from Fick's second law, where diffusivity is also a function of temperature, and it serves another factor that controls the drug release rate.

Simon [52] studied the release flux through a planar membrane with a temperature gradient imposed to a concentration gradient. The steady-state flux was given by

$$J = \frac{C_A D \exp\left(-\frac{(E_s + E_d)(T_0 - T_s)}{RT_0 T_S}\right)}{L} \tag{5.61}$$

where E_s and E_d are overall energy of salvation and activation energy for diffusion through the polymer, respectively. T_0 is the temperature at which diffusivity is D and T_s is the temperature at the donor–membrane interface, assuming linear temperature gradient at steady-state. All other parameters are the same as defined in other equations.

Partition/Solubility Oriented

In the porous description of the solute transportation process, partition is a measure of the concentration difference in pores and the bulk solution, and it is inherently considered in the mathematical treatment. However, in the nonporous description, diffusion and partition are considered two separate steps. Before the diffusion step, the very first step in the release mechanism is a partition step, where drug molecules dissolve in the membrane phase. Although partition of proteins is an intensively studied topic in protein purification, in the area of controlled drug release, intentional control of partition does not draw much interest. However, as the solution–diffusion model suggests, both partition and diffusion affect the effective diffusion coefficient of the solute and hence determine the rate of release through the membrane. Since partition coefficient is a measure of the drug relative solubility in membrane as compared with the aqueous solution, the key of this route is to control the solubility of drug in the membrane phase. Therefore, a solid understanding of the thermodynamics of solution–mixture is a must.

Thermodynamics, which originated during the nineteenth century, were originally applied to describe heat energy. After J. Willard Gibbs, who generalized the thermodynamics, a wide variety of phenomena both physical and chemical were successfully described by thermodynamic approaches. Thermodynamic description is eventually an energy approach; to discuss thermodynamics involved in solution–mixture, we start by defining a system under consideration. A solution could be considered as a homogeneous open system, in which matters and energy are allowed to exchange with the surroundings. In a homogeneous open system, the total energy change dU is given by

$$dU = TdS - PdV + \sum_i \mu_i dn_i$$

$$\mu_i = \left(\frac{\partial U}{\partial n_i} \right)_{S,V,n_j}$$

(5.62)

n_i refers to all mole numbers of the components in the system.

The first term describes energy change due to heat exchange, the second term is energy change due to the work done to the system, and the last term accounts for the change in energy from matter exchange. μ_i is defined as chemical potential of component i.

By rearrangement of T, S, P, and V in the above equation, we have different energy terms:

$$dH = TdS + VdP + \sum_i \mu_i dn_i$$

$$dA = -SdT - PdV + \sum_i \mu_i dn_i$$

(5.63)

$$dG = -SdT + VdP + \sum_i \mu_i dn_i$$

H is the enthalpy of the system, A is the Helmholtz energy, and G is the Gibbs energy. By definition

$$H = U + PV$$

$$A = U - TS \tag{5.64}$$

$$G = U + PV - TS = H - TS = A + PV$$

So that

$$\mu_i \equiv \left(\frac{\partial U}{\partial n_i}\right)_{S,V,n_j} = \left(\frac{\partial H}{\partial n_i}\right)_{S,P,n_j} = \left(\frac{\partial A}{\partial n_i}\right)_{T,V,n_j} = \left(\frac{\partial G}{\partial n_i}\right)_{T,P,n_j} \tag{5.65}$$

In all homogeneous open systems

$$SdT - VdP + \sum_i \mu_i dn_i = 0 \tag{5.66}$$

To obtain the expression for chemical potential, we first start from the chemical potential for a pure, ideal gas.

$$\left(\frac{\partial \mu_i}{\partial P}\right) = v_i \tag{5.67}$$

v_i is the molar volume of component i; and by the ideal gas law:

$$v_i = \frac{RT}{P} \tag{5.68}$$

And integrate at constant temperature:

$$\mu_i - \mu_i^0 = RT \ln \frac{P}{P_0} \tag{5.69}$$

This is the chemical potential change from isothermal process (P to P_0). For an ideal gas, its partial pressure is proportional to its mole fraction in the system.

For a nonideal substance (gas, liquid, solid), whose intermolecular interaction is not negligible, at constant temperature:

$$\mu_i - \mu_i^0 = RT \ln \frac{f_i}{f_i^0} \tag{5.70}$$

where f is called fugacity. For ideal gas, f is equal to pressure, and for ideal gas mixture, f_i is equal to its partial pressure. The ratio f/f_0 is the activity of the component denoted as a. The physical meaning of activity is an indication of how active a substance is relative to its standard state.

The change in Gibbs free energy of ideal solution is

$$\Delta G_{mix} = \Delta H_{mix} - T\Delta S_{mix} \tag{5.71}$$

To extend Gibbs free energy to real solution, an excess term is added to the ideal equation. The excess term is defined by the difference of real Gibbs free energy in mixing minus the Gibbs free energy predicted by ideal equation.

$$\mu_i - \mu_i^0 = RT \ln \gamma_i x_i = RT \ln x_i + RT \ln \gamma_i \tag{5.72}$$

Compare it with the ideal solution, the last term is an excess chemical potential, since the partial molar Gibbs free energy is the chemical potential, the partial molar excess Gibbs free energy is

$$\left(\frac{dg^E}{dn_i} \right)_{P,T,n_{j \neq i}} = RT \ln \gamma_i$$

$$\gamma_i \equiv \frac{a_i}{x_i} \tag{5.73}$$

And the total excess Gibbs free energy is given by

$$g^E = RT \sum x_i \ln \gamma_i \tag{5.74}$$

Equilibrium Condition of Partition

The governing condition of partition at the equilibrium state is equal in chemical potential of all components. In the simplest case, pressure and temperature are constants in the system. Recall the equilibrium condition of fugacity, which is equivalent to activity equity; the solubility of a component in phase 2 is given by

$$x_{i,2} = \frac{\gamma_{i,1}}{\gamma_{i,2}} x_{i,1} \tag{5.75}$$

$\frac{\gamma_{i,1}}{\gamma_{i,2}}$ is known as the partition coefficient as discussed in the previous section. Hence, in order to reduce drug partition into membrane, it is equivalent to increase the solute activity coefficient in the membrane.

Partition of Protein in Aqueous Two-Phase Systems

Chemical potential equilibrium can be illustrated in an aqueous two-phase system (ATPS), which is widely used for protein purification. An ATPS will be formed if a thermodynamically incompatible substance is added into an aqueous medium and above some minimum concentrations [53]. Protein separation can be achieved by adding proteins in ATPS because they will prefer one phase to another (partitioning into one phase). The protein partitioning is influenced by a few factors: pH, type of buffers, ionic strength, temperature, and the phase-forming solution.

Since ion in the protein solution redistributes until equilibrium is established, an electrostatic potential exists at the interface. The chemical potential of protein at a constant temperature and pressure is therefore also a function of ions in the solution

$$\mu_p = \mu_p^0 - \frac{Z_p}{Z_\gamma}\mu_\gamma^0 + RT\ln x_p\gamma_p - RT\frac{Z_p}{Z_\gamma}\ln\gamma_\gamma + Z_iF\varphi \tag{5.76}$$

F is Faraday's constant, z is net surface charge, and φ is electric potential. Subscript p denotes protein and r denotes a reference ion in the solution. At equilibrium, the partition of protein from top to the bottom is

$$\ln K_p = \ln\frac{x_B}{x_A} = \ln\frac{\gamma_p^A}{\gamma_p^B} - \frac{Z_p}{Z_\gamma}\left[\ln\left(\frac{a_\gamma^A}{a_\gamma^B}\right)\right] \tag{5.77}$$

And partition coefficient of reference ion is

$$\ln K_{p,r} = \ln\frac{x_{\gamma,B}}{x_{\chi,A}} = -\frac{Z_\gamma F}{RT}\Delta\varphi \tag{5.78}$$

Partition of Protein in Hydrogel Membrane

In ATPS, pressure is equal in two phases; however, in the hydrogel membrane (commonly used as coating in drug delivery systems), a higher pressure is expected because of the rigidity of the polymer structure, and therefore, the reference state of chemical potential in the membrane is at a higher pressure compared to aqueous phase

$$\mu_p^B = \mu_{\text{pure p}}^B(T,P+\pi) + RT\ln a_p^B \tag{5.79}$$

$$\mu_p^A = \mu_{\text{pure p}}^A(T,P+\pi) + RT\ln a_p^A \tag{5.80}$$

For a pure incompressible liquid $\left(\dfrac{\partial\mu}{\partial P}\right)_T = v$, so

$$\mu_p^B = \mu_{\text{pure p}}^B(T,P) + \pi v_p + RT\ln a_p^B$$

and

$$\mu_{\text{pure p}}^B = \mu_{\text{pure p}}^A \tag{5.81}$$

By applying equilibrium condition

$$\mu_p^A = \mu_p^B \tag{5.82}$$

Therefore

$$\pi = \left(RT \ln \frac{a_p^A}{a_p^B} \right) / v_p \tag{5.83}$$

Thus, partition coefficient is

$$\ln K_p = \ln \frac{\gamma_p^A}{\gamma_p^B} - \frac{\pi v_p}{RT} \tag{5.84}$$

This equation suggests that the higher the osmotic pressure in the membrane, the lower the partition coefficient from aqueous phase to the membrane.

In most experiment setups, ions are present in the buffer solution; therefore, an electrostatic potential exists at the interface, at equilibrium, and the protein partition coefficient is given by

$$\ln K_p = \ln \frac{x_B}{x_A} = \ln \frac{\gamma_p^A}{\gamma_p^B} - \frac{Z_p}{Z_\gamma} \left[\ln \left(\frac{a_\gamma^A}{a_\gamma^B} \right) \right] - \pi v_p \tag{5.85}$$

To alter the partition of protein drug in membrane, the ion concentration is set to be constant (factor that is not controlled); therefore, by increasing solute activity coefficient and/or increase osmotic pressure in the membrane, drug partition is reduced, and vice versa.

To figure out what are the factors that affect activity coefficient and how they affect it, we need the mathematical models to express activity coefficient in solution.

Excess Function and Activity Coefficient (for Nonelectrolytes)

In the previous section, it can be seen that if the activity coefficient of a component in a system can be calculated, its partition coefficient will be known. Moreover, to calculate the activity coefficient, excess Gibbs free energy (excess function) is needed. In this section, different models of excess function and activity coefficient will be reviewed; therefore, factors that affect activity coefficient, thus partition coefficient, can be understood.

Gibbs free energy of a solution is determined by an entropy term and an enthalpy term; if we assume heat of mixing is zero, molecules are of the same size, and the intermolecular force of different molecules is identical, the Gibbs free energy is solely contributed by entropy change (athermal solution). An idealized description of solution is the liquid lattice theory, in which a solution is considered as a regular array in space, and solvent and solute molecules are located in the lattice sites. (First introduced by Flory and Huggins [36]).

In this model, coordination number z (nearest neighbors) is between 6 and 12 depending on the type of packing. For typical liquids at ordinary condition, z is close to 10.

By ignoring the size difference of solute and solvent, if the distribution of molecules is totally random, the total change in Gibbs free energy is given by

$$\frac{\Delta G}{RT} = (N_1 \ln \Phi_1 + N_2 \ln \Phi_2) \tag{5.86}$$

where

$$\Phi_1 = \frac{N_1}{N_1 + N_2} \quad \Phi_2 = \frac{N_2}{N_1 + N_2}$$

N_1 is number of solvent molecules, and N_2 is the number of solute molecules; therefore, total number of lattice site is $N_1 + N_2$. The excess Gibbs free energy in this case is zero, corresponding to ideal solution.

Wilson Model

Wilson [54] considered interaction between molecules in a mixing (Figure 5.8) and proposed a new expression for excess Gibb's free energy. In his derivation, the interaction between molecules surrounding a central molecule is considered based on the random distribution of molecules described by Flory and Huggins. The models derived based on this assumption are called "local composition models."

In a binary system, the mole fraction of molecule 2 around molecule 1 and the mole fraction of molecule 1 around molecule 1 are assumed to be related by:

$$\frac{x_{21}}{x_{11}} = \frac{x_2 \exp(-g_{21}/RT)}{x_1 \exp(-g_{11}/RT)} \tag{5.87}$$

g's are energies of interaction between molecules, and x_i is the overall mole fraction in the mixture. For athermal mixtures, the excess Gibbs free energy is

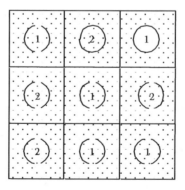

FIGURE 5.8
Local composition lattice.

$$g^E = -x_1 \ln(x_1 + \Lambda_{12}x_2) - x_2 \ln(x_2 + \Lambda_{21}x_1)$$

$$\ln \gamma_1 = -\ln(x_1 + \Lambda_{12}x_2) + x_2 \left(\frac{\Lambda_{12}}{x_1 + \Lambda_{12}x_2} - \frac{\Lambda_{21}}{\Lambda_{21}x_1 + x_2} \right)$$

$$\ln \gamma_2 = -\ln(x_2 + \Lambda_{21}x_1) - x_1 \left(\frac{\Lambda_{12}}{x_1 + \Lambda_{12}x_2} - \frac{\Lambda_{21}}{\Lambda_{21}x_1 + x_2} \right)$$

$$\Lambda_{12} = \frac{v_2}{v_1} \exp\left(-\frac{g_{12} - g_{11}}{RT} \right) \tag{5.88}$$

$$\Lambda_{21} = \frac{v_1}{v_2} \exp\left(-\frac{g_{21} - g_{22}}{RT} \right)$$

where v_i is the molar liquid volume of a pure component. Interaction energy is in fact temperature dependent; however, it does not vary much over moderate temperature range.

The corresponding multicomponent equations are

$$\frac{g^E}{RT} = -\sum_{i=1}^{m} x_i \ln\left(\sum_{j=1}^{m} x_j \Lambda_{ij} \right) \tag{5.89}$$

where

$$\Lambda_{ij} = \frac{v_j}{v_i} \exp\left(-\frac{g_{ij} - g_{ii}}{RT} \right)$$

$$\Lambda_{ji} = \frac{v_i}{v_j} \exp\left(-\frac{g_{ji} - g_{jj}}{RT} \right)$$

$$\ln \gamma_k = -\ln\left(\sum_{j=1}^{m} x_j \Lambda_{kj} \right) + 1 - \sum_{i=1}^{m} \frac{x_i \Lambda_{ik}}{\sum_{j=1}^{m} x_j \Lambda_{ij}} \tag{5.90}$$

Nonrandom, Two-Liquid Model

The Wilson's model is based on the random mixing description of Renon and Prausnitz [55] pursued the original Wilson's model and introduced a term describing nonrandomness of the mixing

$$\frac{x_{21}}{x_{11}} = \frac{x_2 \exp(\alpha_{12}g_{21}/RT)}{x_1 \exp(\alpha_{12}g_{11}/RT)} \tag{5.91}$$

α_{12} indicates randomness of the mixture, and zero means completely random. α_{12} varies from 0.2 to 0.47; a typical choice is 0.3 [57].

$$\frac{g^E}{RT} = x_1 x_2 \left(\frac{\tau_{21} G_{21}}{x_1 + x_2 G_{21}} + \frac{\tau_{12} G_{12}}{x_2 + x_1 G_{12}} \right) \tag{5.92}$$

where

$$\tau_{12} = \frac{g_{12} - g_{22}}{RT} \qquad \tau_{21} = \frac{g_{21} - g_{11}}{RT}$$

$$G_{12} = \exp(-\alpha_{12}\tau_{12}) \qquad G_{12} = \exp(-\alpha_{12}\tau_{21})$$

Activity coefficient derived from nonrandom, two-liquid model is:

$$\ln \gamma_1 = x_2^2 \left[\tau_{21} \left(\frac{G_{21}}{x_1 + x_2 G_{21}} \right)^2 + \frac{\tau_{12} G_{12}}{\left(x_2 + x_1 G_{12} \right)^2} \right]$$

$$\ln \gamma_2 = x_1^2 \left[\tau_{12} \left(\frac{G_{12}}{x_2 + x_1 G_{12}} \right)^2 + \frac{\tau_{21} G_{21}}{\left(x_1 + x_2 G_{21} \right)^2} \right] \tag{5.93}$$

g_{ij} is the energy parameter of i–j interaction as before.

Multicomponent equations:

$$\frac{g^E}{RT} = \sum_{i=1}^{m} x_i \frac{\displaystyle\sum_{j=1}^{m} \tau_{ji} G_{ji} x_j}{\displaystyle\sum_{l=1}^{m} G_{li} x_l} \tag{5.94}$$

where

$$\tau_{ji} = \frac{g_{ji} - g_{ii}}{RT}$$

$$G_{ji} = \exp(-\alpha_{ji}\tau_{ji}) \qquad (\alpha_{ij} = \alpha_{ji})$$

$$\ln \gamma_i = \frac{\displaystyle\sum_{j=1}^{m} \tau_{ji} G_{ji} x_j}{\displaystyle\sum_{l=1}^{m} G_{li} x_l} + \sum_{j=1}^{m} \frac{x_j G_{ij}}{\displaystyle\sum_{l=1}^{m} G_{lj} x_l} \left(\tau_{ij} - \frac{\displaystyle\sum_{r=1}^{m} x_r \tau_{rj} G_{rj}}{\displaystyle\sum_{l=1}^{m} G_{lj} x_l} \right) \tag{5.95}$$

Universal Quasi-Chemical Theory

The previous models are applicable to the case in which solute and solvent are of the same size. For nonrandom solution containing nonelectrolyte molecules of different sizes, the model universal quasi-chemical theory (UNIQUAC) was developed based on the same local composition description [56]. In UNIQUAC equation, excess Gibbs free energy has two parts, a combinatorial part that describes the dominant entropic contribution and a residual part that is due primarily to short-range intermolecular forces that induce enthalpy contribution. The combinatorial part is affected only by the composition, sizes, and shapes of the molecules of pure component.

$$\frac{g^E}{RT} = \left(\frac{g^E}{RT}\right)_{combinatorial} + \left(\frac{g^E}{RT}\right)_{residual} \tag{5.96}$$

For binary:

$$\left(\frac{g^E}{RT}\right)_{combinatorial} = x_1 \ln\frac{\Phi_1^*}{x_1} + x_2 \ln\frac{\Phi_2^*}{x_2} + \frac{z}{2}\left(x_1 q_1 \ln\frac{\theta_1}{\Phi_1^*} + x_2 q_2 \ln\frac{\theta_2}{\Phi_2^*}\right)$$

$$\left(\frac{g^E}{RT}\right)_{residual} = -x_1 q_1' \ln\left(\theta_1' + \theta_2'\tau_{21}\right) - x_2 q_2' \ln\left(\theta_2' + \theta_1'\tau_{21}\right)$$

coordination number z=10

segment fraction

$$\tag{5.97}$$

$$\Phi_1^* = \frac{x_1 r_1}{x_1 r_1 + x_2 r_2} \qquad \Phi_2^* = \frac{x_2 r_2}{x_1 r_1 + x_2 r_2}$$

area fraction

$$\theta_1 = \frac{x_1 q_1}{x_1 q_1 + x_2 q_2} \qquad \theta_2 = \frac{x_2 q_2}{x_1 q_1 + x_2 q_2}$$

$$\theta_1' = \frac{x_1 q_1'}{x_1 q_1' + x_2 q_2'} \qquad \theta_2' = \frac{x_2 q_2'}{x_1 q_1' + x_2 q_2'}$$

R, q, and q' are pure-component molecular-structure constants. q' is the surface of interaction, and q is the geometric external surface [58]. In the original derivation of Abrams and Prausnitz [56], q' and q were not distinguished, but for water and lower alcohols (for water, $r = 0.92$, $q = 1.4$, $q' = 1$ [58]), they are different. Only for fluids other than water and lower alcohols, $q = q'$.

$$\tau_{12} = \exp\left(-\frac{g_{12} - g_{22}}{T}\right)$$

$$\tag{5.98}$$

$$\tau_{21} = \exp\left(-\frac{g_{21} - g_{11}}{T}\right)$$

where τ_{ij} is an adjustable parameter that accounts for energy interaction.

Activity coefficients are given by

$$\ln\gamma_1 = \ln\frac{\Phi_1^*}{x_1} + \frac{z}{2}q_1\ln\frac{\theta_1}{\Phi_1^*} + \Phi_2^*\left(l_1 - \frac{r_1}{r_2}l_2\right) - q_1'\ln(\theta_1' + \theta_2'\tau_{21}) + \theta_2'q_1'\left(\frac{\tau_{21}}{\theta_1' + \theta_2'\tau_{21}} - \frac{\tau_{12}}{\theta_2' + \theta_1'\tau_{12}}\right)$$

$$\ln\gamma_2 = \ln\frac{\Phi_2^*}{x_2} + \frac{z}{2}q_2\ln\frac{\theta_2}{\Phi_2^*} + \Phi_2^*\left(l_2 - \frac{r_2}{r_1}l_1\right) - q_2'\ln(\theta_2' + \theta_1'\tau_{12}) + \theta_1'q_2'\left(\frac{\tau_{12}}{\theta_2' + \theta_1'\tau_{12}} - \frac{\tau_{21}}{\theta_1' + \theta_2'\tau_{21}}\right)$$

$$(5.99)$$

where

$$l_1 = \frac{z}{2}(r_1 - q_1) - (r_1 - 1)$$

$$l_2 = \frac{z}{2}(r_2 - q_2) - (r_2 - 1)$$

Multicomponent equations:

$$\frac{g_{combinatorial}^E}{RT} = \sum_{i=1}^{m} x_i\ln\frac{\Phi_i^*}{x_i} + \frac{z}{2}\sum_{i=1}^{m} q_i x_i\ln\frac{\theta_i}{\Phi_i^*}$$

$$\frac{g_{residual}^E}{RT} = \sum_{i=1}^{m} q_i' x_i\ln\left(\sum_{j=1}^{m}\theta_j'\tau_{ji}\right)$$

$$(5.100)$$

where

$$\Phi_i^* = \frac{r_i x_i}{\sum\limits_{j=1}^{m} r_j x_j} \qquad \theta_i = \frac{q_i x_i}{\sum\limits_{j=1}^{m} q_j x_j} \qquad \theta_i' = \frac{q_i' x_i}{\sum\limits_{j=1}^{m} q_j' x_j}$$

$$\tau_{ij} = \exp\left(-\frac{g_{ij} - g_{jj}}{T}\right) \quad \text{and} \quad \tau_{ji} = \exp\left(-\frac{g_{ji} - g_{ii}}{T}\right)$$

Coordination number z is set to 10.

$$\ln\gamma_i = \ln\frac{\Phi_i^*}{x_i} + \frac{z}{2}q_i\ln\frac{\theta_i}{\Phi_i^*} + l_i - \frac{\Phi_i^*}{x_i}\sum_{j=1}^{m} x_j l_j$$

$$- q_i'\ln\left(\sum_{j=1}^{m}\theta_j'\tau_{ji}\right) + q_i' - q_i'\sum_{j=1}^{m}\frac{\theta_j'\tau_{ji}}{\sum\limits_{k=1}^{m}\theta_k'\tau_{kj}}$$

$$(5.101)$$

where

$$l_j = \frac{z}{2}\left(r_j - q_j\right) - \left(r_j - 1\right)$$

The first three terms are derived from the combinatorial contribution, and the rest of the three terms are from the residual part of the excess free energy.

Although r does not correspond to the exact size of molecules, it measures the relative size of the solute over solvent. The relative size of the solute dramatically affects the solute activity coefficient. The solute with a bigger size is more sensitive to composition, whereas the solvent activity coefficient is independent of the solute size as long as protein solutes are concerned.

UNIQUAC Functional-Group Activity Coefficients

The interaction between molecules is accounted by the residual part of UNIQUAC model. By considering the interaction between functional groups of the molecules in the mixture, the residual part of UNIQUAC model could be calculated from each functional group of the molecule by

$$\ln \gamma_i^R = \sum_k n_k^{(i)}\left[\ln \Gamma_k - \ln \Gamma_k^{(i)}\right] \tag{5.102}$$

where $n_k^{(i)}$ is the number of groups of type k in molecule I, Γ_k is the group residual activity coefficient, and $\Gamma_k^{(i)}$ is the residual activity coefficient of group k in a reference solution containing only molecules of type i.

$$\ln \Gamma_k = Q_k\left[1 - \ln\left(\sum_m \Theta_m \tau_{mk}\right) - \sum_m \left(\frac{\Theta_m \tau_{km}}{\sum_n \Theta_n \tau_{nm}}\right)\right]$$

$$\Theta_m = \frac{Q_m x_m}{\sum_n Q_n x_n} \tag{5.103}$$

$$\tau_{mn} = \exp\left(-\frac{a_{mn}}{T}\right)$$

$$Q_k = \frac{A_{wk}}{2.5 \times 10^9}$$

A_{wk} is the group surface area. a_{mn} is the group interaction parameter and can be found in the literature [59]. From this model, the activity coefficient can be estimated by structure analysis of the components in the system from available experimental data. This model is widely known as UNIQUAC Functional-group activity coefficients, or UNIFAC model.

The combinatorial part is given by [65]

$$\ln \gamma_i^C = 1 - \phi_i + \ln \phi_i - \frac{z}{2} q_i \left(1 - \frac{\phi_i}{F_i} + \ln \left(\frac{\phi_i}{F_i} \right) \right)$$

$$\phi_i = \frac{r_i}{\sum_j r_j x_j}, \; F_i = \frac{q_i}{\sum_j r_j x_j} \tag{5.104}$$

r and q can also be estimated by

$$r_i = \sum_k v_k^{(i)} R_k \qquad q_i = \sum_k v_k^{(i)} Q_k$$

$$R_k = \frac{V_{wk}}{15.17} \tag{5.105}$$

R_k and Q_k are the van der Waals group volume and surface area, respectively, and their value can also be found in literature [59].

Polymer Solution

In the delivery of macromolecules, there are specific issues to be considered: first of all, the solute and solvent molecules are of different sizes; second, they are chemically dissimilar; and third, proteins are usually charged. Hence, the solution equations for nonelectrolytes are not completely applicable to polymer solution (protein solution). Recall from the UNIQUAC model that excess Gibbs free energy is composed of a combinatorial term, which accounts for the entropy of mixing, and a residual term, which accounts for the enthalpy of mixing. We start by considering the entropy contribution of a polymer solution; this is because of the huge difference in size and shape between solvent and solute. By applying Lattice model again, assume athermal solution behavior and consider that polymer is composed of r segments, each having the same size as that of a solvent molecule. Change in Gibbs free energy is

$$\frac{G^c}{RT} = (N_1 \ln \Phi_1^* + N_2 \ln \Phi_2^*)$$

where

$$\Phi_1^* = \frac{N_1}{N_1 + rN_2} \qquad \Phi_2^* = \frac{N_2}{N_1 + rN_2} \tag{5.106}$$

N_1 is number of solvent molecules and N_2 is the number of solute molecules; therefore, total number of lattice site is $N_1 + rN_2$.

r, according to the definition, is the ratio of the molecular volumes of the polymer and the solvent. As in the UNIQUAC model, the ratio of surface area of the polymer and the solvent gives q, and q/r is a measure of polymer shape.

Flory-Huggin's Model

The partial molar excess Gibbs free energy is

$$\frac{g^E}{RT} = x_1 \ln\left[1 - \Phi_2^*\left(1 - \frac{1}{r}\right)\right] - x_2 \ln\left[r - \Phi_2^*(r - 1)\right] \tag{5.107}$$

and

$$\ln \gamma_1 = \ln\left[1 - \left(1 - \frac{1}{r}\right)\Phi_2^*\right] + \left(1 - \frac{1}{r}\right)\Phi_2^* \tag{5.108}$$

For large value of r, the activity coefficient of the solvent is independent of r.

Since a real polymer solution is not athermal, the interaction between molecules plays important roles. To account for the enthalpy contribution, an intermolecular interaction parameter, χ, which is also known as Flory–Huggins interaction parameter, is introduced. The activity coefficient then becomes

$$\ln \gamma_1 = \ln\left[1 - \left(1 - \frac{1}{r}\right)\Phi_2^*\right] + \left(1 - \frac{1}{r}\right)\Phi_2^* + \chi\Phi_2^{*2} \tag{5.109}$$

where

$$\chi = \frac{w}{kT}$$

If r is the ratio of molar volume

$$\chi = \frac{v_1}{RT}(\delta_1 - \delta_2)^2 \tag{5.110}$$

UNIQUAC-Based Description for Polymer Solution

In polymer solution, where charged species are present, that is, protein solution and geometric distribution of molecules, intermolecular forces are very different from the uncharged solution (nonelectrolyte). For the geometric distribution, because of electrostatic repulsion, ions with the same charge are far apart, so in consideration of the local composition, only neutral and counterions are present in the neighborhood. Therefore, the combinatorial excess free energy becomes [60]

$$\frac{g^E_{combinatorial}}{RT} = \sum_{i=1}^{m} x_i \ln \frac{\Phi_i^*}{x_i} + \frac{z}{2}\sum_{i=1}^{m} q_i x_i \ln \frac{\theta_i}{\Phi_i^*} + \sum_{i=1}^{n} q_i x_i \left[\ln a_{ii} + \sum_{\substack{j=1 \\ j \neq i}}^{n} \theta_j \ln\left(\frac{a_{ji}}{aii}\right)\right]$$

$$a_{ii} = \frac{1}{\sum \theta_j \tau_{ji}} \tag{5.111}$$

$$a_{ji} = \tau_{ji} a_{ii}$$

a is the nonrandom factor, which is similar to nonrandom, two-liquid model. Notice that the first two terms are the same as UNIQUAC model; therefore, this model is known as the UNIQUAC-NRF model. The combinatorial activity coefficient is expressed as

$$\ln \gamma_{i,combinatorial} = \ln\left(\frac{\Phi_i^*}{x_i}\right) + \frac{zq_i}{2}\ln\left(\frac{\theta_i}{\Phi_i^*}\right) + l_i - \left(\frac{\Phi_i^*}{x_i}\right)\sum_{j=1}^{n}\left(x_j l_j\right) + q_i$$

$$+ \left[1 + \ln a_{ii} - \sum_{\substack{j=1 \\ j\neq i}}^{n}\theta_j a_{ij} + \left(1-\theta_j\right)\ln\left(\frac{a_{ij}a_{ji}}{a_{ii}a_{jj}}\right) - \frac{1}{2}\sum_{\substack{k=1 \\ k\neq i}}^{n}\sum_{\substack{l=1 \\ l\neq k \\ l\neq i}}^{n}\theta_k\theta_l \ln\left(\frac{a_{lk}a_{kl}}{a_{ll}a_{kk}}\right)\right] \quad (5.112)$$

Charging of species in the solution does not only influence geometric distribution of components in the solution, but more importantly, the electrostatic interaction contributes to excess enthalpy, which is denoted as long-range interaction contribution, whereas short-range contribution can be taken from the residual part of the UNIQUAC.

$$\left(\frac{g^E}{RT}\right)_{residual} = \left(\frac{g^E}{RT}\right)_{long\text{-}range} + \left(\frac{g^E}{RT}\right)_{short\text{-}range} \quad (5.113)$$

Hence, the total activity coefficient of species *i* is

$$\ln \gamma_i = \ln \gamma_{i,long\text{-}range} + \ln \gamma_{i,short\text{-}range} + \ln \gamma_{i,combinatorial} \quad (5.114)$$

The electrostatic contribution to the excess Gibbs energy was suggested by Fowler and Guggenheim electrostatic interactions [60]

$$\ln \gamma_{i,long\text{-}range} = -\frac{Az_i^2 I^{1/2}}{1+bI^{1/2}} \quad (5.115)$$

I is the ionic strength of the mixture, which is expressed in terms of molarity of species *i*.

$$I = \frac{1}{2}\sum_{i=1}^{n} m_i z_i^2 \quad (5.116)$$

z is the absolute charge number of ionic species and *b* is a constant that depends on sizes of the components. For the protein with a size of 4 nm, *b* was taken as 15 $(kg\ mol^{-1})^{1/2}$ [61] and *A* is the Debye–Huckel constant for a given system:

$$A = 1.327757 \times 10^5 d^{0.5}/(DT)^{1.5} \quad (5.117)$$

For water,

$$A = 1.131 + 1.335 \times 10^{-3} \times (T - 273.15) + 1.164 \times 10^{-5} \times (T - 273.15)^2 \quad (5.118)$$

For neutral species [60, 62, 63],

$$\ln \gamma_n^{LR} = \frac{2Av_n d}{b^3} \left[1 + bI^{1/2} - (1 + bI^{1/2})^{-1} - 2\ln(1 + bI^{1/2}) \right]$$

$$= \frac{2AM_w}{1000b^3} \left[1 + bI^{1/2} - (1 + bI^{1/2})^{-1} - 2\ln(1 + bI^{1/2}) \right] \tag{5.119}$$

where v is the molar volume and d is the density of the mixture.

The activity coefficient calculated from the above equation is in the unit of molarity (mole/kilogram solvent), to convert it to mole fraction used in consistent to previous equations:

$$\ln \gamma_{\text{mole-fraction}} = \ln \gamma_{\text{molarity}} - \ln \left(1 + \frac{vM_w m}{1000} \right) \tag{5.120}$$

Free-Volume Contribution

In polymer solution, free-volume effects are not negligible; therefore, an extra term is introduced [64]

$$\ln \gamma_i = \ln \gamma_i^R + \ln \gamma_i^C + \ln \gamma_i^{FV} \tag{5.121}$$

The combinatorial part of UNIFAC model is sometimes given in another form [65]:

$$\ln \gamma_i^C = 1 - \phi_i + \ln \phi_i - \frac{z}{2} q_i \left(1 - \frac{\phi_i}{F_i} + \ln \left(\frac{\phi_i}{F_i} \right) \right)$$

$$\phi_i = \frac{r_i}{\sum r_j x_j}, F_i = \frac{q_i}{\sum_j r_j x_j} \tag{5.122}$$

q_i and r_i are calculated as in UNIFAC model.

Residual part is given as the same as UNIFAC, and the free-volume contribution is

$$\ln \gamma_i^{FV} = 3c_i \ln \left[\frac{v_i^{-1/3} - 1}{v_m^{-1/3} - 1} \right] - c_i \left[\left(\frac{\bar{v}_i}{\bar{v}_m} - 1 \right) \left(1 - \frac{1}{v_i^{-1/3}} \right)^{-1} \right]$$

$$\bar{v}_i = \frac{v_i}{v_i^*} = \frac{v_i}{15.17br_i} \tag{5.123}$$

where v_i is the molar volume, v_i^* is the hard core molar volume, b is the proportionality constant, and c is also a constant depending on the type of molecules involved in the system.

Modeling of Charged Solute Partitioning in Hydrogel

The simplest model describing partition of protein into gel is at infinitely dilute solute concentration, and the gel is considered as randomly distributed straight cylindrical fibers. Considering the space occupied by the fibers and the probability of finding a solute in the membrane, the partition coefficient of solute is given by [66]

$$K_p = \exp\left[-\phi_p\left(1 + \frac{a_s}{a_p}\right)\right] \tag{5.124}$$

This partition coefficient is contributed by the size-exclusion effect of membrane. By considering long-range interactions between solute and fibers (electrostatic interaction), from the probability of finding a solute in the gel, different models [66] were derived since the first publication of Ogston in 1958.

Partition of solute could be contributed by nonelectrostatic and electrostatic forces between solutes and the membrane. By considering only steric effect for nonelectrostatic effect, a more rigorous model describing solute partition in hydrogel was established [67,68]. The total partition coefficient is

$$K_p = K_{p\text{-non}} + K_{p\text{-elec}} \tag{5.125}$$

Steric effect refers to size exclusion of solute by highly swollen hydrogels. Schnitzer's uniform-pore model agrees well with experimental data [68]

$$
\begin{aligned}
K_{p\text{-non}} &= (1-\phi_p)\left(1 - \frac{r_s}{r_p}\right) & r_s \le r_c \\
K_{p\text{-non}} &= 0 & r_s > r_c
\end{aligned} \tag{5.126}
$$

The pore radius of the nonporous membrane is taken to be one-half of the mesh size.

The contribution by electrostatic interaction can be derived from chemical potential equilibrium condition.

Chemical potentials of all components in the solution and hydrogel must be equal.

$$\mu_{i,\text{membrane}} = \mu_{\text{bulk}} \tag{5.127}$$

The equilibrium equation can be rewritten as before

$$\mu_i^0 + RT \ln\left(\gamma_{i,\text{bulk}} x_{i,\text{bulk}}\right) = \mu_i^0 + v_i \pi + RT \ln\left(\gamma_{i,\text{membrane}} x_{i,\text{membrane}}\right) \tag{5.128}$$

The osmotic pressure in the membrane is calculated based on gel elasticity.

$$\pi_{\text{elastic}} = -C_{\text{cross}} RT \left(\frac{\phi_p}{\phi_{p,\text{synthesis}}}\right)^{1/3} \tag{5.129}$$

C_{cross} is the concentration of cross-links (mol/m^3).

After substituting in the equilibrium equation

$$\ln(\gamma_{i,bulk}x_{i,bulk}) = -C_{cross}v_i\left(\frac{\phi_p}{\phi_{p,synthesis}}\right)^{1/3} + \ln(\gamma_{i,membrane}x_{i,membrane})$$

(5.130)

Since the solution and the membrane are electrically neutral, if proteins are charged, there must be some counterions to balance the surface charge. Therefore, we consider a protein as an ion pair. Depending on the pH of the solution, proteins will have different net charges and therefore different types of counterions (Table 5.1). The chemical potential for protein ion pairs could be written as a sum of chemical potentials contributed by cations and anions, and the above equation could be written as:

$$\ln[\gamma'_{p,bulk}x_{p,bulk}] = -C_{cross}v_p\left(\frac{\phi_p}{\phi_{p,synthesis}}\right)^{1/3} + \ln[\gamma'_{p,membrane}x_{p,membrane}]$$

(5.131)

where

$$\gamma'_p = \left(\gamma_p^{z_c}\gamma_c^{z_p}\right)^{1/(z_p+z_c)}$$

Where γ_p is the activity coefficient of a charged protein, γ_c is the activity of counterion. z_p is the number of charges on one protein molecule, and z_c is the number of charges on one counterion, which is equal to unity.

$$\ln\left[\frac{\gamma'_{p,bulk}x_{p,bulk}}{\gamma'_{p,membrane}x_{p,membrane}}\right] = -C_{cross}v_p\left(\frac{\phi_p}{\phi_{p,synthesis}}\right)^{1/3}$$

(5.132)

TABLE 5.1

Net Charge of BSA

Parameter	Ion Concentration	Value
Net charge	$I = 1.0$ mol/L	+20 at pH 4.0
		−13.5 at pH 6.0
		−18.4 at pH 7.0
		−22.9 at pH 8.0
	$I = 0.15$ mol/L	−20.4 at pH 7.4
		−9.1 at pH 5.4
		+4.5 at pH 4.7

Source: Jin et al., *Journal of Colloid and Interface Science*, 304, 77–83, 2006. With permission.

therefore

$$K_{p\text{-elec}} = \frac{x_{p,\text{membrane}}}{x_{p,\text{bulk}}} = \frac{\gamma'_{p,\text{bulk}}}{\gamma'_{p,\text{membrane}}} \frac{1}{\exp\left(-C_{\text{cross}}v_p\left(\dfrac{\phi_p}{\phi_{p,\text{synthesis}}}\right)^{1/3}\right)}$$

The protein net charge can be calculated by [61]

$$PNC = \sum_{i+}\left(n_{i+} \times \frac{10^{pK_{i+}-pH}}{10^{pK_i-pH}+1}\right) + \sum_{i-}\left(n_{i-} \times \frac{10^{pH-pK_{i-}}}{10^{pH-pK_{i-}}+1}\right) \tag{5.133}$$

$i+$ are the basic groups in the protein and $i-$ are the acid groups in the protein.

In this case, the polymer is taken to be a cylinder of the uniform surface charge density. This description is often refereed as cell model polyeletrolyte solutions.

$$\gamma_{counterion} = \frac{0.7X/\left(\varsigma z_{cn}\right)+1}{X+1}$$
$$\gamma_{coion} = \frac{0.7X/(\varsigma z_{co})+1}{0.53X/(\varsigma z_{co})+1} \tag{5.134}$$

X is the ratio of the concentration of charged monomers to the concentration of salt in the hydrogel, $\varsigma = l_B/b$, where l_B is the Bjerrum length, which is equal to 7.14 Å in water at room temperature, and b is the axial length per unit charge (2.52 Å for poly-N-isoprolacrylamide). Z is the valences of ions. Counterion means the charge opposite to the hydrogel, co-ion means the ion that has a charge identical to that of the hydrogel. For the case of BSA, the valence of charged BSA at different pH can be found in the work of Lin et al. [69], and those values are used in the calculation in Appendices A and B.

Since the only intermolecular interaction in consideration of this model is electrostatic interaction between charged species, and the activity coefficient of charged ion in the membrane was derived by ignoring the interaction between mobile ions (consider only ion–polymer interaction), the activity coefficient of charged ions in the bulk solution should therefore also ignore mobile ion interactions, which implies that the bulk solution shall be treated as an ideal solution ($\gamma'_{p,\text{bulk}} = 1$). Hence, the partition caused by protein–polymer interaction is

$$\ln K_{p\text{-elec}} = \ln \frac{x_{p,\text{membrane}}}{x_{p,\text{bulk}}} = -\ln \gamma'_{p,\text{membrane}} + C_{\text{cross}}v_p\left(\frac{\phi_p}{\phi_{p,\text{synthesis}}}\right)^{1/3} \tag{5.135}$$

The fraction of ionized monomer (HA type) is obtained by using

$$pH - pK_a - \log_{10}\left(\frac{\alpha}{1+\alpha}\right) = 0 \tag{5.136}$$

The average pK_a of the hydrogel can be estimated by plotting swelling vs. pH and take the pH of the inflection point. Also, α is the fraction of charged monomers.

For amine ionizable groups,

$$pH - pK_a + \log_{10}\left(\frac{\alpha}{1+\alpha}\right) = 0 \tag{5.137}$$

Recent progress has enabled researchers to model a more complicated case for the purpose of controlling drug release rate. Shang et al. [70] proposed a method to tailor the chemical potential equilibrium at the donor–membrane interface. Their method works as follows: a certain amount of the solute molecule is first immobilized in the membrane. The immobilized solute could contribute to the overall chemical potential of solute in the membrane; hence, the amount of free solute molecules from donor that could partition into the membrane is reduced. It is because that less amount of solute molecules is needed to balance its chemical potential in the donor because of the contribution of immobilized ones. In conventional thermodynamics, all components in a system are considered independent (Equation 5.65). However, in practice, the amount of one component could affect the amount of the other, which means dependence shall be considered. The infinitesimal expression of Gibb's free energy equation (Equation 5.63) is reconfigured in the following way to handle the "dependent" case: in a general scenario, two dependent substances (A and B) in the membrane are grouped together, represented by a combined chemical potential ($\mu_{M,grouping}$), and the total concentration of solute molecules in the membrane ($C_{M,grouping} = C_{M,A} + C_{M,B}$), where $C_{M,A}$ and $C_{M,B}$ are the concentrations of A and B in the membrane, and they are dependent; subscript M denotes membrane. Mathematically, the above description writes

$$dG = -SdT + VdP + (\mu_{M,A}dC_{M,A} + \mu_{M,B}dC_{M,B}) + \sum_{i=3}\mu_i dC_i \tag{5.138}$$

and

$$\mu_{M,grouping}dC_{M,grouping} = \mu_A dC_A + \mu_B dC_B \tag{5.139}$$

where S is entropy.

Hence, the combined chemical potential is

$$\mu_{M,grouping} = \mu_{M,A}\left(\frac{dC_{M,A}}{dC_{grouping}}\right)_{T,P,n_{i>2}} + \mu_{M,B}\left(\frac{dC_{M,B}}{dC_{grouping}}\right)_{T,P,n_{i>2}} \tag{5.140}$$

and let

$$\alpha = \left(\frac{dC_{M,A}}{dC_{M,grouping}}\right)_{T,P,n_{i>2}} \quad \text{and} \quad \beta = \left(\frac{dC_{M,B}}{dC_{M,grouping}}\right)_{T,P,n_{i>2}} \tag{5.141}$$

At chemical potential equilibrium, it is assumed that the combined chemical potential in the membrane is balanced by the chemical potential of substance A in the donor:

$$\mu_{M,grouping} = \mu_{D,A} \tag{5.142}$$

Subscript D denotes donor. Substituting the expressions for chemical potential into the above equation:

$$\mu_{M,0} + RT \ln(\gamma_{M,grouping} C_{M,grouping}) = (\mu_{M,0} + RT \ln(\gamma_{M,A} C_{M,A}))\alpha$$

$$+ (\mu_{M,0} + RT \ln(\gamma_{M,B} C_{M,B}))\beta = \mu_{D,0} + RT \ln(\gamma_{D,A} C_{D,A}) \tag{5.143}$$

where μ_0 is the reference chemical potential and γ is the activity coefficient.

Therefore, the concentration ratio of substance A in membrane and donor is

$$\frac{C_{M,A}}{C_{D,A}} = \left[\frac{\exp\left(\dfrac{\mu_{D,o} - \mu_{M,o}}{RT}\right) \gamma_{D,A}}{C_{D,A}^{\alpha-1} \gamma_{M,A}{}^{\alpha} (\gamma_{M,B} C_{M,B})^{\beta}} \right]^{\frac{1}{\alpha}} \quad \text{for} \quad C_{M,B} > 0 \tag{5.144}$$

Now consider the partition control scheme: Let A stand for the free drugs and B for the immobilized ones of same type as A. Assuming the donor is an infinite source of A; thus, $C_{A,D}$ is constant. The concentration ratio derived in Equation 5.144 is therefore the partition coefficient of free drugs (K_{eff}):

$$K_{eff} = \left[\frac{\exp\left(\dfrac{\mu_{D,o} - \mu_{M,o}}{RT}\right) \gamma_{D,free}}{C_{D,free}^{\alpha-1} \gamma_{M,free}{}^{\alpha} (\gamma_{M,immob} C_{M,immob})^{\beta}} \right]^{\frac{1}{\alpha}} \quad \text{for} \quad C_{M,immob} > 0 \tag{5.145}$$

where $\mu_{D,0}$, $\mu_{M,0}$, R, T, and $\gamma_{D,free}$ are constants at a given donor condition, and the activity coefficients of the free and the immobilized molecules in the membrane are related through

$$\gamma_{M,immob} = b\gamma_{M,free} \tag{5.146}$$

This is because the free drugs constantly undergo random movement in the membrane, but when they are immobilized through a spacer, they can move in a similar fashion as free drug molecules only within a distance defined by the length of the spacer. Factor b takes this restriction into account. Inserting Equation 5.146 into Equation 5.145 gives rise to

$$K_{eff} = \left[\frac{\exp\left(\dfrac{\mu_{D,o} - \mu_{M,o}}{RT}\right) \gamma_{D,free}}{C_{D,free}^{\alpha-1} \gamma_{M,free} (b C_{M,immob})^{\beta}} \right]^{\frac{1}{\alpha}} \quad \text{for} \quad C_{M,immob} > 0 \tag{5.147}$$

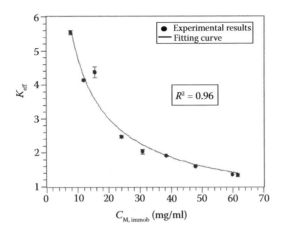

FIGURE 5.9
Partition–coefficient curve.

The partition coefficient equation was successfully fitted to experimental data as shown in Figure 5.9 [70].

Another approach to control release rate by partition/solubility control is to alter pH values of the microenvironment of the coating so as to tailor the protein solubility in it. It is widely known that basic drugs have higher solubility in acidic environment and vice versa, and only dissolved drug can be released. Hence pH modifiers (fumaric, tartaric, adipic, glutaric, and sorbic acid) have been added into the coating for release rate control [71].

Erosion Controlled

In a biodegradable coating configuration, there are a couple of mechanisms that the release rate can be tailored: (1) dense coating so that drug can only be released upon degradation of the coating; (2) coarse coating, in which the drug has a smaller but noticeable diffusivity; and (3) drug containing coating that drug can be released from the coating when degradation occurs. In situation (1), the coating serves as a complete diffusion barrier so that solution–diffusion model discussed in the previous section is no longer valid. The control over release rate is pulsatile: as long as the coating completely covers the drug carrier, there is no drug being released. Once the carrier is exposed to the external environment, the release rate will not be significantly affected by the residual coating left on the surface. In situation (2), the release behavior is more complicated. The coating serves as a solution-diffusion coating with two exceptions: thickness and pore size change with time. As more coating is degraded, thickness of the coating might change, and when the cross-links are hydrolyzed, the pore size is increased, so that drug diffusivity and partition coefficient are both affected. In situation (3), release rate is solely determined by the degradation rate and the drug loading level.

Diffusion is again an important factor to affect the rate of degradation: reagents need to enter the matrix to hydrolyze the cross-links; on the other hand, products of the hydrolysis reaction need to diffuse out to facilitate the reaction toward degradation. Besides diffusion, degradation kinetics affects the overall degradation rate as well.

Degradation Kinetics

In a lot of degradable polymers, degradation happens when ester bond is cleaved. Water molecules contact with the amorphous region of the ester backbone and degradation occurs. This is a random process catalyzed by the presence of acid, therefore the degradation rate increases as the reaction proceeds due to the production of acid during the degradation process [72]. Because the amorphous phase is more easily hydrolysized, the degradation rate of the amorphous coating is usually higher than the semi crystalline ones [73]. Degradation could occur from the surface or simultaneously across the coating (bulk erosion). In certain coatings such as PLGA, in which water diffusion rate is much faster than degradation, the degradation is a bulk erosion process. Since degradation mode depends on both water diffusion and degradation rate, it is expected that the degradation mode also relies on geometry: there will be a critical dimension, lower than which coating would exhibit surface erosion behavior.

Diffusion in a Degrading Coating

As more degradation occurs, polymer chains become shorter, and they start to diffuse out, which reduces the density of the coating and increases its porosity. Due to the increased porosity, the diffusivity of the drug in the degradation layer will be greater. Therefore, a bulk erosion coating can be considered as a film with a variable drug diffusion constant; whereas a surface erosion coating can be considered to be composed of two regions: a denser region with defined diffusivity and a degrading region with variable diffusivity (Figure 5.10) [74]. Although the diffusivity of the drug in the dense region is considered fixed, however, its thickness reduces with respect to time.

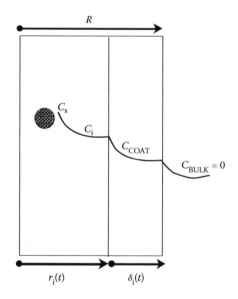

FIGURE 5.10
Drug distribution in a degrading coating. (From Arosio et al., *Polymer International*, 57, 912–920, 2008. With permission.)

Therefore to predict the release behavior of drug molecules, the variable diffusivity needs to be studied with respect to the degree of degradation. The time dependent diffusivity in a degrading region is studied by Porter [116]:

$$D(t) = D(t = 0) + \{[D_{water} - D(t = 0)] \times W(t) \times [100\% - CRSTL(t)]\} \tag{5.148}$$

where $W(t)$ is the film's weight loss at time t, and $CRSTL(t)$ is the coating's degree of crystallinity.

Prabhu and Hossainy [75] used numerical simulation to study the degradation and drug release behavior simultaneously. The time-dependent diffusivity was given as an exponential function with respect to the concentration of the degrading polymer in the system.

Another type of degradation kinetics is ion exchange. Ion-exchange microspheres are polymeric microspheres formed by electrostatic attraction between oppositely charged polymers. The microsphere can be degraded in electrolyte solutions when electrolytes from a solution replace the polymer in the microsphere (hence the name ion exchange). Ionic drugs can be easily loaded, and its release is controlled by two factors: diffusion of the drug and degradation of the microsphere. Besides diffusion barrier, coating can be used to block electrolytes from entering the microspheres to slow down the degradation process [76]. Coated ion-exchange formulation offers a better release rate controllability. In such a configuration, the release rate is controlled by (1) drug diffusivity in the matrix and (2) drug diffusivity in the coating. The overall release profile depends on the limiting step only. If (1) is the rate-limiting step, the core/matrix swells upon contacting with water; hence the drug diffusivity in the matrix gradually increases. Moreover, the net flux is governed by both Brownian motion and electric coupling of ionic flux. It was shown that swelling of the matrix did not have significant effect on the release profile, but the ionic flux affects the release rate more significantly [77].

Osmotic Pressure Controlled

When a semipermeable coating is applied to a drug containing core, only water molecules are allowed to diffuse into the core, but the core materials and the drug are retained inside; therefore, the pressure inside the core will increase. If orifices are drilled in the coating, the content in the core will be pushed out due to the hydrodynamic pressure built up by water uptake.

The release kinetics of osmotic pressure controlled system can be described by the following equation [78]:

$$\frac{dM_t}{dt} = \frac{AP_W \Delta \pi C_d}{l} \tag{5.149}$$

where the left-hand side of the equation is the release rate of the drug. A is the surface area of the device, P_W is the water permeability of the coating, $\Delta \pi$ is the osmotic pressure gradient across the membrane, l is the thickness of the coating, and C_d is the drug concentration in the core.

As can be seen from the equation, surface area and thickness of the coating are device parameters that can be easily applied. However, water permeability and osmotic pressure are dependent on the membrane materials and osmotic agents used in the system, respectively.

Coating Materials and Techniques

Both synthetic and natural polymers have been used in coating to control the release rate. Different methods can be applied to coat a particular polymer on different substrates (films, tablets, granules, etc.). Some of the commonly used materials are summarized, followed by techniques to coat those materials.

Coating Materials

Collagen

Collagen is a major constituent of connective tissue and a major structure protein of any organ. It readily self-assembles into higher-order structures (i.e., fibers) in physiological solutions [79]. Cross-linking of collagen can be achieved by various reactants, and the degradation of collagen network can be controlled by cross-linking density [80]. Collagen can be obtained from various sources in different forms.

Gelatin

Gelatin is a natural polymer derived from collagen, and its electric properties can be easily tailored according to preparation conditions [81]. The most commonly used gelatin in pharmaceutical industry is capsules, but it is widely used as coating material as well. The popularity of using gelatin as a coating material for drug delivery systems is largely because of its biodegradability (100% reabsorbable in vivo) and biocompatibility (no antigenicity) [82]. Degradation of gelatin happens in a few different ways: (1) dissolution and (2) enzymatic degradation. Dissolution of gelatin occurs when hydration of the gelatin coating is high if the molecules are not cross-linked. Alternatively, gelatin can be cross-linked when carboxyl group and free amines of adjacent molecules are condensed. The cross-linking can be induced by water-soluble carbodiimide (such as N,N-(3-dimethylaminopropyl)-N 8-ethyl carbodiimide and N-hydroxysuccinimide) and aldehyde (i.e., glutaraldehyde and formaldehyde) to form hydrogel [83]. Degradation of cross-linked gelatin occurs when peptide bonds are cleaved. By altering cross-linking density, degradation time can be tailored from days to months [84].

Alginate

Alginate is a family of un-branched polysaccharides isolated from brown algae found in coastal water. Alginate is composed of two monomers, namely β-D-mannuronic acid (M) and α-L-guluronic acid (G), linked by one to four glycoside bounds. It is found that the G-monomer and M-monomer join together in a blockwise fashion.

Cross-linking of alginate can be achieved in the presence of di/trivalent ions. It has been found that Ca^{2+} and Sr^{2+} mainly form GG linkage, whereas Zn^{2+} can form GG, MM, and GM linkages [85]. The flexibility of alginate in aqueous solutions is in the order:

MG > MM > GG [86]. Therefore, alginate gels with higher G content will have higher mechanical strength and higher porosity. There gels are more stable in monovalent solution [87].

Chitosan

Chitosan is a natural polymer obtained by alkaline deacetylation of chitin, and it is a copolymer of β-1,4-linked 2-acetamido-2-deoxy-D-glucopyranose and 2-amino-2-deoxy-D-glucopyranose. As compared to alginate, chitosan is positively charged. Chitosan is a weak base and is soluble only in a dilute acidic solution. Similar to synthetic polymer PEG, chitosan is found to show mucoadhesive properties [88], which make chitosan a good candidate for oral delivery. Because of its solubility and charge, chitosan is often dissolved in acetic acid, and the chitosan solution is extruded dropwise to aqueous counterion solutions, to form chitosan gels [89]. The drug loading efficiency is positively correlated to chitosan concentration in the precursor solution, whereas lower drug release is observed for chitosan with higher molecular weight [88]. Chitosan is susceptible to glycosidic hydrolysis by microbial enzymes in the colon [90]; hence, chitosan is a good candidate for colon-targeted delivery.

Cellulose and Its Derivatives

Hydroxypropyl methylcellulose (HPMC) is a water-soluble cellulose derivative. It offers good mechanical strength and easy processing as a coating material [91]. Although it is widely used for taste masking in oral dosages, its application in release rate control is fairly common in practice. HPMC can be casted into films, and the film can be coated onto different formulations. HPMC can be coated by direct compression from powder form as well [92].

Polyvinyl-Based Polymers

Polyvinyl acetate (PVAc) is a water insoluble polymer, whereas PVA, which is a hydrolysis product of PVAc, is water soluble. PVAc is highly ductile (elongate to 200%–300% without failure [93]), which makes it a good candidate for drug coating because it ensures the coating integrity and reduces the risk of film rupture. Kollicoat® SR 30D is a commercially available product that is a 30% aqueous dispersion of polyvinyl acetate stabilized by polyvinylpyrrolidone. It can be made into film or coating easily at low temperature (18°C [94]); hence, no thermal treatment is needed when used as a coating material. When the film is in contact with gastrointestinal fluid, polyvinylpyrrolidone dissolves so that pores are created in the coating for sustained release [95]. Kollicoat1 SR 30D is known as one of the aqueous colloidal polymer dispersions for the manufacturing of pH-independent sustained release drug delivery systems [77].

Ethylene vinyl acetate is a copolymer containing the semicrystalline polyethylene and amorphous vinyl acetate, and these are commonly used as rate-controlling membranes in drug delivery devices [96]. Because higher diffusivity is observed at lower crystallinity, higher VA content increases diffusivity of the drug in the ethylene vinyl acetate polymer.

Acrylate-Based Materials

Poly(methylmethacrylate) is a commonly used polymer in biomedical applications owing to its good mechanical property and biocompatibility. Different Eudragit L30 D-55 (anionic copolymer of methacrylic acid and ethylacrylate [1:1]) is a commonly used enteric coating (dissolves above 6.0 [97]). The recommended coating level for Eudragit L30 D-55 to achieve enteric properties is in the range of 4- to 6-mg polymer per cm^2 surface area of the core [98] Eudragit FS 30 D is an anionic copolymer of methyl acrylate, methyl methacrylate, and methacrylic acid. Eudragit SL and RL series are widely used in sustained release coating in pharmaceutical industry.

Polyethylene Glycol

PEG is a water-soluble polymer, which has two hydroxyl groups at the end of the linear structure. It exists in a wide range of molecular weight from a few hundred to tens of thousands of Dalton. It is one of the most popular biomaterials because of its low toxicity. PEG has been widely used to modify other materials in biomedical applications for better solubility, prolonged circulation time in the circulation system, and adhesion to mucosa. The process of conjugating PEG onto other polymer is known as PEGylation [99].

Polyesters

Poly-lactic acid (PLA) and poly lactic-*co*-glycolic acid (PLGA) are Food and Drug Administration–approved biodegradable polyesters. Poly ε-caprolactone is degradable polyester, which does not generate acid during degradation and has a slower degradation rate as compared to PLA and PLGA [100].

Coating Techniques

Coatings are usually applied in aqueous or organic solutions; however, solvent-free coating technologies are used as well. Different coating techniques can be found in both laboratories and industry.

Fluid Bed

Fluid bed coating is one of the most commonly used coating techniques. In this technique, fluidized particle by turbulent air is coated by an atomized spray to produce a uniform coating; however, it is limited to big particles, ranging from 0.5 to 1.2 mm [101]. This is because smaller particles cannot have a stable fluidization state in the conventional fluid bed [102]. The parameters to control the coating are as follows: (1) inlet temperature and speed, (2) bed temperature, (3) spray rate, and (4) spray solution composition and distance. The size restriction is because interparticular force overtakes gravitational force, which negatively affects the flow properties so as to prevent forming a uniform coating [103]. There are different types of fluid-bed systems, which can be classified by the type of the spray: top spray, bottom spray (Wurster), and tangential spray. In the top spray configuration, air is blown upward; coating materials are sprayed from the top of the chamber. In bottom spray configuration, air is blown upward as well; however, air flow is stronger in the center of the chamber. A Wurster insert is installed above the air distribution plate, and it ensures that particles are lifted upward in the center and fall outside the insert. When particles return to the bottom from the outside of the insert, they are blown upward again. The spraying is down in the center, whereas particles are lifted upward. Particles will be dried when they return back to the bottom. This process will be repeated for several times until the desired thickness is achieved. After coating is applied, curing is needed for a uniform coating to be formed. Hamed and Sakr [104] studied the effect of plasticizer and curing temperature on drug release behavior: higher plasticizer level decreases the glassy transition temperature; hence, a complete coating can be formed with a lower curing temperature. It was also found that a suitable curing time is needed to complete the film forming process, which reduces the drug release rate; however, if curing time is too long, drug in the core will migrate to the coating, which results in a burst release. One of the most commonly encountered problems in fluid-bed coating is agglomeration, which is caused by liquid bridges between particles [105]. The formation of liquid bridges depends on the coating solution and the size of the spray mist. It was found that adding NaCl could reduce the particle agglomeration due to the reduction of viscosity of the coating solution by salting-out effect [106]. A smaller mist size is preferred to suppress agglomeration, which can be realized by a smaller spray–particle distance, a higher inlet temperature, and higher fluidization air volume [139]. Similar to fluid bed, pan coater is commonly used in pharmaceutical research and industry for film coating. In a pan coater, tablets are placed on a bed rather than being fluidized in the fluid-bed coating system. Coating materials are still applied by spray, and the tablets are tumbled to ensure complete coating on the tablets.

Compression Coating

Coating can be applied to the core by direct compression of the coating materials. Coating materials are first introduced into a mold, and then the core is placed in the mold. Additional coating materials are fed into the mold to cover the core. The compression is done by two punches at a given pressure to form the coating. Lin et al [107] used compression coating technique to coat ethylcellulose on an inorganic drug. Two compression forces were evaluated: inner-core compression force and the coating compression force. It was found that at a constant coating compression force (300 kg/m^2), a higher inner-core compression force could slow the dissolution of the drug, whereas at a constant inner-core compression force (200 kg/m^2), a higher coating compression force results in a longer lag time. Besides ethylcellulose, another commonly used polymer in compression coating is acrylic-based polymers (marketed under the brand of Kollicoat and Eudragit). The common problem encountered in compression coating is the damage to the coating due to high compression force. Dashevsky and coworkers [108] observed that drug was released faster with a higher compression force.

Plasticizer Dry Coating

Coating polymers and plasticizer are sprayed onto the core materials from different nozzles simultaneously. The coated polymer is then cured at elevated temperature (above glassy transition temperature) to form a uniform coating. The function of the added plasticizer is to lower the glass transition temperature of the coating material. Cellulose derivatives can be easily coated onto particles using this method [109]. It has been observed that an increase in moisture could increase the coating quality in terms of smoothness and integrity [110].

Hot–Melt

For the hot–melt coating technique, the coating material is applied to the core at molten state, and the coating is formed upon cooling. It has been suggested that the melting temperature of the coating material to be around 85°C because the molten coating material is usually kept at 40–60°C higher than the melting temperature before spraying so that the overall operating temperature does not go beyond 150°C. The suggested spray rate for a uniform coating is at 30 g/min. To ensure good coverage of the core, it has been reported that the optimal size of the core shall be 0.1–0.75 mm in diameter [111].

Supercritical Fluid Coating

The supercritical state is defined as a state where both the pressure and temperature of a substance are greater than its critical pressure and critical temperature [112]. Carbon dioxide is the most commonly used supercritical solution for industrial applications because of its moderate critical pressure (72 bar) and critical temperature (31.1°C) [113]. The supercritical fluid coating works as follows: coating materials are dissolved in the supercritical solution in a high-pressure vessel; insoluble core particles are dispersed in the supercritical solution as well. A rapid expansion of volume of the vessel decreases the pressure quickly, and supercritical solution becomes less "supercritical"; hence, the dissolved coating material precipitates and coats onto the core particles. It is apparent that a key requirement of the supercritical solution coating technique is that the coating material and the core particles must have different solubility in the supercritical solution. Cosolvent can be added into the supercritical solution to enhance the solubility of either coating material or the core.

Electrospinning

Electrospinning can be used for coating preparation. The distinct feature of electrospun coating is that it is composed of fibers down to the size of submicron in diameter. In this process, a high voltage (in the order of kilovolts) is applied across the spinning solution (usually in a syringe) and a collector (distance between them is altered to reach different electric field strength). The spinning solution is directed to the collector by the high electric field and syringe pump. Yu et al. [114] used the electrospinning to fabricate a polyvinylpyrrolidone fiber film that exhibits a fast dissolving process. Drug can be simultaneously loaded into the film by adding drug molecules into the spinning solution.

Another technique that uses electrostatic force is known as electrostatic spray powder coating. Instead of using solution, in the electrostatic spray powder coating method, dry powders of the coating material are charged at a high voltage (100 kV) [115], and the substrate is grounded. The powder is carried by the air though an electrostatic powder gun to the substrate. Once the powders are coated onto the substrate by electrostatic force, the coating material is molten by heat so as to complete the coating process. The resistivity of the core has to be less than 10^9 Ω m, whereas the resistivity of the powder should be more than 10^{11} Ω m [116]. A key parameter in this technique is the powder size of the coating material, with 30–100 μm being the optimal.

Precipitation Method

Precipitation coating method has been widely used for many different materials. Core is dispersed in coating precursor solution. Precipitation of the precursor is induced by pH, adding antisolvent or using supersaturation solution. Xu and Czernuszka [117] used precipitation method to coat PLGA microspheres with a layer of HA for release rate control. PLGA suspended water was added into a supersaturated solution of HA precursor. HA would precipitate and deposit on the PLGA microspheres, and the onset of the experiment would induce a drop in pH. It was reported that a more negative surface facilitated

HA nucleation; hence, negatively charged PLGA was used in their study. The precipitation occurs in the following manner: The drop in pH and Ca^{2+} activity triggered the simultaneous addition of two titrants containing PO_4^{3-} and Ca^{2+} ions to keep the reaction solution at a constant high supersaturation. By this means, the ionic activities of the two ions were maintained at a fixed level. The same coating method has been applied to liposomes as well [118]. Most recently, a biomimetic method has been utilized to coat minerals onto microspheres [119]. The biomimetic method uses a simulated body fluid to mimic physiological HA formation process. When incubating the seeding materials (microspheres for instance) in the simulated body fluid, a layer of HA will be formed onto the surface of the seeding at 37°C in a duration of a few days.

Drug Delivery Systems with Coating

Coating as both drug carrier and rate controller is widely used in biomedical devices, such as stents, scaffold [120], microneedles [121], and microparticles (drug containing coating on a magnetic microparticle for targeting [122]). However, in most devices with drug containing coating, burst release is usually observed (majority of the drug is released during the first few hours). The reason for the burst release is largely due to the quick release of the drug entrapped near the surface of the coating. When a drug containing film is coated on the surface of biomedical devices (i.e., drug eluting stent), it also suffers from burst release; hence, it may be difficult to sustain the release. A practical approach to enhance the long-term effectiveness of a drug-containing film/matrix is to capsulate it with another layer, which is essentially a reservoir–membrane system as well [123]. Venkatraman and Boey [124] reviewed several reservoir–membrane systems in the application of cardiology stents. In one of the applications where drug is supposed to be released over a longer period, a drug-free coating is applied on the surface of the drug-containing layer (Figure 5.11). Since drug molecules have to pass through an extra layer, its release rate is supposed to be reduced; otherwise, a faster release profile can be found in a design that has no drug-free layer.

Sriamornsak and Kennedy [125] studied the alginate and pectin coating in controlling the release of a few water insoluble drugs. The drug pellets were prepared by blending drug, cellulose, and calcium acetate. Pellets were coated by solution coating of pellets in an alginate/pectin solution and cross-linking of alginate/pectin on the surface of pellets with soluble calcium acetate. It was found that the alginate/pectin coating lowered the release rate by four- to six-folds, regardless of the type of the drug, whereas the release rate was slowest for drugs having low water solubility.

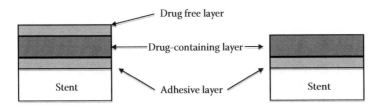

FIGURE 5.11
Multilayer-coated stent.

For charged coatings, the release behavior depends on the polarity and thickness of the coating. Zhou and coworkers [126] coated PLGA microspheres with electrolytes of different polarities. Their findings were that the release rate of charged molecules decreased with increases in coating thickness, but layer thickness had little effect on neutral molecules. The outer layer polarity had a more prominent effect on the drug release rate because the charging state of the coating is determined by the outermost layers. Molecules with opposite charge compared to the outermost layer had slower release rate due to the strong binding.

Schwartz et al. [108] studied the effect of coating level on the release kinetics. It was summarized that four different mechanisms might exist for different coating levels [127]:

(1) Thin and uneven coatings: transport of the drug through flaws, cracks, and imperfections within the matrix or uncoated systems

(2) Thin and even coatings: transport of the drug through a network of capillaries filled with release media

(3) Thick and hydrogel: transport of the drug through a hydrated swollen film

(4) Thick and more rigid film: transport of the drug through barriers or nonporous coatings, which are determined by the permeability of drug in the film

As the coating level (measured by the weight of the coating) gradually increased, the drug release rate was reduced. A faster release at lower coating levels was attributed to the incomplete/discontinuous coating. When coating level was high, more of the core surface was covered by the coating material until the whole surface was covered. Core–shell structure has been used in particulate formulations for release rate control. Winey et al. [128] studied the chitosan-coated PLGA nanoparticles and found that the burst release was dramatically reduced even with a single layer of coating by physical absorption. Lee et al. studied the effect of plasticizers on the release profile. Plasticizers are used in coating preparation to alter its mechanical and thermal properties (glass transition temperature, free volume, brittleness). It was found that the hydrophilicity of the plasticizer itself does not significantly affect the release profile if they were retained inside the coating, but the hydrophilic plasticizer could easily leash out from the coating [129].

Kaplan et al. [130] used layer-by-layer assembly of silk onto alginate and PLGA microspheres. The assembly was driven by hydrophobic interaction between silk and the microspheres. It has been shown that the release of model drugs is more linear and last for a longer period after coating with silk (Figure 5.12).

Dual-layer coating is also used to alter the release rate of drugs. Dashevsky et al. [94] coated a drug containing core with Kollicoat SR 30 D as a release rate limiting layer. A PVA layer is applied in between the core and Kollicoat coating to prevent hydrophobic drug from partitioning into the outer layer during coating and storage. It has been shown that drug release rate can be easily controlled by the coating levels (measured by the weight percentage of coating in the formulation).

In coated microspheres, the release rate of drugs is mainly determined by the coating, whereas the core serves as nothing but a reservoir. If the core can be removed, a microcapsule will be formed for loading hydrophilic drugs. Li [131] used $CaCO_3$ microspheres as a template and coated it with poly-L-lysine hydrobromide and chondrotin sulfate sodium salt (CS) through layer-by-layer assembly. The core was then dissolved in disodium ethylenediaminetetraacetic acid. However, this configuration shows a pH-dependent loading behavior because the assembly is driven by an electrostatic force; hence, the wall of the

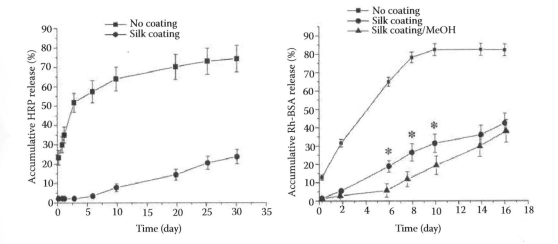

FIGURE 5.12
Release of HRP-encapsulated PLGA microspheres with/without silk coating (left); release of Rh-BSA encapsulated alginate microspheres with/without silk coating and further treatment with methanol (MeOH; right). (From Bose, S., Bogner, R.H., *Pharmaceutical Development and Technology*, 12, 115–113, 2007. With permission.)

microcapsule is strongly charged. Therefore, it is dependent on the charge of the drug to give rise to different loading efficiencies. If bovine serum albumin is used as a model drug, its loading efficiency was found the highest at pH 3.8.

When a matrix is cross-linked, its cross-linking is usually done throughout the polymer matrix; but local alternation of cross-linking density (such as surface cross-linking) can be used to modify overall release rate. This configuration is more like a core–shell system, where the cross-linked surface behaves like a coating. Brazel et al. [132] reported surface cross-linked poly-2-hydroxyethyl methacrylate (PHEMA) disks, where cross-linking of the PHEMA is only induced at the surface by controlling the contacting time between cross-linking agent and the matrix. It is shown that a much longer sustained release profile can be achieved at a suitable cross-linking density (Figure 5.13, left). It is worth noting that a similar effect can be achieved by changing the PHEMA concentration during preparation (Figure 5.14). But most interestingly, a delayed release profile was found for a high PHEMA concentration hydrogel with a high surface cross-linking density (Figure 5.13, right): drug is only released after an initial silent period. A delayed formulation is beneficial for oral delivery because it takes hours for the delivery system to reach small intestine and colon. Moreover, it solved the burst release problem. The surface cross-linking approach has been applied to PVA hydrogels for delayed and sustained release as well [133].

Kennedy et al. [134] studied the effect of drug solubility on the release behavior of calcium polysaccharide gel (such as alginate gel) coated pellets: low solubility drugs and gels with higher cross-linking density resulted in the lowest release rate; however, specific drug–polymer interaction might change the general rules.

Besides the diffusivity and solubility of the drug in the coating, the location of the drug in the coating has a dramatic effect on the release behavior as well. This is because the location of the drug determines the distance it has to travel before it is released. The location of the drug in the coating can be controlled if solvent evaporation method is used. In the evaporation method, polymer and drug are dissolved in an organic solvent and then the solution is casted onto the substrate. Drying of the casting solution is needed to form a coating. It has been proved that evaporation rate and concentration of casting solution

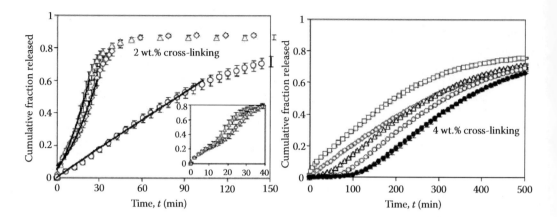

FIGURE 5.13
PHEMA, 20%, with different amount of crosslinking concentration (left); 40% PHEMA with different amount of crosslinking (right; the intermediate curves between the two boundaries are 1, 2, and 3 wt.%). (From Luque de Castro et al., *Analytical Supercritical Fluid Extraction* ed., Springer-Verlag, New York, 1994. With permission.)

determine the location of the drug in the coating [135]: a low concentration and slower evaporation rate result in a segmentation of the polymer and drug, whereas a high concentration and faster evaporation rate make the drug distribute more evenly in the coating.

More often than not, achieving the desired coating property is difficult by a single material; a feasible approach to overcome this problem is to blend two or more types of polymers together. The property of the coating can be easily altered by varying polymer: polymer blend ratio [136]. For diffusion-controlled systems, the diffusivity of the drug can be easily manipulated by blending different types of polymers with distinct water infinity. The drug diffusion rate will be higher if the concentration of the higher water-soluble polymer is higher in the blend. Lehman [137] studied the blending of Eudragit® RL and Eudragit RS for release rate control and found out that a faster release rate was achieved

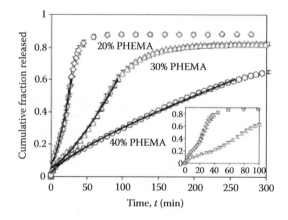

FIGURE 5.14
Proxyphylline release from PHEMA matrix with different concentration. (From Luque de Castro et al., *Analytical Supercritical Fluid Extraction* ed., Springer-Verlag, New York, 1994. With permission.)

by more Eudragit RL because it is more hydrophilic. Together with HPMC, Wei Wu et al. [138] added lactose to form a coating by compression coating technique. Lactose readily dissolves out when in contact with water, leaving a diffusion path for drug to be released. Therefore, a faster release and shorter lag time were observed for higher lactose content, but a linear release profile was observed regardless of lactose content. A similar idea is widely used for polyvinyl-based polymers to alter the drug release rate. It is rather a common practice to blend hydrophobic polymers with hydrophilic polymers such as cellulose derivatives to tailor drug release behavior (Table 5.2). Besides the fact that blendings of different polymers could affect the overall hydrophilicity of the coating, the hydrophilic constitutes could dissolve and leach out from the coating when in contact with the body fluid, hence leaving diffusion channels for the core material to be released [139]. Hence, both porous and nonporous descriptions of the diffusion process are needed to describe the drug release behavior of certain coatings.

In practice, release rate in erosion controlled drug delivery system is mainly controlled by degradation rate of the coating. Therefore, most research has been devoted to design polymers with different degradation rates. Mather and coworkers [140] studied the release behavior of a family of nanostructured hybrid polyurethanes, which was synthesized by covalently connecting polyhedral oligosilsesquioxane thermoplastic polyurethanes and biodegradable soft segments of poly-D,L-lactide/caprolactone copolymer with incorporation of PEG. It was found out that the release rate could be easily tailored from half a day to 90 days by altering the polymer structure.

HPMC can be used as both matrix and coating materials. Uncoated HPMC usually shows a linear release profile (zero-order release profile), and its release rate can be reduced by applying Eudragit RS 30D coating at different levels: the higher the coating level, the smaller the release rate is. Drug molecules can be dispersed in the core and coating at the same time (dual-drug loaded) to have more complex release profiles. It was reported that at moderate coating levels, a biphase release profile is observed with a faster release rate in the first few hours followed by a slower release rate [141]. Maroni and coworkers [142] manufactured insulin tablets coated with HPMC. It was found that the insulin tablets could be manufactured by an industrial method: direct compression without loss of functionality. Because the major challenge in oral insulin delivery (and other acidic sensitive drugs, such as Omeprazole) is to protect the insulin from degradation until it reaches the

TABLE 5.2

Cellulose Derivatives as Coating Materials

Polymer	Property
Methylcellulose (MC)	Soluble in cold water
Ethylcellulose	Soluble in organic solvents, but insoluble in water. Used to realize sustained release formulation. Used together with water-soluble celluloses to alter the release behavior
Hydroxyethylcellulose (HEC)	Soluble in water
Methyl hydroxyethylcellulose (MHEC)	Soluble in water
Hydroxypropyl cellulose (HPC)	Soluble in water, but tacky when dried
HPMC	Soluble in water, alcohols, and halogenated hydrocarbons

Source: Gibson, M., Pharmaceutical Preformulation and Formulation: A Practical Guide From Candidate Drug Selection to Commercial Dosage Form, 2007.

small intestine, the HMPC could serve as a protection layer, which gradually dissolves with time in the gastrointestinal tract. The time required for the HPMC coating to be completely degraded (lag time) can be controlled by the coating level. The design objective is to make sure that the lag time coincides with the time needed to deliver the tablet to the small intestine. It was shown that the lag time can be modulated from zero to 150 min by HPMC coatings. The coatings that help the medicine to reach the small intestine are collectively known as enteric coatings. Aqueous methacrylic acid copolymer dispersion (Eudragit L 30D-55) is commonly used to form enteric coatings. The coating forms compact structure in acidic environment, hence prevents direct contact between the ingredients and acid, but quickly dissolves in basic condition found in the small intestine. However, the challenge of this approach is that basic drugs could migrate into the enteric coatings and be degraded during storage. To solve this problem, subcoating/buffer is required to separate the drug and the enteric coating. He et al. [143] constructed multilayer structure and made of a salt layer and an HPMC layer to be the buffer. The salt layer enhanced the stability of the drug but had no effect on the release rate. HPMC layer controls the release rate when the enteric layer dissolves. The overall shell life of the formulation was reported to be 2 years. Among different commercially available HPMC, it was reported that the lag time decreases according to Methocel K4M > E50 > E5 [144].

A recent design of biodegradable coating was reported by Murphy and coworkers [145]. Biodegradable ceramics, hydroxyapatite, was coated on a biodegradable PLGA microsphere by biomimetic process. Since most protein drugs are charged, they can be bound strongly to the mineral coating by electrostatic attraction so that proteins cannot escape from it. It has been shown that protein release was controlled by the degradation of the mineral coating, and burst release was not observed in their design since degradation was a time-dependent process.

Since PLA or PLGA is biodegradable, they can be casted into films and can be coated onto drug pellets using a hot template ((120°C, 1 h, 1 MPa) to alter release behavior. The PLA-coated drug pellets showed a biphase release profile: a quick release due to partition of the drug in the film during preparation and a slow linear release over days governed by degradation [146]. Schmidmaier et al. [73] reported on poly(D,L-lactide)–coated osteosynthetic implants, loaded with growth factors, and found that the incorporated growth factor can be gradually released in a month, and the coated implant could sustain a higher load than the bare metal implant. Degradation rate of PLA can be increased by incorporating PEG due to decreased acidity [147]. To minimize the burst release with increased degradation rate, another coating can be applied onto the PLG-g-PEG film.

More advanced erosion-controlled designs are available. Degradable/water-soluble coating can be applied to the amorphous solid formulation widely used in oral delivery. The coating could stabilize the amorphous formulation and meanwhile control the rate of dissolution of the solid formulation by its degradation/dissolution rate. Eudragit L100, an ionic polymer, has been used in such designs [148]. The ion exchange dissolves the Eudragit L100 coating, and the amorphous core is quickly dissolved after the coating is gone.

The general configuration of an osmotic pressure-driven drug delivery system is a semipermeable coating on a drug containing core. When contacting with water, the osmotic pressure drives water into the formulation and the pressure inside the formulation is increased. Drug is then pushed out through orifices in the membrane due to the elevated pressure. A lag time is usually observed, and the release of the drug is linear. The coating can be asymmetric: the coating is composed of a semipermeable polymer with discrete channels [149]; therefore, there is no need to create orifices for drug to be released. Another configuration of the osmotic pressure-driven drug delivery system is known as push–pull systems [150]. A piece of hydrogel is loaded in a chamber surrounded by a semipermeable membrane. When water is driven into the chamber, the hydrogel swells and pushes the drug out of the chamber. Multicompartment of osmotic pressure-driven system can be fabricated to deliver different types of drugs simultaneously. To generate a large osmotic pressure gradient across the membrane, osmotically active ingredients, that is, sodium and potassium chloride [151], and sucrose are added into the compartment. Cellulose acetate is widely used to prepare semipermeable membrane, and water-soluble polymers such as PEG are commonly used as a leachable component to form the orifices for the drug to be released [152]. A similar concept was adopted by Pan et al. [153]. In their system, a coating made of Eudragit L100 protects the system from acidic environment of the stomach, and it dissolves in the small intestine. A semipermeable membrane is made from cellulose acetate and chitosan. In the small intestine, although water is allowed to enter the core through the semipermeable membrane, there are no orifices for the drug to be released. The chitosan in the semipermeable membrane is eventually degraded by the microflora in the colon; hence, the semipermeable membrane becomes porous and allows the drug to be released driven by osmotic pressure.

Summary

Drug release rate control by coating technology can be a target at different control mechanisms, namely, diffusion, erosion, and osmotic pressure. Understanding of those mechanisms is critical to choose suitable materials and coating techniques for the purpose of release rate control. For diffusion-controlled coatings, diffusivity and partition coefficients are two key parameters, which can be affected by some common factors, such as cross-linking density, hydrophilicity, and specific binding; however, partition-specific control method (drug immobilization in the coating) is available as well. The ability to control diffusivity and partition coefficients separately is beneficial to a more precise release rate control. In the erosion and osmotic pressure coatings, diffusion plays a critical role in determining the final release rate as well because it affects the degradation rate and osmotic pressure.

References

[1] L. Shang, S. Zhang, S.S. Venkatraman, and H. Du, Physiological insights of pharmacokinetics and host response for drug delivery system design, *Biomaterials and Engineering* (ISBN 0-87849-480-4), edited by W. Ahmed, N. Ali, A. Öchsner, Trans Tech Publications, Switzerland, 419–472 (chapter 11), 2007

[2] T. Yoshida, H. Tasaki, A. Maeda, M. Katsuma, K. Sako, and T. Uchida, Optimization of salting-out taste-masking system for micro-beads containing drugs with high solubility, *Chemical and Pharmaceutical Bulletin* 56 (11) (2008) 1579–1584

[3] M. Cerea, W. Zheng, C.R. Young, and J.W. McGinity, A novel powder coating process for attaining taste masking and moisture protective films applied to tablets, *International Journal of Pharmaceutics* 279 (2004) 127–139

[4] B. Ziaie, A. Baldi, M. Lei, Y. Gu, and R.A. Siegel, Hard and soft micromachining for BioMEMS: review of techniques and examples of applications in microfluidics and drug delivery, *Advanced Drug Delivery Reviews* 56 (2004) 145–172

[5] J.W. McBain and T.H. Liu, Diffusion of electrolytes, non-electrolytes and colloidal electrolytes, *Journal of the American Chemical Society*, 53 (1931) 59–74

[6] W.A. Rogers, R.S. Buritz, and D. Alpert, Diffusion coefficient, solubility, and permeability for Helium in glass, *Journal of Applied Physics*, 25 (1954) 868–875

[7] B.-H. Chen and D.J. Lee, Slow release of drug through deformed coating film: effects of morphology and drug diffusivity in the coating film, *Journal of Pharmaceutical Sciences* 90 (2001) 1478–1496

[8] A. Einstein, *Investigations on the Theory of the Brownian Movement*, edited by R. Furth, Dover, New York (1956)

[9] J.S. Vrentas and C.M.M. Vrentas, Transport in nonporous membranes, *Chemical Engineering Science* 57 (2002) 4199–4208

[10] J.D. Ferry, Statistical evaluation of sieve constrains in ultrafiltration, *Journal of General Physiology*, 20 (1926) 95–104

[11] W.M. Deen, Hindered transport of large molecules in liquid-filled pores, *AIChE Journal* 33 (1987) 1409–1425

[12] A.K. Wright and M.R. Thompson, Hydrodynamic structure of bovine serum albumin determined by transient electric birefringence, *Biophysics Journal* 15 (1975) 137

[13] I.L. Anderson and R.J.A. Quinn, Restricted transport in small pores. A model for steric exclusion and hindered particle motion, *Biophysics Journal* 14 (1974) 957

[14] E.M. Renkin, Filtration, diffusion, and molecular sieving through porous cellulose membrane, *Journal of General Physiology* 38 (1954) 225–243

[15] C.N. Satterfield, C.K. Colton, and W.H. Pitcher Jr., Restricted diffusion in liquids within fine pores, *AIChE Journal* 19 (1973) 628–635

[16] W.B. Russel, Brownian motion of small particles suspended in liquids, *Annual Review of Fluid Mechanics* 13 (1981) 425–455

[17] H. Brenner and L.J. Gaydos, The constrained Brownian movement of spherical particles in cylindrical pores of comparable radius, *Journal of Colloid and Interface Science* 58 (1977) 312–356

[18] E.N. Lightfoot, J.B. Bassingthwaighte, and E.F. Grabowski, Hydrodynamic models for diffusion in microporous membranes, *Annals of Biomedical Engineering* 4 (1976) 78–90

[19] M. Ladero, A. Santos, and F. Garcia-Ochoa, Hindered diffusion of proteins and polymethacrylates in controlled-pore glass: An experimental approach, *Chemical Engineering Science* 62 (2007) 666–678

[20] H.C. Hamaker, The London–van der Waals attraction between spherical particles, *Physica* 10 (1937) 1058–1072

[21] R. Tadmor, The London–van der waals interaction energy between objects of various geometries, *Journal of Physics: Condensed Matter* 13 (2001) L195–L202

[22] J. Shao and R.E. Baltus, Hindered diffusion of dextran and polyethylene glycol in porous membranes, *AIChE Journal* 46 (2000) 1149–1156

[23] P.C. Hiemenz and R. Rajagopalan, *Principle of Colloid and Surface Chemistry*, 3rd ed., Macrel Dekker, New York (1997)

[24] S. Bhattacharjee and A. Sharma, Apolar, polar, and electrostatic interactions of spherical particles in cylindrical pores, *Journal of Colloid and Interface Science* 187 (1997) 83–95

[25] F.G. Smith III and W.M. Deen, Electrostatic effects on the partitioning of spherical colloids between dilute bulk solution and cylindrical pores, *Journal of Colloid and Interface Science* 91 (1983) 571–590

[26] W.W. Graessley, Polymer chain dimensions and the dependence of viscoelastic properties on concentration, molecular weight and solvent power, *Polymer* 21 (1980) 258–262

[27] K.H. Keller, E.R. Canales, and S. II Yum, Tracer and mutual diffusion coefficients of proteins, *Journal of Physical Chemistry* 75 (1971) 379–387

[28] J. Shao and E. Baltus, Effect of solute concentration on hindered diffusion in porous membranes, *AIChE Journal* 46 (2000) 1307–1316

[29] G.K. Batchelor, Brownian diffusion of particles with hydrodynamic interaction, *Journal of Fluid Mechanics* 74 (1976) 1

[30] B.D. Fair and A.M. Jamieson, Effect of electrodynamic interactions on the translational diffusion of bovine serum albumin at finite concentration, *Journal of Colloid and Interface Science* 73 (1980) 130–135

[31] M. Sami Selim and M.A. Al-Naafa, Brownian diffusion of hard spheres at finite concentrations, *AIChE Journal* 39 (1993) 3–16

[32] R. Krishna and J.A. Wesselingh, The Maxwell–Stefan approach to mass transfer, *Chemical Engineering Science* 52 (1997) 861–911

[33] T.R. Noordman and J.A. Wesselingh, Transport of large molecules through membranes with narrow pores: The Maxwell–Stefan description combined with hydrodynamic theory, *Journal of Membrane Science* 210 (2002) 227–243

[34] T. Yamaguchi, S. Nakao, and S. Kimura, Plasma-graft filling polymerization: preparation of a new type of pervaporation membrane for organic liquid mixtures, *Macromolecules* 24 (1991) 5522–5527

[35] J.G. Wijman, and R.W. Baker, The solute-diffusion model: A review, *Journal of Membrane Science* 107 (1995) 1–21

[36] P.J. Flory, *Principles of Polymer Chemistry*, Cornell University Press, London, 1953 (chapter XII)

[37] M.H. Cohen and D. Turnbuli, Molecular transport in liquids and glasses, *Journal of Chemical Physics* 31 (1959) 1164–1169

[38] B. Amsden, Solute diffusion within hydrogels. Mechanisms and models, *Macromolecules* 31 (1998) 8382–8395

[39] H. Yasuda, L.D. Ikenberry, and C.E. Lamaze, Permeability of solutes through hydrated polymer membranes: Part II, Permeability of water soluble organic solutes, *Die Makromoleculare Chemie* 125 (1969) 108–118

[40] H. Yasuda, C.E. Lamaze, and L.D. Ikenberry, Permeability of solutes through hydrated polymer membranes: Part I. Diffusion of sodium chloride, *Die Makromoleculare Chemie* 118 (1968) 19–35

[41] H. Yasuda, A. Peterlin, C.K. Colton, K.A. Smith, and E.W. Merrill, Permeability of solutes through hydrated polymer membranes: Part III. Theoretical background for the selectivity of dialysis membranes, *Die Makromolekulare Chemie* 126 (1969) 177–186

[42] N.A. Peppas and C.T. Reinhart, Solute diffusion in swollen membranes: Part I. A new theory, *Journal of Membrane Science* 15 (1983) 275–287

[43] C.T. Reinhart and N.A. Peppas, Solute diffusion in swollen membranes: Part II. Influence of crosslinking on diffusive properties, *Journal of Membrane Science* 18 (1984) 227–239

[44] R.A. Robinson and R.H. *Stokes, Electrolyte Solutions*, second revised edition, Dover Publications, ICN, Mineola, NY, 2002

[45] T. Canal and N.A. Peppas, Correlation between mesh size and equilibrium degree of swelling of polymeric networks, *Journal of Biomedical Materials Research* 23 (1989) 1183–1193

[46] M. Tanya, A.M. Ende, and N.A. Peppas, Transport of ionizable drugs and proteins in Crosslinked poly (acrylic acid) and poly(acrylic acid-*co*-2-hydroxyethylmethacrylate) hydrogels. I. Polymer characterization, *Journal of Applied Polymer Science* 59 (1996) 673–685

[47] S.R. Lustig and N.A. Peppas, Solute diffusion in swollen membranes: IX. Scaling laws for solute diffusion in gels, *Journal of Applied Polymer Science* 36 (1988) 735–747

[48] N.N. Peppas, H.J. Moynihan, and L.M. Lucht, The structure of highly crosslinked poly(2-hydroxyethyl methacrylate) hydrogels, *Journal of Biomedical Materials Research* 19 (1985) 397–411

[49] R.W. Korsmeyer, S.R. Lustig, and N.A. Peppas, Solute and penetrant diffusion in swellable polymers: I. Mathematical modeling, *Journal of Polymer Science: Polymer Physics Edition* 24 (1986) 395–408

[50] R.W. Korsmeyer, E. Von Meerwall, and N.A. Peppas. Solute and penetrant diffusion in swellable polymers: II. Verification of theoretical models, *Journal of Polymer Science: Polymer Physics Edition* 24 (1986) 409–434

[51] S.R. Lustig and N.A. Peppas, Solute and penetrant diffusion in swellable polymers: VII. A Free volume–based model with mechanical relaxation, *Journal of Applied Polymer Science* 33 (1987) 533–549

[52] L. Simon, Analysis of heat-aided membrane-controlled drug release from a process control perspective, *International Journal of Heat and Mass Transfer* 50 (2007) 2425–2433

[53] P.P. Madeira, X. Xu, J.A. Teixeria, and E.A. Macedo, Prediction of protein partition in polymer/salt aqueous two-phase systems using the modified Wilson model, *Biochemical Engineering Journal* 24 (2005) 147–155

[54] G.M. Wilson, Vapor–liquid equilibrium: XI. A new expression for the excess free energy of mixing, *Journal of American Chemistry Society* 86 (1964) 127–130

[55] H. Renon and J.M. Prausnitz, Local compositions in thermodynamic excess functions for liquid mixtures, *AIChE Journal* 14 (1968) 135–144

[56] D.S. Abrams and M. Prausnitz, Statistical thermodynamics of liquid mixtures: A new expression for the excess Gibbs energy of partly or completely miscible systems, *AIChE Journal* 21 (1975) 116–128

[57] J.M. Prausnitz, R.N. Lichtenthaler, and E. Gomes de Azevedo, *Molecular Thermodynamics of Fluid-Phase Equilibrium*, 3rd edition, Prentice Hall, New Jersey, 1999 (chapter 6)

[58] S. Denis and J.M. Prausnitz, Statistical thermodynamics of liquid mixtures: A new expression for the excess Gibbs energy of partly or completely miscible systems, *AIChE Journal* 21 (1975) 116–128

[59] A. Fredenslound, R.L. Jones, and J.M. Prausnitz, Group-contribution estimation of activity coefficients in nonideal liquid mixtures, *AIChE Journal* 21 (1975) 1086–1099

[60] A. Haghtalab and B. Mokhtarani, On extension of UNIQUAC-NRF model to study the phase behavior of aqueous two phase polymer–salt systems, *Fluid Phase Equilibria* 180 (2001) 139–149

[61] J.A.P. Coutinho and F.L.P. Pessoa, A modified extended UNIQUAC model for proteins, *Fluid Phase Equilibria* 222–223 (2004) 127–133

[62] Y.-T. Wu, D.-Q. Lin, and Z.-Q. Zhu, Thermodynamics of aqueous two-phase systems—the effect of polymer molecular weight on liquid–liquid equilibrium phase diagrams by the modified NTRL model, *Fluid Phase Equilibria* 147 (1998) 25–43

[63] A. Haghtalab and B. Mokhtarani, The UNIFAC-NRF activity coefficient model based on group contribution for partitioning of proteins in aqueous two phase (polymer + salt) systems, *Journal of Chemical Thermodynamics* 37 (2005) 289–295

[64] T. Oishi and J.M. Prausnitz, Estimation of solvent activities in polymer solutions using a group-contribution method, *Industrial and Engineering Chemistry Process Design and Development* 17 (1978) 333–339

[65] H.O. Paksoy, S. Ornektekin, B. Balcl, and Y. Demirel, The performance of UNIFAC and related group contribution models: Part I. Prediction of infinite dilution activity coefficients. *Thermochimica Acta* 287 (1996) 235–249

[66] K.K.S. Buck, N.I. Gerhardt, S.R. Dungan, and R.J. Philips, The effect of solute concentration on equilibrium partitioning in polymeric gels, *Journal of Colloid and Interface Science* 234 (2001) 400–409

[67] A.P. Sassi, H.W. Blanch, and J.M. Prausnitz, Phase equilibria for aqueous protein/polyelectrolyte Gel systems, *AIChE Journal* 42 (1996) 2335–2353

[68] J. Wu, A.P. Sassi, H.W. Blanch, and J.M. Prausnitz, Partitioning of proteins between an aqueous solution and a weakly-ionizable polyelectrolyte hydrogel, *Polymer* 37 (1996) 4803–4808

[69] L. Jin, Y.-X. Yu, and G.-H. Gao, A molecular-thermodynamic model for the interactions between globular proteins in aqueous solutions: Applications to bovine serum albumin (BSA), lysozyme, α-chymotrypsin, and uno-gamma-globulins (IgG) solutions, *Journal of Colloid and Interface Science* 304 (2006) 77–83

[70] L. Shang, S. Zhang, H. Du, and S.S. Venkatraman, A novel approach for the control of drug release rate through hydrogel membrane: II. Thermodynamic modelling of the partition control scheme, *Journal of Membrane Science* 321 (2008) 331–336

[71] C. Guthmann, R. Lipp, T. Wagner, and H. Kranz, Development of a novel osmotically driven drug delivery system for weakly basic drugs, *European Journal of Pharmaceutics and Biopharmaceutics* 69 (2008) 667–674

[72] H. Antheunis, J.-C. van der Meer, M. de Geus, W. Kingma, and C.E. Koning, Improved mathematical model for the hydrolytic degradation of aliphatic polyesters, *Macromolecules* 42 (2009), 2462–2471

[73] G. Schmidmaier, B. Wildemann, A. Stemberger, N.P. Haas, and M. Raschke, Biodegradable poly(D,L-lactide) coating of implants for continuous release of growth factors, *Journal of Biomedical Materials Research* 58 (2001) 449–455

[74] P. Arosio, V. Busini, G. Perale, D. Moscatelli, and M. Masi, A new model of resorbable device degradation and drug release—part I: zero order model, *Polymer International* 57 (2008) 912–920

[75] S. Prabhu and S. Hossainy, Modeling of degradation and drug release from a biodegradable stent coating, *Journal of Biomedical Materials Research Part A* 80A (2007) 732–741

[76] Z. Liu, X.Y. Wu, J.R. Ballinger, and R. Bendayan, Synthesis and characterization of surface-hydrophobic ion-exchange microspheres and the effect of coating on drug release rate, *Journal of Pharmaceutical Sciences* 89 (2000) 807–817

[77] S.H. Jeong, N.H. Berhane, K. Haghighi, and K. Park, Drug release properties of polymer coated ion-exchange resin complexes: Experimental and theoretical evaluation, *Journal of Pharmaceutical Sciences* 96 (2007) 618–632

[78] S.M. Herbig, J.R. Cardinal, R.W. Korsmeyer, and K.L. Smith, Asymmetric-membrane tablet coatings for osmotic drug delivery, *Journal of Controlled Release* 35 (1995) 127–136

[79] D. Olsen, C. Yang, M. Bodo, R. Chang, S. Leigh, J. Baez, D. Carmichael, M. Perälä, E.-R. Hämäläinen, M. Jarvinen, and J. Polarek, Recombinant collagen and gelatin for drug delivery, *Advanced Drug Delivery Reviews* 55 (2003) 1547–1567

[80] C.H. Lee, A. Singla, and Y. Lee, Biomedical applications of collagen, *International Journal of Pharmaceutics* 221 (2001) 1–22

[81] S. Young, M. Wong, Y. Tabata, and A.G. Mikos, Gelatin as a delivery vehicle for the controlled release of bioactive molecules, *Journal of Controlled Release* 109 (2005) 256–274

[82] W.J.E.M. Habraken, L. de Jonge, J.G.C. Wolke, L. Yubao, A.G. Mikos, and J.A. Jansen, Introduction of gelatin microspheres into an injectable calcium phosphate cement, *Journal of Biomedical Materials Research Part A* 87A (2008) 643–655

[83] C.M. Ofner III and W.A. Bubnis, Chemical and swelling evaluations of amino group crosslinking in gelatin and modified gelatin matrices, *Pharmaceutical Research* 13 (1996) 1821–1827

[84] A.J. Kuijpers, P.B. van Wachem, M.J.A. van Luyn, J.A. Plantinga, G.H.M. Engbers, J. Krijgsveld, S.A.J. Zaat, J. Dankert, and J. Feijen, *In vivo* compatibility and degradation of crosslinked gelatin gels incorporated in knitted Dacron, *Journal of Biomedical Materials Research* 51 (2000) 136–145

[85] P. Aslani and R.A. Kennedy, Studies on diffusion in alginate gels: 1. Effect of crosslinking with calcium or zinc ions on diffusion of acetaminophen, *Journal of Controlled Release* 42 (1) (1996) 75–82

[86] O. Smidsrod, The relative extension of alginates having different chemical composition, *Carbohydrate Research* 27 (1973) 107–118

[87] W.R. Gombotz and S.F. Wee, Protein release from alginate matrices, *Advanced Drug Delivery Reviews* 31 (1998) 267–285

[88] V.R. Sinha, A.K. Singla, S. Wadhawan, R. Kaushik, R. Kumria, K. Bansal, and S. Dhawan, Chitosan microspheres as a potential carrier for drugs, *International Journal of Pharmaceutics* 274 (2004) 1–33

[89] J. Berger, M. Reist, J.M. Mayer, O. Felt, and R. Gurny, Structure and interactions in chitosan hydrogels formed by complexation or aggregation for biomedical applications, *European Journal of Pharmaceutics and Biopharmaceutics* 57 (2004) 35–52

[90] L.-F. Fan, W. He, Y.-Z. Chang, B. Xiang, Q. Du, F. Wang, M. Qin, and D.-Y Cao, Studies of chitosan/Kollicoat SR 30D film-coated tablets for colonic drug delivery, *International Journal of Pharmaceutics* 375 (2009) 8–15

[91] S.P. Li, S.A. Martellucci, R.D. Bruce, A.C. Kinyon, M.B. Hay, and J.D. Higgins III, Evaluation of the film-coating properties of a hydroxyethyl cellulose/hydroxypropyl methylcellulose polymer system, *Drug Development and Industrial Pharmacy* 28 (2002), 389–401

[92] T. Ugurlu, M. Turkoglu, U. Soyogul Gurer, and B. Gurbuz Akarsu, Colonic delivery of compression coated nisin tablets using pectin/HPMC polymer mixture, *European Journal of Pharmaceutics and Biopharmaceutics* 67 (2007) 202–210

[93] S. Ensslin, K.P. Moll, K. Paulus, and K. Mäder, New insight into modified release pellets—internal structure and drug release mechanism, *Journal of Controlled Release* 128 (2008) 149–156

[94] A. Dashevsky, K. Wagner, K. Kolter, and R. Bodmeier, Physicochemical and release properties of pellets coated with Kollicoat® SR 30 D, a new aqueous polyvinyl acetate dispersion for extended release, *International Journal of Pharmaceutics* 290 (2005) 15–23

[95] M. S. Bordaweka and H. Zia, Evaluation of polyvinyl acetate dispersion as a sustained release polymer for tablets, *Drug Delivery* 13 (2006) 121–131

[96] P. Tallury, N. Alimohammadi, and S. Kalachandra, Poly(ethylene-*co*-vinyl acetate) copolymer matrix for delivery of chlorhexidine and acyclovir drugs for use in the oral environment: Effect of drug combination, copolymer composition and coating on the drug release rate, *Dental Materials* 23 (2007) 404–409

[97] N. Huyghebaert, A. Vermeire, and J.P. Remon Alternative method for enteric coating of HPMC capsules resulting in ready-to-use enteric-coated capsules European, *Journal of Pharmaceutical Sciences* 21 (2004) 617–623

[98] F. Liu, R. Lizio, U.J. Schneider, H.-U. Petereit, P. Blakey, and A.W. Basit, SEM/EDX and confocal microscopy analysis of novel and conventional enteric-coated systems, *International Journal of Pharmaceutics* 369 (2009) 72–78

[99] J.M. Harris and R.B. Chess, Effect of pegylation on pharmaceuticals, *Nature Reviews Drug Discovery* (2003) 214–221

[100] S. Aishwarya, S. Mahalakshmi, and P. Kumar Sehgal, Collagen-coated polycaprolactone microparticles as a controlled drug delivery system, *Journal of Microencapsulation* 25(2008) 298–306

[101] Lai Wah Chan, Xiaohua Liu and Paul Wan Sia Heng, Liquid phase coating to produce controlled-release alginate microspheres, *Journal of Microencapsulation* 22 (2005) 891–900

[102] Y. Chen, J. Yang, A. Mujumdar, and R. Dave, Fluidized bed film coating of cohesive Geldart group C powders, *Powder Technology* 189 (2009) 466–480

[103] H. Ehlers, H. Räikkönen, O. Antikainen, J. Heinämäki, and J. Yliruusi, Improving flow properties of ibuprofen by fluidized bed particle thin-coating *International Journal of Pharmaceutics* 368 (2009) 165–170

[104] E. Hamed and A. Sakr, Effect of curing conditions and plasticizer level on the release of highly lipophilic drug from coated multiparticulate drug delivery system, *Pharmaceutical Development and Technology* 8 (2003) 397–407

[105] H. Yuasa, T. Nakano, and Y. Kanaya, Suppression of agglomeration in fluidized bed coating. II. Measurement of mist size in a fluidized bed chamber and effect of sodium chloride addition on mist size, *International Journal of Pharmaceutics* 178 (1999) 1–10

[106] H. Yuasa, T. Nakano, and Y. Kanaya, Suppression of agglomeration in fluidized bed coating: I. Suppression of agglomeration by adding NaCl, *International Journal of Pharmaceutics* 158 (1997) 195–201.

[107] K.-H. Lin, S.-Y. Lin, and M.-J. Li, Compression forces and amount of outer coating layer affecting the time-controlled disintegration of the compression-coated tablets prepared by direct compression with micronized ethylcellulose, *Journal of Pharmaceutical Sciences* 90 (2001) 2005–2009

[108] A. Dashevsky, K. Kolter, and R. Bodmeier, Compression of pellets coated with various aqueous polymer dispersions, *International Journal of Pharmaceutics* 279 (2004) 19–26

[109] Y. Luo, J. Zhu, Y. Ma, and H. Zhang, Dry coating, a novel coating technology for solid pharmaceutical dosage forms, *International Journal of Pharmaceutics* 358 (2008) 16–22

[110] N. Pearnchob and R. Bodmeier, Coating of pellets with micronized ethylcellulose particles by a dry powder coating technique, *International Journal of Pharmaceutics* 268 (2003) 1–11

[111] S. Bose and R.H. Bogner, Solventless pharmaceutical coating processes: A review, *Pharmaceutical Development and Technology* 12 (2007) 115–131

[112] B. Subramaniam, R.A. Rajewski, and K. Snavely, Pharmaceutical processing with supercritical carbon dioxide, *Journal of Pharmaceutical Sciences* 86 (8) (1997) 885–890

[113] M.L. Luque de Castro, M. Valcarcel, and M.T. Tena, *Analytical Supercritical Fluid Extraction* ed. Springer-Verlag, New York (1994)

[114] D.-G. Yu, X.-X. Shen, C. Branford-White, K. White, L.-M. Zhu, and S.W. Annie Bligh, Oral fast-dissolving drug delivery membranes prepared from electrospun polyvinylpyrrolidone ultra-fine fibers, *Nanotechnology* 20 (2009) 1–9

[115] M.P. Grosvenor, *The physicomechanical properties of electrostatically deposited polymers for use in pharmaceutical powder coating*, University of Bath, Bath, UK, 330 (1991)

[116] S.C. Porter, Principles and application of dry powder deposition coating technology, AAPS Pharmaceutical Processing Conference, New Jersey, June 2003

[117] Q. Xu and J.T. Czernuszka, Controlled release of amoxicillin from hydroxyapatite-coated poly(lactic-*co*-glycolic acid) microspheres, *Journal of Controlled Release* 127 (2008) 146–153

[118] Q. Xu, Y. Tanaka, and J. T. Czernuszka, Encapsulation and release of a hydrophobic drug from hydroxyapatite coated liposomes, *Biomaterials* 28 (2007) 2687–2694

[119] L. Jongpaiboonkit, T. Franklin-Ford, and W.L. Murphy, Mineral-coated polymer microspheres for controlled protein binding and release, *Advanced Materials* 21 (2009) 1960–1963

[120] H.-W. Kim, J. Knowles, and H.-E. Kim, Hydroxyapatite/poly(e-caprolactone) composite coatings on hydroxyapatite porous bone scaffold for drug delivery, *Biomaterials* 25 (2004) 1279–1287

[121] H.S. Gill and M.R. Prausnitz, Coating formulations for microneedles, *Pharmaceutical Research*, 24 (2007) 1369–1380

[122] B. Gaihre, M. Seob Khil, D.R. Lee, and H.Y. Kim, Gelatin-coated magnetic iron oxide nanoparticles as carrier system: Drug loading and *in vitro* drug release study, *International Journal of Pharmaceutics* 365 (2009) 180–189

[123] Q. Guo, S. Guo, and Z. Wang, A type of esophageal stent coating composed of one 5-fluorouracil-containing EVA layer and one drug-free protective layer: In vitro release, permeation and mechanical properties, *Journal of Controlled Release* 118 (2007) 318–324

[124] S. Venkatraman and F. Boey, Release profiles in drug-eluting stents: Issues and uncertainties, *Journal of Controlled Release* 120 (2007) 149–160

[125] P. Sriamornsak and R.A. Kennedy, Effect of drug solubility on release behavior of calcium poly-saccharide gel-coated pellets, *European Journal of Pharmaceutical Sciences* 32 (2007) 231–239

[126] J. Zhou, S. Moya, L. Ma, C. Gao, and J. Shen, Polyelectrolyte coated PLGA Nanoparticles: templation and release behavior, *Macromolecular Bioscience* 9 (2009) 326–335

[127] G.H. Zhang, J.B. Schwartz, and R.L. Schnaare, Bead coating: 1. change in release kinetics (and mechanism) due to coating levels, *Pharmaceutical Research* 8 (1991) 331–335

[128] A. Budhian, S.J. Siegel, and K.I. Winey, Controlling the in vitro release profiles for a system of haloperidol-loaded PLGA nanoparticles, *International Journal of Pharmaceutics* 346 (2008) 151–159

[129] T.W. Kim, C.W. Ji, S.Y. Shim, et al., Modified release of coated sugar spheres using drug-containing polymeric dispersions, *Archives of Pharmacal Research* 30 (2007) 124–130

[130] X. Wang, E. Wenk, X. Hu, G.R. Castro, L. Meinel, X. Wang, C. Li, H. Merkle, and D.L. Kaplan, Silk coatings on PLGA and alginate microspheres for protein delivery, *Biomaterials* 28 (2007) 4161–4169

[131] Q. Zhao and B. Li, pH-controlled drug loading and release from biodegradable microcapsules, *Nanomedicine: Nanotechnology, Biology, and Medicine* 4 (2008) 302–310

[132] L. Wu and C.S. Brazel, Surface crosslinking for delayed release of proxyphylline from PHEMA hydrogels, *International Journal of Pharmaceutics*, 349 (2008) 1–10

[133] X. Huang, B.L. Chestang, and C.S. Brazel, Minimization of initial burst in poly(vinyl alcohol) hydrogels by surface extraction and surface-preferential crosslinking, *International Journal of Pharmaceutics*, 248 (2002) 183–192

[134] P. Sriamornsak and R.A. Kennedy, Effect of drug solubility on release behavior of calcium polysaccharide gel-coated pellets, *European Journal of Pharmaceutical Sciences* 32 (2007) 231–239

[135] M. Zilberman and A. Malka, Drug controlled release from structured bioresorbable films used in medical devices—a mathematical model, *Journal of Biomedical Materials Research Part B Applied Biomaterials* 89B (2009) 155–164

[136] F. Siepmanna, J. Siepmann, M. Walther, R.J. MacRae, and R. Bodmeier, Polymer blends for controlled release coatings, *Journal of Controlled Release* 125 (2008) 1–15

[137] K. Lehmann, In Wasser dispergierbare, hydrophile Acrylharze mit abgestufter Permeabilität für diffusionsgesteuerte Wirkstoffabgabe aus Arzneiformen, *Acta Pharmacological Technology* 32 (1986) 146–152

[138] B. Wu, N. Shun, X. Wei, and W. Wu, Characterization of 5-fluorouracil release from hydroxypropylmethylcellulose compression-coated tablets, *Pharmaceutical Development and Technology* 12 (2007) 203–210

[139] F. Sadeghi, J. L. Ford, M.H. Rubinstein, and A.R. Rajabi-Siahboomi, Study of drug release from pellets coated with surelease containing hydroxypropylmethylcellulose, *Drug Development and Industrial Pharmacy* 27 (2001) 419–430

[140] Q. Guo, P.T. Knight, and P.T. Mather, Tailored drug release from biodegradable stent coatings based on hybrid polyurethanes, *Journal of Controlled Release* 137 (2009) 224–233

[141] B.-J. Lee, S.-G. Ryu, and J.-H. Cui, Controlled release of dual drug-loaded hydroxypropyl methylcellulose matrix tablet using drug-containing polymeric coatings, *International Journal of Pharmaceutics* 188 (1999) 71–80

[142] A. Maroni, M. Dorly Del Curto, M. Serratoni, A.L. Zema, A. Foppoli, A. Gazzaniga, and M.E. Sangalli, Feasibility, stability and release performance of a time-dependent insulin delivery system intended for oral colon release, *European Journal of Pharmaceutics and Biopharmaceutics* 72 (2009) 246–251

[143] H.E. Wei, L.-F. Fan, Q. Du, B. Xiang, C.-L. Li, M. Bai, Y.-Z. Chang, and D.-Y. Cao, Design and *in vitro/in vivo* evaluation of multi-layer film coated pellets for omeprazole, *Chemical and Pharmaceutical Bulletin* 57 (2009) 122–128

[144] L. Zema, A. Maroni, A. Foppoli, L. Palugan, M.E. Sangalli, and A. Gazzaniga, Different HPMC viscosity grades as coating agents for an oral time and/or site-controlled delivery system: an investigation into the mechanisms governing drug release, *Journal of Pharmaceutical Sciences* 96 (2007) 1527–1536

[145] L. Jongpaiboonkit, T. Franklin-Ford, and W.L. Murphy, Mineral-coated polymer microspheres for controlled protein binding and release, *Advanced Materials* 21 (2009) 1960–1963

[146] Y.M. Kim, J.-O. Lim, H.-K. Kim, S.-Y. Kim, and J.-P. Shin, A novel design of one-side coated biodegradable intrascleral implant for the sustained release of triamcinolone acetonide, *European Journal of Pharmaceutics and Biopharmaceutics* 70 (2008) 179–186

[147] Y.-Y. Huang, T.-W. Chung, T.-W. Tzeng, A method using biodegradable polylactides:polyethylene glycol for drug release with reduced initial burst, *International Journal of Pharmaceutics* 182 (1999) 93–100

[148] C. Fan, R. Pai-Thakur, W. Phuapradit, L. Zhang, H. Tian, W. Malick, N. Shah, and M. Serpil Kislalioglu, Impact of polymers on dissolution performance of an amorphous gelleable drug from surface-coated beads, *European Journal of Pharmaceutical Sciences* 37 (2009) 1–10

[149] M.T. am Ende and L.A. Miller, Mechanistic investigation of drug release from asymmetric membrane tablets: effect of media gradients (osmotic pressure and concentration), and potential coating failures on in vitro release, *Pharmaceutical Research* 24 (2007) 288–297

[150] R.K. Verma, D. Murali Krishna, and S. Garg, Formulation aspects in the development of osmotically controlled oral drug delivery systems, *Journal of Controlled Release* 79 (2002) 7–27

[151] C. Guthmann, R. Lipp, T. Wagner, and H. Kranz, Development of a novel osmotically driven drug delivery system for weakly basic drugs, *European Journal of Pharmaceutics and Biopharmaceutics* 69 (2008) 667–674

[152] Y. Bi, S. Mao, L. Gan, Y. Li, C. Wang, N. Xu, Y. Zheng, Q. Cheng, and S. Hou, A controlled porosity osmotic pump system with biphasic release of theophylline, *Chemical and Pharmaceutical Bulletin* 55 (2007) 1574–1580

[153] H. Liu, X.-G. Yang, S.-F. Nie, L.-L. Wei, L.-L. Zhou, H. Liu, R. Tang, and W.-S. Pan, Chitosan-based controlled porosity osmotic pump for colon-specific delivery system: Screening of formulation variables and in vitro investigation, *International Journal of Pharmaceutics* 332 (2007) 115–124

[154] M. Gibson, Pharmaceutical Preformulation and Formulation: A Practical Guide From Candidate Drug Selection to Commercial Dosage Form, Informa, USA, 2007.

6

Release-Controlled Coatings

James Zhenggui Tang and Nicholas P. Rhodes

CONTENTS

Introduction 260
Matrix Materials 261
   Polymer-Based Matrix 261
      Nonerodible Polymeric Matrix 262
      Erodible Polymer Matrix 266
   Inorganic-Based Matrix 269
      Ceramic-Coated Tacrolimus-Eluting Stent 269
      Yukon Drug-Eluting Stent 270
      Janus Carbostent™ 270
      Axxion Paclitaxel-Eluting Stent 270
      Genous™ Endothelial Progenitor Cell Capturing Stent 270
   Fully Erodible Metallic and Polymer Stents 271
      Fully Polylactic Acid Stent 271
      Biocorrodible Metallic Stents 272
Structures and Forming Techniques 272
   Passive Coating 275
   Active Coatings 276
      A Single Layer Reservoir 276
      Multiple-Layer Reservoir 278
      Intra-Built Holes 279
      Intra-Built Cavity 279
      Surface-Built Micro- and Nanoporous Membrane 280
   Top Coat 280
   Coating Techniques 280
      Dip Coating 280
      Spray Coating 281
      Ink-Jet Technology 282
Controlled Release 283
   Local Drugs 284
   Controlled Release 287
      Diffusion-Controlled Release 288
      Dissolution/Degradation-Controlled Release 290
Perspectives of Release-Controlled Coatings 292
References 295

Introduction

Atherosclerosis is a cardiovascular disease of the arteries, which harden and become narrower. It is caused by plaque build-up and results in blood vessel narrowing and blood flow reduction. The clinical symptoms are heart attack, stroke, and in extreme cases, death. In 1977, Dr. Andreas Gruentzig, a German cardiologist, performed the first coronary angioplasty (clearing the stenosed lumen of the coronary artery) on an awake human in Zurich (De Jaegere et al., 1994; King and Schlumpf, 1993). From a 10-year follow-up of the original series of percutaneous transluminal coronary angioplasties performed in Zurich, there was an overall survival rate of 89.5% in 133 patients. However, restenosis after plain balloon angioplasty occurred as frequently as one-third to one-half of the cases (Gottsauner-Wolf et al., 1996).

Coronary artery stents were introduced as a step to reduce restenosis rates and prevent abrupt vessel closure. The first elective coronary stent implantation was performed in 1986 by Dr. Jacques Puel in France to prevent restenosis after plain balloon angioplasty (Cook and Windecker, 2009). By 1999, stents were used in 84% of percutaneous coronary interventions (PCI). However, the use of stenting was always accompanied by the risk of stent thrombosis after implantation. As a precaution, aspirin was given in conjunction with dipyridamole, sulfapyrazone, and oral anticoagulation (acenocoumarin) for up to 6 months. The major limitation of PCI in bare-metal stenting is neointimal hyperplasia, an exaggerated healing response resulting from vessel trauma due to the angioplasty and the physical damage caused by the stent against the vascular endothelial layer (Kukreja et al., 2008), leading to restenosis.

Intimal injury from stenting results in increased smooth muscle cell proliferation and migration (Deconinck et al., 2008; Tesfamariam, 2008). However, stents alone induce less neointimal proliferation (one-quarter) than balloon angioplasty (more than one-third). Because of the use of thrombogenic metallic materials, stenting has another major limitation in addition to in-stent restenosis, namely, late thrombosis (Caves and Chaikof, 2006). To address these issues, interventional cardiologists defined the concept of an active stent, targeting on each step of the restenosis process: platelet thrombosis, inflammation, smooth muscle cell migration, and smooth muscle cell proliferation. Anti-inflammatory, antimigratory, antiproliferative, and pro-healing drugs were all of interest in the control of in-stent thrombosis and restenosis.

Drug-eluting stents (DES) were introduced in 2002 by Cordis Corporation, a Johnson & Johnson company with the CYPHER™ stent. This is an expandable, slotted, stainless steel tube, with a drug (sirolimus) contained within a thin polymer coating on its surfaces. DES are considered a local drug delivery system, resulting in higher concentrations of drug at the target site (Acharya and Park, 2006), minimizing the risk of systemic toxicity, and having the possibility of controlled drug release (Deconinck et al., 2008). Using DES can reduce neointimal proliferation to less than 10% of that of bare-metal stents.

DES consist of three major components:

(1) A stent platform to scaffold the vessel

(2) A drug to inhibit neointimal growth

(3) A matrix material to deliver the drug with controlled release kinetics

Release-controlled coatings are a concept derived from drug elution. It generally refers to the structural part of DES for controlled release and simply refers to the primary matrix/

drug component. In this chapter, release-controlled coatings are categorized as polymer-based, inorganic-based, and matrix-free. Under each category, the primary matrix materials will be described in terms of materials, structures and forming techniques, and release kinetics. With the introduction of individual cases, the perspectives of release-controlled coatings will be discussed.

Matrix Materials

The materials used for fabricating the matrix of stents, indicated in the constructive triangle for DES (Figure 6.1), have undergone continuous and rapid development since 2002. Traditional, simple, nonerodible polymers have been replaced by erodible, inorganic-based systems.

Polymer-Based Matrix

Synthetic and natural polymers that are biocompatible and biodegradable are widely used in medical and surgical applications. Among these, nonerodible polymers, such as acrylic polymers or copolymers and erodible polymers, such as polylactic acid (PLA) and poly(lactide-*co*-glycolide) (PLGA), are used as the matrix materials for loading drugs onto coronary stents (Raval et al., 2007). As a reservoir for the controlled release of drugs, the polymer-based matrix materials that first received FDA approval were nonerodible. The sirolimus-eluting CYPHER stent (Cordis, Warren, NJ) consists of a stainless steel platform coated with a nonerodible polymer (poly(ethylene-*co*-vinyl acetate) [PEVA] and

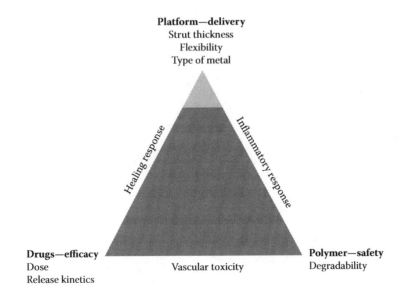

FIGURE 6.1
Constructive triangle for DES.

poly(*n*-butyl methacrylate) [PBMA]) containing 140 µg/cm² sirolimus (Kukreja et al., 2008). The paclitaxel-eluting TAXUS™ stent (Boston Scientific, Natick, MA) incorporates a stainless steel platform with a nonerodible polymer coating (polystyrene-*b*-isobutylene-*b*-styrene [SIBS]) combined with 100 µg/cm² of paclitaxel (Kukreja et al., 2008). The strength of the nonerodible polymers in both CYPHER and TAXUS stents lies in their ability to prevent restenosis in a diverse range of patients. However, both cause significant delay in arterial healing manifested by persistent fibrin deposition and poor endothelialization when compared to instances of bare metal stent implantation (Finn et al., 2007). Consequently, more biocompatible matrix materials have been introduced. These include the nonerodible phosphorylcholine (PC) and erodible polyesters such as PLGA, PLA, poly-L-lactide (PLLA), and poly-D,L-lactide (PDLLA) (Raval et al., 2007).

Nonerodible Polymeric Matrix

The market for commercially available DES is currently dominated by stents with nonerodible polymer matrices (Kukreja et al., 2008; Fishell et al., 2009). Table 6.1 shows the DES drug delivery systems using these matrices. Phosphorylcholine is the only natural polymer among a number of synthetic polymers that have proven track records in stenting applications.

Polymer Blends

The CYPHER sirolimus-eluting coronary stent (CYPHER stent) is a combination product comprising two regulated components: a device (a stent system) and a drug product (a formulation of sirolimus in a polymer coating). The CYPHER stent was the first DES to receive both the Conformité Européenne (CE) mark and FDA approval in April 2002 and 2003, respectively (Daemen and Serruys, 2007). The stent, under the name of Bx Velocity (manufactured by Cordis Corporation/Johnson & Johnson), is used to treat lesions 30 mm in length or smaller and with a reference diameter of 2.25–4 mm. The stent material is electropolished stainless steel (316L), laser cut from seamless tubing in a sinusoidal pattern. The designed strut thickness is 140 µm (Nakazawa et al., 2009). The usable length of the stent placement system is either 145 cm for RAPTOR™ over-the-wire or 137 cm for RAPTORRAIL® Rapid Exchange. Polymer blend PEVA/PBMA is used as the matrix material for loading sirolimus, which it achieves using a mixture at a ratio of 67% polymer and 33% sirolimus. The molecular formula of sirolimus is $C_{51}H_{79}NO_{13}$ with a molecular weight of 914.2 g/mol and is contained within the drug reservoir layer at a density of 140 µg/cm², 80% of which is released in 30 days (Kukreja et al., 2008).

PEVA and PBMA have proven track records as controlled release polymers (Rhodes and Porter, 1998). PEVA (Figure 6.2) is produced by copolymerization of ethylene and vinyl acetate (VA). With increasing proportion of the polar comonomer VA, the products change from modified polyethylene to a rubberlike product. Commercially available PEVA

TABLE 6.1

DES Drug Delivery Systems Using a Nonerodible Polymer Matrix

Stent Design	Drug (Dose)	Matrix (Ratio)	Manufacturer
Cypher	Sirolimus (1.4 µg/mm²)	PEVA + PBMA	Cordis
Taxus	Paclitaxel (1.0 µg/mm²)	SIBS (Translute)	Boston Scientific
Xience V	Everolimus (1.0 µg/mm²)	Fluoropolymer	Abbott Vascular
Endeavor	Zotarolimus (1.6 µg/mm²)	Phosphorylcholine	Medtronic

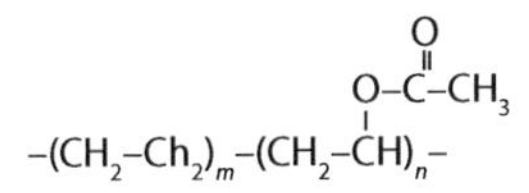

$$
\begin{array}{c}
\text{O} \\
\| \\
\text{O–C–CH}_3 \\
| \\
-(\text{CH}_2-\text{Ch}_2)_m-(\text{CH}_2-\text{CH})_n-
\end{array}
$$

FIGURE 6.2
Chemical structure of PEVA.

copolymers have a VA concentration between 10% and 50%, in the form of beads, pellets, granules, and so on (typically, 12%, 14%, 18%, 25%, or 33%) (Chudzik et al., 2001). PEVA copolymers with low percent VA become increasingly insoluble in typical solvents, whereas those with higher percent VA become decreasingly durable. PBMA is a homopolymer of monomer (Figure 6.3) with a molecular weight range from 200 to 320 kDa. These products vary in viscosity, solubility, and form.

Block Copolymers

The TAXUS Express[2] and TAXUS Express[2] Atom Paclitaxel-eluting coronary stent systems are device/drug combination products comprising two regulated components: a device (Express Coronary Stent System, Boston Scientific, USA) and a drug product (a formulation of paclitaxel contained in a polymer coating). The stent is manufactured by Boston Scientific (Natick, MA) and is used to treat lesions 28 mm or smaller in length with reference diameter ranging from 2.25 to 4 mm. The stent material is a 316L surgical grade stainless steel with a design strut thickness of 132 µm (Nakazawa et al., 2009). The usable length of the stent delivery systems is 140 cm for TAXUS Express[2] Monorail and 135 cm for the TAXUS Express[2] over-the-wire systems. The drug/polymer coating consists of paclitaxel (the active ingredient) and Translute™ polymer carrier (the inactive matrix). The molecular formula of paclitaxel is $C_{47}H_{51}NO_{14}$ with a molecular weight of 853.91 g/mol. The polymer carrier is loaded with 1 µg/mm^2 paclitaxel in a slow release formulation and coated over the stent with a maximum nominal drug content of 282 µg on the largest stent (4.00 × 32 mm).

The only inactive ingredient in the TAXUS Express stent is SIBS, a tri-block copolymer composed of styrene and isobutylene units built on 1,3-di(2-methoxy-2-propyl)-5-*tert*-butylbenzene and sold under the trade name of Translute (Figure 6.4). It is a hydrophobic, elastomeric copolymer with an M_n (number average molecular weight) of 80,000–130,000 g/mol, and a polydispersity index of 1.0–2.0. The polymer is mixed with the drug paclitaxel and then applied to the stents, without a primer or topcoat layer, over the entire stent surface (i.e., both luminal and abluminal). The structural formula for the polymer is shown below.

The SIBS polymer used on the TAXUS stent is a form of rubber, an adhesive compound with elastomeric properties. SIBS is a biologically inactive and biostable compound that retains the drug on the stent, provides relatively uniform drug delivery, prevents mechanical disruption during processing and deployment, and has a relatively long shelf life

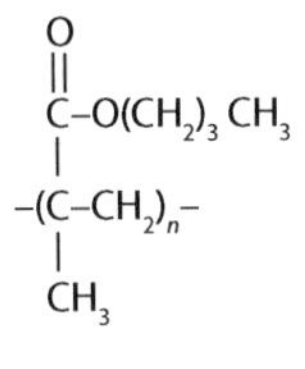

$$
\begin{array}{c}
\text{O} \\
\| \\
\text{C–O(CH}_2)_3\text{ CH}_3 \\
| \\
-(\text{C–CH}_2)_n- \\
| \\
\text{CH}_3
\end{array}
$$

FIGURE 6.3
Chemical structure of PBMA.

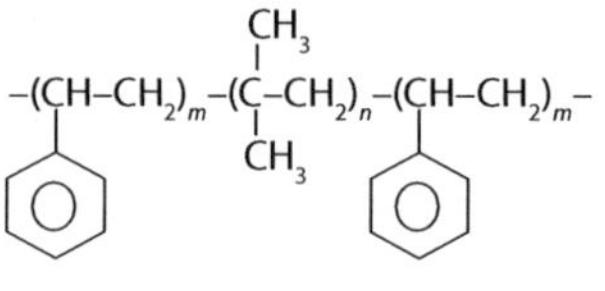

$$-(CH-CH_2)_m-(C-CH_2)_n-(CH-CH_2)_m-$$

with CH_3 methyl groups on the central carbon and phenyl rings on the outer units.

FIGURE 6.4
Chemical structure of SIBS.

(Fishell et al., 2009). Unlike the CYPHER stent, TAXUS stent retains at least 90% of the drug on the polymer after elution of the initial 10% during the first few months.

Fluoropolymer

The XIENCE™ V Everolimus-eluting coronary stent system (XIENCE V or XIENCE V EECSS) is a device/drug combination product consisting of either the MULTI-LINK VISION® Coronary Stent System or the Multi-Link Mini Vision® Coronary Stent System coated with a formulation containing Everolimus as the active ingredient, embedded in a nonerodible polymer. The stent has a reference diameter of 2.5–4.0 mm and is used to treat lesions 28 mm in length or smaller, marketed under the names of XIENCE V Rapid-Exchange EECSS and XIENCE V over-the-wire EECSS. The stent material is a medical-grade L605 cobalt chromium (CoCr) alloy with a design strut thickness of 81 μm (Nakazawa et al., 2009). The usable length of the delivery system is 143 cm for both (rapid exchange and over-the-wire) delivery systems. The drug Everolimus is a novel, semisynthetic macrolide immunosuppressant, synthesized by chemical modification of rapamycin (sirolimus). The molecular formula of Everolimus is $C_{53}H_{83}NO_{14}$ with a molecular weight of 958.224 g/mol. The nonerodible polymer is loaded with 100 μg/cm^2 of Everolimus and has a maximum nominal drug content of 181 μg on the stent (4.0 × 28 mm).

The inactive ingredients comprise PBMA (Figure 6.3), a polymer that adheres to the stent and acts as the drug coating, and poly(vinylidene fluoride-*co*-hexafluoropropylene) (PVDF-HFP) (Figure 6.5) as the stent matrix layer containing Everolimus. PVDF-HFP is a nonerodible semicrystalline random copolymer with an M_w of 254,000–293,000 Da. This copolymer is mixed with Everolimus (83%:17% w/w polymer/Everolimus) and applied to the entire PBMA-coated stent surface as a conformal coating. The drug is loaded at a density of 100 μg/cm^2 for all product sizes. No topcoat layer is used.

Phospholipid Polymer

The Endeavor® Zotarolimus-Eluting Coronary Stent on an over-the-wire or Multi-Exchange® II (MX2) stent delivery system is a device/drug combination product with a reference diameter of 2.5–3.5 mm that is used to treat lesions of 27 mm in length or smaller. The stent material is an F-562 CoCr alloy with a design strut thickness of 91 μm (Nakazawa et al., 2009). The drug delivery system consists of a PC coating in a conformal layer with Zotarolimus at a density of 1.6 μg/mm^2 (Udipi et al., 2007). Zotarolimus, also named ABT-

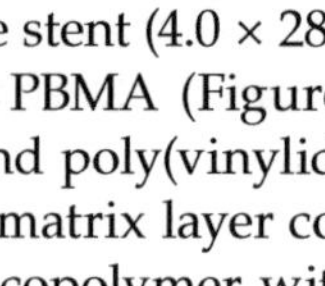

$$-(C-C)_m-(C-C)_n-$$

with H and F substituents, and CF_3 on the hexafluoropropylene unit.

FIGURE 6.5
Chemical structure of (PVDF-HFP).

578, is a semisynthetic derivative of rapamycin, with a molecular formula of $C_{52}H_{79}N_5O_{12}$ and molecular weight of 966.21 g/mol. Phosphorylcholine consists of a copolymer of methacryloylphosphorylcholine and lauryl methacrylate (LMA) (Acharya and Park, 2006).

Phosphorylcholine is a zwitterionic phospholipid found on the outer surface of red blood cell membranes (Lewis, 2006) carrying both positive and negative charges, yet overall electrically neutral. One consequence of the charged nature of the headgroup is its propensity to form a large hydration shell around it, estimated to comprise 12–19 water molecules per headgroup. In the late 1970s, workers in Japan were successful in developing a process for producing a polymerizable phospholipid-like monomer based on methacrylate chemistry. The groups of Nakabayashi and Ishihara have studied materials based on 2-methacryloyloxyethyl phosphorylcholine (MPC) with respect to their interfacial, solution, and bulk properties, and more recently, to drug delivery.

In parallel to the work in Japan, a family of MPC polymers were developed and commercialized by Biocompatibles UK Ltd. This range of materials is described as PC Technology™ and has been approved and used in the manufacture of a variety of medical devices. Among these, PC1036 and PC2028 are used to encapsulate drugs for coronary stents such as Biodiv Ysio® stent (stainless steel) and Endeavor™ stent (chromium cobalt alloy).

PC1036 (Figure 6.6) and PC2028 (Figure 6.7) are hydrogels with hydrophobic alkyl cocomponents that aid in the formation of coherent films and result in good adhesion to a variety of substrates used in medical device manufacturing. These polymers carry a silyloxyalkyl cross-linking group that is capable of thermal cross-linking after application of the coating. This controllable cross-linking provides a method of varying the interstitial space between polymer chains, and hence the free-water content, through which the drug may diffuse.

Endeavor Resolute stents use a proprietary biocompatible polymer called BioLinx™, a unique blend of three polymers: a hydrophilic C19 polymer, water-soluble polyvinyl pyrrolidinone (PVP), and a lipophilic/hydrophobic C10 polymer (Udipi et al., 2007). The C10 polymer stimulates controlled drug release, the C19 polymer provides enhanced biocompatibility and is helpful in drug elution, and PVP increases the initial drug burst and enhances the elution rate (Daemen and Serruys, 2007). Like the PC polymer, it is also designed to be biomimetic and confer the same biocompatibility as the Endeavor stent's PC while extending the duration of drug exposure in the vessel. Developed by Medtronic scientists, BioLinx is the first polymer created specifically for use on a DES. Extensive

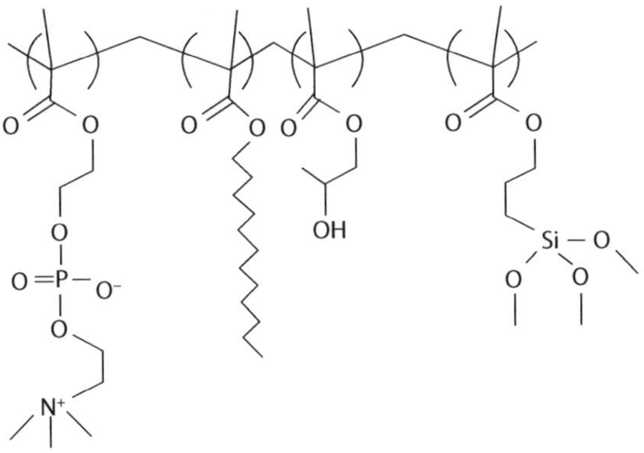

FIGURE 6.6
Cross-linkable PC coating (1), PC1036.

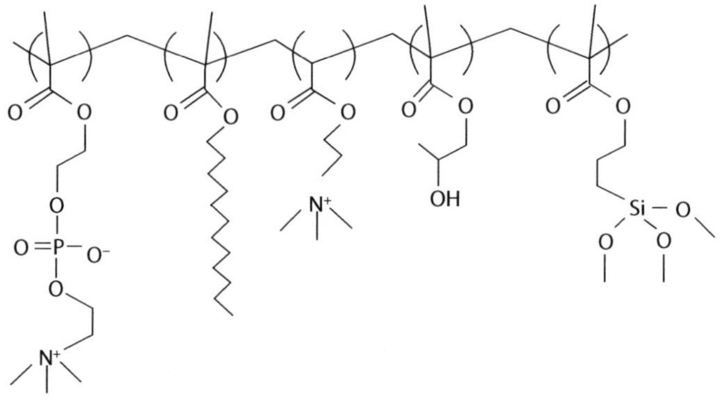

FIGURE 6.7
Cross-linkable PC coating (2), PC2028.

preclinical studies have established that the polymer has good biocompatibility with blood, endothelial, and smooth muscle cells.

Erodible Polymer Matrix

Erodible polymer matrix materials mainly include PLGA (Figure 6.8) and PLA families (Figure 6.9) (Vert, 2009). PLGA is a family of copolymers of lactic acid with glycolic acid in different ratios. Park (1995) summarized seven members of the PLGA polymers in terms of suppliers, the ratio of lactic acid/glycolic acid, weight average molecular weight, and glass transition temperature (T_g) of microspheres of the products. Drugs, such as paclitaxel and dexamethasone, have been encapsulated in PLGA (Kumari et al., 2010). PLA is a family of homopolymers of lactic acid in either L or D handedness. Poly-L-lactic acid (Figure 6.9) is supplied in two forms (Lincoff et al., 1997; von Recum et al., 1995), high molecular weight (in the range 82,500–321,000 Da) and low molecular weight forms (in the range 7600 to 80,000 Da). Low molecular weight PLLA (80 kDa) is associated with an intense inflammatory reaction, whereas only minimal inflammation has been observed with implants of high molecular weight (321 kDa) PLLA. Poly-D,L-lactide is a blend of poly(D-lactic acid) (PDLA) and PLLA in varying ratios (Figure 6.9). The thermal and mechanical properties of PLLA and PDLLA are summarized in the review by Fan et al. (2009). Poly-L-lactide is a semicrystalline polymer with a melting point in the range of 173–178°C, whereas PDLLA is an amorphous polymer of the racemic mixture of PLLA and PDLA. Both have similar glass transition temperature in the range of 50–65°C.

Polylactide

DES using PLA as a matrix material are summarized in Table 6.2. Among these, Biolimus A9 is the more common drug component. Biolimus A9 is a highly lipophilic, semisynthetic ana-

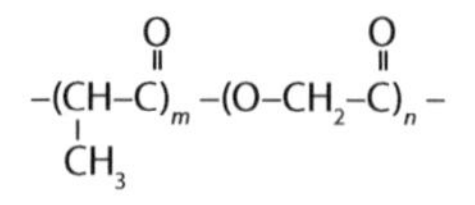

$$-(CH-C)_m-(O-CH_2-C)_n-$$

FIGURE 6.8
Chemical structure of PLGA.

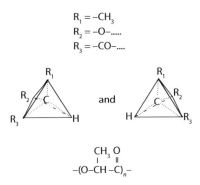

$R_1 = -CH_3$
$R_2 = -O-.....$
$R_3 = -CO-....$

and

$$CH_3 \ O$$
$$-(O-CH-C)_n-$$

FIGURE 6.9
Chemical structure of PLLA and PDLA.

logue of sirolimus having an alkoxy-alkyl group replacing hydrogen at position 42-O. The molecular formula of Biolimus A9 is $C_{55}H_{87}NO_{14}$ with a molecular weight of 986.29 g/mol.

The Devax Axxess™ Biolimus A9® (Devas; Irvine, CA) eluting bifurcation stent system is a proprietary self-expanding Nitinol stent specifically engineered for the treatment of coronary and vascular bifurcation lesions. Nitinol is an alloy composed of 55 wt.% nickel and balance titanium. It is well known for its unusual shape memory effect. Controlled release of Biolimus A9 is achieved after encapsulation in PLA and application onto the surface of Nitinol stents. Bifurcation lesions account for approximately 20–30% of all PCI. The Devax Axxess Plus™ stent was the first of these dedicated bifurcation stents designed to elute an antirestenotic drug (Chen and Sheiban, 2009).

Biosensors use Biolimus A9 and PLA on a highly flexible stainless steel stent, designed for enhanced deliverability, on its BioMatrix drug-eluting Coronary Stent System. This DES is used to treat lesions 28 mm or smaller in length, and has a reference diameter of 2.5–3.5 mm. The stent material is 316L VM stainless steel with a strut thickness of 112 μm (Nakazawa et al., 2009). The S-stent™, code-named BioFlex™ (Biosensor International, Singapore), is the bare-metal stent which is the basis of the BioMatrix DES, is coated with a primer layer of Parylene (Grabow et al., 2009), and forms the metal backbone of the BioMatrix™ DES. The S-Stent platform has wider struts and more uniform geometry to optimize the release of antirestenosis drugs using a proprietary asymmetrical coating process. The drug delivery system differs from CYPHER and TAXUS stents by having the drug/polymer application solely onto the abluminal surface (the surface facing the arterial wall) of the stent (Windecker et al., 2008), comprising PLA mixed with Biolimus A9 at a concentration of 15.6 μg/mm stent length. The BioMatrix concept is also licensed by Terumo (Japan) and marketed as the Nobori stent (Grabow et al., 2009).

The EXCEL from JW Medical Systems, China, also has a sirolimus and PLA drug-delivery system covering a laser-cut, 316L stainless steel, open cell design stent with strut thickness

TABLE 6.2

DES Using PLA as a Matrix Material

Stent Design	Drug	Polymer
Axxess	Biolimus A9	PLA
BioMatrix (Nobori)	Biolimus A9	PLA
Excel	Sirolimus	PLA

of 119 μm (Doyle and Holmes, 2009). The PLA is abluminally coated and contains sirolimus at a range of 195–376 μg per stent.

Poly(Lactide-co-Glycolide)

PLGA is an erodible copolymer of lactic acid and glycolic acid. It is found in diverse applications over a range of compositions, the different monomer ratios significantly influencing the physical and chemical properties of the copolymer. DES using PLGA as the matrix material include the Medstent™ stent from Conor MedSystem and the NEVO stent from Cordis Corporation (Table 6.3). Although it employs the reservoir (RES) technology from the Conor Medsystems Medstent™, the Cordis NEVO metal stent uses a different form of PLGA, uses a different drug, and has a different design of CoCr architecture.

The Conor stent uses paclitaxel mixed with the PLGA covering a metallic stent. The Conor stents originally were constructed from 316 stainless steel, but the subsequent design uses a CoCr alloy with multiple intra-strut wells (Kukreja et al., 2008). A single cell of the Conor stent has intra-strut-built wells and the ductile hinge allows full deployment of the stent without deformation of the wells containing the drug (Serruys et al., 2005). The stainless steel stent had a strut thickness of 127 μm (Serruys et al., 2005), and the CoCr alloy stent has a thinner strut thickness. The molecular formula of paclitaxel is $C_{47}H_{51}NO_{14}$ with a molecular weight of 853.91 g/mol. The paclitaxel/PLGA combination is injected into each hole using an automated microjet system with a drug loading in the range 10–30 μg. Studies have suggested that this dose released over a 10-day period is ineffective in reducing in-stent neointimal proliferation, but shows significant benefit when released over 30 days.

The NEVO™ sirolimus-eluting stent (Cordis Corporation) is fabricated from CoCr alloy and also uses a drug delivery system based on PLGA (Otake et al., 2009). It utilizes the same reservoir system (RES) that Conor Medsystems uses, with hundreds of small reservoirs or holes in the stent struts into which the drug–polymer mixture is loaded. The NEVO RES-I stent is used to treat lesions 28 mm or smaller in length, and has a reference diameter of 2.5–3.5 mm. The design allows drug delivery from a surface that is 75% bare metal upon insertion. The system contains 166 μg sirolimus (Fishell et al., 2009).

Erodible Polymer Blends

The Infinnium paclitaxel-eluting stent (Sahajanand Medical, India) is constructed using four erodible polymers over a surgical grade 316L stainless steel Millennium Matrix® stent, laser cut from seamless tubing in a snaking pattern. The Infinnium stent is used to treat lesions 39 mm or smaller in length and has a reference diameter of 2.5–4 mm with a strut width and thickness of 110 and 80 μm, respectively. The usable length of the delivery system is 135 cm. The matrix material is a combination of PLLA, poly-D,L-lactide-co-glycolide, poly-L-lactide-co-caprolactone, and PVP that is applied in multiple layers to provide programmed drug release. The polymer coating is 5 μm thick with 50–500 μg paclitaxel over the stent length (Table 6.4).

TABLE 6.3

DES Using PLGA as a Matrix Material

Stent Design	Drug	Polymer
CoStar	Paclitaxel	PLGA
Nevo	Sirolimus	PLGA

TABLE 6.4

DES Using Erodible Polymer Blends

Stent Design	Drug	Polymer
Infinnium	Paclitaxel	PLLA + PLGA + PVP
Supralimus-Core	Sirolimus	PLLA + PLGA + PVP

The Supralimus-Core Sirolimus-eluting stent (Sahajanand Medical) is a device/drug product system that consists of sirolimus, an erodible polymer, and a surgical grade L605 CoCr alloy stent. The stent is used to treat lesions 40 mm or smaller in length with reference diameter from 2.5 to 3.5 mm. The metal stent has a strut thickness of 60 μm and the usable length of the delivery system is 140 cm. The delivery system has a thickness of 5–6 μm that is made of two layers: a base layer containing the drug and a top protective layer without drug for a programmed biphase drug release.

Inorganic-Based Matrix

By completely removing polymer matrix materials, manufacturers have developed systems for introducing inorganic-based matrix drug reservoirs directly onto the metal surfaces through processes such as surface deposition. To avoid drug elution into the blood, abluminal surface coating is generally employed.

Ceramic-Coated Tacrolimus-Eluting Stent

Jomed International, recently acquired by Abbott Vascular, developed a thin ceramic coating of 300–500 nm onto a 316L stainless steel stent (Jomed, Rangendingen, Germany) for drug elution (Wieneke et al., 2003). The metal stent has a length of 16 mm, a surface area of 91.81 mm^2, and a strut diameter of 120 μm. The porous ceramic membrane is made in two steps. First the bare metal stent was coated with a thin layer of aluminum using a specially designed vapor deposition process (anodic arc discharge, involving evaporation and ionization of metal vapor), which is then electrically converted into a nanoporous ceramic–alumina using a bath of 2% oxalic acid in cold water (0°C). Pores formed during the process in the range of 5–15 nm are used for carrying the drug. Drug loading is achieved by dipping the stents into a defined solution of 3 mg tacrolimus in 1 mL methanol with subsequent drying steps. The nanoporous ceramic membrane controlled the release of 75% tacrolimus in 2 to 3 days (Table 6.5).

TABLE 6.5

DES with Inorganic Drug Delivery Systems

Stent Design	Drug	Matrix
Axxion	Paclitaxel	None
Janus Flex	Tacrolimus	None
Yukon	Sirolimus	None
Genus	Anti-CD34	None

Yukon Drug-Eluting Stent

The Translumina Yukon® CC stent (Translumina, Hechingen, Germany) is a microporous, onsite-coated, sirolimus-eluting stent composed of drug reservoir machined directly into the stent using mechanical means. The stent also has a strut thickness of 87 mm. With 100% pore coverage, the surface micropores have an average depth of approximately 2 µm with approximately 1 million pores/cm^2. This unique structure allows polymer-free coating of sirolimus using a proprietary coating device (Mehilli et al., 2006). The equipment comprises a drug reservoir, spraying system, and a cartridge, into which a mounted stent is positioned. This mobile machine can complete the entire drug application within 10 min. Freshly coated Yukon Sirolimus-eluting stents are used to treat lesions 40 mm or smaller in length with reference diameter from 2.0 to 3.5 mm.

Janus Carbostent™

The Janus CarboStent™ is manufactured by Sorin, Europe's largest cardiovascular diseases technology company. The Janus™ flex stent is a matrix-free tacrolimus-eluting stent. The stent material is an AISI 316 LVM stainless steel with Carbofilm™ coating for reduced risk of thrombolic events. The metallic stent has a strut thickness of 110 µm, a slotted tube multicellular architecture with characteristic deep grooves on its external surface, which are loaded with drug. The amount of drug loaded into the grooves is significantly higher than that in a polymeric film (2.3 µg/mm^2), and none of the drug is lost into the bloodstream. The maximum concentration of tacrolimus in the endothelial wall is reached during the first day after implantation, reducing to a steady state after 10 days. Fifty percent of the loaded drug is released after 28 days. This stent is used to treat lesions 31 mm or smaller in length with reference diameter from 2.5 to 4.0 mm.

Axxion Paclitaxel-Eluting Stent

Biosensors' Axxion paclitaxel-eluting stent is a polymer-free stent that received its CE Mark in July 2005 (Fishell et al., 2009). The stent is laser cut from a 316L LVM stainless steel tube with multicellular slots with stent rings connected by U-shaped links that are positioned between successive rings. The thickness of the strut is 117 µm. The stent surface is coated with a thin, uniform film of a semisynthetic glycocalix (Calix) through a covalent bonding process. The glycocalix coating is designed to mimic the carbohydrate chain–coated surface of endothelial cells. Paclitaxel is spray coated to the abluminal surface of the coated stent, directly applied to the Calix-coated surface with a drug dose of 2.5 µg/mm^2. Calix is inert and permanently preventing inflammation, platelet activation, and immunological responses, and facilitates reendothelialization.

Genous™ Endothelial Progenitor Cell Capturing Stent

The Genous Bio-engineered R stent™ stent is a 316L stainless steel stent with a covalently coupled polysaccharide matrix coating (OrbusNeich Medical Technologies; Fort Lauderdale, FL) (Beijk et al., 2009). Using asymmetrical coating, a murine monoclonal antihuman CD34t antibody is applied onto the luminal surface. The anti-CD34t antibodies specifically adhere to circulating endothelial progenitor cells, bone marrow–derived cells that are thought to be responsible for postnatal neoangiogenesis and the arterial repair response. The Genous stent received a CE mark in August 2005. The Genous stent is designed to attract endothelial progenitor cells and form an endothelial layer that provides protection against thrombosis and modulates restenosis.

Fully Erodible Metallic and Polymer Stents

High molecular weight PLLA (321 kDa) has been used to fabricate a full polymeric stent. This polymer was selected because of minimal inflammation after implantation. High molecular weight PLLA is the platform material for both the Igaki–Tamai drug-free stent and the bioabsorbable vascular solution Everolimus-eluting stent. The other erodible material for constructing degradable stents is tyrosine-derived polycarbonate that was used to make the REVA stent (REVA Medical, San Diego, CA). The polycarbonate REVA stent is radio-opaque, permitting direct visualization under standard fluoroscopy.

Two biocorrodible materials, iron and magnesium, have been used to manufacture coronary stents. Iron is a necessary trace element used by almost all living organisms. The plasma protein, transferrin, which circulates in the blood, binds excess iron found within the circulation. Iron is a transition metal with an atomic weight of 55.845 g/mol. Magnesium is an important element required for the utilization of adenosine-5'-triphosphate, which exists in cells as a chelate of adenosine-5'-triphosphate and magnesium ions. Magnesium is an alkaline earth metal and has a standard atomic weight of 24.3 g/mol. The metallic stent of interest is the absorbable metal stent, constructed from magnesium.

Fully Polylactic Acid Stent

The Igaki–Tamai stent manufactured by Kyoto Medical Planning Company (previously Igaki Medical Planning Company) is a coil stent made of PLLA monofilament (molecular mass = 183 kDa) with a zigzag helical design. This drug-free stent is the first bioabsorbable stent to obtain a CE mark in November 2007 (Daemen and Serruys, 2007; Kukreja et al., 2008). This biodegradable stent combines the features of a thermal self-expandable and a balloon-expandable stent. Although it spontaneously expands at 37°C, deployment of the Igaki–Tamai stent requires the use of a balloon containing a heated contrast agent (Tamai et al., 2000). The Igaki–Tamai stent, which has a strut thickness of 240 μm, and is used to treat lesions 36 mm or smaller in length with reference diameter ranging from 5.0 to 8.0 mm. Although pioneering in its design, the mechanical properties of the Igaki–Tamai stent render it unattractive for widespread clinical application (Griffiths et al., 2004) (Table 6.6).

The bioabsorbable vascular solution stent manufactured by Guidant (Indianapolis, IN) is the first fully absorbable DES, consisting of bioabsorbable PLA containing Everolimus (98 μg/cm^2) (Daemen and Serruys, 2007) with a strut thickness of 159 μm. Although the stent is radiolucent, it contains two platinum markers at each end to allow identification on both conventional and noninvasive angiography. The mechanical properties appear favorable: acute recoil (the difference in mean diameter during and after balloon dilatation) is

TABLE 6.6

Fully Erodible Stents

Stent Design	Drug	Polymer
Igaki–Tamai	None	PLLA
Bioabsorbable vascular solution	Everolimus	PDLLA
Absorbable metal stent	None	None

similar to a CoCr Everolimus-eluting stent (6.9% vs. 4.9%). During trials, it was reported to have degraded with no inflammation and positive remodeling at 2 years after implantation (Nakazawa et al., 2009).

Biocorrodible Metallic Stents

Two biocorrodible materials, iron and magnesium, have been evaluated in animal studies. The NOR-I stent is a slotted tube design constructed from pure iron (>98.8%), with a strut thickness of 100–120 μm. They were used to treat lesions 10 mm in length with reference diameter of 2.5–3.5 mm. Quantitative angiography at follow-up showed a 40% loss of perfused lumen between 10 and 35 days caused by corrosion of the stent. Strut thickness biocorrosion had begun at 35 days, and it was estimated by extrapolation that this would be complete by 98 days. Magnesium is an attractive material for further evaluation as its degradation generates an electronegative, and therefore thrombosis-resistant surface (Griffiths et al., 2004). A magnesium stent made of magnesium alloy, AE21, also contains 2% aluminum and 1% rare earth metals (Ce, Pr, Nd), and has a slotted tube design, having an uneven strut thickness of 150–200 μm. The magnesium stent appears to have scaffolding properties, radial strength, and thickness of the delivery system similar to those of first-generation metallic stents. This metal stent induces rapid endothelialization, has low thrombogenicity, and a degradation time of 2–3 months.

Biotronik has recently developed the Lekton Magic coronary stent, constructed from a magnesium alloy (WE43) also containing zirconium (<5%), yttrium (<5%), and rare earths (<5%), and is balloon-expandable. This stent has a novel design characterized by circumferential noose-shaped elements connected by unbowed cross-links along its longitudinal axis. In vitro studies have indicated that the stent undergoes biocorrosion within 2 months. Although the stent is completely radiolucent, accurate positioning during deployment is possible because of the two radio-opaque markers at the balloon ends (Eggebrecht et al., 2005).

Structures and Forming Techniques

Controlled-released coatings for DES are not simply a continuous layer of matrix materials used for the sustained release of specific drugs. They vary with the design of the stent platform. DES are still at the stage of trial and modification. The basic structures of the stent platform are prepared using micro- and nanofabrication technologies (Caves and Chaikof, 2006).

The basic stent structure is the tubular slotted structure of the flexible metallic stent. It is manufactured by laser cutting a tube of either the 316L surgical grade stainless steel, medical grade L605 CoCr alloy or Nitinol alloy (Menown et al., 2005). Lasers can be used through either the direct write method or masked-projection method. In both methods, the laser is pulsed at 1 kHz or faster, allowing the substrate to briefly cool between exposure and avoiding melting. Each pulse typically removes 0.1–0.5 μm of metal. Polymers and metals can be readily cut with channels as thin as 50–100 μm. A conductive substrate can be machined with feature sizes as small as 25 μm.

The second basic stent structure is the rectangular strut defined by strut thickness and width. The laser cut surface is electropolished and cleaned before adding protective coatings. Without preparing additional architecture for asymmetrical coating, the first generation of DES has a continuous layer of the drug/matrix coating covering the whole stent surface. The strut thickness of the DES varies with the mechanical properties of the stent material. The fully absorbable PLLA and biocorrosive magnesium stents have the largest strut thicknesses, ranging from 150 to 240 μm. Stainless steel stents have median strut thicknesses ranging from 110 to 140 μm. Finally, CoCr alloy stents, the strongest stent platform material, have strut thicknesses ranging from 60 to 90 μm. The stent structure can be defined as luminal (interior) and abluminal (exterior) surfaces (Figure 6.10b). The abluminal surface is against the wall of the blood vessel and the luminal surface is in contact with the flow of the bloodstream.

The third basic structure is the combination of holes and hinges (Kukreja et al., 2008). The intra-built holes are used to load drugs either with or without matrix materials. The housing structure for holes is much stronger than the hinge structure. The flexibility of the stent is a function of the ductility of the hinge structure without deformation of the holes, preventing the matrix from extruding out. Figure 6.11a shows the hole-and-hinge structure of the CoStar stent.

The fourth basic structure is the intra-built deep grooves for drug loading, such as in the Janus stent (Figure 6.11b) (Acharya and Park, 2006). The grooves are cut on the abluminal surface of the stent. Drugs are loaded in these cavities and delivered directly to the contacting vessel wall. No drugs are directly eluted into the bloodstream. Both holes and

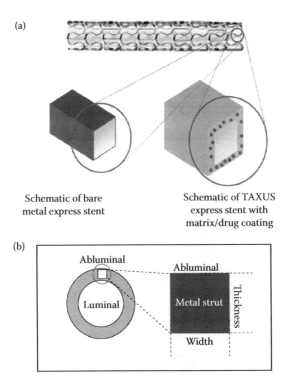

(a)

Schematic of bare metal express stent

Schematic of TAXUS express stent with matrix/drug coating

(b)

Abluminal

Luminal

Abluminal

Metal strut

Thickness

Width

FIGURE 6.10
Tubular and rectangular structures of bare metal stent. (Reproduced with permission from HMP Communications LLC. Chadwick, D.R., *Cath. Lab. Dig.*, 14, 1.1, 2006.) (a) Express stent with and without coating. (b) Cross section of tubular and rectangular structures.

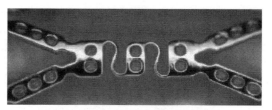

(a) CoStar holes-and-hinges structure

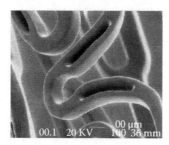

(b) Janus intra-built deep grooves

FIGURE 6.11
Intra-built reservoirs–holes (a) and grooves (b). (a) CoStar holes-and-hinges structure. (Reproduced with permission from Elsevier Ltd. Kukreja et al., *Pharmacol. Res.*, 57:171–180, 2008.) (b) Janus intra-built deep grooves. (Reproduced with permission from HMP Communications LLC. Chadwick, D.R., *Cath. Lab. Dig.*, 14, 1.1, 2006.)

grooves provide the feasibility of delivering multiple drugs in a noncontinuous coating. It minimizes the unnecessary delivery of drugs and matrix materials into the bloodstream.

The fifth basic structure is the nonpreferential porous structure made from mechanical machining (Mehilli et al., 2006) or the selective oxidative itching (Wieneke et al., 2003). The former produces a microporous membrane, and the latter introduces nanoporous structure. The porous membrane can be made using the stent surface directly or using an additional layer, such as aluminum (Figure 6.12).

Using the metal stent platform for controlled release of drugs or recruitment of endothelial progenitor cells, DES have three or fewer coating layers to create the active surface.

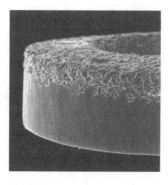

FIGURE 6.12
Porous top surface of the BioFreedom experimental stent. (Reproduced with permission from Prof. Dr. Grube.)

The first layer is passive for surface protection, the bridging layer for the coupling of active agents, and the transition layer for good adhesion. This layer is sometimes deleted from the coating specification. The second layer is the matrix for drug loading and controlled release. In a drug-free stent, only active agents are incorporated in this layer. The final layer is the top coating, which is often used to minimize the burst release and sustain the long-term release for a significant duration. It is a drug-free layer of matrix material.

Passive Coating

Table 6.7 summarizes the compositions of major elements in alloys for coronary stents. DES with FDA approval are manufactured from 316L stainless steel. Stainless steel and small amounts of nickel, chromium molybdenum, and other contaminants tend to produce a foreign body reaction when implanted in human coronary arteries (Colombo and Airoldi, 2003). Passive coatings (Figure 6.13) have been introduced to provide a biologically inert barrier between the stent surface, circulating blood, and endothelial wall. These coatings are a thin, continuous layer of gold, heparin, carbon, silicon carbide, titanium-nitride-oxide, or PC (Menown et al., 2005). The Janus CarboStent (Bartorelli et al., 2003) consists of an integral Carbofilm coating combined with the capability to load and release the antirestenotic drug from deep sculptures on the external surface of the stent. Phosphorylcholine-coated BiodiVsio Stent (Menown et al., 2005) has the capacity to load and release the rapamycin analogue ABT-578. A similar coating is found on the CYPHER stent, which has a prime layer of Parylene C.

The Parylene C layer on the Cypher stent is formed by chemical vapor deposition following the Gorham process (Figure 6.14) (Chang et al., 2007), which has three main stages: vaporization, pyrolysis, and deposition. Briefly, dichloro-di(*p*-xylylene) is first vaporized at 150°C at 1 Torr, then pyrolyzed at 690°C and 0.5 Torr to form chloro-*p*-xylylene, the monomer of Parylene C. At 25°C and 0.1 Torr, this monomer condenses onto the device surface to form the final Parylene C film. The thickness of the film is determined by the amount of dimer fed into the furnace: 1 g of dimer adds 0.5 μm to the thickness of the Parylene C film (Wright et al., 2007).

Parylene C (Figure 6.15) is a member of the Parylene family (Fortin and Lu, 2004). The basic member of the series, Parylene N (poly-*para*-xylylene), is a completely crystalline material. In 1947, *para*-xylylene was first identified as the gaseous precursor for the formation of parylene film, followed by the use of di-*para*-xylylene, the dimer, for more efficient deposition of parylene film, the so-called Gorham process. Parylene C is the most widely used dimer and provides a useful combination of properties, plus a very low permeability to moisture, chemicals, and other corrosive gases. It is used in a conformal layer, pinhole-free coating. The material is applied at 5 μm/h in a thickness of 0.100–76 μm in a single operation. Because of its unique properties, Parylene C conforms to virtually any shape, including sharp edges, crevices, points, or flat and exposed internal surfaces.

TABLE 6.7

Compositions of Major Elements in Alloys for Coronary Stents

Alloy	Iron (%)	Cobalt (%)	Nickel (%)	Chromium (%)	Tungsten (%)	Titanium (%)
316 L Stainless steel	60–65		12–14	17–18		
L605 CoCr	<3	50	10	20	15	
Nitinol			55			45

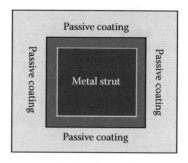

FIGURE 6.13
Passive coating around an alloy strut.

Carbofilm coatings are pure carbon with a polycrystalline structure nearly identical to that of pyrolytic carbon (Kutryk and Serruys, 2003), which has been used for years to coat prosthetic heart valves. Carbofilm is deposited in a high vacuum at room temperature to obtain stable bonds, which results in permanent adhesion of an extremely thin film of the coating to the substrate. The film comprises diamond-like carbon that is amorphous, with high hydrogen content (20–60%) and good hemocompatibility.

Active Coatings

Use of stents is often associated with early thrombus formation on strut surfaces, acute inflammation, development of granulation tissue, giant cell infiltration, smooth muscle cell proliferation, and extracellular matrix synthesis (Virmani and Farb, 1999). Passive coatings generally fail to prevent in-stent restenosis, and therefore the concept of active coatings that, in addition to being simply protective, provide thromboresistance, reduce local inflammation, and minimize tissue proliferation (Menown et al., 2005). The active coating can be applied onto the bare metal stent surface either simply by physical attachment or by chemically bonding to the device. It forms either a single layer or a multiple layer drug delivery system.

A Single Layer Reservoir

The first FDA-approved (2004) DES having a single layer reservoir for drug release was the Boston TAXUS stent. The Biosensors Axxion received a CE mark in 2005 followed by the Medtronic Endeavor in 2007. They all feature as a single-layer reservoir for drug release without a drug-free topcoat (Figure 6.16). The TAXUS DES uses a sticky proprietary polymer (Translute), which physically holds paclitaxel firmly in the matrix material (Colombo et al., 2003) whereas the synthetic glycocalix of the Axxion DES holds paclitaxel electrostatically.

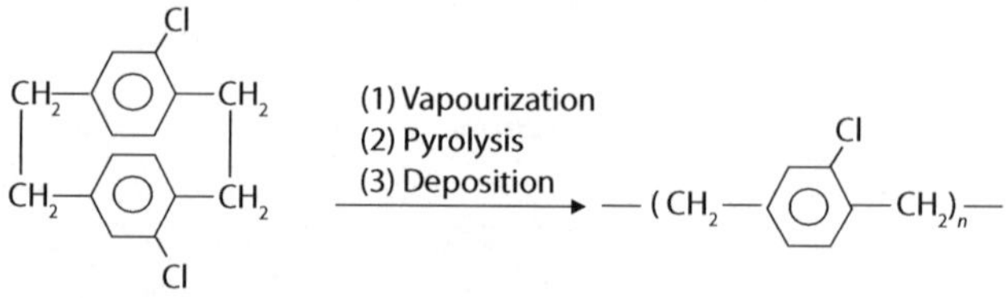

FIGURE 6.14
Route of polymerization for Parylene C: (left) dimer and (right) Parylene C polymer.

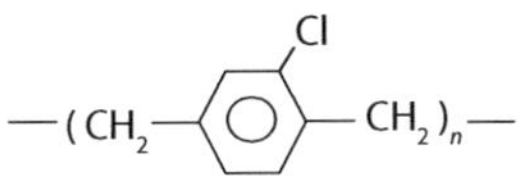

$$-\left(CH_2-\underset{\bigcirc}{\bigotimes}-CH_2\right)_n-$$

FIGURE 6.15
Chemical structure of Parylene C.

For the TAXUS stent, three formulations of matrix/drug mixtures allow for fast, moderate, and slow release; profiles are 35:65, 25:75, and 8.8:91.2, respectively (Acharya and Park, 2006). All formulations have the same dose of 1 µg/mm². For the fast release formulation, the burst release occurs in the first day followed by slow release over the next 10 days. In clinical applications, the rate of release profoundly affects the outcome, with less benefit derived from the fast-releasing formulation of the Cypher stent (Sousa et al., 2003), so only moderate and slow release formulations are manufactured. The single layer has a thickness of 16 µm, which elutes paclitaxel over a period of about 90 days.

The PC polymer drug carrier on ZoMaxx stents, known simply as PC-1036, is composed of the polymers, MPC, LMA, hydroxypropyl methacrylate (HPMA), and trimethoxysilyl-propyl methacrylate (TSMA) in the ratios of MPC_{23}, LMA_{47}, $HPMA_{25}$, and $TSMA_5$. This PC Zotarcrolimus-eluting system provides a 30-day controlled release with approximately 60% of the total released in the first week, an additional 20% in the second week, and the last 20% in the last 2 weeks (Chevalier et al., 2008). Phosphorylcholine-based polymer generally binds the metal stent surfaces through the phospho-rich coordination layer (Figure 6.17).

Vascular endothelium has a surface covering of glycocalyx (Vogel et al., 2000), a 0.4- to 0.5-µm-thick layer of negatively charged polysaccharide strands from selectins, proteoglycans, and glycosaminoglycans (VanTeeffelen et al., 2007). Degradation of glycocalyx structures has been observed after the addition of inflammatory and atherogenic stimuli. A synthetic glycocalyx has been produced using a polyethylene glycol-lipid to create a mobile polymer brush (Cuvelier et al., 2004) as a hemocompatible protective barrier. The layer is covalently bound to the activated implant surface (Horres et al., 2004; Meng et al., 2009). The surfaces to be coated are degreased and aminolyzed with 3-aminopropyltriethoxysilane. The heparin-like component of the synthetic glycocalyx is coupled with the aminolyzed stent covalently, leaving the carbohydrate backbone fragments on the surface of the stent, creating a nonthrombogenic surface.

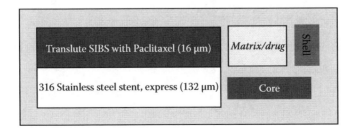

FIGURE 6.16
A single-layer structure of TAXUS paclitaxel delivery system.

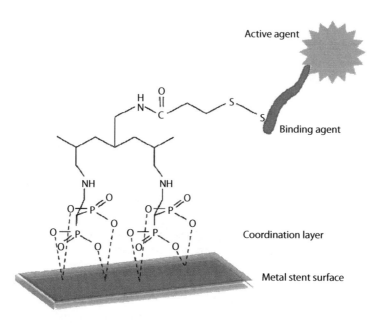

FIGURE 6.17
Phosphorylcholine-based copolymers used for drug release coatings.

Multiple-Layer Reservoir

The Cordis CYPHER Sirolimus stent has a matrix coating consisting of three layers: the primer Parylene C layer (2 μm thick), the matrix/drug layer, and the matrix only topcoat layer (Figure 6.18). After coating with Parylene C, the matrix/drug layer, which is 10 μm thick, is applied, onto which a drug-free 0.6-μm layer of PBMA is added, which minimizes the burst release (Acharya and Park, 2006).

In experiments reported by Morice et al. (2002), a prolonged release of sirolimus demonstrated from a three-layer system, with 80% being released over 30 days through a drug-free polymer top coat.

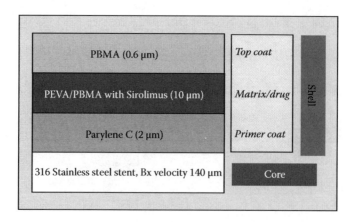

FIGURE 6.18
Three-layer structure of the CYPHER sirolimus delivery system.

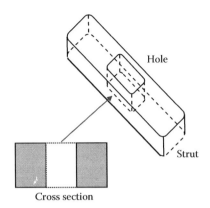

FIGURE 6.19
An in-stent built hole (honeycombed) structure of matrix/drug coating in a Conor stent.

Intra-Built Holes

The Conor Medsystems stent has numerous holes (in a honeycomb arrangement) on each strut. Each hole is filled with a mixture of drug and biodegradable polymer in a solvent, using a piezoelectric microdispenser. The loading process is repeated on each hole as many as 22 times, in the case of PLGA/paclitaxel in dimethyl sulfoxide (DMSO) (Finkelstein et al., 2003). This controlled-release coating (Figure 6.19) has a limited exposed surface area for drug release.

Intra-Built Cavity

The Janus CarboStent has deep grooves on the outer stent surface that are used to hold tacrolimus (Acharya and Park, 2006). The stent surface is first treated with an integral carbofilm coating, which is known to render the stent surface nonthrombogenic when in contact with blood. The deep grooves (Figure 6.20) can load more drugs than other DES in the similar size range, and the polymer-free drug can be loaded with promising release profile.

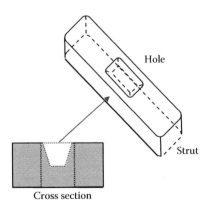

FIGURE 6.20
In-stent built cavity (deep grooves) of polymer-free drug coating in a Janus CarboStent.

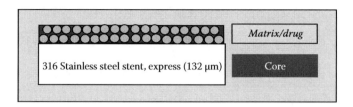

FIGURE 6.21
Micro- and nanoporous ceramic coating loaded with drug.

Surface-Built Micro- and Nanoporous Membrane

Combining physical vapor deposition of aluminum with oxalic acid oxidation, a nanoporous ceramic (alumina/aluminum oxide/Al_2O_3) membrane has been produced for loading tacrolimus (Wieneke et al., 2003). The ceramic coating is relatively thin (1 μm) with tacrolimus loaded in a dip coating process in methanol (Figure 6.21).

Top Coat

The reason for applying a layer of top coat is to minimize the burst release of the active ingredient in a fast delivery system such as the CYPHER Sirolimus-eluting stent. It is simply a drug-free layer of matrix. In view of the problems caused by polymeric matrices, new DES seldom use top coats (Deconinck et al., 2008; Kukreja et al., 2008; Nakazawa et al., 2009).

Coating Techniques

The active ingredients, dominantly drugs, are applied onto stent surfaces using two major techniques: dip coating and spray coating. Dip coating provides a nonpreferential layer to any part of the open stent surface. It is considered an inferior technique for a matrix that is polymer-based because of bridging and imperfect coating of tight spaces. Spray coating produces a thinner layer with better surface quality. It is considered as a superior technique for manufacturing DES. Embracing the technical advances in micro- and nanofabrication, dip and spray coating techniques have their own advantages in preparing new generation of DES. As DES are moving in the direction of polymer-free devices, dip coating is probably the simplest and cheapest forming process, requiring low technical input in a preclinical treatment. When DES require preferential delivery of the active ingredients, spray coating is advantageous in abluminal coating of functionalized devices. In addition, ink-jet technology is an emerging process for acquiring a layer of a preferential coating.

Dip Coating

Dip coating is a simple process used for coating bare metal stents, both surface-modified or not. The matrix/drug mixture is mixed into a dilute solution and then the bare metal stent dipped into it, then often allowed to air-dry. The thickness of the coating layer is controlled mixture concentration and chemical cross-linking (Juan et al., 2009). Cordis coat the combination of PEVA, PBMA, and sirolimus by successive dipping and air-drying of the stent in a solution of THF a controlled number of times (Wolf et al., 2008). Coating of tacrolimus onto ceramic stents is achieved by dipping in a 3-mg/mL solution of the drug in methanol with subsequent drying steps (Wieneke et al., 2003), with quantification using high-pressure liquid chromatography.

Spray Coating

Different spray coating processes differ in the way in which fine droplets are formed. Two atomizing techniques are employed in spray-coating stents: ultrasonic atomization, which creates droplets with a diameter of 18 μm, and compressed air atomization, which mixes the coating material at the tip of a 0.3-mm nozzle.

Ultrasonic Spray Process

Ultrasonic spray nozzles are ideally suited for coating arterial stents because they are capable of producing low flow rates, precisely shaped spray patterns, low-velocity delivery, and relatively small drops. The operating frequency of the ultrasonic nozzles is 120 kHz, which yields a median drop diameter ($D_{N0.5}$) in the order of 18 μm when using water. Once the solution of the mixture of matrix/drug is atomized, the velocity of the spray is typically 0.25–0.4 m/s compared with 10–20 m/s for standard pressure atomizing nozzles. The sprayed liquid consists of the matrix/drug solution at approximately 0.5–2% by weight. The solvent typically has a high vapor pressure so that drying occurs quickly. The flow rate and spray coating process can be optimized by varying the rotational speed and the distance between the spray and the stent. The sprayed liquid flows better during contact with the stent surface if performed in a nitrogen environment.

In a typical ultrasonic spraying process, copolymers of methacrylates were prepared in one recipe of *n*-butyl methacrylate (BMA, 60 parts) and VA (40 parts) with 0.6 wt.% 2,2'-azobisisobutyronitrile (AIBN). In another recipe, *n*-hexyl methacrylate (48 parts), *N*-vinyl pyrrolidinone (27 parts), and VA (25 parts) have been used (Udipi et al., 2008). These polymers and Zotarolimus (65:35 weight ratio) were dissolved in chloroform at a concentration of 1% and filtered to 0.2 μm for coating. The polymer/drug chloroform solution was ultrasonically sprayed onto Parylene C-primed Driver® stent before mounting and sterilization with ethylene oxide.

Airbrush Spray Process

Airbrushes have three main features: the trigger, feed, and mix. Briefly, trigger controls the amount of the inlet and outlet of the coating materials. The feed system is a reservoir where the coating materials are stored for atomization, and the mix point is the tip of the airbrush where coating materials mix with compressed air and create a finer atomized "mist." This technique is generally used for painting and recently employed for spray coating stents.

Poly(ethylene carbonate) (PEC) synthesized by Novartis Pharma AG has a weight average molecular weight of 242 kDa and a polydispersity of 1.90 (Unger et al., 2007). 1% (w/w) PEC in dichloromethane is sprayed onto Parylene N coated stents at a distance of 5 cm using an airbrush (Model Aero-pro Classic 10; Hansa, Oststeinbek, Germany) followed by drying under vacuum for 2 days at room temperature.

Collagen has been delivered as a coating using an airbrush spray process (Chen et al., 2005). Briefly, the aqueous collagen (3 mg/mL) was loaded into an air brush with a 0.3-mm nozzle (Rich AS-3; Japan) that was controlled by a linear motor (Figure 6.23). The stent was mounted on a PTFE mandrill driven by a rotator. The aqueous collagen in the air brush was then spray-coated onto the surface of the mounted stent layer by layer (0.4 mL of aqueous collagen per layer before drying in air for 24 h). Rhodamine 6G (a red dye, 200 ppm)

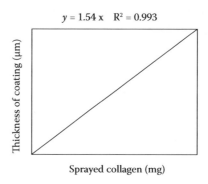

FIGURE 6.22
Relationship between thickness of collagen coated onto a stent and amount of collagen sprayed by an air brush.

was added into the aqueous collagen to visualize the uniformity of the coating. To prevent dissolution of the collagen coating, aqueous genipin (0.4 mL, 5% by w/v) solution (containing 70% ethanol by v/v) was directly spray-coated onto the collagen-coated stent. The cross-linking process occurs in a sealed tube at 37°C for 1 day. By repeating this procedure three times followed by air drying for 24 h, the thickness of collagen layer was found to be proportional to the quantity of collagen sprayed (Figure 6.22), an 8-μm collagen coating was prepared using approximately 5 mg collagen in a spray coating process (Figure 6.23).

Ink-Jet Technology

The fundamental principles of reagent jetting are described and summarized below (Tarcha et al., 2007). During the jetting process, a capillary chamber is filled with reagent solution. By applying voltages to the wall of the capillary, a distortion is caused, resulting in capillary expansion and pressure drop, and the drawing-in of more reagents into the capillary. When the voltage is released and the capillary returns to its original volume, a droplet is expelled through the print nozzle orifice (Figure 6.24). Ink-jet printing technology can dispense spheres of fluid with diameter of 15–200 μm (2 pL to 5 nL) at rates of 1 MHz for continuous droplets (continuous mode jetting) and 1 Hz to 25 kHz for single

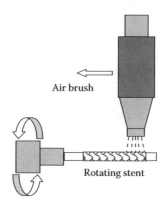

FIGURE 6.23
Schematic illustration of spray-coating equipment used in the study.

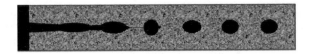

FIGURE 6.24
Formation of droplets in an ink-jet printing process.

droplets on demand (drop-on-demand jetting). In a continuous mode ink-jet printer, pressurized fluid is forced through an orifice, typically 50–80 μm in diameter, to form a liquid jet. In a drop-on-demand ink-jet printer, the fluid is maintained at an ambient pressure, and a transducer is used to create a drop only when needed (Figure 6.23).

Matrix Free Ink-Jet Printing

Using ink-jet printing, fenofibrate was dissolved in isobutanol at a concentration of 20 mg/mL. The ink-jet microdispenser was programmed to jet 21,900 droplets and aimed to deliver a target dosage of 150 μg per stent tube. Analysis of the stent demonstrated a coating of 140.0 ± 2 μg (Figure 6.24).

Jet Spray Process

Jet spraying has been used to coat microporous stent surfaces with sirolimus (Wessely et al., 2005). Sirolimus (0.75%) in ethanol was sprayed onto sandblasted 316L stainless steel stents. The stent surface is dried by removing the ethanol with pressured air. The coating process could be repeatedly run for the purpose of increasing drug dosage.

Controlled Release

Restenosis has been a major limitation of angioplasty since its introduction in 1978, but it can be controlled by administering effective agents to the stented artery (Faxon, 2002). The absence of a clear overview of the complete pathophysiology of restenosis has hampered progress in precise treatment options. In the early 1980s, it was largely thought that platelets and thrombi were the primary factors responsible for restenosis. Subsequent studies demonstrated the important role of smooth muscle cell proliferation. However, the importance of inflammation and extracellular matrix turnover is now recognized as a key component of the condition. However, the most important observation has been the critical role of vascular remodeling in restenosis (Lafont and Topol, 1997). By eliminating this phenomenon, the pharmacological approach has been largely simplified by allowing the primary treatment focus to reduce smooth muscle cell proliferation (Farb et al., 1999). In this way, the immediate postoperative period (less than 2 weeks) is associated with the appearance of fibrin, platelets, and acute inflammatory cells, followed by the emergence of a neointima containing smooth muscle cells. In longer-term stents (>30 days after implant), success was characterized by neointimal growth within the stent and was not influenced by artery or stent size.

The choice of drugs in the treatment of restenosis and the manner in which they are administered is of considerable interest. Systemic drugs with bare metal stents are cheap and applicable to blood vessels of a broad range of sizes. However, patients have to tolerate the systemic toxicity. Local delivery of drugs through release from stents brings with it minimal toxicity, but with higher cost and restriction to the sizes of the blood vessels that can be treated. Eight drugs have been demonstrated to be effective in systemic delivery. These agents include probucol, the antioxidant AG1-1067, cilostazol, troglitazone, valsartan, pemirolast, and folic acid. Three families of drugs have been incorporated onto the stents for local targeted release. These are sirolimus analogues, calcinuerin inhibitors, and paclitaxel. Drugs for systemic and local delivery are different in terms of molecular weight and size (Figure 6.25).

Efforts aimed at the pharmacological prevention of restenosis should be considered in the light of drug efficacy, appropriateness of drug regimen, and method of administration. A reliable measure of the efficacy of antirestenotic therapy is the reduction in in-stent diameter 6 to 9 months postoperatively, which corresponds to the degree of neointima formation. As shown in Figure 6.26, the antirestenotic effect of commercially available DES is reproducibly more profound than with oral treatment regimens (Schömig et al., 2005). Local delivery is able to administer high dose in the first 10 days and treat the early events for neointimal formation.

Later on in this section, we will describe the release profiles of locally delivered drugs. The delivery systems will be defined in terms of loading efficiency and release profiles.

Local Drugs

Local drugs can be categorized mainly as sirolimus analogues, calcinuerin inhibitors, and paclitaxel (Kukreja et al., 2008). Sirolimus analogues include sirolimus, everolimus, biolimus, and zotarolimus. These analogues have a macrocyclic lactone comprising 35 groups, with an mTOR binding site from macrocyclic positions 14–21 and an FKBP binding site from macrocyclic positions 25–29. The analogue structures are generated by varying the pendent R group at the 4-cyclohexyl-1 attached to macrocyclic position 3 (Figure 6.27). The structures of the R groups of the analogues are described in Figure 6.28.

Sirolimus (formerly known as rapamycin) is a lipophilic, potent immunosuppressive agent that was developed by Wyeth-Ayerst Laboratories and approved by the FDA for the prophylaxis of renal transplant rejection in 1999 (Sousa et al., 2001). It binds to FK506-binding protein 12 (FKBP12) and subsequently mTOR and thereby blocks the cell cycle at the G1 to S phase transition (Figure 6.31), the major effect required to inhibit smooth muscle cell migration and proliferation (Kukreja et al., 2008; Marx and Marks, 2001).

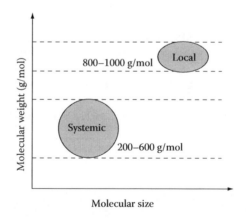

FIGURE 6.25
Differences in molecular weights of antirestenotic drugs.

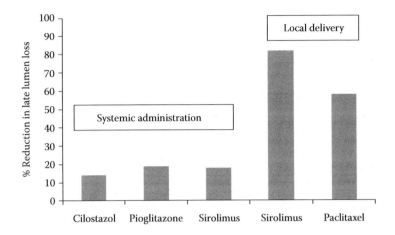

FIGURE 6.26
Percent reduction in late lumen loss by systemic or local pharmacological delivery.

Everolimus is the second derivative of the Limus family. It is a sirolimus analogue with an ethyl addition at the R group. Although no modification of the mTOR binding domain is effected, Everolimus-eluting stents have been described as having a more rapid endothelialization in rabbit iliac arteries when compared with sirolimus-, zotarolimus-, or paclitaxel-eluting stents (Daemen and Serruys, 2007).

Biolimus A9 is a highly lipophilic sirolimus analogue that inhibits T cell and smooth muscle cell proliferation. The Biolimus A9 eluting BioMatrix stent showed significantly less late lumen loss in the Biolimus arm compared with the Taxus arm (Daemen and Serruys, 2007).

Zotarolimus (ABT-578; Abbott Pharmaceuticals, Abbott Park, IL) is the third variety of the Limus family. Zotarolimus has been shown in experiments in pigs to have a smaller impact on the function of endothelial cells after stent placement compared to both Cypher and Taxus implantation (Haraguchi et al., 2006).

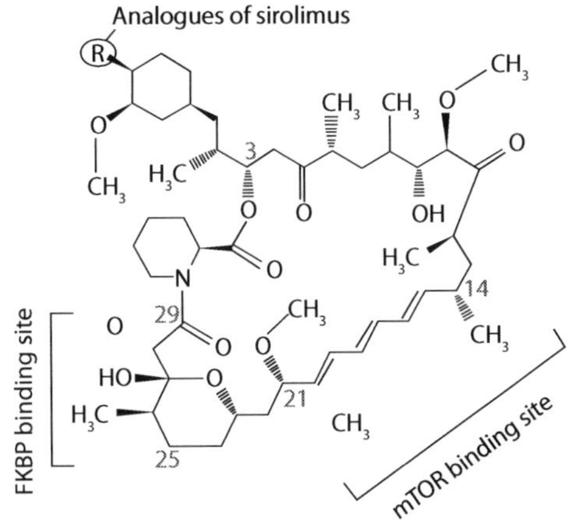

FIGURE 6.27
Macrocyclic lactone structure of sirolimus analogues.

Sirolimus	OH
Everolimus	OCH_2CH_2OH
Biolimus	OCH_2CH_2OR
Zotarolimus	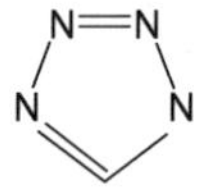

FIGURE 6.28
Structures of R groups of sirolimus analogues.

Calcinuerin inhibitors have two members, tacrolimus and pimecrolimus. This family has a macrolide comprising 27 elements. The two differ in the pendent R group at the 4-cyclohexyl-1 attached to macrocyclic position 3 and the structure at position 8 (Figure 6.29) (Billich et al., 2004). The R group of pimecrolimus is chloride with an ethyl at position 8 whereas tacrolimus has a derivative of hydroxyl group for an R group, with a propenyl at position 8. In contrast to sirolimus analogues, the macrolide has no lactone structure but a hydroxyl group at the macrocyclic point 5. The macrolide does not possess the 6-carbon mTOR binding site but has the characteristic Limus FKBP-binding site at macrocyclic positions 16–22.

Pimecrolimus does not block mTOR and inhibits to a much lesser degree the endothelial cell proliferation (Zollinger et al., 2006). Tacrolimus is water-insoluble and isolated from *Streptomyces tsukubaensis*. It is also sold as Prograf, a drug widely used to prevent allograft rejection after organ transplantation. Tacrolimus is a noncytotoxic T-cell inhibitor, which holds cells at G_0 in the cell cycle. It inhibits smooth muscle cell proliferation more potently and has less effect on endothelial cells compared to sirolimus (Hofma et al., 2006; Steffel et al., 2005).

Paclitaxel is a diterpenoid with a taxane skeleton (Figure 6.30). It is highly lipophilic with a molecular weight of 853.9 Da (Duda et al., 2003). The drug promotes the stabilization of microtubules, which inhibits the action of cell division during all phases, but has the most significant effect at the M phase (Figure 6.31), disrupting SMC migration and

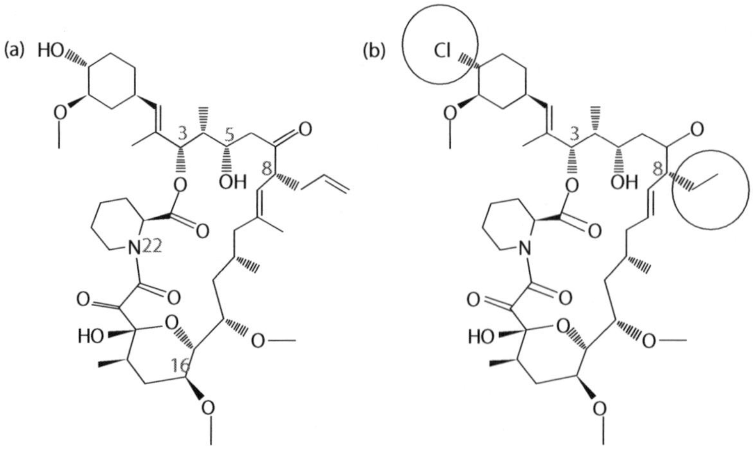

FIGURE 6.29
Structure of macrolide in calcinuerin inhibitors: (a) tacrolimus and (b) pimecrolimus.

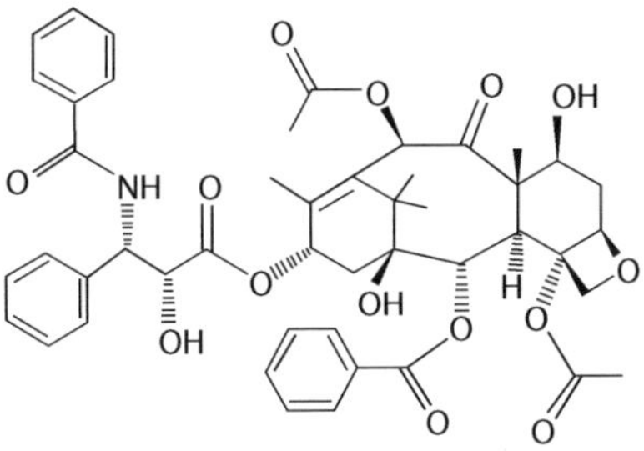

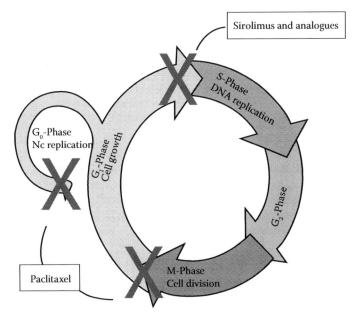

FIGURE 6.30
Structure of paclitaxel.

proliferation through centrosomal impairment (Kukreja et al., 2008; Abal et al., 2003). It is a strong antiproliferative and was first used as an anticancer drug (Daemen and Serruys, 2007). However, it is potentially cardiotoxic, and the dose at which paclitaxel can be delivered safely has yet to be resolved (Am. Soc. Health Syst. Pharm. 1989; Rowinsky and Donehower, 1995).

Controlled Release

The controlled release coating generally comprises two materials, the active pharmaceutical and the matrix, although in some cases the drug is coated onto the stent alone. In this section, we will describe the controlled release characteristics of polymer-based matrices. Nonpolymeric reservoirs will be discussed later in the chapter (Figure 6.31).

Methods of controlled release can be broadly classified into physical and chemical mechanisms in terms of the nature of the interaction between the drug and the matrix (Acharya et al., 2006). When the drug is mixed with the matrix using physical means, the

FIGURE 6.31
Effects of sirolimus analogues and paclitaxel on the cell cycle.

noncovalently bonded drug molecules diffuse through the matrix and become released into the environment. The release kinetics can be controlled by the drug delivery system itself and follows physical factors. Adjusting the parameters of the matrix, such as drug miscibility, ionic charges of the matrix, and degradation rate of the delivery system, can predetermine drug release kinetics. Conversely, delivery systems comprising covalently bound drug and matrix molecules (prodrugs) require chemical modification to effect release, either chemical or enzymatic degradation. The process of prodrug formation is, of course, more complicated. For this reason, physical mechanisms have been used most widely. They can be highly effective in controlling drug release kinetics.

Diffusion-controlled drug release is managed using two different methods: a reservoir system and a matrix system. In the reservoir devices, a small pool of active agent is covered with a thin polymer layer which functions as a rate-controlling membrane. One exemplar of this delivery system is the Cordis CYPHER sirolimus stent. At the steady state, drug release remains constant giving zero-order release. In the matrix (or monolithic) systems, the drug is usually dispersed inside the polymer matrix, and the drug is released without a rate-controlling barrier layer. An exemplar of this is the Boston TAXUS DES. The release rate decreases over time because of an increase in diffusion distance during elution, resulting in nonzero-order release.

Drug release kinetics becomes critical when the therapeutic index is low. This index is the ratio of the maximum safe concentration (C_{max}) and the minimum effective concentration (C_{min}). Thus, careful control of the release characteristics can improve the likelihood of therapeutic benefit.

Dissolution or degradation-controlled drug release is based on the disappearance of the polymer comprising the matrix or encapsulating the drug reservoir. Water-soluble polymers dissolve rather quickly and do not meet the requirements of sustained release (months). Therefore, biodegradable polymers, such as PGA, PLA, and PCL are more widely used, and have been effective in the development of DES. A typical example of these is the BioMatrix BiolimusA9-Eluting system, in which biodegradable PLA is used.

Diffusion-Controlled Release

Drug delivery systems using nonerodible polymers as the matrix materials for drug loading and release exploit diffusion-controlled release. Drug delivery systems are formed in either single or multiple layer reservoirs, exemplar systems being Taxus and Cypher DES, respectively.

Single-Layer Reservoir Diffusion-Controlled System

The Taxus stent manufactured by Boston Scientific employs Translute polymer, which is SIBS (Figure 6.4), a triblock copolymer, for sustained delivery of paclitaxel, which is released directly without diffusing through a rate-controlling membrane, and thus the Taxus stent is also a diffusion-controlled matrix system. It forms a single-layer reservoir and the release profile at the steady state after the initial burst release can be described as zero order (Figure 6.32) (Acharya and Park, 2006). The paclitaxel/translute ratio for fast, moderate, and slow release profiles are 35:65, 25:75, and 8.8:91.2, respectively, the latter being used clinically. The release profile of matrix devices containing excess drug over the dissolved drug is described by the following equation:

$$M = S[DC_s(2A - C_s)t]^{1/2}$$

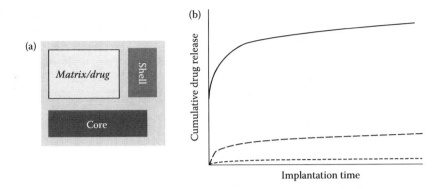

FIGURE 6.32
(a) Core–shell structure of Taxus stent; shell is a single-layer reservoir without top coat. (b) Paclitaxel release profile over 10 days from single-layer reservoir. Three curves represent release at fast, moderate, and slow release profiles (from top to bottom).

where M is the mass of drug released, S is the surface area available for drug delivery, D is the diffusion coefficient, C_s is the solubility of the drug in the polymer matrix, A is the total drug concentration (i.e., total of dissolved and dispersed drug), and t is time. If A is substantially larger than the solubility of the drug in the polymer matrix (C_s), then the equation becomes:

$$M = S[2DC_sAt]^{1/2}$$

Paclitaxel in the single-layer reservoir is contained at 100 μg/cm² (0.117 μmol/cm²), less than 10% of which is released in 10 days. This is unlike the Cypher stent, which shows a sustained release of as much as 50% in 10 days (Ranade et al., 2001). In a patient study ($n = 1314$) at 9 months, restenosis rates were 7.9% compared to 26.6% for bare metal stents (Stone et al., 2004).

Multiple-Layer Reservoir Diffusion-Controlled System

Cordis Corp.'s Cypher stent uses PEVA and PBMA. The combined polymers are mixed with sirolimus at a ratio of 67:33 and applied to the stent as the base coat (drug reservoir layer). This coating is then covered with another thin layer of PBMA. The presence of the topcoat makes the Cypher stent a diffusion-controlled reservoir device in a multiple-layer reservoir. The release profile at the steady state after the initial burst release can be described as zero-order release (Figure 6.33) (Leon et al., 2003), described by the following equation:

$$M = SDK\frac{\Delta C}{h}\left(t + \frac{h^2}{3D}\right)$$

where M is the total amount of drug released, S is the surface area available for drug delivery, D is the diffusion coefficient of drug through the rate-controlling membrane, K is the partition coefficient of drug to the rate-controlling membrane, ΔC is the concentration gradient (which is the same as the saturated drug concentration in the drug reservoir), h is the thickness of the rate-controlling membrane, and t is the time for drug release. The term $h^2/3D$ accounts for the initial burst before reaching steady state release.

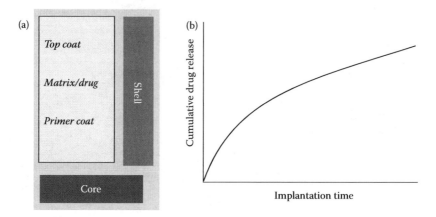

FIGURE 6.33
(a) Core-shell structure of Cypher stent (multiple-layer reservoir); (b) sirolimus release profile over 30 days from multiple-layer reservoir.

Sirolimus in the multiple-layer reservoir is contained at 140 µg/cm² (0.153 µmol/cm²), 80% of which is released in 30 days (Kukreja et al., 2008). Almost half of the total amount (56 µg/cm²) is released within the first week with a similar quantity following zero-order release over 3 weeks (Figure 6.33). The remaining sirolimus (approximately 20% or 28 µg/cm²) is more slowly released.

In a recent review, Venkatraman and Boey (2007) described the in vitro release kinetics of two sirolimus DES, both slow (trilayer) and fast (bilayer) release formulations. The difference in release rates is obtained by merely coating a drug-free top layer onto the drug reservoir layer to create the slow-release formulation. In the fast-release formulation, the entire amount of sirolimus (~140 µg/cm²) was released within 15 and 90 days for the slow release, whose steep initial burst release was moderated by application of the top coat.

A patient study (*n* = 1058) showed that restenosis rates at 8 months were 8.9% compared with 36.3% for bare metal stents (Moses et al., 2003).

Dissolution/Degradation-Controlled Release

Drug delivery systems using erodible polymers as matrix materials for drug loading and controlled release follows a modified controlled release mechanism. The delivery systems are formed in a honeycomb (intra-built holes) or groove (intra-built cavity) structures. Exemplar DES are the Conor and Janus CarboStent, respectively.

Honeycombed (Intra-Built Holes) Matrix Delivery System

The MedStent manufactured by Conor Medsystems (Figure 6.34) has numerous holes on its struts, each filled with a mixture of drug and biodegradable polymer (paclitaxel and PLGA) using a piezoelectric microdispenser (Finkelstein et al., 2003). The paclitaxel release profile can be easily controlled through modification of the degradation kinetics of PLGA by changing the ratio of LA and glycolic acid and the polymer molecular weight. Compared with diffusion-controlled release, dissolution/degradation-controlled release does not follow the zero-order release profile after the initial burst release. When the polymer matrix

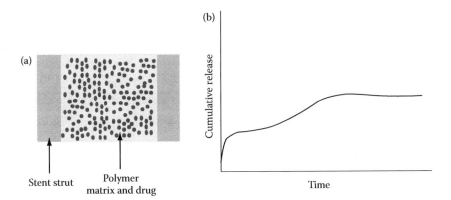

FIGURE 6.34
(a) Intra-built holes of Conor stent.

absorbs water at around 10 days, it starts to degrade rapidly (because of autoaccelerated degradation of PLGA), introducing relatively fast release during the second week.

Deep Groove (Intra-Built Cavity) Matrix-Free Delivery System

The Janus CarboStent is a unique stent characterized by deep grooves, or sculptures, on the outer stent surface that are used to hold tacrolimus (Bartorelli et al., 2003). The stent surface is first treated with an integral carbofilm coating, which is known to render the stent surface nonthrombogenic. The deep sculptures on the surface increase the drug loading capability up to five times in comparison to other DES of similar size. The grooves can be filled with a polymer matrix mixed with a drug, although this stent is used clinically with the drug alone (2.3 µg/mm^2 tacrolimus). It is observed that the maximum concentration of tacrolimus in the endothelial wall is reached in approximately 3 days, which falls thereafter to a steady-state concentration after 10 days (Figure 6.35). Fifty percent of the loaded drug has been released after 28 days.

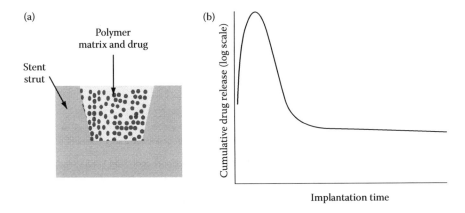

FIGURE 6.35
(a) Intra-built cavity for matrix-free dissolution release in Janus CarboStent; (b) in vivo tacrolimus release profile over 30 days as measured by concentration in vascular tissue.

Perspectives of Release-Controlled Coatings

In 2001, >500,000 angioplasties were performed in the United States, more than double the number of coronary artery bypass graft surgeries (American Heart Association, 2003). In Europe, the reported number of coronary stenting procedures was 395,000 in 2000 (Balmer et al., 2005), stents being applied to 71% of coronary angioplasties. In patients who undergo conventional balloon angioplasty without stenting, >40% of patients develop restenosis within 6 months of the procedure (Fischman et al., 1994). Clinical trials have shown that stenting reduces the occurrence of restenosis by 30% compared with angioplasty alone (Fischman et al., 1994; Serruys et al., 1994). In 2002–2003, DES were approved by regulatory bodies in Europe and the USA after initial studies showed a dramatic reduction in rates of restenosis compared with bare metal (Morice et al., 2002; Moses et al., 2003; Stone et al., 2004, 2005). Using DES, neointimal proliferation can be reduced further to less than 10%.

Controlled release coatings are the format used in DES, generally comprising a polymeric matrix material and drug mixture. However, one challenge in polymeric matrix stents is the onset of late stent thrombosis, in the causation of which the polymer matrix materials are often implicated. Coronary stents are foreign bodies that can trigger platelet adhesion and activation of the coagulation cascade. However, high-pressure implantation generally causes some vessel injury, including exposure of the thrombogenic subintima, media, and atherosclerotic plaque components to blood. Studies (Kukreja et al., 2008) have shown that healing takes place over an extended period (Figure 6.36), including thrombosis (14 days), inflammation (90 days), smooth muscle cell migration/proliferation (more than 3 months from day 14), extracellular matrix production (3 until 15 months), and extracellular matrix reabsorption (post 1-year event).

The reason that late stent thrombosis is claimed to be a matrix material–induced event is that all the drugs from DES are released within 1 year, with only polymer matrix remaining. Together with the bare metal, polymer matrix is likely to be the component responsible for late stent thrombosis. More biocompatible materials have demonstrated better clinical performance than conventional nonerodible polymer matrix stents (e.g., Cypher and Taxus).

The first perspective of the released controlled coatings is to improve the biocompatibility of the polymer matrix or coating materials in order to target the post-1-year late stent thrombosis. Although not fully accepted by the FDA, erodible polymers such as PLA and PLGA are still used as matrix materials in new DES, such as the Axxess Plus stent (Devax), a nitinol (nickel–titanium) self-expanding thin strut stent, coated with abluminal PLA and

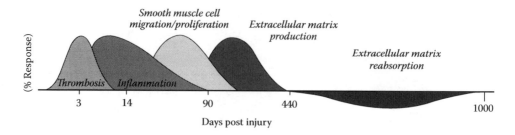

FIGURE 6.36
Typical vessel healing response following bare-metal stent implantation. (Reproduced with permission from Elsevier Ltd. Kukreja et al., *Pharmacol. Res.*, 57, 171–180, 2008.)

biolimus A9 (Grube et al., 2008). However, the second-generation Endeavor ZES stent uses PC to achieve better biocompatibility.

The second perspective is modification of the existing drug regimens that suppress the smooth muscle cell migration and proliferation in the first 3 months after implantation. Two antiproliferative agents, paclitaxel (Honda et al., 2001; Liistro et al., 2002) and sirolimus (Degertekin et al., 2002), have now been widely used in humans with promising results. Its short cellular residence time (1 h), along with reversible antiproliferative activity, suggests that it should be formulated in sustained-release dosage form (Alexis et al., 2004).

Owing to their lipophilic properties, both sirolimus and paclitaxel easily penetrate cells leading to their retention in arterial tissue (Finn et al., 2005; Gummert et al., 1999; Suzuki et al., 2001). Eluting drug in the first 3 months (Table 6.8) suppresses the growth of smooth muscle cells and therefore reduces the rate of restenosis by approximately 80%. Consequently, the use of DES has been swiftly embraced with market penetration of up to 90% in certain countries.

Given the ubiquitous expression of cell-cycle regulatory proteins, it is conceivable that agents released from DES do not only affect proliferation and migration of VSMCs, but also of endothelium. Indeed, sirolimus can inhibit endothelial cell proliferation (Steffel et al., 2005) and migration (Matter et al., 2006) in vitro. Similarly, paclitaxel reduces endothelial cell proliferation and migration through interaction with cell-cycle regulators and, at least in part, through induction of apoptosis (Parry et al., 2005).

In animal models, the time course of reendothelialization after stent implantation varies in different species. In pigs, the extent of reendothelialization is similar for DES and bare metal stenting after 28 days (Suzuki et al., 2001). However, delayed endothelial healing occurs in a rabbit iliac overlapping stent model after implantation of both sirolimus and paclitaxel DES compared to bare metal (Finn et al., 2005). In humans, near complete reendothelialization seems to occur after 3–4 months after bare metal stent implantation (Farb et al., 2003), compared to delayed arterial healing and poor reendothelialization in DES found at autopsy (Joner et al., 2006). Hence, there is clear evidence that the current generation of DES may significantly impair reendothelialization.

In an in vitro study of coronary arterial smooth muscle cells and endothelial cells, it was found that sirolimus reversibly inhibited proliferation of both smooth muscle and endothelial cells in nanomolar concentrations regardless of the duration of exposure (Parry et al., 2005). In contrast, 2-day exposure of paclitaxel on smooth muscle cells was weak with, but 5 days elicited almost complete not reversible cellular inhibition in the low nanomolar range.

TABLE 6.8

Drugs Released from Delivery System on Stents

Stent	Matrix	Drug	Loading Efficiency ($\mu g/cm^2$)	Percentage of Release (%)	Length of the Period (Days)
CYPHER	PEVA/PBMA	Sirolimus	140	80	30
TAXUS	SIBS	Paclitaxel	100	10	90
XIENCE V	Fluoropolymer	Everolimus	100		
Conor	PLGA	Paclitaxel			30

Note: PEVA, poly(ethylene-co-vinyl acetate); PBMA, poly(*n*-butyl methacrylate); SIBS, polystyrene-*b*-isobutylene-*b*-styrene; PLGA, poly(lactide-*co*-glycolide).

Ideally, the released drug should inhibit neointimal hyperplasia by inhibition of one or more of platelet activation, acute inflammation, smooth muscle cell proliferation or migration, extracellular matrix production, angiogenesis, and vascular remodeling, yet preserve vascular healing (van der Hoeven et al., 2005; Sousa et al., 2003) and allow reendothelialization of the injured vessel wall. This seems not to be the case in the current generation of DES.

It has been shown that neointimal growth after bare metal stent implantation in humans peaks at 6–9 months before decreasing slowly for up to 3 years (Kimura et al., 1996), raising the question of the specific timing of antiproliferative drugs, so as to have less negative effect on artery healing.

An alternative approach, concentrating on healing as opposed to cellular inhibition, is used in the Genous endothelial progenitor cell capture stent (OrbusNeich Medical Technologies). This stent appears effective in stable patients (Aoki et al., 2005; Duckers et al., 2007a, 2007b) and also in the setting of acute myocardial infarction (Co et al., 2008).

The third perspective of the released controlled coatings is restructuring of the coating using micro- and nanofabrication techniques. The intention is to minimize the amount of polymer matrix or completely remove it from the release system (Jeffrey et al., 2006). Two new stents, the Janus CarboStent (Sorin Biomedica Cardio S.p.A., Via Crescentino, Italy) and the Conor MedStent (Conor Medsystems, Inc., Menlo Park, CA), contain microfabricated reservoirs for drug release. Both designs contain more drug than first-generation DES and release it specifically toward the vascular wall. In the case of the Janus design, the drug is loaded directly into the sculptures with no polymer matrix. The Conor stent releases the drug from a fully degradable PLGA matrix. This design permits drug release on both the abluminal and adluminal sides of the strut for the controlled containment and elution of multiple drugs.

Nanotextured coatings that enhance cell adhesion can improve the endothelialization of stent struts, and therefore reduce late thrombosis. Local delivery of nanoparticles, combined with ionic or antibody targeting, may allow sustained, high-concentration therapy required to prevent restenosis without reduction in healing.

The last perspective of the released controlled coatings is the complete resorption of the stent within a year, either with or without drugs (Zilberman and Eberhart, 2006). The rationale is to support vessel opening only during its healing process. During resorption, stent mass and strength decreases with time, the mechanical load gradually being transferred to the surrounding tissue. PLLA, PGA, PCL, and PDLLA are the most frequently used aliphatic poly(α-hydroxy-acids) for preparing bioresorbable stents (Eberhart et al., 2003; Nguyen et al., 2004; Kohn and Langer, 2000). The Igaki/Tamai stent is a bioresorbable balloon-expandable design based on PLLA monofilament (Tamai et al., 1999, 2000; Zilberman et al., 2002; Nuutinen et al., 2002; Saito et al., 2002). Animal studies demonstrated that it reduced stenosis in a pig from 64% to 19% at 2 weeks, compared to PLLA knitted type stent (Tsuji et al., 1998). It induced minimal neointimal hyperplasia, whereas moderate to severe neointimal hyperplasia was observed in knitted PLLA stents. The PLLA coil stents also exhibited long-term biocompatibility with minimal inflammatory response after 16 weeks (Tamai et al., 1999; Tsuji et al., 2001).

Other fully erodible stents are reported on trial, and one of these uses just magnesium. It is foreseen that fully erodible stent could be a choice for patients in the future. Release-controlled coatings are likely to become more sophisticated with the ability to provide multiple drug delivery. This is likely to be an evolution of the current coronary stenting devices with release-controlled coatings or drug delivery systems.

References

Abal M, Andreu JM, Barasoain I. 2003. Taxanes microtubule and centrosome targets, and cell cycle dependent mechanisms of action. *Curr Cancer Drug Targets* 3:193–203.

Acharya G and Park K. 2006. Mechanisms of controlled drug release from drug-eluting stents. *Adv Drug Deliv Rev* 58:387–401.

Alexis F, Venkatraman SS, Rath SK, Boey F. 2004. In vitro study of release mechanisms of paclitaxel and rapamycin from drug-incorporated biodegradable stent matrices. *J Control Release* 98:67–74.

American Heart Association. 2003. Heart Disease and Stroke Statistics—2004 Update. Dallas, TX: American Heart Association.

Am. Soc. Health Syst. Pharm. 1989. AHFS Drug Information, pp.1075–1086. Bethseda, MD: Am. Soc. Health Syst. Pharm.

Aoki J, Serruys PW, van Beusekom H et al. 2005. Endothelial progenitor cell capture by stents coated with antibody against CD34: The HEALING-FIM(Healthy Endothelial Accelerated Lining Inhibits Neointimal Growth-First In Man) registry. *J Am Coll Cardiol* 45:1574–1579.

Balmer F, Rotter M, Togni M et al. 2005. Percutaneous coronary interventions in Europe 2000. *Int J Cardiol* 101:457–463.

Bartorelli AL, Trabattoni D, Fabbiocchi F et al. 2003. Synergy of passive coating and target drug delivery: The tacrolimus-eluting Janus Carbostent. *J Interv Cardiol* 16(6):499–505.

Beijk MAM, Klomp M, Verouden NJW et al. 2009. Genous™ endothelial progenitor cell capturing stent vs the Taxus Liberté stent in patients with de novo coronary lesions with a high-risk of coronary restenosis: a randomized, single-centre, pilot study. *Eur Heart J* in press.

Billich A, Aschauer H, Aszódi A et al. 2004. Percutaneous absorption of drugs used in atopic eczema: pimecrolimus permeates less through skin than corticosteroids and tacrolimus. *Int J Pharm* 269:9–35.

Caves JM and Chaikof EL. 2006. The evolving impact of microfabrication and nanotechnology on stent design. *J Vasc Surg* 44:1363–1368.

Chang TY, Yadav VG, De Leo S et al. 2007. Cell and protein compatibility of Parylene-C surface. *Langmuir* 23:11718–11725.

Chadwick DR. 2006. The smaller contenders for the DES market. *Cath Lab Digest* 14:1.1.

Chen MC, Liang HF, Chiu YL et al. 2005. A novel drug-eluting stent spray-coated with multi-layers of collagen and sirolimus. *J Control Release* 108:178–189.

Chen SL and Sheiban I. 2009. Dedicated bifurcation stents strategy. *Interv Cardiol* 4:70–72.

Chevalier B, di Mario C, Neumann FJ et al. 2008. A randomized, controlled, multicenter trial to evaluate the safety and efficiency of Zotarcrolimus-versus paclitaxel-eluting stents in de novo occlusive lesions in coronary arteries: The ZoMaxx I trial. *J Am Coll Cardiol Intv* 1:524–532.

Chudzik SJ, Anderson AB, Chapp RA et al. 2001. Kloke TM: Bioactive agent release coating. United States Patent, Patent No. US 6214901B1, April 10, 2001.

Co M, Tay E, Lee CH et al. 2008. Use of endothelial progenitor cell capture stent (Genous Bio-Engineered R Stent) during primary percutaneous coronary intervention in acute myocardial infarction: Intermediate- to long-term clinical follow-up. *Am Heart J* 155:128–132.

Colombo A and Airoldi F. 2003. Passive coating: The dream does not come true. *J Invas Cardiol* 15(10):566–567.

Colombo A, Drzewiecki J, Banning A et al. 2003. Randomized study to assess the effectiveness of slow-and moderate-release polymer-based paclitaxel-eluting stents for coronary artery lesions. *Circulation* 108:788–794.

Cook S and Windecker S. 2009. Early stent thrombosis: Past, present, and future. *Circulation* 119:657–659.

Cuvelier D, Vezy C, Viallat A et al. 2004. Mimicking cell/extracellular matrix adhesion with lipid membranes and solid substrates: Requirements, pitfalls and proposals. *J Phys Condens Matter* 16:S2427–S2437.

Daemen J and Serruys PW. 2007. Drug-eluting stent update 2007: Part I. A survey of current and future generation drug-eluting stents: Meaningful advances or more of the same? *Circulation* 116:316–328.

Deconinck E, Sohier J, De Scheerder I et al. 2008. Pharmaceutical aspects of drug eluting stents. *J Pharm Sci* 97:5047–5060.

Degertekin M, Serruys PW, Foley DP et al. 2002. Persistent inhibition of neointimal hyperplasia after sirolimus-eluting stent implantation: Long-term (up to 2 years) clinical, angiographic, and intravascular ultrasound follow-up. *Circulation* 106:1610–1613.

de Jaegere P, Serruys PW, van Es GA et al. 1994. Recoil following Wiktor stent implantation for restenotic lesions of coronary arteries. *Cathet Cardiovasc Diagn* 32(2):147–156.

De Jaegere PP, De Feyter PJ, Van der Giessen WJ et al. 1994. Intracoronary stents: A review of the experience with five different devices in clinical use. *J Interv Cardiol* 7(2):117–128.

Doyle B and Holmes Jr DR. 2009. Next generation drug-eluting stents: Focus on bioabsorbable platforms and polymers. *Med Devices Evidence Res* 2:47–55.

Duckers HJ, Silber S, de Winter R et al. 2007a. Circulating endothelial progenitor cells predict angiographic and intravascular ultrasound outcome following percutaneous coronary interventions in the HEALING-II trial: Evaluation of an endothelial progenitor cell capturing stent. *EuroIntervention* 3:67–75.

Duckers HJ, Soullié T, den Heijer P et al. 2007b. Accelerated vascular repair following percutaneous coronary intervention by capture of endothelial progenitor cells promotes regression of neointimal growth at long term follow-up: Final results of the Healing II trial using an endothelial progenitor cell capturing stent (Genous R stent)™. *EuroIntervention* 3:350–358.

Duda SH, Poerner TC, Wiesinger B et al. 2003. Drug-eluting stents: Potential applications for peripheral arterial occlusive disease, *J Vasc Interv Radiol* 14:291–301.

Eberhart RC, Su SH, Nguyen KT et al. 2003. Bioresorbable polymeric stents: Current status and future promise. *J Biomater Sci Polym Ed* 14(4):299–312.

Eggebrecht H, Rodermann J, Hunold P et al. 2005. Images in cardiovascular medicine. Novel magnetic resonance-compatible coronary stent: The absorbable magnesium-alloy stent. *Circulation* 112(18):e303–e304.

Fan W, Johnson DM, Feldman MD. 2009. Metallic stents coated with bioabsorbable polymers, an overview of polymer technology as a drug-carrier mechanism. *Cardiac Interv* Jun/July: 42–49.

Farb A, Burke AP, Kolodgie FD et al. 2003. Pathological mechanisms of fatal late coronary stent thrombosis in humans. *Circulation* 108:1701–1706.

Farb A, Sangiorgi G, Carter AJ et al. 1999. Pathology of acute and chronic coronary stenting in humans. *Circulation* 99:44–52.

Faxon DP. 2002. Systemic drug therapy for restenosis "Déjà Vu all over again." *Circulation* 106:2296–2298.

Finkelstein A, McClean D, Kar S et al. 2003. Local drug delivery via a coronary stent with programmable release pharmacokinetics. *Circulation* 107:777–784.

Finn AV, Kolodgie FD, Harnek J et al. 2005. Differential response of delayed healing and persistent inflammation at sites of overlapping sirolimus- or paclitaxel-eluting stents. *Circulation* 112:270–278.

Finn AV, Nakazawa G, Joner M et al. 2007. Vascular responses to drug eluting stents: Importance of delayed healing. *Arterioscler Thromb Vasc Biol* 27:1500–1510.

Fischman DL, Leon MB, Baim DS et al. 1994. The Stent Restenosis Study Investigators. A randomized comparison of coronary-stent placement and balloon angioplasty in the treatment of coronary artery disease. *N Engl J Med* 331:496–501.

Fishell TA, Dishmon D, Elhaddi A et al. 2009. The perfect drug-eluting stent: Goals for stent, polymer, and drug development. *Cardiac Interv Today* June/July:29–35.

Fortin JB and Lu TM. 2004. *Chemical Vapour Deposition Polymerization: The Growth and Properties of Parylene Thin Films*. Kluwer Academic Publishers, Boston USA.

Gottsauner-Wolf M, Moliterno DJ, Lincoff AM et al. 1996. Restenosis—an open file. *Clin Cardiol* 19(5):347–356.

Grabow N, Martin DP, Schmitz KP et al. 2009. Absorbable polymer stent technologies for vascular regeneration. *J Chem Technol Biotechnol* 26 Oct 2009 online (http://www3.interscience.wiley .com/cgi-bin/fulltext/122662738/PDFSTART).

Griffiths H, Peeters P, Verbist J et al. 2004. Future devices: Bioabsorbable stents. *Br J Cardiol (Acute Interv Cardiol)* 11:AIC 80–AIC 84.

Grube E, Sievert H, Hauptmann KE et al. 2008. Novel drug eluting stent system for customised treatment of coronary lesions: CUSTOM I feasibility trial 24 month results. *EuroIntervention* 4(1):71–76.

Gummert JF, Ikonen T, Morris RE. 1999. Newer immunosuppressive drugs: A review. *J Am Soc Nephrol* 10:1366–1380.

Haraguchi G, Pruitt S, Brodeur A et al. 2006. Increased expression of eNOS by Endeavor zotarolimus-eluting stents compared to other DES in porcine coronary artery implants. *Am J Cardiol* 98(Suppl):32–33.

Hofma SH, van der Giessen WJ, van Dalen BM et al. 2006. Indication of long-term endothelial dysfunction after sirolimus-eluting stent implantation. *Eur Heart J* 27:166–170.

Honda Y, Grube E, de la Fuente LM et al. 2001. Novel drug-delivery stent: Intravascular ultrasound observations from the first human experience with the QP2-eluting polymer stent system. *Circulation* 104:380–383.

Horres R, Linssen MK, Hoffmann M et al. 2004. Medical products comprising a haemocompatible coating, production and use thereof. US Patent US2004/0234575 A1, Nov 25, 2004.

Jeffrey SC, Andreyka JB, Bernhardt SX et al. 2006. Development and properties of beta-glucuronide linkers for monoclonal antibody–drug conjugates. *Bioconjug Chem* 17(3):831–840.

Joner M, Finn AV, Farb A et al. 2006. Pathology of drug-eluting stents in humans: Delayed healing and late thrombotic risk. *J Am Coll Cardiol* 48:193–202.

Juan AS, Bala M, Hlawaty H et al. 2009. Development of a functionalized polymer for stent coating in arterial delivery of small interfering RNA. *Biomacromolecules* 10:3074–3080.

King 3rd SB, Schlumpf M. 1996. Ten-year completed follow-up of percutaneous transluminal coronary angioplasty: The early Zurich experience. *J Am Coll Cardiol* 22(2):353–360.

Kimura T, Yokoi H, Nakagawa Y et al. 1996. Three-year follow-up after implantation of metallic coronary-artery stents. *N Engl J Med* 334:561–566.

Kohn J, Langer R. 2000. Bioresorbable and bioerodible materials. In *Biomaterials Science—An Introduction to Materials in Medicine*, ed. BD Ratner, AS Hoffman, FJ Schoen, JE Lemons, 64–73. New York, NY: Academic Press.

Kukreja N, Onuma Y, Daemen J et al. 2008. The future of drug-eluting stents. *Pharmacol Res* 57:171–180.

Kumari A, Tadav SK, Yadav SC. 2010. Biodegradable polymeric nanoparticles based drug delivery systems. *ColloidsSurf B Biointerfaces* 75:1–18.

Lafont A, Topol E. 1997. *Arterial Remodeling: A Critical Factor in Restenosis*. Boston, MA: Kluwer Academic Publishers.

Leon MB, Abizaid A, Moses JW. 2003. *The CYPHER™ Stent: A New Gold Standard in the Treatment of Coronary Artery Disease*. New York, NY: The Cardiovascular Research Foundation, 90 pp.

Lewis AL. 2006. PC technology™ as a platform for drug delivery, from combination to conjugation. *Expert Opin Drug Deliv* 3(2):289–298.

Lincoff M, Furst M, Ellis M et al. 1997. Sustained local delivery of dexamethasone by a novel intravascular eluting stent to prevent restenosis in the porcine coronary injury model. *J Am Coll Cardiol* 29:808–816.

Liistro F, Stankovic G, Di Mario C et al. 2002. First clinical experience with a paclitaxel derivate-eluting polymer stent system implantation for in-stent restenosis: Immediate and long-term clinical and angiographic outcome. *Circulation* 105:1883–1886.

Marx SO, Marks AR. 2001. Bench to bedside: The development of rapamycin and its application to stent restenosis. *Circulation* 104(8):852–855.

Matter CM, Rozenberg I, Jaschko A et al. 2006. Effects of tacrolimus or sirolimus on proliferation of vascular smooth muscle and endothelial cells. *J Cardiovasc Pharmacol* 48:286–292.

Mehilli J, Kastrati A, Wessely R et al. 2006. Randomised trial of a nonpolymer-based rapamycin-eluting stent versus a polymer-based paclitaxel-eluting stent for the reduction of late lumen loss. *Circulation* 113(2):273–279.

Meng S, Liu Z, Shen L et al. 2009. The effect of a layer-by-layer chitosan-heparin coating on the endothelialization and coagulation properties of a coronary stent system. *Biomaterials* 30:2276–2283.

Menown I, Lowe R, Penn I. 2005. Passive stent coatings in the drug-eluting era. *J Invas Cardiol* 17:222–228.

Morice M-C, Serruys PW, Sousa JE et al. 2002. A randomized comparison of a sirolimus eluting stent with a standard stent for coronary revascularization. *New Engl J Med* 346:1773–1780.

Moses JW, Leon MB, Popma JP et al. 2003. Sirolimus-eluting stents versus standard stents in patients with stenosis in a native coronary artery. *New Engl J Med* 349:1315–1323.

Nakazawa G, Finn AV, Kolodgie FD et al. 2009. A review of current devices and a look at new technology: Drug-eluting stents. *Expert Rev Med Devices* 6(1):33–42.

Nguyen K, Su SH, Zilberman M et al. 2004. Biomaterials and stent technology. In *Tissue Engineering and Novel Delivery Systems*, ed. M Yaszemski, D Trantolo, KU Lewandrowski, V Hasirci, D Altobelli, D Wise, 5, 107–130. New York, NY: Marcel Dekker.

Nuutinen JP, Valimaa T, Clerc C . 2002. Mechanical properties and in vitro degradation of bioresorbable knitted stents. *J Biomater Sci Polym Ed* 13(12):1313–1323.

Otake H, Shimohama T, Tsujino I et al. 2009. Abstract 4156: Comparison of sirolimus-eluting NEVO™ stents with paclitaxel-eluting CoStar™ Stents and paclitaxel-eluting Taxus Liberte™ stents: Insights from intravascular ultrasound analysis of the Res-elution I and CoStar II trials. *Circulation* 120: S915.

Park TG. 1995. Degradation of poly(lactic-*co*-glycolic acid) microspheres: Effect of copolymer composition. *Biomaterials* 16:1123–1130.

Parry TJ, Brosius R, Thyagarajan R et al. 2005. Drug-eluting stents: Sirolimus and paclitaxel differentially affect cultured cells and injured arteries. *Eur J Pharmacol* 524:19–29.

Ranade K, Shue WH, Hung YJ et al. 2001. The glycine allele of a glycine/arginine polymorphism in the beta2-adrenergic receptor gene is associated with essential hypertension in a population of Chinese origin. *Am J Hypertens* 14(12):1196–1200.

Ranade S, Miller KM, Richard RE et al. 2004. Physical characterization of controlled release of paclitaxel from the TAXUS Express™ drug-eluting stent. *J Biomed Mater Res* 71A:625–634.

Raval A, Choubey A, Engineer C et al. 2007. Novel biodegradable polymeric matrix coated cardiovascular stent for controlled drug delivery. *Trends Biomater Artif Organs* 20(2):131–141.

Rhodes CT and Porter SC. 1998. Coatings for controlled release drug delivery systems. *Drug Dev Ind Pharm* 24(12):1139–1154.

Rowinsky EK, Donehower RC.1995. Drug therapy: Paclitaxel (Taxol). *N Engl J Med* 332:1002–1014.

Saito Y, Minami K, Kobayashi M et al. 2002. New tubular bioabsorbable knitted airway stent: Biocompatibility and mechanical strength. *J Thorac Cardiovasc Surg* 123:161–167.

Schömig A, Kastrati A, Wessely R. 2005. Prevention of restenosis by systemic drug therapy. Back to the future? *Circulation* 112:2759–2761.

Serruys PW, de Jaegere P, Kiemeneij F et al. 1994. The Benestent Study Group. A comparison of balloon-expandable-stent implantation with balloon angioplasty in patients with coronary artery disease. *N Engl J Med* 331:489–495.

Serruys PW, Sianos G, Abizaid A et al. 2005. The effect of variable dose and release kinetics on neointimal hyperplasia using a novel paclitaxel-eluting stent platform: The Paclitaxel In-Stent Controlled Elution Study (PISCES). *J Am Coll Cardiol* 46:253–260.

Sousa JE, Costa MA, Abizaid A et al. 2001. Lack of neointimal proliferation after implantation of sirolimus-coated stents in human coronary arteries: A quantitative coronary angiography and three-dimensional intravascular ultrasound study. *Circulation* 103:192–195.

Sousa JE, Serruys PW, Costa MA. 2003. New frontiers in cardiology. Drug-eluting stents: Part 1. *Circulation* 107:2274–2279.

Steffel J, Latini RA, Akhmedov A et al. 2005. Rapamycin, but not FK-506, increases endothelial tissue factor expression: Implications for drug-eluting stent design. *Circulation* 112:2002–2011.

Stone GW, Ellis SG, Cox DA et al. 2004. A polymer-based, paclitaxel eluting stent in patients with coronary artery disease. *New Engl J Med* 350:221–231.

Stone GW, Ellis SG, Cannon L et al. 2005. the TAXUS V Investigators. Comparison of a polymer-based paclitaxel-eluting stent with a bare metal stent in patients with complex coronary artery disease: A randomized controlled trial. *JAMA* 294:1215–1223.

Suzuki T, Kopia G, Hayashi S et al. 2001. Stent-based delivery of sirolimus reduces neointimal formation in a porcine coronary model. *Circulation* 104:1188–1193.

Tamai H, Igaki K, Kyo E et al. 2000. Initial and 6-month results of biodegradable poly-L-lactic acid coronary stents in humans. *Circulation* 102:399–404.

Tamai H, Igaki K, Tsuji T et al. 1999. A biodegradable poly-L-lactic acid coronary stent in porcine coronary artery. *J Interv Cardiol* 12:443–449.

Tarcha PJ, Verlee D, Hui HW et al. 2007. The application of ink-jet technology for the coating and loading of drug-eluting stents. *Ann Biomed Eng* 35 (10):1791–1799.

Tesfamariam B. 2008. Drug release kinetics from stent device-based delivery systems. *J Cardiovasc Pharmacol* 51:118–125.

Tsuji T, Tamai H, Kyo E. 1998. The effect of PLLA stent design on neointimal hyperplasia. *J Cardiol* 32:235A.

Tsuji T, Tamai H, Igaki K et al. 2001. Biodegradable polymeric stents. *Curr Interv Cardiol Rep* 3:10–17.

Udipi K, Melder RJ, Chen M et al. 2007. The next generation Endeavor Resolute stent: Role of the BioLinx™ polymer system. *EuroIntervention* 3:137–139.

Udipi K, Chen M, Cheng P et al. 2008. Development of a novel biocompatible polymer system for extended drug release in a next-generation drug eluting stent. *J Biomed Mater Res* 85A: 1064–1071.

Unger F, Westedt U, Hanefeld P et al. 2007. Poly(ethylene carbonate): Athermoelastic and biodegradable biomaterial for drug eluting stent coatings? *J Control Release* 117:312–321.

van der Hoeven BL, Pires NMM, Warda HM et al. 2005. Drug eluting stents: Results, promises and problems. *Int J Cardiol* 99:9–17.

VanTeeffelen JW, Brands J, Stroes ES et al. 2007. Endothelial glycoc lyx: Sweet shield of blood vessels. *Trends Cardiovasc Med* 17:101–105.

Venkatraman S and Boey F. 2007. Release profiles in drug-eluting stents: Issues and uncertainties. *J Control Release* 120:149–160.

Vert M. 2009. Degradable and bioresorbable polymers in surgery and in pharmacology: Beliefs and facts. *J Mater Sci MM* 20:437–446.

Virmani R, Farb A. 1999. Pathology of in-stent restenosis. *Curr Opin Lipidol* 10:499–506.

Vogel J, Sperandio M, Pries AR et al. 2000. Influence of the endothelial glycocalyx on cerebral blood flow in mice. *J Cereb Blood Flow Metab* 20:1571–1578.

von Recum HA, Cleek RL, Eskin SG et al. 1995. Degradation of polydispersed poly(L-lactic acid) to modulate lactic acid release. *Biomaterials* 16:441–447.

Wessely R, Hausleiter J, Michaelis C et al. 2005. Stent system that allow for dose-adjustable, multiple, and on-site stent coating. *Arterioscler Thromb Vasc Biol* 25:748–753.

Wieneke H, Dirsch O, Sawitowski T et al. 2003. Synergistic effects of a novel nanoporous stent coating and tacrolimus on intima proliferation in rabbits. *Catheter Cardiovasc Interv* 60:399–407.

Windecker S, Serruys PW, Wandel S et al. 2008. Biolimus-eluting stent with biodegradable polymer versus sirolimus-eluting stent with durable polymer for coronary revascularization (LEADERS): A randomized non-inferiority trial. *Lancet* 372:1163–1173.

Wolf KV, Zong Z, Meng J et al. 2008. An investigation of adhesion in drug-eluting stent layers. *J Biomed Mater Res* 87A:272–281.

Wright D, Rajalingam B, Selvarasah S et al. 2007. Generation of static and dynamic pattered co-cultures using microfabricated parylene-C stencils. *Lab Chip* 7:1272–1279.

Zilberman M, Eberhart RC. 2006. Drug-eluting bioresorbable stents for various applications. *Annu Rev Biomed Eng* 8:153–180.

Zilberman M, Eberhart R, Schwade N. 2002. In vitro study of drug loaded bioresorbable films and support structures. *J Biomater Sci Polym Ed* 13:1221–1240.

Zollinger M, Waldmeier F, Hartmann S et al. 2006. Pimecrolimus: Absorption, distribution, metabolism, and excretion in healthy volunteers after a single oral dose and supplementary investigations in vitro. *Drug Metab Dispos* 34:765–774.

7

Orthopedic and Dental Implant Surfaces and Coatings

Racquel Z. LeGeros, Paulo G. Coelho, David Holmes,
Fred Dimaano, and John P. LeGeros

CONTENTS

Introduction 301
Implant Surfaces—Basics 303
Basic Research Methods for Implant Surface Evaluation 304
    Biocompatibility of Biomaterials..304
    In Vitro Testing..305
    In Vivo Testing 306
    Clinical Evaluation of Implant Surfaces 309
    Implant Retrieval Analysis 310
Surface Treatments to Modify Implant Topography... 310
    Surface Roughening by Grit-Blasting with Abrasives.. 314
    Surface Modifications by Laser Texturing 314
    Surface Modifications Using Chemical Methods 314
Bioactive Surface Coatings 315
    Plasma-Sprayed HA Coatings 316
    Alternatives to Plasma-Spray Technique of Depositing Calcium Phosphate Coating....... 320
Surface Treatments to Introduce Osteoinductivity 324
Surface Treatments and Coatings with Antibacterial Properties 325
Summary and Conclusion 325
Acknowledgments... 326
References... 326

Introduction

Replacement of missing or diseased hard tissues (teeth and bones) has become a common procedure in medicine and dentistry. Materials employed in the manufacture of orthopedic and dental implants include metals and metal alloys, ceramics, polymers, and composites (e.g., metal/metal, ceramic/ceramic, metal/ceramic, ceramic/polymer) (Ratner et al., 2004). The different metals and metal alloys employed in the commercial manufacture of orthopedic and dental implants include cobalt–chromium–molybdenum (Co–Cr–Mo) alloy, stainless steel, commercially pure titanium (cpTi), Ti alloy (Ti_6Al_4V), tantalum (Black, 1994; Christie, 2002; Ratner et al., 2004; Williams, 1981). CpTi and Ti alloys have become the metals of choice, especially for dental implants, because of their desirable properties that include corrosion resistance, biocompatibility, strength, and the presence of a reactive Ti oxide surface layer (Brunette et al., 2001; Faria et al., 2008; Lemons, 2004; Park et al., 2008; Steinmann, 1998; Williams, 1981).

Ideally, a successful orthopedic or dental implant should have a long-term skeletal fixation with the host bone (see reviews by Albrektsson and Wenneberg, 2004; Coelho et al., 2009; Stevens et al., 2008) and be free of later complications, especially microbial infection (Garvin and Hannsen, 1995; Mombelli, 1997; Zimmerli et al., 2004). A considerable number of investigations have focused on modifying the implant surface, especially dental implants, to enhance bone contact or bone anchorage, defined as osseointegration (Albrektsson and Wenneberg, 2004; Coelho et al., 2009; Narayanan et al., 2008; Stevens et al., 2008). Fewer studies, especially on dental implants, have focused on implant surface treatments that would prevent bacterial adhesion, growth, and colonization (Das et al., 2008; Shi et al., 2008; Tabanella et al., 2009; Zhao et al., 2009). Even fewer studies have addressed both osseointegration and antibacterial property in the same implant.

The term "osseointegration" was originally introduced by Brannemark (1969, 1977) to describe "a close implant–bone contact at the light microscopic level." However, at the electron microscopic level, nonmineralized fibrous interface is observed between the cpTi or Ti alloy and the host bone (Daculsi et al., 1995) as shown in Figure 7.1. Such fibrous tissue interface is a weak one and when subjected to micromotion may lead to implant loosening and eventual implant failure. To enhance osseointegration, several surface modifications have been developed especially for dental implants (Albrektsson and Wenneberg, 2004; Coelho et al., 2009; Narayanan et al., 2008; Stevens et al., 2008). These modifications can be classified into two general categories: (1) surface treatments to modify topography and (2) deposition of bioactive surface coatings, such as by deposition of calcium phosphate coatings (Figure 7.1).

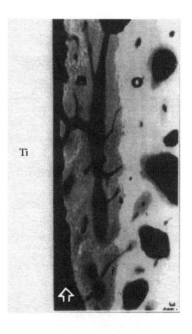

FIGURE 7.1
SEM image showing a gap (occupied by fibrous tissue) between Ti alloy implant surface and host bone indicating absence of true osseointegration. (From Daculsi et al., *Scan. Microsc.*, 4, 309–314, 1995. With permission.)

Studies on surface treatments to prevent bacterial infection have been reviewed by Das et al. (2008) and Zhao et al. (2009).

This chapter presents a critical appraisal of basic methods employed in implant research and a review of studies on implant surface treatments that modify topography, introduce bioactivity, and introduce antibacterial property, incorporating published reviews and past and current studies by the authors.

Implant Surfaces—Basics

The implant–bone interface can be visualized at macroscopic and molecular levels (Kasemo and Lausmaa, 1988). In case of Ti or Ti alloy (Ti_6Al_4V) implants, the metal substrate is covered by the always present surface oxide, TiO_2, to which protein molecules from the biologic liquid attach themselves (Figure 7.2). The nature of the biomolecular layer determines

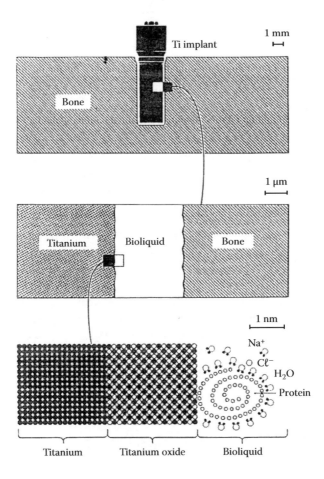

FIGURE 7.2
Ti implant and bone interface at the tissue, cellular, and atomic levels. (From Kasemo, B., Lasumaa, J., *Int. J. Oral Maxillofac. Implants*, 3, 247–239, 1988. With permission.)

the cell response (proliferation, differentiation) that would eventually lead to bone formation. For this reason, the microarchitecture of the surface (topography, roughness, etc.) and its chemical composition are important determinants of the response of the biologic system to the implant.

Immediately after implant placement, a series of events occur between the host and the surface of the implants (Lemons, 2004). This sequence of events includes the initial interaction between blood and the implant surface, where proteins and ligands are dynamically adsorbed onto and released from the implant surface, through an inflammatory process, which is followed by initial bone formation around the implant (modeling), and through several remodeling cycles, where bone surrounding the implant achieves its highest degree of organization and mechanical properties (Lemons, 2004). Because of the dynamic nature of the bone–biomaterial interface as a function of implantation time, endosseous dental implant biomaterials must have short- and long-term biocompatible and biofunctional properties (Coelho et al., 2009).

From the point of view of physics, a surface may be defined as the sudden interruption of the atomic arrangement. This sudden interruption results in differences between surface and bulk electronic properties, leading to different physico/chemical behavior between the two regions of the material. Therefore, from a theoretical standpoint, different modification methods utilized for implant surface engineering may lead to different and unique surface properties (Kittel, 1995). These different physico/chemical properties can potentially lead to changes in the host-to-implant response. New surface treatments should be tested as new biomaterials. As examples, the alteration of surface topography or the incorporation of bioactive ceramics as coatings have been investigated and utilized on a large scale by implant dentistry practitioners with no or limited surface characterization (Lemons, 2004; Coelho et al., 2009).

Despite the extensive literature accumulated over the past decades concerning the host/ biomaterial response, several considerations should be taken into account concerning the complex effects of endosseous dental implants surface modifications during and after the process of osseointegration. Biological considerations, such as biocompatibility and osseoconductivity of the implant, should be addressed. In addition, specific surface effects on initial bone healing kinetics and mechanical properties evolution as implantation time elapses in vivo, as well as the in vivo stability of the surface (often regarded as one of the leading factors of long-term osseointegration) should be hierarchically investigated to more fully evaluate implant therapy surgical and/or prosthetic protocol modifications.

A hierarchical approach, where in vitro testing followed by laboratory animal research leads to subsequent controlled prospective and/or retrospective clinical trials, is often neglected before new biomaterials are commercially introduced. Therefore, treatment protocol changes, such as a decrease in the time allowed for osseointegration of immediate/ early loaded dental implants, have often followed empirical rationales.

Basic Research Methods for Implant Surface Evaluation

Biocompatibility of Biomaterials

Before clinical trials, new biomaterials (including surface modifications) should undergo in vitro and in vivo evaluation. This type of evaluation typically follows a hierarchical approach, where in vitro testing evolves to in vivo laboratory experiments, and then to clinical trials in humans (Lemons, 2004). The hierarchical testing approach is useful in cases where surface modifications are compared with previous surfaces that have successfully been in function for several years. In a simplistic fashion, if the new surface or biomaterial does not have at least equivalent performance when tested in in vitro and in vivo laboratory models, time-consuming complex clinical research protocols may be avoided.

In Vitro Testing

In vitro laboratory models often consist of evaluating the effects of novel surfaces versus control surfaces (in the case of dental implant surfaces, machined or surface-modified cpTi or Ti alloys) on cell cultures (Groth et al., 2005).

Cell culture studies attempt to track cell morphology, adhesion, migration, proliferation, or death as a function of potentially toxic agents derived from the biomaterial (Lemons, 2004). Whereas in vitro cell culture evaluations have been shown to be useful for preliminary evaluation of novel biomaterials biocompatibility related to safety, results obtained in cell cultures have not yet been fully correlated to in vivo performance (Groth et al., 2005; Coelho et al., 2009). Specific to evaluating cellular behavior associated with implant surfaces, cell cultures by no means represent the dynamic in vivo bone/biomaterial environment, and multiple conclusions concerning the potential in vivo behavior based on in vitro cell testing should be taken as speculation. Validation must be based on animal models and subsequent clinical trials. Nonetheless, cell culture has been useful as a first assessment of biocompatibility related to the safety of novel biomaterial designs (Groth et al., 2005).

Implant surface modifications through chemical process may lead to production of leachable products potentially toxic to cells (Nimomya et al., 2001; Santavirta et al., 1999). Direct contact, agar diffusion, and extract dilution are the primary cytocompatibility assays, where standardized procedures enable comparisons and minimize bias. The inclusion of positive and negative controls and the use of established cell lines and standardized protocols published by the U.S. Pharmacopeia, the American Society for Testing and Materials (ASTM), the British Standards Institute (BSI), and International Standards Organization (ISO) rationalize the screening for cytocompatible biomaterials (ISO 10993-5; 1999). It is worthwhile to mention that health organizations in the United States (Food and Drug Administration), Brazil (National Agency of Sanitary Vigilance), Europe, and other countries legally require pharmacopeial assays for regulatory and commercialization of biomaterials and medical devices (Schildhauer et al., 2008; Tamaki et al., 2008). What remains to be fully explored are cell functions, such as adhesion, migration, proliferation, synthesis, and deposition of extracellular matrix chemical compounds using mammalian cells of the tissue/organ relevant to specific applications.

Considering new biomaterials, an understanding of biomaterial-induced cell signaling molecules is strategic for device design. For instance, the role of monocytes/macrophages in foreign body reaction has become evident (Schildhauer et al., 2008; Tamaki et al., 2008), and specific information concerning the osteoblast (Lenz et al., 2008) and osteoclast (Makihira et al., 2007) responses to wear particles and surface topography can be screened in specific in vitro assays of cell signaling molecules. Thus, currently available in vitro assays have increasingly gained popularity in biomedical device designing regarding materials safety.

On the other hand, whereas biomaterials safety is currently tested in in vitro assays, regulatory and scientific governmental agencies, such as the National Institutes of Health in the United States, have expressed interest in developing more complex laboratory-based testing methods. The intent is to develop models that are more representative and predictive of in vivo behavior such as organ cultures presenting similar cellular content and architecture as the host tissue.

The development of bone organ cultures requires the maintenance of three-dimensional bone explants and their cellular and extracellular content in the laboratory setting (Jones et al., 2008). In addition to biological content maintenance in vitro, the physiologic-like maintenance of bone organ cultures has been challenged by difficulties in appropriately reproducing physiologic loading conditions in vitro (Jones et al., 2008). Such difficulties have resulted in the limited use of bone organ culture studies of hard tissue integration, which requires establishment and maintenance of cultures for long periods. However, bone organ cultures have been utilized in other research areas such as the effects of wear particle composition and size in bone inflammatory response (Zhang et al., 2008).

It is acknowledged that despite the current difficulties and limitations provided by in vitro cell and organ cultures, developments will soon result in cell and organ cultures that are more representative of in vivo scenarios. Such developments will expand the in vitro evaluation of biomaterials beyond safety issues, mimicking in vivo testing conditions decreasing the time, cost, and regulatory issues concerning animal research protocols.

In Vivo Testing

After in vitro laboratory testing for the general safety of new biomaterials' surfaces, laboratory in vivo models are the next step in biocompatibility testing complexity.

Various animal models and surgical protocols have been utilized to evaluate the host response to endosseous implants (Coelho et al., 2009). Despite the development of an extensive literature in the field, variations in wound healing and the kinetics of bone healing due to local physiologic properties of different surgical sites and animal species have not been sufficiently characterized to enable direct one-to-one comparisons between animal models or data extrapolation to human clinical scenarios. Nonetheless, animal models are of vital importance when novel biomaterial design is compared with previously investigated designs of known clinical performance.

The most frequently used animals for dental implant research are rats, rabbits, sheep, dogs, pigs, and nonhuman primates. Among the attributes taken into consideration to determine which animal model is most appropriate for a particular research protocol are site similarity to humans under physiologic and pathologic conditions as well as availability of large numbers of specimens over time (Pearce et al., 2007; Lienbschner et al., 2004). Other considerations include acceptability to the society, cost, availability, age, size (multiple implant placement for comparison), tolerance to surgery and captivity, housing, and animal protection acts of different countries (Schimandle et al., 1994). Specific to studies considering the bone–implant interface, bone macrostructure, microstructure, and modeling/remodeling kinetics should be considered while extrapolating results to humans (Schimandle et al., 1994).

Because of its relatively low cost, ease of handling, and a substantial number of previously published data, the rabbit model has been the most utilized for dental implant bone–implant interface studies. The amount of published work is then followed by research protocols utilizing dogs (Pearce et al., 2007; Lienbschner et al., 2004). Detailed information regarding other animal models utilized in bone–implant interface studies can be found elsewhere (Pearce et al., 2007; Lienbschner et al., 2004).

Despite its extensive use in dental implant research, the rabbit model's major drawback includes its size compared with larger animals, such as dogs and sheep, when a number of control and experimental implants are recommended per animal (ISO 10993-6). In addition, the commonly utilized rabbit bones such as tibia and femur are one of the least similar animal models compared to human (Castaneda et al., 2006). Significantly different bone macrostructure (especially when comparing the amount of trabecular bone between human alveolar bone and rabbit long bones), microstructure, kinetics, and cell content are found between rabbit and human. Thus, the extrapolation of results obtained in rabbit studies relative to humans is a challenge and should be carefully performed.

The second most utilized model in musculoskeletal and dental implant research is the canine model (Neyt et al., 1998). Compared with the rabbit model, the canine model is remarkably larger, and different sites with relatively different bone macromorphology and micromorphology are available.

Considering the canine intraoral site, extraction of the four premolars followed by a healing period before implant placement has been commonly employed. Alternative to the intraoral site, the femur and the tibia have also been utilized. Whereas the intraoral site provides a bone microstructure that is morphologically similar to human mandible with respect to cortical-to-trabecular ratio, the tibia and femur sites provide a model where high amounts of trabecular bone are present (Coelho et al., 2009). The elimination of potential complications involved in tooth extraction makes the tibia and femur attractive relative to the dog intraoral sites. In addition, the presence of high amounts of trabecular bone in these long bones is attractive for testing dental implant properties because highly osteo-conductive materials are desirable for regions of low cortical-to-trabecular bone ratios. Specific to dental implant surface research, where most protocols comprise the temporal placement of implants for comparison in physiologically loaded implants, relative differences in osseointegration and biomechanical assessment can be tracked in both mandible and long bones such as the femur and tibia (Coelho et al., 2009).

It has been previously shown that dog along with pig bones are the most similar to human bone composition among the animal models utilized for musculoskeletal research (Aerssens et al., 1998). However, data extrapolation between these large animals and humans is still challenged by the different mineral apposition rates (MAR) encountered at different bones (Aerssens et al., 1998). Another drawback related to larger animal models is the ethical issue of their utilization in medical research, especially concerning the number of animals and operable sites/times per animal.

There are many different animal models, surgical sites, times in vivo, and the lack of a standard control biomaterial (i.e., a standard implant surface) among the many in vivo studies reported in the dental literature. Therefore, direct comparison between previously published results is practically impossible with respect to which implant surface has the best physico/chemical configuration to increase early wound healing kinetics.

Regardless of differences in species and site, it is acknowledged that valuable information may be retrieved from properly designed animal studies. Specific to comparison between different implant surfaces, power analysis should be performed relative to the parameter to be evaluated because this dictates the number of animals to be utilized. Because implant surfaces are expected to increase the host-to-implant response, it is recommended that several implantation times be utilized to establish temporal evolution of the analyzed variables between implant surfaces. The implantation times should be determined from the literature pertinent to each species and site, or from pilot investigations. Regardless of animal model, it is acknowledged that extrapolation of results to human scenarios is a challenge. However, controlled animal studies evaluating temporal changes in the bone–implant interface provide valuable relative comparisons between different implant surfaces.

Measurable indicators of the host/implant response have been utilized in cases where two different surface designs are compared. However, to decrease the degree of speculation with respect to the most critical mechanisms of the host/implant response between different surface designs, the largest possible number of biological response indicators (static and dynamic histomorphometric parameters, plus biomechanical testing) should be evaluated to establish correlations.

Substantial data have been published concerning the temporal evolution of various bone–biomaterial interfaces. Yet, whether the increased mechanical stability of different surfaces is due to an increased mechanical locking of tissue within the surface roughness, increased bone–implant contact, increased surrounding bone density, biologically modified bone bonding, or the interplay between such variables is still controversial or unknown (Lemons, 2004). Often, a combination of factors exists.

In vivo comparisons between different implant surface designs typically have a histomorphometric and/or a biomechanical component. The histomorphometric part of the study typically evaluates static parameters such as the amount of bone-to-implant contact (BIC), bone density, amount and type of cellular content, among others. Less often reported, but not less valuable than the static measurements, dynamic histomorphometric parameters, such as MAR, have also been utilized. The biomechanical testing component usually evaluates the push-out force, pull-out force, or torque-to-interface failure of implants in bone (Coelho et al., 2009).

It has been established that general tissue response to implants, biocompatibility, and osseoconductivity information may be obtained through static histomorphometric measurements. However, any of the previously mentioned parameters alone does not address the tissue healing events that lead to the measured parameters evaluated at a given period in vivo (Coelho et al., 2009). For example, if a given surface results in higher BIC percentage relative to another at early implantation times, it is impossible to determine the relevance of such observation unless extreme differences in BIC values were observed or a series of other supporting histomorphometric and biomechanical parameters were also measured. From a structural perspective, the BIC amount may be overwhelmed by the quality of the structural support, and implants surrounded by less bone with higher magnitude mechanical properties may be more desirable than an implant surrounded by more bone presenting lower magnitude mechanical properties. This concept should be taken into account especially as bone has the ability to model and remodel under microstrain thresholds (bone deformation under a given load), and bone regions of high stress concentrations in the proximity of the implant may be unfavorable if low-magnitude bone mechanical properties exist.

Because BIC has been the most often measured parameter in in vivo investigations, meticulous histomorphologic and biomechanical testing (preferentially nanoindentation along and away from the implant surface) should also be performed to decrease the degree of speculation concerning the benefit of increased BIC for one surface relative to another. In this case, dynamic measurements such as MAR would be desirable to temporally evaluate bone modeling/remodeling kinetics around different implant surfaces. This would provide insight on how different histomorphologic, histomorphometric, and bone mechanical properties evolved as a function of implantation time.

Studies concerning the effect of different surfaces in bone healing kinetics have been successful in indicating relationships between MAR and static parameters such as density (Suzuki et al., 1997). Unfortunately, the literature concerning bone healing dynamics around different implant surfaces is not only sparse but also contradictory. Also, comprehensive studies utilizing both static and dynamic histomorphometric parameters along with biomechanical testing are desirable for better characterization of the evolution of the bone–biomaterial interface around different implant surfaces. This information would decrease the degree of speculation concerning the mechanisms leading to differences in the results.

Ex vivo standard biomechanical tests (torque, pull-out, push-out) usually measure the amount of force or torque to failure of the bone–biomaterial interface surrounding different implant surfaces. Although information concerning the relative degree of biomechanical fixation is obtained, these tests do not provide detailed microscopic information about inherent mechanical properties of the bone–biomaterial interface. In addition, these test methods tend to favor rough implant surfaces, making it a challenge to evaluate different implant surface effects on the evolution of bone healing/mechanical properties.

Recently, nanoindentation studies have successfully evaluated the effect of different surface textures in bone mechanical properties as a function of implantation time (Butz et al., 2005). Although inherent mechanical property measurements made as a function of time may be assessed through nanoindentation, the value of relative changes in modulus and hardness as a function of healing time around implants is still subjective. For example, it is not possible to predict by simple mechanical property assessment over a given loading range, if stress patterns or microstrain threshold for bone maintenance or loss would significantly affect the overall biomechanical response as a function of implant surface and implantation time. Thus, biomechanical experimental designs that take into consideration both the bone mechanical properties and the geometry around the implant (through 3D imaging tools) are desirable for future designing of improved dental implant systems.

Several factors that influence the phenomena of osseointegration remain under active investigation (i.e., implant/biofluid interactions, the elemental chemistry and structure of surfaces, and the overall mechanisms and kinetics of bone response to implants). Therefore, what is needed is careful interpretation of the literature along with definitive characterization of bone physiology and kinetics of healing (MAR, bone mechanical properties) around implants with different surfaces. The evaluation of the highest possible number of host/implant response parameters should be taken into account in future research. This approach would allow a better understanding of bone healing kinetics associated with different implant surfaces, providing an informed design rationale for future implant systems that would deliver reduced osseointegration time frames and minimize failures of immediate/early loaded implants.

Clinical Evaluation of Implant Surfaces

Clinical evaluation comprises the most complex type of device testing, especially the factors associated with the biomaterial per se. Although clinical data collection may illustrate the interaction between human tissues and different implant surfaces, from a statistical standpoint, any data collected from clinical trials should be interpreted with caution. Clinical evaluation of different implant surfaces may be a challenge, as large numbers of subjects must be analyzed in a previously determined statistically validated model, and any deviation from the established protocol may lead to results with low credibility. Both prospective and retrospective studies must be carefully designed with a rigorous number of subjects, inclusion, and exclusion criteria. Because the description of prospective and retrospective studies is beyond the scope of this review, the reader may refer to the articles where this type of study is critically evaluated (Chuang et al., 2001, 2005).

Despite the specific points concerning clinical evaluation of implants, it is important to highlight the need for double-blind studies and for registration of trials in order to mitigate against publication bias, to prevent study duplication, and to evidence gaps in the knowledge base favoring international collaboration. To date, there are only three published randomized controlled double-blinded studies of implant surface treatments. Given that endosseous implants have been in clinical practice for several decades, it is surprising that effectiveness studies in the general practice setting have not been reported. The vast majority of clinical studies are based on outcomes from specialists and medical and university centers.

Implant Retrieval Analysis

The retrieval of previously functional implants is one of the valuable tools for characterizing short- and long-term host–implant interactions as well potential failure mechanisms (Lemons, 2004).

The relative value of implant retrieval analysis is directly related to the amount of information available from patient, clinician, implant therapy modality, and implant system (i.e., lot number). Nonetheless, a lack of knowledge of any of these variables does not limit specific information that can be acquired from retrieved specimens even though limitation of critical information could ultimately lead to erroneous conclusions. For instance, if data concerning the patient medical history and functional habits are not available, it is difficult to relate specific failure mechanisms obtained from retrieval analysis to associated risk factors.

Surface Treatments to Modify Implant Topography

A considerable number of in vitro studies using cell culture has documented that rough surfaces promote greater cell adhesion, proliferation, and differentiation compared with smooth or machined surfaces (Boyan et al., 1998; Brunette, 1988; Cooper et al., 1999; deOliviera and Nanci, 2004; Masaki et al., 2005; Makihira et al., 2007; Ricci et al., 2000). In vivo studies have demonstrated higher bone–implant contact and greater bone volume around the implant with rough surfaces compared to those with smooth or machined surfaces (Buser et al., 1999, 2001; Butz et al., 2006; Frenkel et al., 2002; Klokkevold et al., 1997; Suzuki et al., 1997; Yamamuro et al., 1991).

Commercial and experimental methods to produce surfaces of different implant surface topographies or roughness or modifying the homogeneity or thickness of the TiO_2 layer have included: (1) grit blasting with abrasives (e.g., alumina, silica, Ti oxide, calcium phosphate); (2) treatment with an acid or combination of acids (e.g., HCl, H_2SO_4, HF, HCl/H_2SO_4), with an alkali (NaOH)] or with H_2O_2; (3) anodization; (4) laser-texturing; (5) deposition of metal powder or beads (cpTi, Ti alloy or Co–Cr–Mo alloy) or metallic oxide (TiO_2) coatings by plasma spraying, or arc-oxidation; (6) high temperature fusion (e.g., TiO_2 powder with Ti alloy); or (7) combinations of different methods, such as grit-blasting and acid treatment, alkali treatment and heating (Beatty, 1999; Citeau et al., 2004; Coelho and Lemons, 2009; Coelho et al., 2009; Guo et al., 2007; Ishikawa et al., 1997; Lakstein et al., 2009; LeGeros et al., 1996; LeGeros and LeGeros, 2006; Nishiguchi et al., 2001; Ong and Lucas, 1994; Park et al., 2005, 2008; Ricci et al., 2000; Rohanizadeh

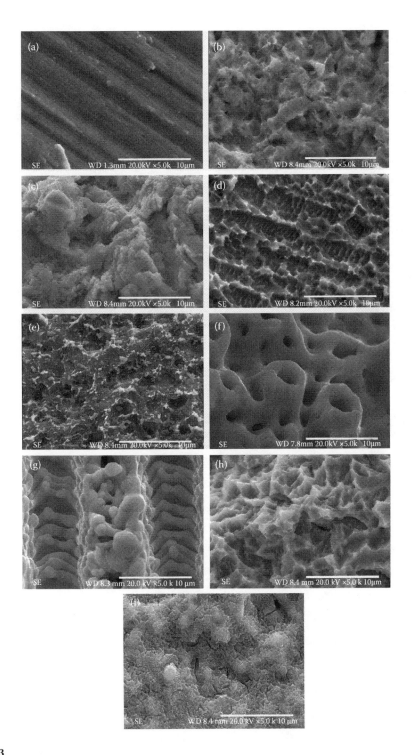

FIGURE 7.3
SEM images of cpTi and Ti alloy surfaces treated by: (a) machining; (b) grit-blasting with apatitic abrasive; (c) grit-blasting with TiO$_2$ then acid-etching with HF; (d) dual acid-etching (HCl/H$_2$SO$_4$); (e) dual acid-etching then depositing with DCD; (f) anodic oxidation; (g) laser-texturing; (h) grit-blasting with alumina abrasive then acid-etching; (i) treating with NaOH. Panels (b) to (g) are surfaces of commercial dental implants. Scale: 10 μm.

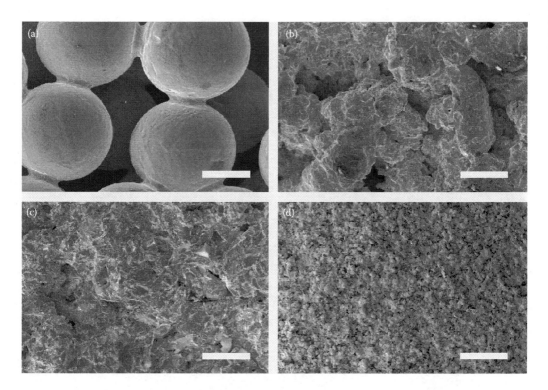

FIGURE 7.4
SEM images of orthopedic implant surfaces: (a) Co–Cr sintered beads; (b) plasma-sprayed cpTi; (c) arc-deposited Ti; (d) plasma-sprayed HA. Scale: 200 μm. (Courtesy of Stryker-Orthopaedics, New Jersey.)

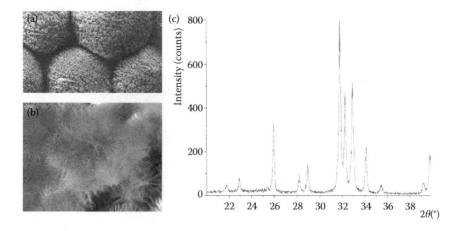

FIGURE 7.5
SEM images (a, b) of Co–Cr beads with precipitated apatite (Peri-Apatite) coating. (c) X-ray diffraction profile of the coating identified as HA. (Courtesy of Stryker-Orthopaedics, New Jersey.)

TABLE 7.1

Surface Treatment on Commercial Dental Implants

Manufacturer	Trade Name	Surface Description
Astra	Tioblast	Grit-blasted, TiO_2/acid-etched
	Osseospeed	Grit-blasted, TiO_2/HF treatment
Biohorizons	RB M	Grit-blasted, apatitic abrasive
	Bio-Lok	Laser-textured
Biomet 3i	Osseotite	Dual acid-etched (HCl/H_2SO_4)
	Nanotite	Dual acid-etched/discrete crystalline (CaP) deposition
Branemark		Machined
Neoss	Biomodal	Grit blasted/acid-etched
m	Proactive	Grit-blasted/acid-etched
Nobel Biocare	TiUnite	Anodic oxidation
ITI/Straumann	SLA	Grit-blasted, Al_2O_3 abrasive/acid-etched
Sybron	RBM	Grit-blasted, apatitic abrasive
Zimmer	MTX	Grit-blasted, apatitic abrasive

et al., 2004, 2005; Salgado et al., 1998; Schupbach; Son et al., 2003; Vercaigne et al., 2000; Wenenberg et al., 1996; Yao and Webster, 2006). The different methods of surface roughening produce different topographies (irregularities, ridges) described in terms of S_a values (the arithmetic mean of the absolute deviation from the mean line over a sampling area) as measured using profilometry. Albrektsson and Wenneberg (2004) defined

TABLE 7.2

Surface Description of Some of the Commercial Orthopedic Implants

Manufacturer	Surface Description
Biomet	Regenerex™: porous Ti alloy
	RoughCoat™: sintered Co–Cr bead porous coating with and without plasma-sprayed HA
DePuy	Oription™: porous coating, porous pure Ti alloy coating
	Purocoat®: porous coating, sintered Co–Cr beads
	Duofix® HA: plasma sprayed HA over Purocoat® coating
Smith & Nephew	Stiktite™: porous three-dimensional asymmetric Ti powder coating
	RoughCoat™: sintered Co–Cr bead porous coating with and without plasma-sprayed HA
Stryker	PureFix™ HA: plasma-sprayed HA
	Peri-Apatite™: solution deposited HA coating that uniformly coats three-dimensional porous ingrowth surfaces
	Plasma-sprayed cpTi with and without PureFix™ HA coating
	Arc-deposited cpTi with PureFix™ HA coating
	Co–Cr sintered beads with Peri-Apatite™ coating
Zimmer	Trabecular Metal™: open cell porous tantalum construct
	CSTi™, Cancellous-Structured Titanium™ coating with and without plasma-sprayed HA coating
	Fiber metal: Ti fiber metal with and without plasma-sprayed HA/TCP coating
	CoCr-beaded ingrowth surfaces

roughness in current dental implants as: "smooth" (S_a = 0.0–0.4 μm), "minimally rough" (S_a = 0.4–1.0 μm), and "rough" (S_a = 2.0 μm and higher). Wennenberg et al. (1995, 1996) have reported that the optimum roughness for increased implant–bone contact has an S_a value of about 1.5 μm; surfaces with roughness above or below this value cause a weaker bone response.

SEM images of some commercial and experimental implants surfaces are shown in Figures 7.3, 7.4, and 7.5, and surface treatments on some commercial orthopedic and dental implants are listed in Tables 7.1 and 7.2.

Surface Roughening by Grit-Blasting with Abrasives

Alumina (Al_2O_3) is commonly used as an abrasive for grit-blasting implants. The surface roughness produced by grit-blasting with alumina depends on the size and shape of the abrasive. Wennenberg et al. (1996) reported that although Ti alloy surface grit-blasted with 75 μm alumina particles elicited higher interfacial bone strength and greater bone contact than that grit-blasted with 25 μm alumina particles, surfaces grit-blasted with larger alumina particles (250 μm) showed lower interfacial bone strength. Thus, although implant surfaces grit-blasted with 75 μm alumina particles elicited higher interfacial bone than those grit-blasted with smaller particle size (25 μm), surfaces grit-blasted with higher particle size (250 μm) showed lower particle size. Studies have also shown that grit-blasting with alumina sometimes leave alumina particle inclusions in the metal substrate even after acid passivation with HNO_3 (Salgado et al., 1998; Szmukler-Montcler et al., 2004). Such alumina inclusion when released in the biologic environment may cause osteolysis or bone loss (Goodman et al., 2006). In comparison, grit-blasting with apatitic abrasive leaves a clean surface (Salgado et al., 1998). Furthermore, as discussed in the section below, grit-blasting with apatitic abrasive may also introduce bioactivity to the implant surface.

Implant surfaces roughened with either TiO_2 or Al_2O_3 abrasives showed similar increased biomechanical fixation (Wennerberg et al., 1995).

Surface Modifications by Laser Texturing

Implant surfaces with laser-textured surfaces (e.g., LaserLok Silhoutte implant, BioLok International) was produced by first grit-blasting with apatitic abrasive, then producing microgrooves with the desired depth and spaces between the grooves (Figure 7.3g). This is accomplished by using a pulsed, computer-controlled Excimer laser system and large area masking techniques. It is reported that such microgrooved surfaces cause orientation of attached cells and inhibition of colonization of fibroblastic cell types that encapsulate smooth substrates, and interfere with new bone formation and growth (Ricci et al., 2000).

Surface Modifications Using Chemical Methods

Acid-etching. Grit-blasting followed by acid-etching with HF is one method of modifying the Ti alloy surface (Figure 7.3b). The dual acid-etching process consists of successively immersing the implant in a 15% HF bath to remove the native Ti oxide layer on the Ti alloy (Ti_6Al_4V) or cpTi implant surface and then etched in a mixture of H_2SO_4/HCl acids (in a 6:1 ratio), then heated at 60–80°C (Beaty, 1999). The surface produced by the dual acid-etch method of a commercial implant is shown in Figure 7.3d).

Alkali treatment. The surface treatment of cpTi or Ti alloy substrates with the NaOH solution first introduced by Kokubo et al. (1996) was modified with subsequent heat treatment at 600°C (Takadama et al., 2001) and results in a surface shown in Figure 7.3i.

Anodic oxidation. The anodization process produces modifications in the microstructure (microporosities) and crystallinity of the Ti oxide layer. The process consists of pontiostatic or galvanostatic anodization of Ti or Ti alloy in strong acids (H_2SO_4, H_3PO_4, HNO_3, HF) at high current density (200 A/m^2) or potential (100 V). This process thickens the Ti surface oxide layer to more than 1000 nm, and the dissolution of this oxide layer along the current convection lines creates micro- or nanopores on the Ti surface (Schupbach et al., 2005) as shown in Figure 7.3f.

Bioactive Surface Coatings

Calcium phosphates (e.g., hydroxyapatite, HA; tricalcium phosphate, β-TCP) and bioactive glasses (e.g., Bioglass) are bioactive and osteoconductive materials (Daculsi and LeGeros, 2008; Hench and Paschall, 1977; Hench and Wilson, 1984; LeGeros, 1988, 1991, 2002, 2008;

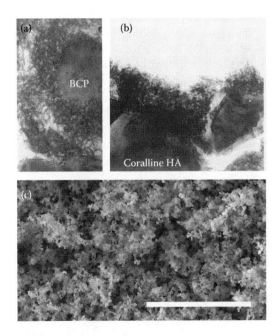

FIGURE 7.6
Formation of apatite on calcium phosphate ceramic (a, b) and treated Ti alloy surface (c) indicating bioactivity.
(a) TEM image of BCP, ceramic after implantation in rabbit; (b) TEM image of coralline HA (coral transformed to apatite) after immersion in calf serum; (c) SEM image after immersion in SBF. Scale on (c): 50 μm. In (a), BCP is an intimate mixture of HA and β-TCP, the large crystal (BCP) is most probably HA because β-TCP is much more soluble than HA and would therefore be preferentially dissolved. (From LeGeros, R.Z., Daculsi, G., *Handbook of Bioactive Ceramics, Vol. II.* CRC Press, Boca Raton, 1990; LeGeros et al., *The Bone-Biomaterial Interface,* University of Toronto Press, Toronto, 1991; LeGeros et al., Apatite, 1, 229–235, 1992; Holmes D.L., Chemical treatment of Ti alloy surfaces: effect on in vitro test for bioactivity, MS thesis, New York University, 2010. With permission.)

LeGeros and Daculsi, 1990; LeGeros and LeGeros, 2008; LeGeros et al., 2008; Osborne and Newesely, 1980).

"Bioactivity," the property that allows the material to directly bond with bone, was first observed and described by Hench et al. (1977) with silica-based bioactive glasses. In vitro, bioactivity is demonstrated by the formation of carbonate apatite on the surfaces of materials after immersion in serum (LeGeros et al. 1991, 1992) or in simulated body fluid (Kokubo et al., 1990) as shown in Figure 7.6. In vitro cell culture studies showed greater cell proliferation and differentiation (gene expression of markers for bone formation) of bone-forming cells on surfaces coated with apatite (Boyan et al., 1998; Brunette, 1988; Cooper et al., 1999; deOliviera and Nanci, 2004; Masaki et al., 2005; DaSilva et al., 2003). In vivo, bioactivity is shown by the formation of the nanocrystals of carbonate apatite associated with the bioactive material (Heughebaert et al., 1988; LeGeros and Daculsi, 1990; LeGeros et al., 1991) as shown in Figure 7.6a.

The bone mineral, idealized as an HA, is a carbonate-substituted apatite or carbonate apatite (LeGeros, 1981). The rationale for using calcium phosphates (especially HA, β-TCP, or biphasic calcium phosphate, BCP—an intimate mixture of HA and β-TCP) as bone substitute material or as coating on implant is the similarity in SEM image showing a gap (occupied by fibrous tissue) between Ti alloy implant surface and host bone indicating absence of true osseointegration (Daculsi et al., 1995) property to bone in terms of composition (mainly calcium and phosphate ions) and in osteoconductive property (which serves as a template for forming new bone). The release of calcium and phosphate ions and subsequent formation of nanoapatite crystals, similar to the nanocarbonate apatite crystals of bone (Figure 7.6a), may be a critical step in bone-bonding of the bioactive ceramic or bioactive coating (LeGeros, 2008). The carbonate apatite layer that forms on the calcium phosphate coating after implantation facilitates the adhesion of proteins on which the osteoprogenitor cells can attach, proliferate, differentiate, and produce extracellular matrix that eventually leads to biomineralization or bone formation (LeGeros, 2008).

Thus, the rationale for depositing calcium phosphate coatings on implants is to provide a bioactive surface that will ensure direct bonding with bone. To improve the adhesion of the coating with the metal substrate, the implant surfaces are first roughened either by acid-etching, grit-blasting, or deposition of a layer of cpTi or TiO$_2$ powder by plasma-spraying or arc deposition.

Plasma-Sprayed HA Coatings

Although by themselves, calcium phosphate ceramics or bioactive glasses have very desirable properties, they are not strong enough to be used in load-bearing areas (deGroot, 1987;

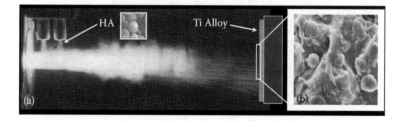

FIGURE 7.7
(a) Representation of the plasma-spray technique for depositing coating on implant. HA beads (inset) are partially melted and partially transformed to different calcium phosphate phases, principally, ACP (From LeGeros et al., *Ceram. Trans.*, 48, 173–189, 1995. With permission.) (b) SEM image of the plasma-sprayed HA surface.

Jarcho, 1981). The rationale for depositing calcium phosphate coatings on metal implants is to combine the strength of the metal and the bioactivity of the calcium phosphate coating. The plasma-spray technique (Figure 7.7) is the most commonly used method for depositing calcium phosphate coating on commercial orthopedic and dental implants that have been either grit-blasted or acid-etched before the deposition of coating (deGroot, 1987; Jarcho, 1992; Lacefield, 1988; Serekian, 1993). Dense HA spherical beads or granules are fed into an electric arc-plasma gas atmosphere. The high temperature (10,000 to 30,000°C) causes the surface of the HA beads or particulates to partially melt and transform to other forms of calcium phosphates, principally a noncrystalline phase, amorphous calcium phosphate (ACP) and small amounts of other crystalline calcium phosphate phases (β-TCP, α-TCP; tetracalcium phosphate, TTCP), and sometimes also calcium oxide, CaO, as shown by the reaction below:

$$\underset{\text{HA source}}{Ca_{10}(PO_4)_6(OH)_2} \rightarrow \underset{\text{HA}}{Ca_{10}(PO_4)_6(OH)_2} + \underset{\text{ACP}}{Ca_x(PO_4)_y} + \underset{\text{β-TCP, α-TCP}}{Ca_3(PO_4)_2} + \underset{\text{TTCP}}{Ca_4P_2O_9}$$

X-ray diffraction analyses of plasma-sprayed HA coatings on orthopedic and dental implants show that the composition of the coating is mainly HA and ACP with varying HA/ACP ratios (LeGeros et al., 1994, 1995, 1998). Variation in the HA/ACP ratios in the coating depends on the extent of melting of the HA, which in turn depends on several operating parameters including distance of the substrate (implant) from the plasma, position of entry (within or outside the nozzle) of the HA particles in the plasma stream, geometry of the substrate, and/or the type of gasses used as the carrier gas (Lacefield, 1988; LeGeros et al., 1998). The plasma-sprayed HA coating is inhomogeneous in composition,

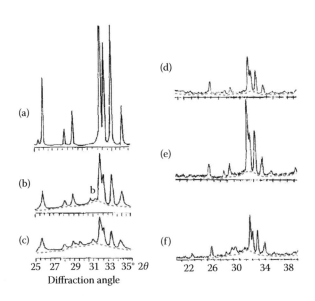

FIGURE 7.8

X-ray diffraction profiles: (a) HA used as the source material for plasma-spraying; (b) outermost layer of the plasma-sprayed coating; (c) coating layer closest to the Ti alloy substrate. In (b) and (c), ACP (area under dotted line) denotes the amorphous phase, ACP. Note that the HA/ACP ratio is higher in the outermost layer. Panels (d), (e), and (f) are x-ray diffraction profiles of plasma-sprayed HA coatings on different commercial dental implants showing variability of the HA and ACP components in the different coatings. (From LeGeros et al., *Ceram. Trans.*, 48, 173–189, 1995. With permission.)

varying in the HA/ACP ratio in the different layers of the coating: the HA/ACP ratio is higher near and at the surface layers compared with the HA/ACP ratio in the layer closest to the substrate (LeGeros et al., 1995) as shown in Figure 7.8. Variability in the HA/ACP ratio was also observed in coatings from different manufacturers (Dalton and Cook, 1995; Gross et al., 2002; LeGeros, 1991; LeGeros et al., 1994, 1995) probably due to differences in parameters used in the plasma-spray procedure. Variability in the coating composition is reflected in the variability of in vitro dissolution properties: the lower the HA/ACP ratio, the higher the dissolution rate (LeGeros et al., 1995; Sun et al., 2002).

Plasma-sprayed HA coatings on commercial implants are usually characterized by their "crystallinity" referring to the percentage of HA phase present in the coating or the percentage of HA present in the crystalline phase as determined by x-ray diffraction analysis. This is not to be confused with "crystallinity" that is used to describe crystal size based on the broadening of the diffraction peaks (Klug and Alexander, 1974). Thus, a coating may be described by a manufacturer as comprising 95% HA (amount present in the crystalline phase: HA/(HA + α-TCP + β-TCP + TTCP) × 100) but may actually only be 30% HA in the total coating (HA/(crystalline phases + amorphous phase, ACP) × 100) (LeGeros et al., 1995).

Plasma-sprayed HA-coated orthopedic and dental implants were reported to have greater osteoconductive properties and provide accelerated skeletal fixation, strong bone–implant interface compared with uncoated implants (Cook et al., 1992; Furlong and Osborne, 1991; Geesink and Hoefnagels, 1995; Jaffe and Scott, 1996; Sanatori et al., 2001; Tanzer et al., 2001; Wang et al., 2006; Wennenberg et al., 1996). Studies comparing survival rates of plasma-sprayed HA coated and uncoated hip implants showed that the HA coating significantly improved the survival rate of the prosthesis (Palm et al., 2002). A study comparing survival rates of uncoated and plasma-sprayed HA-coated hip prostheses at 12 to 16 years showed that the most common cause of revision in the coated group was never due to the coating but due to the severe wear of the polyethylene component, whereas revision in the uncoated prosthesis was due to aseptic loosening of the stem (Chadran et al., 2010).

In addition to providing a bioactive surface, calcium phosphate coating was also shown to minimize the release of potentially harmful ions from the metal substrates. Ducheyne and Healey (1988) demonstrated that apatite-coated implant showed no significant release for the Ti ions and considerably less release of Al ions with time compared with the uncoated substrates.

In spite of the advantages of plasma-sprayed HA-coated implants (greater conductivity, bone contact, interfacial strength compared with uncoated ones), there are some reasons

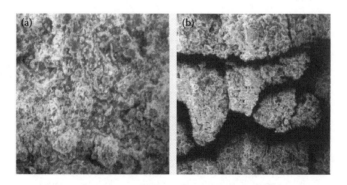

FIGURE 7.9
SEM images of Ti alloy disks before (a) and after (b) exposure to acidic buffer (pH 5, 1 M/L KAc, 37°C). The ACP component was preferentially dissolved making the coating susceptible to delamination.

for concern. Some implant failures due to delamination of the coating and release of particulates from the coating have been observed (Bloebaum et al., 1994; Collier et al., 1993; Fransson et al., 2008; Gross et al., 2002; Lacefield, 1998). This phenomenon may be attributed to the fact that the ACP component of the coating is much more soluble than the HA component and would be preferentially dissolved, resulting in the delamination (Figure 7.9) and release of HA particles (LeGeros, 1983; LeGeros et al., 1998; Ninomiya et al., 2001). Thus, a coating with very high ACP content (i.e., low HA/ACP ratio) could experience premature resorption causing implant loosening leading to implant failure. Variation in the HA/ACP ratios in plasma-sprayed coatings in commercial implants is also reflected in the observed variability in their in vitro dissolution or degradation (LeGeros et al.,

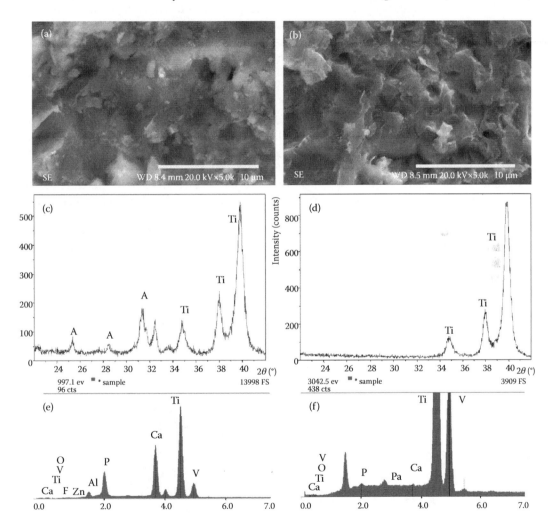

FIGURE 7.10
SEM images (a, b), x-ray diffraction profiles (c, d), and EDS profiles (e, f) of Ti alloy surfaces grit-blasted with apatitic abrasive without (a, c, e) and with (b, d, f) subsequent passivation with HNO_3. Note the presence of apatite, A, in (c) and calcium (Ca) and phosphorus (P) elements in (e) on nonpassivated surfaces. Although the diffraction peaks of apatite are not observed in the XRD profile of the passivated surface (d), its presence is indicated by the Ca and P in the EDS profile (f). (From Holmes, D.L., Chemical treatment of Ti alloy surfaces: effect on in vitro test for bioactivity, MS thesis, New York University, 2010. With permission.)

1995; Sun et al., 2002). The bond between the coating and the bone is a chemical one and, therefore, much stronger than that between the metal substrate and the coating (mechanical or physical bonding) (LeGeros et al., 1995). For this reason, separation of the coating from the substrate (Daculsi et al., 1995) is not a surprising occurrence.

Alternatives to Plasma-Spray Technique of Depositing Calcium Phosphate Coating

In addition to the nonhomogeneous composition of a plasma-sprayed HA coating, the plasma-spray method cannot provide a complete and uniform coverage for implants of complex geometry or porosity because it is a line-of-sight method and subject to shadowing. Because of the disadvantages of the plasma-spray technique in depositing calcium phosphate coatings, several alternative methods of depositing calcium phosphate coatings have been pursued.

Grit-blasting with calcium phosphate abrasives. Ti alloy surfaces grit-blasted with apatitic abrasive showed the presence of apatite in the x-ray diffraction pattern before passivation with HNO_3; to some extent, even after passivation, the presence of calcium and phosphorus elements was observed in the energy dispersive X-ray spectroscopy (EDS) profiles (Figure 7.10). Implanted Ti alloy cylinder showed direct contact with the new bone on the side grit-blasted with apatitic abrasive and fibrous tissue interface on the side grit blasted with alumina abrasive (Figure 7.11), indicating that grit-blasting with apatitic abrasive may introduce bioactive property to the implant (LeGeros and LeGeros, 2006).

Precipitation or biomimetic method of depositing calcium phosphate coating. Calcium phosphate deposition by precipitation on porous Co–Cr-beaded surfaces is used in one commercial orthopedic prosthesis (Table 7.2). This coating (Peri-Apatite), identified as apatite by x-ray diffraction (Figure 7.5), is obtained by precipitation at 80°C from solution containing calcium and phosphate ions (LeGeros, 1991; Zitelli and Higham, 2002). Nanoapatite crystals deposited on dual acid-etched Ti alloy (discrete crystalline deposition [DCD]) as a thin coating on a commercial dental implant demonstrated direct bonding with bone (Mendes et al., 2007).

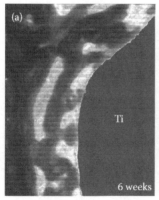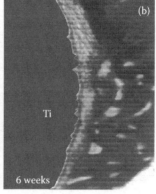

FIGURE 7.11

Microscopic images of Ti alloy rod after implantation. One side (a) of the rod was grit-blasted with apatitic abrasive, the other (b) with alumina abrasive. Direct bone-bonding was observed with side (a), fibrous tissue interface between the Ti rod and the new bone was observed with side (b) indicating that grit-blasting with apatitic abrasive enhanced osseointegration, whereas grit-blasting with alumina did not. (From LeGeros et al., in LeGeros, R.Z., LeGeros, J.P. (eds.) *Bioceramics 11*, Worldwide Scientific Publ, Singapore, pp 181–184, 1996; LeGeros and LeGeros, *Adv. Sci. Technol.*, 49, 203–211, 2006. With permission.)

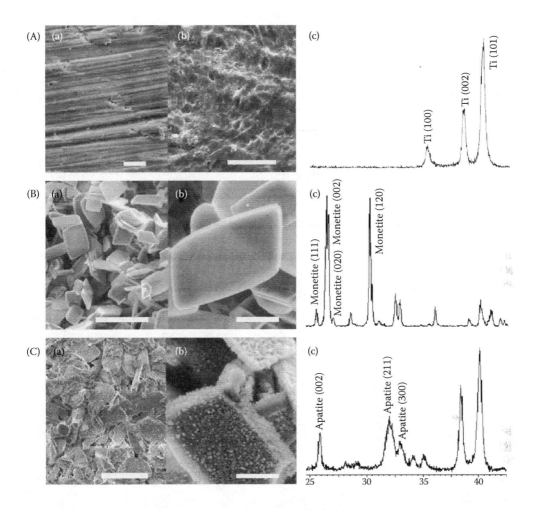

FIGURE 7.12
Deposition of calcium phosphate coating by precipitation. SEM images: (Aa, Ab) before deposition; (Ba, Bb) monetite ($CaHPO_4$) coating formed by precipitation; (Ca, Cb) apatite coating obtained by treatment of B with NaOH causing transformation of monetite to nanocrystals of apatite that followed the outline of the original monetite crystals. Scale: 10 μm for Aa, Ab, Ba, Bb, Ca, Cb; 50 μm for Ba, Ca. X-ray diffraction profiles: (Ac) untreated Ti alloy surface; (Bc) monetite coating; (Cc) apatite coating after transformation of monetite. The monetite coating was thicker than the apatite coating as deduced from the comparative intensities of the Ti diffraction peaks between Bc and Cc. (From Rohanizadeh et al., *J. Biomed. Mater. Res.*, 72A, 428–438, 2005. With permission.)

An experimental precipitation method is by treatment of the Ti alloy with acidic calcium phosphate solution resulting in the form of an acidic calcium phosphate, monetite, $CaHPO_4$, which can be transformed to apatite, if desired, by reacting with NaOH (Figure 7.12) (Rohanizadeh et al., 2005; Rohanizadeh and LeGeros, 2006). If a more reactive coating is desired, the transformation to apatite step can be eliminated. Formation of carbonate apatite after immersion in simulated body fluid (SBF) of the Ti alloy surface pretreated with NaOH (with and without subsequent heating) is another biomimetic method of depositing calcium phosphate (Lakstein et al., 2009; Nishiguchi et al., 2001).

Calcium phosphate coating using modulated electrochemical deposition method. An alternative to plasma-spray method is the electrochemical method of depositing apatite and other calcium phosphates, such as brushite or dicalcium phosphate dihydrate (DCPD), octacalcium phosphate (OCP), or monetite (DCPA) (DaSilva et al., 2001; Kumar et al., 1999; Lin et al., 2003; Narayanan et al., 2008; Shirkanzadeh, 1991).

Adherent OCP coating was obtained on different surfaces (Ti alloy grit-blasted with apatitic abrasive, arc-deposited, acid-etched, and Co–Cr-beaded surfaces) using pulse-modulated electrochemical deposition method (Lin et al., 2003; LeGeros et al., 2004). In this pulse-modulated method, Ti alloy plates were immersed in solution containing calcium phosphate, pH 5 at 60°C. Voltage is applied causing the plates to be negatively charged, thus being able to attract the positive ions (Ca^{2+} and H^+) from the solution; the voltage is discontinued, allowing the now positively charged plates to attract the negative ions (PO_4^3, HPO_4) to react with the Ca^{2+} ions, causing the formation of calcium phosphate (in this case, OCP) on the plates' surfaces. The voltage is alternately applied and discontinued until the desired calcium phosphate coating thickness is achieved. The crystal size of calcium phosphate in the coating can be manipulated by adjusting the current density or the pulse time: the higher the current, the smaller the crystal size; the greater the pulse time, the larger the crystal size (Lin et al., 2003). Using this pulse-modulated electrochemical deposition method, different types of calcium phosphates (e.g., DCPD, DCPA, calcium-deficient apatite, carbonate-substituted apatite, fluoride-substituted apatite, and other substituted apatites or substituted β-TCP), in addition to OCP, can be deposited on Ti alloys or other metals by adjusting the composition, pH, and temperature of the solution (LeGeros, 1991; LeGeros et al., 2004). Figure 7.13 shows coatings of calcium-deficient apatite, carbonate-substituted

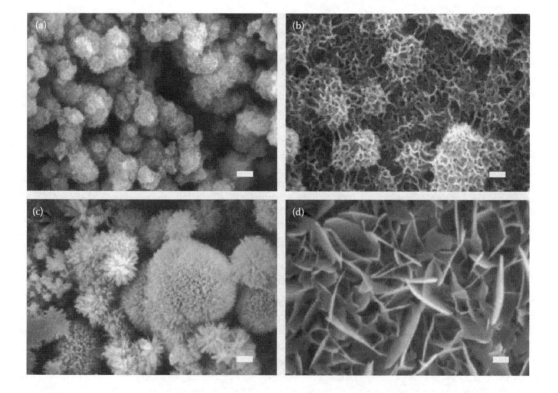

FIGURE 7.13
Deposition of different calcium phosphates on Ti alloy disks using pulse-modulated electrochemical method. SEM images: (a) carbonate-substituted apatite; (b) calcium deficient apatite; (c) fluoride-substituted apatite; and (d) OCP. (From Lin et al., *J. Biomed. Mater. Res.*, 66A, 810–828, 2003. With permission.)

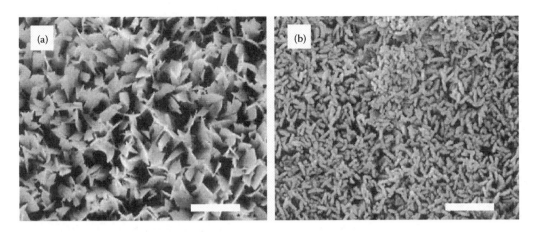

FIGURE 7.14
SEM images showing transformation of OCP (a) to apatite (b). Scale: 10 μm. (From Lin et al., *J. Biomed. Mater. Res.*, 66A, 810–828, 2003. With permission.)

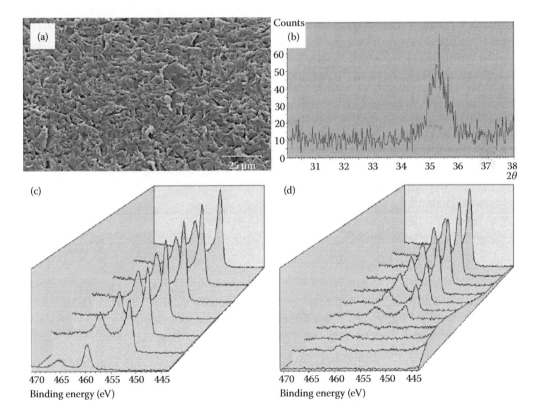

FIGURE 7.15
SEM image (a) and x-ray diffraction profile (b) of coating obtained by ion-beam assisted deposition method. The topography (a) is similar to a grit-blasted and acid-etched surface and the thin calcium phosphate coatings are not always detected depending on its thickness and SEM resolution. (b) Representative thin-film XRD profile of the surface, showing no peak associated with any calcium phosphate phase. (c and d) XPS profiles: increase in Ti peak intensity is a function of etching time for coating thicknesses of (c) 20 to 50 nm and (d) 300–500 nm. (From Coelho, J.E., Lemons, P.G., *J. Biomed. Mater. Res.*, 90, 351–361, 2009. With permission.)

apatite, fluoride-substituted apatite, and OCP on Ti alloy plates. The coating thickness can be adjusted by adjusting the length of the reaction time. The initially formed acidic calcium phosphate (DCPD, DCPA, or OCP) can be transformed to apatite (Figure 7.14) by reaction with NaOH (Kumar et al., 1999; Lin et al., 2003; DaSilva et al., 2001). This method, like the precipitation or biomimetic method, is superior to the plasma-spray method of depositing calcium phosphate coating because it allows deposition of coating with homogeneous composition and allows uniform coverage of the implants, even those with complex geometry or porosity. In addition, because the reaction temperature is low (25°C to 60°C) compared with the plasma-spray method, bioactive molecules can be incorporated into the coating if desired.

Sputtering techniques of depositing calcium phosphate coatings. The ion beam–assisted deposition (IBAD) is a sputtering technique typically involving one or two ion beam sources that impinge on a bioceramic (HA disks) target producing an elemental cloud toward the surface of the metal substrate. This technique provides a coating ranging from a few angstroms to several micrometer thicknesses (Lacefield, 1998). The coating is an ACP coating, which can be transformed to crystalline apatite after heating (Coelho and Suzuki, 2000; Coelho and Lemons, 2009; Ong and Lucas, 1994). Studies by Coelho and Lemons (2009) compared the in vivo performance of implants coated by IBAD sputtering with coating thickness ranging from 30 to 500 nm (Figure 7.15). Implants treated by this technique demonstrated histological and biomechanical performance comparable to plasma-sprayed HA-coated surfaces, both being greater than uncoated surfaces (Coelho and Lemons, 2009).

Magnetron sputtered calcium phosphate coatings also provide an ACP coating. The coating procedure involves the use of RF magnetron sputter unit (e.g., Edwards ESM 100) and HA source (either HA block or a metal substrate with plasma-sprayed HA coating). In one study of such sputtered coating (Jansen et al., 2000), the pressure was 5×10^3 mbar and sputter power of 400 W. The coating was subjected to an additional infrared treatment for 30 s at 425°C to 475°C in air. Animal studies on implants of different coating thickness (0.1, 1.0, and 4.0 μm) showed that the implant with the thickest coating provided the highest interfacial strength compared to the uncoated implants or implants with 0.1 and 1.0 μm coating thickness.

Chemical treatments to provide bioactive surfaces. Hydrothermal treatment of the Ti alloy with calcium solution (10 mmol/L $CaCl_2$) at 200°C for 24 h was reported to give a surface with greater bioactivity and greater bone formation compared to surfaces treated with NaOH and heated (Zhang et al., 2010).

Ti alloy substrates grit blasted with TiO_2 then treated with fluoride solution (HF acid) demonstrated improved biologic response and biomechanical fixation compared with nonfluoride-treated implants (Ellingsen et al., 2004).

Surface Treatments to Introduce Osteoinductivity

"Osteoinductivity" is defined as the property of a material to induce bone formation de novo without the presence of osteogenic factors. A material is described as "osteoinductive" if it is able to form bone in nonbone forming sites (e.g., under the skin, in the muscle). Urist et al. (1967) were the first to conclude that the growth factors present in demineralized bone matrix (DBM), later identified as bone morphogenetic proteins (BMPs), were osteogenic after observing bone formation following implantation of the DBM in nonosseous sites.

Calcium phosphate (CaP) ceramics are generally known to be bioactive and osteoconductive but not osteoinductive. Some CaP ceramics, such as some HA, coralline HA, BCP (Kuboki et al., 1998; LeNihouannen et al., 2005; Ripamonti, 1996; Zhang et al., 1992), and some experimental coatings (e.g., OCP) on Ti alloy implants (Barrere, 2003) have been reported to form bone in nonosseous sites of different animals without the addition of osteogenic factors, whereas other CaP ceramics of the same composition did not show osteoinductive properties. Based on their studies, Habibovic and deGroot (2007) concluded that the macrostructure (e.g., interconnecting macroporosity) and microstructure (microporosity and microroughness) play important roles in "material-directed" osteoinduction. The osteoinduction phenomenon exhibited by some CaP ceramics or coating, but not by others, was attributed to a particular combination of interconnecting macro- and microporosities as well as structural concavities in the CaP ceramic particles or scaffolds that allow the adsorption, entrapment, and concentration of circulating BMPs and/or osteogenic factors and osteoprogenitor cells (Reddi, 2006; Ripamonti et al., 1992) to impart osteoinductive properties to these materials (LeGeros et al., 2008).

Engineered osteoinductive properties can be achieved by grafting growth factors or bioactive peptides to the metal implants or to the calcium phosphate coating of the implant (deBruyn et al., 2008; Liu et al., 2006; Waldeman et al., 2004). Some authors claim that the nanonodular texturing of Ti may provide an osteoinductive surface (Ogawa et al., 2006).

Surface Treatments and Coatings with Antibacterial Properties

The long-term failure rate of dental implants, reported to be between 5% and 10%, is associated with presence of certain bacteria population (Esposito et al., 1998; Tabanella et al., 2008). With regard to orthopedic implants, microbial infection caused by bacterial adhesion and colonization is also a major concern (Darouche, 2003; Shi et al., 2008). Bacterial adhesion and colonization is also a problem with orthodontic brackets (Park et al., 2005) and guided tissue regeneration membranes (Chuo et al., 2007). Some of the recommended strategies to inhibit bacterial growth and development include implantation of zinc ions (Ansilmi et al., 2003; Petrini et al., 2006) or silver or copper (Wan et al., 2007), deposition of zinc-calcium phosphate coatings on metal substrates or membranes (Park et al., 2005; Chou et al., 2007), polypeptide nanocoatings incorporating antibiotics (Jiang and Li, 2009), TiO_2 (anatase form), nanoparticle-chitosan incorporating antibiotic (heparin) or nanosilver (Yuan et al., 2008), and calcium phosphate coatings incorporating antibiotics (Alt et al., 2006; Stigter et al., 2002) or antibacterial agent, such as chlorhexidine (Campbell et al., 2002) and nitric oxide-releasing sol–gel coatings (Nablo et al., 2005). Our current exploratory study showed that surface-treated Ti alloy prevented bacterial colonization (Figure 7.16) (Holmes, 2010).

Summary and Conclusion

The ideal property of orthopedic or dental implants used to replace missing or diseased bones or teeth is long-term stability. Strategies to accomplish this are based on (1) enhancing osseointegration (bone bonding) and (2) preventing microbial infection that could

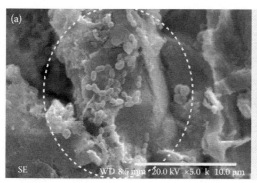
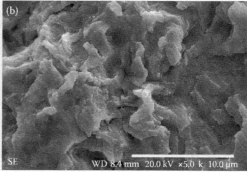

FIGURE 7.16
SEM images of untreated (a) and treated (b) Ti alloy disk after exposure to bacteria. The untreated surface (a) allowed the adhesion and colonization of bacteria, whereas the treated surface (b) prevented it. (From Holmes, D.L., Chemical treatment of Ti alloy surfaces: effect on in vitro test for bioactivity, MS thesis, New York University, 2010. With permission.) Scale: 10 μm.

cause implant loosening or failure. Surface treatments to enhance osseointegration include surface roughening or texturing by physicochemical methods (grit-blasting, acid-etching, alkali treatment) and/or deposition of bioactive coatings (calcium phosphate) or grafting growth factors to the implant or the coating. Prevention of bacterial adhesion and colonization has been accomplished by ion implantation of antibacterial agents (e.g., copper, silver, zinc) and or incorporation of antibiotic or antibacterial agents in implant coatings.

Combining these two strategies is the challenge toward developing the ideal implant.

Acknowledgments

The authors acknowledge the professional collaboration of Drs. R. Rohanizadeh, J. Park, G. Daculsi, S. Lin, A. Chuo, D. Mijares, H. Gu, K Ishikawa, Z. Lei, Y. Kim, and R. Kijkowska for some of the work cited in this chapter. Some of our studies were supported partially by the L. Linkow Implant Research Fund and the Calcium Phosphate Research Fund.

References

Aerssens J, Boonen S, Lowet G, Dequeker J. 1998. Interspecies differences in bone composition, density, and quality: potential implications for in vivo bone research. *Endocrinology* 139:663–670.

Albrektsson T, Wennerberg A. 2004. Oral implant surfaces: Part 1. Review focusing on topographic and chemical properties of different surfaces and in vivo responses to them. *Int J Prosthodont* 17:536–543.

Alt V, Bitschnau A, Osterling J, et al. 2006. The effects of combined gentamicin–hydroxyapatite coating for cementless joint prostheses on the reduction of infection rates in a rabbit infection prophylaxis model. *Biomaterials* 27:4627–4634.

Ansilmi A, LeGeros JP, LeGeros RZ. 2003. Potential for improving the success of implants by zinc coating. *J Dent Res* 82:12.

Barrere F, van der Valk CM, Maijer G, et al. 2003. Osteointegration of biomimetic apatite coating applied onto dense and porous metal implants in femurs of goats. *J Biomed Mater Res Part B: Appl Biomater* 67B:655–665.

Beatty KD. 1999. US Patent No. 5,876,453. Implant surface preparation. March 2.

Black J. 1994. Biological performance of tantalum. *Clin Mater* 16:167–173.

Bloebaum R, Beeks D, Dorr L. 1994. Complications with hydroxyapatite particulate separation in total hip arthroplasty. *Clin Orthop* 298:19–26.

Boyan BD, Batzer R, Kieswetter K, et al. 1998 Titanium surface roughness alters the responsiveness of MG63 osteoblast-like cells to $1,2.5(OH)_2D3$. *J Biomed Mater Res* 39:77–85.

Branemark PI, Adell R, Breine U. et al. 1969. A. Intra-osseous anchorage of dental prostheses. I. Experimental studies. *Scand J Plast Reconstr Surg* 3:81–100.

Branemark PI, Hansson BO, Adell R. et al. 1977. Osseointegrated implants in the treatment of the edentulous jaw. Experience from a 10-year period. *Scand J Plast Reconstr Surg Suppl* 16:1–132.

Brunette DM, Tengvall P, Thompson P. 2001. *Titanium in Medicine*. Springer Verlag, New York.

Brunette DM. 1988. The effects of implant surface topography on the behavior of cells. *Ing J Oral Maxillofac Impl* 3:231–246.

Buser D, Schjenk RK, Steineman S. et al. 1991. Influence of surface characteristics on bone integration of titanium implants. A histomorphometric study in miniature pigs. *J Biomed Mater Res* 25:889–902.

Buser D, Broggini N, Wieland M. et al. 2004. Enhanced bone apposition to a chemically modified SLA titanium surface. *J Dent Res* 83(7):529–533.

Butz F, Aita H, Wang CJ, et al. 2006. Harder and stiffer bone osseointegrated to roughened titanium. *J Dent Res* 85:560–565.

Campbell AA, Song L, Li XS, et al. 2000. Development, characterization and antimicrobial efficacy of hydroxyapatite–chlorhexidine coatings produced by surface-induced mineralization. *J Biomed Mater Res* 33:400–407.

Castaneda S, Largo R, Calvo E, et al. 2006. Bone mineral measurements of subchondral and trabecular bone in healthy and osteoporotic rabbits. *Skeletal Radiol* 35:34–41.

Chadran P, Azzabi M, Miles J, et al. 2010. Furlong hydroxyapatite-coated hip prosthesis vs. the Charnley cemented hip prosthesis. *J Arthoplasty* 25:52–57.

Christie MH. 2002. Clinical applications of trabecular metals. *Am J Orthop* 31:219–230.

Chuang SK, Hatch JP, Rugh J, Dodson TB. 2005. Multi-center randomized clinical trials in oral and maxillofacial surgery: modeling of fixed and random effects. *Int J Oral Maxillofac Surg* 34:341–344.

Chuang SK, Tian L, Wei LJ, Dodson TB. 2001. Kaplan–Meier analysis of dental implant survival: a strategy for estimating survival with clustered observations. *J Dent Res* 80:2016–2020.

Chuo AH, LeGeros RZ, Chen Z, et al. 2007. Antibacterial effect of zinc phosphate mineralized guided bone regeneration membranes. *Implant Dent* 16:89–100.

Citeau A, Guicheux J, Vinatier C, et al. 2005. In vitro biological effects of titanium rough surface obtained by calcium phosphate grit-blasting. *Biomaterials* 26:157–165.

Coelho PG, Lemons JE. 2009. Physico-chemical characterization and *in vivo* evaluation of nanothickness bioceramic depositions on alumina-blasted acid-etched Ti–6Al–4V implant surfaces. *J Biomed Mater Res* 90:351–361.

Coelho P, Granjeiro JM, Romanos GE, et al. 2009. Basic research methods and current trends of dental implant surfaces. *J Biomed Mater Res Part B: Appl Biomater* 88B:579–596.

Collier JP, Suprenant VA, Mayor MB, et al. 1993. Loss of hydroxyapatite coating on retrieved, total hip components. *J Arthroplasty* 8:389–392.

Cook SD, Thomas KA, Dalton JE, et al. 1992. Hydroxylapatite coating of porous implants improves bone ingrowth and interface attachment strength. *J Biomed Mater Res* 26:989–1001.

Cooper LF, Masuda T, Whitson SW, et al. 1999. Formation of mineralizing osteoblast cultures on machined, titanium oxide grit-blasted, and plasma-sprayed titanium surfaces. *Int J Oral Maxilofac Implants* 4:37–47

Daculsi G, LeGeros RZ. 2008. Tricalcium phosphate/hydroxyapatite biphasic ceramics. In: *Bioceramics and Their Clinical Applications*, Kokubo T (ed). Woodhead Publishing, Cambridge, pp. 395–423.

Daculsi G, LeGeros RZ, Deudon C. 1995. Scanning and transmission electron microscopy and electron probe analysis of the interface between implants and host bone. *Scan Microsc* 4:309–314.

Dalton JE, Cook SD. 1995. In vivo mechanical and histological characteristics of HA-coated implants vary with coating vendor. *J Biomed Mater Res* 29:239–245.

Darouche RO. 2003. Antimicrobial approaches for preventing infections associated with surgical implants. *Healthcare Epidemiol* 36:1284–1289.

Das K, Bose S, Bandyopadhyay A, et al. 2008. Surface coatings for improvement o bone cell materials and antimicrobial activities of Ti implants. *J Biomed Mater Res B Appl Biomater* 87:455–460.

DaSilva MHP, Lima JHC, Soares GA, et al. 2001. Transformation of monetite to hydroxyapatite in bioactive coatings on titanium. *Surface Coatings Technol* 137:270–276.

DaSilva MHP, Soares GDA, Elias CN, et al. 2003. In vitro cellular response to titanium electrochemically coated with hydroxyapatite compared to titanium with three different levels of surface roughness. *J Mater Sci Mater Med* 14:511–519.

deBruyn JD, Shakar K, Yuan H, et al. 2008. Osteoinduction and its evaluation. In: *Bioceramics and Their Clinical Applications*, Kokubo T (ed). Woodland Publishing Ltd, London, pp 199–219.

deGroot KC, Wolke JGC, deBieck-Hogervorst JM. 1990. Plasma-sprayed coating of calcium phosphate. In: *Handbook of Bioactive Ceramics, vol. II, Calcium Phosphate and Hydroxyapatite Ceramics*, Yamamuro T, Hench L, Wilson J (eds). CRC Press, Boca Raton, pp 17–25.

deOliveira PT, Nanci A. 2004. Nanotexturing of titanium based surfaces upregulates expression of bone sialoprotein and osteopontin by cultured osteogenic cells. *Biomaterials* 25:403–413.

Ducheyne P, Healey KE. 1988. The effect of plasma-sprayed calcium phosphate ceramic coatings on the metal ion release from porous titanium and cobalt–chromium alloys. *J Biomed Mater Res* 22:1137–1163.

Ellingsen JE, Johansson CB, Wennerberg A, Holmes A. 2004. Improved retention and bone-to-implant contact on the fluoride-modified titanium implant. *Int J Oral Maxillofac Implants* 19:659–666.

Esposito M, Hirsch JM, Lekholm U, et al. 1998. Biological factors contributing to failures of osseointegrated oral implants (II). Etiopathogenesis. *Eur J Oral Sci* 106:721–764.

Faria AC, Rosa AL, Rodrigues RCS, et al. 2008. *In vitro* cytotoxicity of dental alloys and cpTi obtained by casting. *J Biomed Mater Res Part B Appl Biomater* 85B:504–508.

Fransson C, Wennstrom J, Berglundh T. 2008. Clinical characteristics at implants with a history of progressive bone loss. *Clin Oral Implants Res* 19:142–147.

Frenkel SR, Simon J, Alexander H, et al. 2002. Osseointegration on metallic implant surfaces: effects of microgeometry and growth factor treatment. *J Biomed Mater Res* 63:706–713.

Furlong RJ, Osborn JF. 1991. Fixation of hip prostheses by hydroxyapatite ceramic coatings. *J Bone Jt Surg Br* 73:741–745.

Garvin KL, Hanssen AD. 1995. Infection after total hip arthroplasty. Past, present and future. *J Bone Jt Surg Am* 77:1576–1588.

Geesink RG, Hoefnagels NH. 1995. Six-year results of hydroxyapatite-coated total hip replacement. *J Bone Jt Surg Br* 77:534–547.

Goodman SB, Ma T, Chiu R, et al. 2006. Effects of orthopaedic wear particles on osteoprogenitor cells. *Biomaterials* 27:6096–6101.

Gross KA, Berndt CC, Lacono VJ. 1998. Variability of hydroxyapatite coated dental implants. *Int J Oral Maxillofac Implants* 13:601–610.

Gross KA, Ray N, Rekkum M. 2002. The contribution of coating microstructure to degradation and particle release in hydroxyapatite coated prostheses. *J Biomed Mater Res (Appl Biomater)* 63:106–114.

Groth T, Falk P, Miethke RR. 1995. Cytotoxicity of biomaterials: basic mechanisms and in vitro test methods—a review. *ATLA* 1995:790–799.

Guo J, Padilla, RJ, Ambrose W, et al. 2007. The effect of hydrofluoric acid treatment of TiO_2 grit blasted titanium implants on adherent osteoblast gene expression *in vitro* and *in vivo*. *Biomaterials* 8:5418–5425.

Habibovic P, deGroot K. 2007. Ostoinductive biomaterials—properties and relevance to bone repair. *J Tissue Eng Regen Med* 1:25–32.

Hench LL, Paschall HA. 1977. Direct bonding of bioactive glass ceramics to bone and muscle. *J Biomed Mater Res* 4:25–42.

Hench LL, Wilson J. 1984. Surface-active materials. *Science* 226:630–636.

Heughebaert M, LeGeros RZ, Gineste M, et al. 1988. Physico-chemical characterization of deposits associated with HA ceramics implanted in non-osseous sites. *J Biomed Mater Res* 22:354–368.

Holmes DL. 2010. Chemical treatment of Ti alloy surfaces: effect on in vitro test for bioactivity. MS thesis, New York University.

Ishikawa K, Miyamoto Y, Nagayama M, et al. 1997. Blast coating method: new method of coating titanium surface with hydroxyapatite at room temperature *J Biomed Mater Res (Appl Biomater)* 38:129–134.

ISO 10993-5 I. 1999. Biological evaluation of medical devices: Part 5. Tests for cytotoxicity: in vitro methods. International Organization for Standardization, Geneva.

Jaffe WL, Scott DF. 1996. Total hip arthroplasty with hydroxyapatite-coated prostheses. *J Bone Jt Surg Am* A 78:1918–1934.

Jarcho M. 1992. Retrospective analysis of hydroxyapatite development for oral implant applications. *Dent Clin North Am* 36:19–26.

Jiang B, Li B. 2009. Polypeptide nanocoatings for preventing dental and orthopedic device-associated infection: pH induced antibiotic capture, release and antibiotic efficacy. *J Biomed Mater Res Part B Appl Biomater* 88B:332–338.

Jones DB, Broeckmann E, Pohl T, Smith EL. 2003. Development of a mechanical testing and loading system for trabecular bone studies for long term culture. *Eur Cell Mater* 5:48–59; discussion 59–60.

Kasemo B, Lausmaa J. 1988. Biomaterial and implant surfaces: a surface science approach. *Int J Oral Maxillofac Implants* 3:247–259.

Klokkevold PR, Nishimura RD, Adachi M, et al. 1997. Osseointegration enhanced by chemical etching of the titanium surface. A torque removal study in the rabbit. *Clin Oral Implants Res* 8:442–447.

Klug HP, Alexander LE. 1974. *X-ray Diffraction Procedures for Polycrystalline and Amorphous Materials.* 2nd ed. John Wiley & Sons, New York.

Kokubo T, Kushitani H, Sakka S, et al. 1990. Solutions able to reproduce in vivo surface structure changes of bioactive glass ceramic. *J Biomed Mater Res* 24:721–734.

Kokubo T, Miyaki F, Kim M, Nakamura T. 1996. Spontaneous formation of bonelike apatite layer on chemically treated titanium metals. *J Am Ceram Soc* 79:1127–1129.

Kobuki Y, Takita H, Kobayashi D. 1998. BMP-induced osteogenesis on the surface of hydroxyapatite with geometrically feasible and non-feasible structures: topology of osteogenesis. *J Biomed Mater Res* 39:190–199.

Kumar M, Dasarathy HM, Riley C. 1999. Electrodeposition of brushite coatings and its transformation to hydroxyapatite in simulated body fluid. *J Biomed Mater Res* 45:302–310.

Lacefield WR. 1988. Hydroxyapatite coatings. *Ann N Y Acad Sci* 523:72–80.

Lacefield WR. 1998. Current status of ceramic coatings for dental implants. *Implant Dent* 7:315–322.

Lakstein D, Kopelovitch W, Barkay Z, et al. 2009. Enhanced osseointegration of grit-blasted, NaOH-treated and electrochemically hydroxyapatite-coated Ti–6Al–4V implants in rabbits. *Acta Biomater* 5:2258–2269.

LeGeros JP, LeGeros RZ, Burgess A, et al. 1994. X-ray diffraction method for the quantitative characterization of calcium phosphate coatings. In: *Characterization and Performance of Calcium Phosphate Coatings for Implants*, Horowitz E, Parr JE (eds). ASTM STP 1196: 33–42.

LeGeros JP, LeGeros RZ, Lin S. 2004. Method for producing adherent coatings. Patent WO 2004/098436 A3 (18 November 2004).

LeGeros RZ. 1981. Apatites in biological systems. *Prog Crystal Growth Charact* 4:1–45.

LeGeros RZ. 1988. Calcium phosphate materials in restorative dentistry. A review. *Adv Dent Res* 2:164–183.

LeGeros RZ. *Calcium Phosphates in Oral Biology and Medicine. Monographs in Oral Sciences*, Vol. 15. Myers H (ed). S. Karger, Basel, 1991.

LeGeros RZ. 1993. Biodegradation and bioresorption of calcium phosphate ceramics. *Clin Mater* 14:65–88.

LeGeros RZ. 2002. Properties of osteoconductive biomaterials: calcium phosphates. *Clin Orthopaed Rel Res* 395: 81–98.

LeGeros RZ. 2008. Calcium phosphate-based osteoinductive materials. *Chem Rev* 108: 4742–4753.

LeGeros RZ, Daculsi G. 1990. *In vivo* transformation of biphasic calcium phosphate ceramics: Ultrastructural and physicochemical characterizations. In: *Handbook of Bioactive Ceramics, Vol. II*, Yamamuro T, Hench L, Wilson J (eds). CRC Press, Boca Raton, pp 17–28.

LeGeros RZ, LeGeros JP. 2006. In situ characterization of degradation behavior of plasma-sprayed coatings on orthopedic and dental implants. *Adv Sci Technol* 49:203–211.

LeGeros RZ, LeGeros JP. 2008. Hydroxyapatite. In: *Handbook of Bioceramics and their Applications*, Kokubo T (ed). Woodhead Publishing Ltd, London, pp 367–394.

LeGeros RZ, Daculsi G, Orly I, et al. 1991. Substrate surface dissolution and interfacial biological mineralization. In: *The Bone–Biomaterial Interface*, Davies JE (ed). University of Toronto Press, Toronto, pp 76–88.

LeGeros RZ, Orly I, Gregoire M, et al. 1992. Comparative properties and in vitro reactions of HA ceramic and coralline HA. *Apatite* 1:229–235.

LeGeros RZ, LeGeros JP, Kim Y, et al. 1995. Calcium phosphates in plasma-sprayed HA coatings. *Ceram Trans* 48:173–189.

LeGeros RZ, Kim YE, Kijkowska R, et al. 1998. HA/ACP ratios in calcium phosphate coatings on dental and orthopedic implants: effect on properties. In: *Bioceramics 11*, LeGeros RZ, LeGeros JP (eds). Worldwide Scientific Publ, Singapore, pp 181–184.

LeGeros RZ, Daculsi G, LeGeros JP. 2008. Bioactive bioceramics. In: *Orthopedic Biology and Medicine: Musculoskeletal Tissue Regeneration Biological Materials and Methods*, Pietrzak WS (ed). Humana Press, New Jersey, pp 153–181.

Le Guehennec L, Soueidan A, Layrolle P, Amouriq Y. 2007. Surface treatments of titanium dental implants for rapid osseointegration. *Dent Mater* 23:844–854.

Lemons JE. 2004. Biomaterials, biomechanics, tissue healing, and immediate-function dental implants. *J Oral Implantol* 30:318–324.

LeNihouhannen DL, Daculsi G, Gauthier O, et al. 2005. Ectopic bone formation by microporous calcium phosphate ceramic particles in sheep muscles. *Bone* 36:1086–1096.

Lenz R, Mittelmeier W, Hansmann D, et al. 2009. Response of human osteoblasts exposed to wear particles generated at the interface of total hip stems and bone cement. *J Biomed Mater Res A* 88:370–378.

Liebschner MA. 2004. Biomechanical considerations of animal models used in tissue engineering of bone. *Biomaterials* 25:1697–1714.

Lin S, LeGeros RZ, LeGeros JP. 2003. Adherent octacalciumphosphate coating on titanium alloy using a modulated electrochemical deposition method. *J Biomed Mater Res* 66A:810–828.

Liu Y, Li JP, Hunzier, EB, et al. 2006. Incorporation of growth factors into medical devices via biomimetic coatings. *Philos Trans A Math Phys Eng Sci* 64:233–249.

Masaki C, Schneider GB, Zaharias R, et al. 2005. Effects of implant surface microtopography on osteoblast gene expression. *Clin Oral Implants Res* 16:650–656.

Mendes VC, Moineddin R, Davies JE. 2007. The effect of discrete calcium phosphate nanocrystals on bone-bonding to titanium surfaces. *Biomaterials* 28:4748–4755.

Makihira S, Mine Y, Kosaka E, Nikawa H. 2007. Titanium surface roughness accelerates RANKL-dependent differentiation in the osteoclast precursor cell line, RAW264.7. *Dent Mater J* 26:739–745.

Mombelli, A. 1997. Etiology, diagnosis and treatment considerations in peri-implantitis. *Curr Opin Periodontol* 4:127–136.

Nablo BJ, Rodrock AR, Schoenfisch MH. 2005. Nitric oxide-releasing sol–gels as antibacterial coatings for orthopedic implants. *Biomaterials* 26:917–924.

Narayanan R, Seshadri SK, Kwon TY, et al. 2008. Calcium phosphate–based coatings on titanium and its alloys. *J Biomed Mater Res Part B Appl Biomater* 85B:279–299.

Narayanan R, Kwon TY, Kim K-H. 2008. Preparation and characteristics of nano-grained calcium phosphate coatings on titanium from ultrasonicated bath at acidic pH. *J Biomed Mater Res Part B Appl Biomater* 85B:231–239.

Neyt JG, Buckwalter JA, Carroll NC.1998. Use of animal models in musculoskeletal research. *Iowa Orthop J* 18:118–123.

Ninomiya JT, Struve JA, Stelloh CT, et al. 2001. Effects of hydroxyapatite particulate debris on the production of cytokines and proteases in human fibroblasts. *J Orthop Res* 19:621–628.

Nishiguchi S, Kato H, Neo M, et al. 2001. Alkali- and heat-treated porous titanium for orthopedic implants. *J Biomed Mater Res* 54:198–208.

Ogawa T, Ozawa S, Shih JH, et al. 2000. Biomechanical evaluation of osseous implants having different surface topographies in rats. *J Dent Res* 79:1857–1863.

Ogawa T, Saruwatari L, Takeuchi K, et al. 2006. Ti nano-nodular structuring for bone integration and regeneration. *J Dent Res* 87:751–756.

Ong JL, Lucas LC. 1994. Post-deposition heat treatments for ion beam sputter deposited calcium phosphate coatings. *Biomaterials* 15(5):337–341.

Osborne JF, Newesely H. 1980. The material science of calcium phosphate ceramic. *Biomaterials* 1:108–111.

Palm L, Jacobsson SA, Ivarsson I. 2002. Hydroxyapatite coating improves 8- to 10-year performance of the link RS cementless femoral stem. *J Arthoroplasty* 17:172–176.

Park YS, Yi KY, Lee IS, et al. 2005. The effects of ion beam–assisted deposition of hydroxyapatite on the grit-blasted surface of endosseous implants in rabbit tibiae. *Int J Oral Maxillofac Implants* 20:31–38.

Park HS, Lee MH, Bae TS, et al. 2008. Effects of anodic oxidation parameters on a modified titanium surface. *J Biomed Mater Res. Part B: Appl Biomater* 84B:422–429.

Park JH, LeGeros, RZ, LeGeros JP. 2005. Zn–CaP material as potential coating for orthodontic brackets. *J Dent Res* 84:17.

Petrini P, Archioloa CR, Pezzali I, et al. 2006. Antibacterial activity of zinc-modified titanium oxide surface. *Int J Artif Organs* 29:434–442.

Pearce AI, Richards RG, Milz S, et al. 2007. Animal models for implant biomaterial research in bone: a review. *Eur Cell Mater* 13:1–10.

Ratner, BD, Hoffman AS, Schoen FJ, et al. 2004. *Biomaterials Science: An Introduction to Materials in Medicine*. Elsevier Academic Press, Boston.

Reddi AH. 2000. Morphogenesis and tissue engineering of bone and cartilage: inductive signals, stem cells and biomimetic biomaterials. *Tissue Eng* 6:351–359.

Ricci J, Charvel J, Frenkel SR. 2000. Bone response to laser microtextured surfaces. In: *Bone Engineering*, Davies JE (ed). EM² Inc., Toronto, Ont., Chapter 25.

Ripamonti U. 1995. Osteoinduction in porous hydroxyapatite implanted in heterotopic sites of different animal models. *Biomaterials* 17:31–37.

Ripamonti U, Ma S, Reddi AH. 1992. The critical role of geometry of porous hydroxyapatite to delivery system induction of bone by osteogenin, a bone morphogenetic protein. *Matrix* 12:202–212.

Rohanizadeh R, LeGeros RZ, Harsono H, et al. 2005. Adherent apatite coating on titanium substrate using chemical deposition. *J Biomed Mater Res* 72A: 428–438.

Rohanizadeh R, Al-Sadeq M, LeGeros RZ. 2004. Preparation of different forms of titanium oxide on titanium surface: effects of apatite deposition. *J Biomed Mater* Res 71A:343–352.

Rohanizadeh R, LeGeros RZ. 2006. US 2006/0062925 A1.

Salgado T, LeGeros JP, Wang J. 1998. Effect of alumina and apatitic abrasives on implant substrates. In: *Bioceramics 11*, LeGeros RZ, LeGeros JP (eds). World Scientific, Singapore, pp 683–686.

Santavirta S, Takagi M, Gomez-Barrena E, et al. 1999. Studies of host response to orthopedic implants and biomaterials. *J Long Term Eff Med Implants* 9:67–76.

Sanatori FS, Ghera S, Moriconi A, et al. 2001. Results of the anatomic cementless prosthesis with different types of hydroxyapatite coating. *Orthopedics* 24:1147–1150.

Schildhauer TA, Peter E, Muhr G, Koller M. 2009. Activation of human leukocytes on tantalum trabecular metal in comparison to commonly used orthopedic metal implant materials. *J Biomed Mater Res A* 88:332–341.

Schimandle JH, Boden SD. 1994. Spine update. Animal use in spinal research. *Spine* 19:2474–2477.

Schupbach P, Glauser R, Rocci A, et al. 2005. The human bone-oxidized titanium implant interface: a light microscopic, scanning electron microscopic, back-scatter scanning electron microscopic, and energy-dispersive X-ray study of clinically retrieved dental implants. *Clin Implant Dent Rel Res* 7:S37–S43.

Serekian P. 1993. Process application of hydroxyapatite coatings. In: *Hydroxyapatite Coatings in Orthopedic Surgery*, Geesink RGT, Manley MT (eds). Raven Press, Ltd., New York, pp 81–87.

Shi ZL, Chua PH, Neoh KG, et al. 2008. Bioactive titanium implant surfaces with bacterial inhibition and osteoblast function enhancement properties. *Int J Artif Organs* 31:777–785.

Shirkhanzadeh M. 1991. Bioactive calcium phosphate coatings prepared by electrodeposition. *J Mater Sci Lett* 10:1415–1417.

Smith, DF. 1981. *Fundamental Aspects of Biocompatibility*. CRC Press, Boca Raton.

Son W-W, Zhu X, Shin H-I, et al. 2003. In vivo histological response to anodized and anodized/hydrothermally treated titanium implants. *J Biomed Mater Res Part B Appl Biomater* 66B:520–525.

Steinmann SG. 1998. Titanium—the material of choice? *Periodontology* 2000 17:7–21.

Stevens B, Yang Y, Mohandas A, et al. 2008. A review of materials, fabrication methods and strategies used to enhance bone regeneration in engineered bone tissues. *J Biomed Mater Res Part B Appl Biomater* 85B:573–582.

Stigter M, deGroot K, Layrolle P. 2004. Incorporation of different antibiotics into carbonated hydroxyapatite coatings on titanium implants, release and antibiotic efficacy. *J Control Release* 99:127–137.

Sun L, Berndt, CC, Khor KA, et al. 2002. Surface characteristics and dissolution behavior of plasma-sprayed hydroxyapatite coating. *J Biomed Mater Res* 62:228–236.

Sun L, Berndt CC, Gross KA, et al. 2001. Material fundamentals and clinical performance of plasma-sprayed hydroxyapatite coatings: a review. *J Biomed Mater Res B* 58:570–592.

Suzuki K, Aoki K, Ohya K. 1997. Effects of surface roughness of titanium implants on bone remodeling activity of femur in rabbits. *Bone* 21:507–514.

Szmukler-Montcler S, Perrin D, Ahossi V, et al. 2002. Biological properties of acid etched titanium implants: effect of sandblasting on bone anchorage. *J Biomed Mater Res Part B Appl Biomater* 68B:149–159.

Tabanella G, Nowzari H, Slots, J. 2009. Clinical and microbiological determinants of ailing dental implants. *Clin Implant Dent Relat Res* 11:24–36.

Tamaki Y, Sasaki K., Sasaki A, et al. 2008. Enhanced osteolytic potential of monocytes/macrophages derived from bone marrow after particle stimulation. *J Biomed Mater Res B Appl Biomater* 84:191–204.

Tanzer M, Kantor S, Rosenthal L, 2001. Femoral remodeling after porous-coated total hip arthroplasty with and without hydroxyapatite-tricalcium phosphate coating: a prospective randomized trial. *J Arthoplasty* 16:552–558.

Urist MR, Silverman BF, Buring K, et al. 1967. The bone induction principle. *Clin Orthop* 53:243–283.

Vercaigne S, Wolke JG, Naert I, et al. 2000. A histological evaluation of TiO_2-gritblasted and Ca–P magnetron sputter coated implants placed into the trabecular bone of the goat: Part 2. *Clin Oral Implants Res* 11:314–324.

Waldeman B, Bamdad P, Holmer C, et al. 2004. Local delivery of growth factors from coated titanium plate increases osteotomy healing in rats. *Bone* 34:862–868.

Wan YX, Raman S, He F, et al. 2007. Surface modification of medical metals by ion implantation of silver and copper. *Vacuum* 81:114–118.

Wang M. 2003. Developing bioactive composite materials for tissue replacement. *Biomaterials* 24:2133–2151.

Wang H, Eliaz N, Xiang Z, et al. 2006. Early bone apposition in vivo on plasma-sprayed and electrochemically deposited hydroxyapatite coatings on titanium alloy. *Biomaterials* 27: 4192–4203.

Wenneberg A, Alblrektsson T, Lalusmaa J. 1996. Torque and histomorphometric evaluation of cp titanium screws blasted with 25- and 75-micron sized particles of Al_2O_3. *J Biomed Mater Res* 30:251–260.

Williams DF. 1981. Titanium and titanium alloys. In: *Biocompatibility of Clinical Implant Materials, Vol. 1*, Williams DF (ed). CRC Press, Boca Raton, pp 9–44.

Yamamuro T, Takagi T. 1991. Bone-bonding behavior of biomaterials with different surface characteristics under load-bearing conditions. In: *The Bone–Materials Interface*. Toronto University Press, Toronto, pp 406–414.

Yao C, Webster TJ. 2006. Anodization: a promising nano-modification technique of titanium implants for orthopedic application. *J Nanosci Nanotechnol* 6:2682–2692.

Yuan W, Ji J, Fu J, et al. 2008. A facile method to construct hybrid multilayered films as a strong and multifunctional antibacterial coating. *J Biomed Mater Res Part B Appl Biomater* 84B:556–563.

Zhang L, Ayukawa Y, LeGeros RZ, et al. 2010. Tissue-response to calcium-bonded titanium surface. *J Biomed Mater Res Part A* 95A:33–38.

Zhang C, Tang T, Ren W, et al. 2008. Influence of mouse genetic background on wear particle-induced in vivo inflammatory osteolysis. *Inflamm Res* 57:211–215.

Zhao L, Chu PK, Zhang Y, et al. 2009. Antibacterial coatings on titanium implants. *J Biomed Mater Res B Appl Biomater* 91:470–480.

Zimmerli W, Trampu Z, Ochsner PE. 2004. Prosthetic joint infections. *N Engl J Med* 351:1645–1654.

Zittelli J, Higham P. 2000. A novel method for solution deposition of hydroxyapatite onto three dimensionally porous metallic surfaces: peri-apatite HA. *Mater Res Soc Symp Proc* 599:117–128.

8

Piezoelectric Zinc Oxide and Aluminum Nitride Films for Microfluidic and Biosensing Applications

Yong Qing Fu, J. K. Luo, A. J. Flewitt, A. J. Walton, M. P. Y. Desmulliez, and W. I. Milne

CONTENTS

Introduction 336
Acoustic Wave Biosensors 336
Acoustic Wave-Based Microfluidics...340
Selection of Bulk Materials or Thin Films...341
Requirement for ZnO or AlN Films for Sensing and Microfluidic Applications 343
ZnO Film 344
　　ZnO Film Deposition 344
　　Film Texture 349
　　　　Self-Texture and Wave Mode..349
　　　　Interlayer or Buffer Layer...350
　　　　Epitaxial Growth..350
　　　　Oxygen Ion Bombardment...351
　　PE Properties of Sputtered ZnO Films 352
　　　　Substrate Effect 352
　　　　Film Thickness Effect 352
　　　　Other Factors..354
　　MEMS Processing of ZnO Films 355
　　Functionalization of ZnO Surface for Biosensing...356
AlN Films 356
　　AlN Film Deposition...357
　　AlN Film Texture and Substrate Effect...358
　　PE Properties of Sputtered AlN Films 359
　　MEMS Processing of AlN Films...362
　　Functionalization of AlN Surface for Biosensing 362
Thin Film Acoustic Devices for Biosensor Applications 363
　　SAW Biosensor...363
　　Lamb Biosensor 364
　　FBAR Biosensor 364
Thin Films for Microfluidic Applications 366
　　SAW Mixer and Pump..366
　　SAW Heating/Droplet Ejector 369
　　SAW Particle Manipulation 370
Membrane-Based Microfluidics Devices 371
Future Trends for ZnO and AlN Devices for Lab-on-a-Chip.................................372

Summary 373
Acknowledgments 373
References... 374

Introduction

Acoustic wave technologies and devices have been commercially exploited for more than 60 years in industrial applications ranging from communications, automotive, to environmental sensing (Ballantine et al., 1996; Hoummady et al., 1997). When an alternating electric field is applied to an interdigital transducer (IDT) on a piezoelectric (PE) material, an acoustic wave is generated. The wave can propagate in a direction perpendicular to the surface of the material into the bulk (bulk acoustic wave [BAW]) or along the surface of the material (surface acoustic wave [SAW]). This PE effect is manifested in either a Rayleigh mode (vertical and surface normal) or as a shear wave (horizontal in-plane) (Galipeau et al., 1997). Table 8.1 lists several common acoustic wave modes and their related devices. The most commonly used BAW device is the Quartz Crystal Microbalance (QCM), which is generally made of quartz sandwiched between two electrodes. A SAW propagating within a thin surface layer, which has a lower acoustic velocity than that of the PE substrate, is called a Love wave and such devices are typically operated in the shear horizontal (SH) wave mode. Waves propagating in a thin plate with a thickness much less than the acoustic wavelength are called a flexural plate or Lamb waves (Luginbuhl et al. 1997). This chapter reviews the progress related to the application of PE ZnO and AlN thin films in microfluidics and biosensors.

Acoustic Wave Biosensors

Most acoustic wave devices can be used as sensors because they are sensitive to mechanical, chemical, or electrical perturbations on the surface of the device (Lucklum and

TABLE 8.1

Comparison of Different Acoustic Wave Microsensors

Name	QCM	Rayleigh SAW	SH-SAW	FPW	Love Wave	Film Bulk Acoustic Resonator (FBAR)
Mode	Thickness shear bulk mode	Rayleigh wave	Shear wave	Lamb Wave	SH-SAW	Bulk wave
Gas	✓	✓	✓	✓	✓	✓
Liquid	✓✓	×	✓✓	✓	✓✓	✓
Normal frequency	5–20 MHz	20–500 MHz		kHz to lower MHz		>GHz
Sensitivity (cm^2/g)	10–100	100–1000	10–500	100–1000	20–2000	1000–10,000
Example	AT-cut quartz	ST-cut Quartz 120°C LiNbO$_3$	36YX LiTaO$_3$ ST-cut quartz ZX-LiNbO$_3$	Si$_3$N$_4$/ZnO membrane	SiO$_2$/ ST-Quartz, ZnO/LiTaO$_3$	ZnO and AlN membrane

Hauptmann, 2003; Grate et al., 2003). Acoustic wave sensors have the advantage that they are versatile, both sensitive and reliable, being able to detect not only mass/density changes but also viscosity, wave functions, elastic modulus, conductivity, and dielectric properties. They have many applications in the monitoring of pressure, moisture, temperature, force, acceleration, shock, viscosity, flow, pH levels, ionic contaminants, odor, radiation, and electric fields (Shiokawa and Kondoh, 2004; Wohltjen et al., 1997). Recently, there has been an increasing interest in acoustic wave-based biosensors to detect traces of biomolecules through specific bioreactions with biomarkers. These include DNA, proteins (enzymes, antibodies, and receptors), cells and tissues (microorganisms, animal and plant cells, cancer cells, etc.), viruses, as well as the detection of chemical substances through specific chemical absorption layers (Cote et al., 2003; Kuznestsova and Coakley, 2007; Teles and Fonseca, 2003). By detecting the traces of associated molecules, it is possible to diagnose diseases and genetic disorders, prevent potential bioattachment, and monitor the spread of viruses and pandemics (Vellekoop, 1998; Shiokawa and Kondoh, 2004; Gizeli, 1997). Compared with other common biosensing technologies, such as surface plasmon resonance (SPR), optical fibers, and sensors based on field effect transistors or cantilever-based detectors, acoustic wave-based technologies have the combined advantages of simple operation, high sensitivity, small size, and low cost, with no need for bulky optical detection systems (Lange et al., 2008).

The commonly reported acoustic wave-based biosensor is QCM (see Figure 8.1a) (Markx, 2003), which can be operated in a liquid environment using a thickness shear-mode. Advantages of QCM include (1) simplicity in design and (2) a high Q factor. Problems associated with QCM biosensors include low detection resolution due to the low-operating frequency in the range of 5–20 MHz and a large base mass, a thick substrate (0.5–1 mm) and large surface area (>1 cm^2) which cannot be easily scaled down.

Because the SAW-based biosensors have their acoustic energy confined within a region about one wavelength from the surface, the base mass of the active layer is roughly 1 order of magnitude smaller than that of the QCM. Therefore, the sensitivity of the SAW devices increases dramatically compared with that of the QCM (see Table 8.1). The longitudinal or Rayleigh mode SAW device (Figure 8.1b) has a substantial surface-normal displacement that rapidly dissipates the acoustic wave energy into the liquid, leading to excessive damping, and hence poor sensitivity and noise. Waves in a SH-SAW device (Figure 8.1c) propagate in an SH mode and, therefore, do not easily radiate acoustic energy into the liquid (Barie and Rapp, 2001; Kovacs and Venema, 1992); hence, the device maintains a high sensitivity in liquids. Consequently, SH-SAW devices are particularly well suitable for biodetection, especially for "real-time" monitoring. In most cases, Love wave devices (Figure 8.1d) operate in the SH wave mode with the acoustic energy trapped within a thin waveguide layer (typically submicrometers). This enhances the detection sensitivity by more than 2 orders of magnitude when compared with a SAW device owing to their much reduced base-mass (Josse et al., 2001; Mchale, 2003). They are therefore frequently employed to perform biosensing in liquid conditions (Lindner, 2008; Kovacs et al., 1992; Jacoby and Vellekoop, 1997).

In a manner similar to a SAW device, Lamb wave devices (Figure 8.1e) on a membrane structure have been used for biosensing in liquid (Muralt et al., 2005). The wave velocity generated in the flexural plate wave (FPW) or Lamb wave is much smaller than those in liquids, which minimizes the dissipation of wave energy into the liquid. The detection mechanism is based on the relative change in magnitude induced by the perturbation on the membrane and not on the resonant frequency shift. Therefore, the sensitivity of these devices increases as the membrane thickness becomes thinner (Nguyen and White, 2000;

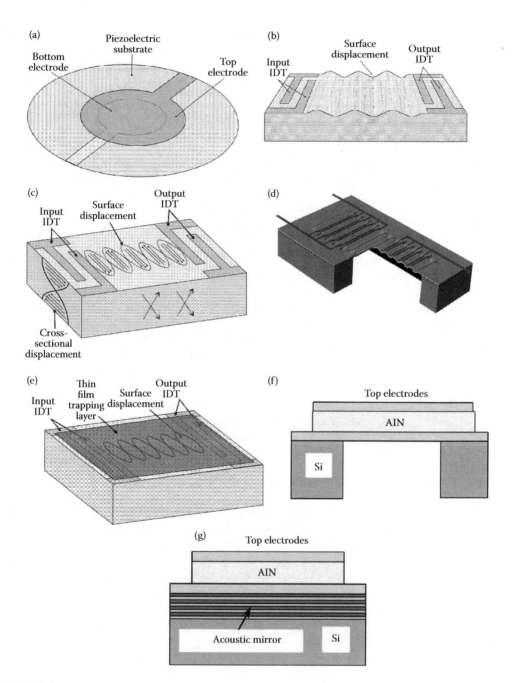

FIGURE 8.1
Illustration of different types of acoustic wave devices: (a) QCM; (b) Rayleigh wave SAW; (c) SH wave; (d) Lamb Wave; (e) Love mode wave; (f) membrane-based FBAR; (g) reflector based FBAR. (From Marx, K.A. *Biomacromolecules*, 4, 1099, 2003; Durdag, K., *Sens. Rev.*, 28, 68–73, 2008; Nguyen, A.H., White, R.M. *J. Micromech. Microeng.*, 2, 169–174, 2000. With permission.)

Luginbuhl et al., 1998). The main drawback of the Lamb wave biosensor is that there is a practical limit on the minimum film thickness as the thin film becomes more fragile.

A newly emerged but promising acoustic wave device for high-sensitivity biodetection is the film bulk acoustic resonator (FBAR) device (Figure 8.1f). Similar to the QCM, an FBAR device consists of a submicrometer thick PE film membrane sandwiched between two metallic layer electrodes (Ruby, 2007). Owing to the much reduced thickness, the FBAR device operates at high frequencies, up to a few GHz (see Table 8.1).

The frequency shift Δf due to mass loading Δm of an acoustic wave device has been described by Buttry and Ward (1992).

$$\Delta f = \frac{2\Delta m f_o^2}{A\sqrt{\rho\mu}}$$

(8.1)

where A, ρ, μ, and f_o are the area, density, shear modulus, and intrinsic resonant frequency, respectively. Because of the much-reduced base mass and high operation frequency, the attachment of a small target mass can cause a large frequency shift—typically a few MHz. This makes the signal easily detected using simple electronic circuitry. Figure 8.2 summarizes the sensitivity range for different types of resonators according to their normal operational frequency ranges (Rey-Mermet et al., 2004). The advantages of the FBAR devices include (1) the ability to fabricate the device using standard complementary metal-oxide-semiconductor (CMOS) processing and compatible materials allowing integration with CMOS control circuitry and (2) the significantly reduced size and sample volume. These features together with the intrinsic high sensitivity make the FBAR technology ideal for highly sensitive real-time diagnostic biosensor arrays, which provide quantitative results at a competitive cost. However, for the membrane-based FBAR design, the membrane fragility and the difficulty in its manufacture are significant issues that have yet to be fully addressed.

In addition to the membrane-based FBAR structure, there is another common FBAR structure that uses an acoustic mirror deposited between the PE layer and the substrate (see Figure 8.1g). The acoustic mirror is composed of many quarter-wavelength layers of alternating high and low acoustic impedance films. Because of the high impedance ratio of the acoustic mirror, the acoustic energy is only reflected and confined inside the top PE layer, thus maintaining an excellent resonant bandwidth. This design has a better

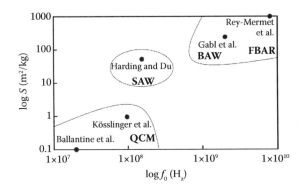

FIGURE 8.2
Sensitivity range for different types of resonators according to their common applied frequency ranges. (From Rey-Mermet at al., *IEEE Trans. Ultrason. Ferroelectr. Freq. Control*, 51, 1347, 2004. With permission.)

mechanical robustness and a simpler process control compared with the membrane-based structures. Also, cheap substrates, such as glass or plastics can be used, thus, the cost can be reduced. Table 8.1 compares the properties of the microsensors fabricated from different acoustic wave devices.

Acoustic Wave-Based Microfluidics

Microfluidic (liquid samples and reagents) manipulation, mixing, and biochemical reaction at the microscale are extremely difficult because of the low Reynolds number flow conditions (Nguyan and Wu, 2005). Acoustic wave technologies are particularly well suited to mixing and as a result are an attractive option for microfluidics applications (Luo et al., 2009). Taking the SAW device as one example, Rayleigh-based SAW waves have a longitudinal component that can be coupled with a medium in contact with the surface of the device. This coupling- or friction-driven effect can transport the media, for example, a solid slider on the surface during wave propagation as shown in Figure 8.3a, although the displacement of the traveling Rayleigh wave is only about 20 nm or less (Kuribayashi and Kurosawa, 2000). When liquid (either in bulk or droplet form) exists on the surface of a SAW device, the energy and momentum of the acoustic wave are coupled into the fluid with a Rayleigh angle, following Snell's law of refraction (see Figure 8.3b) (Wixforth, 2004; Shiokawa et al., 1989). The Rayleigh angle, θ, is defined by

$$\theta = \sin^{-1}\left(\frac{v_l}{v_s}\right) \tag{8.2}$$

where v_l and v_s are the velocities of the longitudinal wave in solid and liquid. The energy and the momentum of the longitudinal wave radiated into the liquid can be harnessed for liquid pumping and mixing. A net pressure gradient, P, forms in the direction of the propagation of the acoustic wave and efficiently drives the liquid (Rotter et al., 1999), according to the relation:

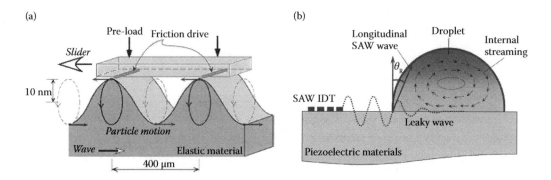

FIGURE 8.3
(a) Principle of SAW motor. (From Kuribayashi, M., and Kurosawa, M., *Ultrasonics*, 38, 15–19, 2000. With permission.) (b) Interaction between propagating SAW and a liquid droplet causing acoustic streaming inside droplet.

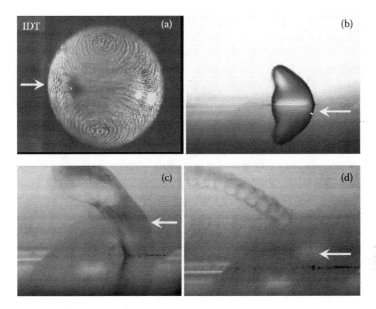

FIGURE 8.4
SAW microfluidics based on a hydrophobically treated LiNbO$_3$ device: (a) SAW streaming pattern; (b) droplet pumping; (c) droplet jumping from surface; (d) droplet ejection.

$$P = \rho_0 v_s^2 \left(\frac{\Delta \rho}{\rho_0} \right)^2 \qquad (8.3)$$

where ρ_0 is the liquid density and $\Delta \rho$ is the slight density change due to the acoustic pressure. The generated acoustic pressure can create significant acoustic streaming in a liquid and result in liquid mixing, pumping, ejection and atomization (Newton et al., 1999) (see Figure 8.4, for examples). This pressure facilitates rapid liquid movement and also internal agitation that speed up biochemical reactions, minimize nonspecific biobinding, and accelerate hybridization reactions in protein and DNA analysis, which are commonly used in proteomics and genomics (Toegl et al., 2003; Wixforth et al., 2004). SAW-based liquid pumps and mixers (Tseng et al., 2006; Sritharan et al., 2006), droplet positioning and manipulation (Sano et al., 1998), droplet ejection and atomization systems (Chono et al., 2004; Murochi et al., 2007), and fluidic dispenser arrays (Strobl et al., 2004) have been proposed and developed. They have distinct advantages: a simple device structure, no moving parts, electronic control, high speed, programmability, manufacturability, remote control, compactness, and high frequency response (Renaudin et al., 2006; Togle et al., 2004; Franke and Wixforth, 2008).

Selection of Bulk Materials or Thin Films

Acoustic wave devices can be used for both biosensing and microfluidics applications, which are two of the major components for lab-on-a-chip systems. Therefore, it is attractive to develop lab-on-chip biodetection platforms using acoustic wave devices because this integrates the functions of microdroplet transportation, mixing, and biodetection. To date, most of the acoustic devices have been made from bulk PE materials, such as quartz (SiO_2), lithium tantalate ($LiTaO_3$), lithium niobate ($LiNbO_3$), and sapphire (Al_2O_3). These bulk materials are expensive, and are less easily integrated with electronics for control and signal processing. PE thin films, such as PZT, ZnO, and AlN, have good PE properties, high electromechanical coupling coefficient, and high sensitivity and reliability (Pearton et al., 2005). They can be grown in thin film form on a variety of substrates, which include silicon, making these materials promising for integration with electronic circuitry, particularly for devices aimed for one-time use, low-price, and mass production (Muralt, 2008). It is suggested that this approach is likely to be the future of acoustic wave-based lab-on-a-chip biosensing devices.

ZnO, AlN, and PZT are the three dominant PE thin film materials which can be integrated into micro-electro-mechanical systems (MEMS) and microelectronics processers. Gallium arsenide (GaAs), silicon carbide (SiC), polyvinylidene fluoride (PVDF), and its copolymers are less common thin film PE materials (see Table 8.2). Among these, PZT has the highest PE constant and electromechanical coupling coefficient. However, for biosensing applications, PZT films have disadvantages, such as higher acoustic wave attenuation, lower sound wave velocities, poor biocompatibility, and, worst of all, the requirement for extremely high temperature sintering and high electric field polarization that make them largely unsuitable for integration with electronics (see Table 8.2).

TABLE 8.2

Comparison of Common PE Materials

Materials	ZnO	AlN	PZT	Quartz	128° Cut LiNbO$_3$	36° Cut LiTaO$_3$	PVDF
Density (g/cm³)	5.61	3.3	7.8	2.64	4.64	7.45	1.79
Moulus (GPa)	110–140	300–350	61	71.7		225	0.16
Hardness	4–5 GPa	15 GPa	7–18 GPa	Moh's 7	Moh's 5 Knoop 800–1000	70–110 Knoop 700–1200	Shore D75–85
Refractive index	1.9 to 2.0	1.96	2.40	1.46	2.29	2.18	1.42
Piezo-constant d33 (pC/N)	12	4.5, 6.4	289–380, 117	2.3 (d11)	19–27	21	35
Coupling coefficient, k	0.15–0.33	0.17–0.5	0.49	0.0014	0.23	0.2	0.12–0.2
Effective coupling coefficient, k^2 (%)	1.5–1.7	3.1–8	20–35	8.8–16	2–11.3	0.66–0.77	2.9
Acoustic velocity by transverse (m/s)	6336 (2650)	11050 (6090)	4500 (2200)	5960 (3310)	3970	3230–3295	2600
Dielectric constant	8.66	8.5–10	380	4.3	85 (29)	54 (43)	6–8
Coefficient of thermal expansion (CTE, ×10⁻⁶)	4	5.2	1.75	5.5	15	−16.5	42–75

The Rayleigh wave phase velocity in AlN is much higher than that of ZnO, which indicates that AlN is better for high frequency and high sensitivity applications (Lee et al., 2004). AlN is a hard material with a bulk hardness similar to quartz and is also chemically stable to attack by atmospheric gases at temperatures less than 700°C. However, the deposition of AlN films and their texture control is more difficult compared with that for ZnO. ZnO shows a higher PE coupling than AlN, and it is much easier to control the film stoichiometry, texture, and other properties (Jagadish and Pearton, 2006). Zinc oxide is biosafe and, therefore, there are no toxic effects for biomedical applications that immobilize and modify biomolecules (Kumar and Shen, 2008). Other PE films are either too expensive, such as GaAs and SiC, or too weak in their PE effect, for example, PE-polymers (Chu et al., 2003; Muthukumar et al., 2001). This chapter will focus on the applications of ZnO- and AlN-based acoustic wave devices for microfluidics and biosensing applications.

Requirement for ZnO or AlN Films for Sensing and Microfluidic Applications

For the successful integration of ZnO or AlN films with acoustic wave biosensing and microfluidic applications, there are several basic film requirements/specifications that must be met. These properties include (Fu et al., 2010):

(1) Microstructure considerations:
- Strong texture
- High crystal quality and low defects
- Uniformity in film microstructure and thickness
- Smooth surface and low roughness
- Good stoichiometry (Zn/O or Al/N ratio)

(2) Good PE properties:
- High frequency and large acoustic velocity
- High electromechanical coupling coefficient, k^2
- Low acoustic loss
- High quality factor, Q
- Good thermal or temperature stability (low thermal coefficient of frequency or velocity)

(3) Fabrication requirements:
- Compatibility with MEMS or CMOS technology
- Easy deposition on different substrates and complex shapes
- High deposition rate
- Low cost and mass production
- Reproducibility/high yield
- Low film stress/good adhesion to substrates

(4) Microfluidics and biosensing:

- High sensitivity and selectivity
- Stability of performance
- High pumping/mixing efficiency
- Easy functionalization of surfaces for immobilization of antibodies
- Biocompatibility

The following sections will focus on the recent progress covering the above issues for both the ZnO and AlN films.

ZnO Film

ZnO Film Deposition

Many different methods have been used to prepare ZnO films. These include the sol–gel process (Wang et al., 2006; Shinagawa et al., 2007; Kamalasanan and Chandra, 1996), molecular beam deposition (Nakamura et al., 2000), chemical vapor deposition (CVD) (Smith et al., 2003; Minami et al., 1994), organometallic chemical vapor deposition (MOCVD) (Gorla et al., 1999; Zhang et al., 2004; Park et al., 2001), and sputtering (Maniv and Zangvil, 1978; Wu et al., 1998; Hachigo et al., 1994; Sundaram and Khan, 1997), molecular beam epitaxy (MBE) (Look et al., 2002; Chen et al., 1998), pulsed laser deposition (PLD) (Narayan et al., 1998; Liu et al., 2003), and filtered vacuum arc deposition (FCVA) (Wang et al., 2003; Goldsmith, 2006). The main advantage of MBE is its precise control over the deposition parameters and in situ diagnostic capabilities. For ZnO thin film deposition by MBE, Zn metal and O_2 are usually used as the source materials, and the deposition is performed at a high temperature ranging from 800 to 1000°C. In the PLD method, high-power laser pulses are used to evaporate material from a target surface such that the stoichiometry of the material is preserved in the process. As a result, a supersonic jet of particles (plume) is directed normal to the target surface, and the ablated species condense on the substrate, which is located opposite to the target. The main advantages of PLD are its ability to create high-energy source particles, permitting high-quality film growth at potentially low substrate temperatures (typically ranging from 200 to 800°C) in high ambient gas pressures in the 10^{-5} to 10^{-1} Torr range. CVD technology is also important for ZnO film growth because it not only gives rise to high-quality films but also is applicable to large-scale production. However, the high temperature is a potential issue for the CVD method, although plasma-enhanced CVD (PECVD) and MOCVD do enable lower temperatures to be used. One of the most popular deposition techniques for the ZnO film is sputtering (DC sputtering, radio frequency, RF magnetron sputtering, and reactive sputtering). When compared with sol–gel and chemical vapor deposition, magnetron sputtering is a preferred method because of its low cost, simplicity, and low operating temperature. ZnO films can be deposited at a controlled substrate temperature either by sputtering from a high-purity ZnO target or by sputtering a Zn target in an Ar and O_2 gas mixture. Table 8.3 compares the different deposition methods for the ZnO films.

From an MEMS fabrication point of view, RF magnetron reactive sputtering is one of the best methods, with good reproducibility and compatibility with planar device fabrication

TABLE 8.3

Comparison of Different Types of Deposition Methods

	Sputtering	CVD and MOCVD	Laser Ablation	MBE	Sol–Gel	FCVA
Deposition rate	medium (a few nm/s)	Low (0.2 to a few nm/s)	Low (0.1 to 0.4 nm/s)	Very low	High	High (0.2–15 nm/s
Compatibility with MEMS processing	Good	OK	Poor	Poor	Good	Poor
Temperature	25 to 400°C	300 to 900°C	200 to 600°C	300 to 800°C	25 to 100°C	Below 400°C
Quality	Good	Good	Good	Excellent	Poor	Good
Cost	Slightly cost	Medium	Medium	High	Cheap	Medium
Deposition size	Large area	Large area	Small size	Medium	Large area	Small size

technology (Dang et al., 2007). In this section, we will focus on the texture and acoustic wave properties of sputtered ZnO films (Table 8.4).

The microstructure, texture, and PE properties of the sputtered ZnO films are normally affected by sputtering conditions such as plasma power, gas pressure, substrate, temperature, and film thickness. During sputtering, the energetic ion bombardment has significant effects on the stoichiometry, size, shape and orientation of ZnO crystals, intrinsic stress, defects, electrical and optical properties, as well as the surface and cross-section

TABLE 8.4

Summary of Velocity of ZnO Films on Different Substrates

Substrate Materials	Substrate Materials	Structure	Lattice Difference (%)	Velocity (m/s)	Temperature Expansion Coefficient (10^{-6} K^{-1})
ZnO	ZnO	HCP		2724	2.9 (4.751)
ZnO/Si	Si (111)	Cubic	41.3	2653	3
ZnO/Pt	Pt (111)	Cubic	1.8	2684	8.8
ZnO/Au	Au (111)	Cubic	2.5		14
ZnO/SiO$_2$	Quartz			4200	13.2 (a)/7.1c
Sapphire	Al$_2$O$_3$ (0001)	HCP	31.8	4000–5750	7.3 (18.1)
ZnO/LiNbO$_3$	LiNbO$_3$ (0001)	HCP			14.8 (4.1)
ZnO/sapphire	sapphire (0001)	HCP	31.8		8.4 (5.3)
ZnO/GaN	GaN	HCP	1.8		3.17
ZnO/AlN	AlN	HCP	4.1	4522,	5.3 (4.1)
ZnO/DLC	DLC	Amorphous		5000–7000	
ZnO/ Nanocrystalline diamond				8500	1.18
ZnO/Diamond	Diamond (111)	Cubic		10,000–12,000	1.18
ZnO/AlN/ diamond	ZnO/AlN/ diamond			12,200	

Note: Most data are from SAW devices; data are only used for comparison, as velocity is related to thickness, thus comparison of velocities is not meaningful unless film thickness is similar.

morphologies. Figure 8.5 shows the cross-sectional SEM images of the ZnO film for different film thicknesses. Columnar grains of ZnO can be observed that are perpendicular to the surface. This is because ZnO crystals typically grow as long hexagonal rods along the c-axis, which results in columnar grain structures. c-Axis ZnO structures are the preferred structures for SAW devices used for microfluidics, as these normally require a wave displacement perpendicular to the surface. X-ray diffraction (XRD) spectra of the ZnO films of different thickness indicate that most of the films have a single peak at 34.2° which corresponds to the diffraction from the (002) plane of the ZnO. Atomic force microscopy (AFM) images of samples grown under different conditions are shown in Figure 8.6. The surface roughness values for these films are approximately of the order of tens of nanometers, indicating that the films are reasonably smooth. Both grain sizes and roughness increase with thickness. The sputtered ZnO films show significant compressive stress that is made up of both the intrinsic and thermal components and presents a major challenge to the SAW devices. The thermal stress is related to the difference between the deposition temperature and operational temperature of the devices. However, the main cause of internal stress in ZnO film is compressive and is significantly greater than the thermal stress with typical values of 1 GPa. This internal compressive stress is a consequence of the high-energy ion bombardment on the film surface, which can be decreased significantly with

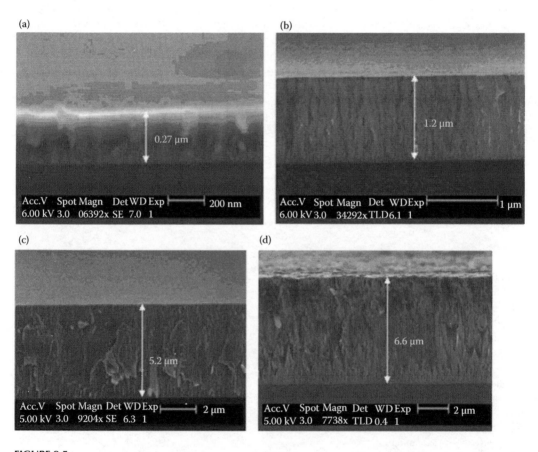

FIGURE 8.5
SEM images of cross section of ZnO films of different thickness. (a) 0.27 μm; (b) 1.2 μm; (c) 5.2 μm; and (d) 6.6 μm. (From Du, X.Y., PhD thesis, University of Cambridge, 2008. With permission.)

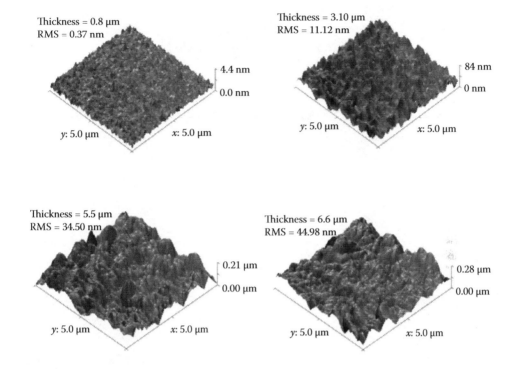

FIGURE 8.6
AFM images of surface morphologies for different thicknesses. (From Du, X.Y., PhD thesis, University of Cambridge, 2008. With permission.)

post-deposition annealing that reduces the number of defects by providing the thermal activation energy required for the defects states to move to a lower-energy crystalline phase.

The effects of the processing parameters, such as the sputtering gas pressure, RF power, total flux density, bias voltage, and substrate temperature, have been successfully described using modified Thornton models (Kluth et al., 2003). Figure 8.7a and b shows two examples of the modified Thornton zone model using a total energy flux density, E_Φ, instead of the commonly used gas pressure (Kluth et al., 2003; Tvarozek et al., 2007). The total energy flux density E_Φ (W/m^2) can be expressed by the parameters of RF power, deposition rate, voltage on target, gas pressure, and substrate bias voltages. The ratio of the total energy flux density E_Φ and its minimum value $E_{\Phi min}$, specified by the sputtering mode and the geometrical arrangement of the sputtering ZnO, can clearly describe the effects of RF power, gas pressure, and substrate voltages (see Figure 8.7a).

Several general conclusions about the effects of sputtering parameters on the growth of ZnO thin films are summarized as follows:

(1) Higher plasma or bias powers result in a higher deposition rate because the deposited particles have higher kinetic energies. However, the film surface roughness can increase significantly at a higher power, due to ion bombardment.

(2) Low gas pressure generally results in a dense and fine grain film. Higher gas pressure can result in porous, columnar films with rough surfaces (Zhu et al., 2000).

(3) The O_2/Ar ratio is a critical parameter, and a sufficient oxygen partial pressure is needed to maintain the stoichiometry of the ZnO films.

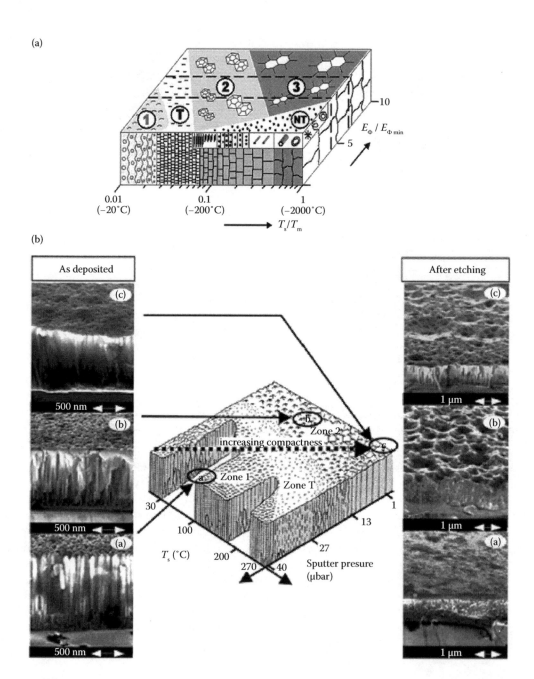

FIGURE 8.7
(a) Crystalline structure zone model of sputtered ZnO thin films: Zone 1—porous structure of tapered amorphous or crystalline nanograins separated by voids, Zone T—dense polycrystalline structure of fibrous and nanocrystalline grains, Zone 2—columnar grain structure, Zone 3—single-crystal micrograin structure, Zone NT—nanostructures and nanoelements. (From Tvarozek et al., *Thin Solid Films*, 515, 8756–8760, 2007. With permission.) (b) Modified Thornton model describes correlation between sputter parameters (sputter pressure and substrate temperature), structural film properties, and etching behavior of RF sputtered ZnO: Al films on glass substrates. (Kluth et al., *Thin Solid Films*, 442, 80, 2003. With permission.)

(4) ZnO thin films can be deposited at low temperature (<200°C), which is compatible with post-processing on CMOS circuitry. However, high-temperature deposition enhances the atom mobility, decreases the defects, promotes film adhesion to the substrate, improves film texture, quality, and increases grain size, resulting in compact and dense film structure.

(5) The sputtered film normally exhibits a good PE effect. Thus, post-deposition poling to obtain a good PE effect can be unnecessary.

Film Texture

The film texture of the ZnO film is crucial for the PE and acoustic wave properties of the acoustic devices with the substrate having significant influence on nucleation, growth, texture, acoustic wave velocity/frequency, and electromechanical coupling coefficient of the ZnO acoustic wave devices.

Self-Texture and Wave Mode

ZnO normally crystallizes in a hexagonal or wurtzite type crystalline structure (Özgür et al., 2005) (see Figure 8.8), which is dominated by three crystal planes: (0001), (10$\bar{1}$0), and (11$\bar{2}$0), with surface energy density of 0.099, 0.123, and 0.209 eV/Å^2, respectively (Fujimura et al., 1993). The (0001) plane has the lowest surface-free energy. Therefore, under equilibrium, if there is no epitaxy between the film and substrate, or without any external energy source, the films exhibit self-texture and grow along the (0001) orientation on both crystalline and amorphous substrates (Koch et al., 1997). However, as the film thickness increases, other orientation peaks may appear and become stronger (Lee et al., 1998). Excess Zn during film growth can cause the deterioration of the ZnO film crystallinity (Chiu and Liu, 2003). The O_2/Ar gas ratio and gas pressure also have significant effects on the film stress and texture.

ZnO SAW devices with a (0001) film texture can be used for sensing in air or gaseous environments. However, many biosensors need to detect chemical reactions in a liquid

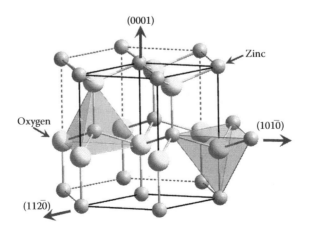

FIGURE 8.8
ZnO crystalline structure–Wurtzite structure with directions of (0001), (11$\bar{2}$0), and (10$\bar{1}$0) indicated. Lattice constants are a = 3.25 Å and c = 5.2 Å (http://upload.wikimedia.org/wikipedia/commons/8/8e/Wurtzite_poly hedra.png).

environment. For biosensing in liquids, it is necessary to generate an SH mode wave, where the wave displacement is within the plane of the crystal surface (Kadoka and Miura, 2002; Yanagitani et al., 2005). For the generation of such a SH wave, other film textures such as $(11\bar{2}0)$ and $(10\bar{1}0)$ are necessary (Yanagitani et al., 2004). Theoretical predictions indicate that (1) (002), (004) oriented ZnO films generate a pure longitudinal mode; (2) (100), (110), (200), (211), (300), and (220) oriented films a pure shear mode wave; (3) (101), (102), (103), (112), (201) oriented films a combination of longitudinal and shear mode waves (Wu et al., 2008).

Interlayer or Buffer Layer

An amorphous ZnO intermediate layer is normally formed before the growth of the crystalline ZnO layer on substrates, such as Ni, Cu, Si, Ti, Ni and glass, and this layer is about 10- to 50-nm thick depending on the type of substrates (Koch et al., 1997; Yoshino et al., 2000). Self-textured (0001) ZnO films slowly grow on this amorphous layer, which is probably the reason why the ZnO films deposited on Ni, Cu, and Cr substrates show poor texture. No such amorphous interlayer has been observed on Au, Ru, Pt, Al, and sapphire substrates (Kim et al., 2006; Matsuda et al., 2008), and the ZnO films deposited on these substrates show good (0001) orientation. Buffer layers are frequently used to enhance the film crystalline quality and texture, as reported for AlN, MgO, Al_2O_3, GaN, DLC, SiO_2, and so on (see Table 8.5) (Lee et al., 2004; Yoshino, 2009; Jung et al., 2004), and these buffer layers can also be used to promote the epitaxial growth of ZnO films.

Epitaxial Growth

Epitaxial growth on different substrates can lead to dissimilar ZnO orientations. The growth of ZnO can be attributed to the competition between the lowest surface free energy

TABLE 8.5

Summary of Velocity of AlN Films on Different Substrates

Substrate Materials	Substrate Materials	Structure	Lattice Difference (%)	Velocity (m/s)	Temperature Expansion Coefficient (10^{-6} K^{-1})
AlN/Si	Si (111)	Cubic		5000–5050	3
AlN/Al	Al (001)	Cubic	23.15		23.1
AlN/Pt	Pt (110)	Cubic	3		8.8
AlN/Au	Au (111)	Cubic			14
AlN/W	W (110)				
AlN/Mo			0.87		4.8
AlN/SiO$_2$	Quartz				13.2/7.1
AlN/Sapphire	Al$_2$O$_3$ (0001)	HCP		6000	8.4 (5.3)
AlN/LiNbO$_3$	LiNbO$_3$ (0001)	HCP			7.3 (18.1)
AlN/SiC	SiC (0001)	HCP	31.8	6500–7500	
AlN/GaN	GaN	HCP			
AlN/ZnO	ZnO (001)	HCP	4.1		2.9 (4.751)
AlN/DLC	DLC	Amorphous			
AlN/Diamond	Diamond (111)	Cubic		10,000–12,000	1.18

(0001) of ZnO and the closest lattice mismatch between the ZnO growth plane and the substrate plane (see Table 8.4) (Jo and Koo, 2009). However, this significantly depends on the deposition methods and substrate materials. MBE, PLD, MOCVD, and sputtering have frequently been used to grow the ZnO epitaxial films (Peruzzi et al., 2004; Triboulet and Perriere, 2003), whereas the common substrates for epitaxial growth of the ZnO film include quartz, sapphire, LiNbO$_3$, SrTiO$_3$, diamond, and MgO.

Oxygen Ion Bombardment

During ZnO sputtering, a directional oxygen ion beam, placed at an angle toward the substrate surface, plays an important role in changing the ZnO film texture from (0001) into (10$\bar{1}$0) or (11$\bar{2}$0) because of an ion channeling effect (Yanagitani and Kiuchi, 2007). The ZnO films with these two textures can excite a shear acoustic wave without a longitudinal wave (Mitsuyu et al., 1980). A prerequisite for the significant oxygen ion bombardment effect is a low gas pressure which contributes to a longer mean free path for the oxygen ion bombarding the film surface. ZnO films at different positions on the substrate under plasma also show different crystal orientations (see Figure 8.9) (Petrov et al., 1984), which can simply be explained by the oxygen ion bombardment angle under the target.

In summary, a (0001) film texture is relatively easy to obtain for sputtered ZnO films. To obtain other types of film texture, the following methods can be employed:

(1) Epitaxial growth on a specific substrate using a suitable deposition method

(2) Control of the sample position under the plasma (Miyamoto et al., 2006)

(3) Use of an additional anode near the substrate, which can have an apparent orientating effect on the growing films (Wang and Lakin, 1983)

(4) Substrate tilting with a set angle to create an oblique incidence of the particles on the growing film

(5) Use of an external oxygen ion source and control the oxygen ion bombardment during film growth

(6) Use of a shutter which can be positioned between the target and substrate to only allow oblique particles to be incident on substrate surface (Link et al., 2006)

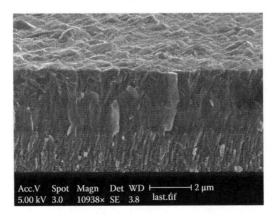

FIGURE 8.9
SEM cross-section morphologies of inclined ZnO films deposited using magnetron sputtering method.

PE Properties of Sputtered ZnO Films

Substrate Effect

The acoustic velocity of a ZnO film significantly depends on the substrates used for growth, with substrates with a large acoustic velocity, resulting in a large acoustic velocity in the film. Therefore, by selecting a substrate with a high acoustic velocity, the wave velocity in the ZnO SAW devices can be increased accordingly. For example, the acoustic velocity of bulk ZnO is 2724 m/s, increasing to 4522 m/s for ZnO/AlN and reaching up to 12,200 m/s for a ZnO/AlN/diamond substrate (Lamara et al., 2004; Hakiki et al., 2007). Table 8.4 summarizes the acoustic velocities of the ZnO films on different substrates. Among them, AlN, DLC, nanodiamond films, and diamond are regarded as the best substrate materials to provide a dramatic increase in acoustic wave velocities associated with ZnO films (Mortet et al., 2008; Lim et al., 2001; Lamara et al., 2004). As discussed before, the increase in resonant frequency is beneficial for the sensitivity of the acoustic wave sensors.

Film Thickness Effect

The acoustic velocity depends significantly on the ZnO film thickness for both ZnO-based SAW and FBAR devices and is discussed in more detail below.

(1) ZnO SAW devices

The ZnO film thickness effect for a ZnO/Si SAW device can be summarized as follows (Auld, 1973; Du et al., 2008):

(a) For a SAW device made on a very thin ZnO film (less than a few hundreds of nanometers), the acoustic wave can penetrate much deeper into the substrate as the thin film thickness is normally much less than one wavelength. In this case, the energy of a SAW device is largely dissipated in the substrate where the wave predominantly propagates. Thus, the wave velocity of the SAW approaches the Rayleigh velocity of the substrate material, as shown in Figure 8.10a.

(b) When the ZnO film thickness is increased, the acoustic velocity gradually changes to that of ZnO film (about 2724 m/s). Therefore, by varying the thickness of the ZnO film, the phase velocity of the acoustic wave can vary between the acoustic velocities of the surface PE layer and the substrate material. However, there is normally a cutoff thickness, below which no wave mode can be detected, because of the low electromechanical coupling coefficient for a very thin ZnO film.

(c) A Rayleigh-type wave (called the fundamental mode) can be generated when the film is thin. With increasing film thickness, a higher-order acoustic wave mode known as the Sezawa wave can be obtained. A Sezawa mode is realized from a layered structure in which the substrate has a higher acoustic velocity than the overlying film (Armstrong and Crampm, 1973). This wave exhibits a larger phase velocity (higher resonant frequency) than the Rayleigh wave for a fixed thickness (see Figure 8.11) and is thus desirable for high-frequency applications (Takagaki et al., 2000; Talbi et al., 2004). In a similar manner to that of Rayleigh wave, the resonant frequency and the phase velocity of the Sezawa wave decrease with film thickness.

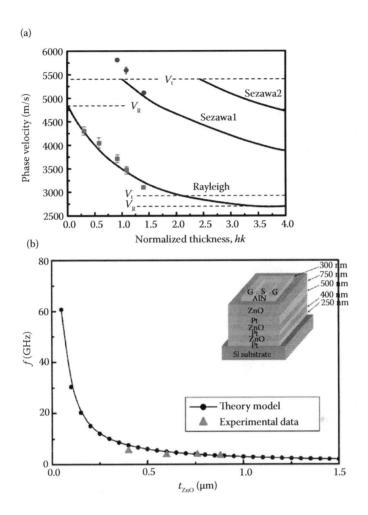

FIGURE 8.10
(a) Phase velocities for Rayleigh and Sezawa modes on different thickness of ZnO film. A film normalized thickness, hk, is used to describe film thickness effect ($k = 2\pi/\lambda$: wave vector, h: film thickness). (From Du, X.Y., PhD thesis, University of Cambridge, 2008. With permission.) (b) Resonant frequency of ZnO FBAR devices vs. film thickness. (From Yan et al., *Appl. Surf. Sci.*, 90, 9372–9380, 2007. With permission.)

(d) For the ZnO/Si SAW devices, the metallization ratio (ratio of thickness of metal and ZnO film) of the IDTs affects the generation of the guided mode and its harmonics. For example, if the metallization ratio changes from 0.5 to 0.4 (or to 0.7) in the ZnO/Si devices, many higher-order odd harmonic waves, such as the 3rd or 5th Rayleigh mode harmonic, or 3rd Sezawa mode harmonic can be realized together with the fundamental one (Brizoual et al., 2006, 2008). These higher mode harmonic waves can reach frequencies of a few GHz using conventional photolithography that potentially makes it unnecessary to use high acoustic velocity substrate materials (such as diamond) or advanced lithography processes (such as e-beam or deep-UV lithography) to make IDTs with submicron arm widths.

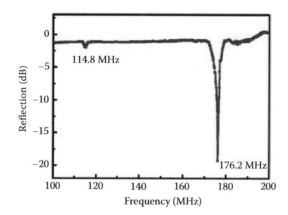

FIGURE 8.11
Rayleigh and Sezawa modes in frequency response of delay line for a ZnO SAW device with thickness of ZnO film of microns. (From Du, X.Y., PhD thesis, University of Cambridge, 2008. With permission.)

(2) ZnO FBAR devices

For ZnO FBAR devices, the resonant frequency depends on (1) the thickness and material type of the electrode; (2) the thickness ratio of the PE and electrode layers; (3) the material and thickness of the interlayer or buffer layer (Pham et al., 2008). With the decrease in ZnO film thickness the frequency generally increases significantly, with an example shown in Figure 8.10b (Yan et al., 2007; Tay et al., 2004). However, there is a practical minimum thickness limitation for the ZnO film. If the film is too thin, the frequency changes dramatically with variation in thickness which makes it more difficult to manufacture devices with a set specification.

Other Factors

For ZnO acoustic wave devices, the most frequently used electrode material is aluminum. However, the lifetime of the Al electrode in aqueous media is limited because of significant corrosion effects. The other common electrode materials include Au, Ni, W, Cu. The electromechanical coupling coefficient (k^2) of the ZnO/substrate acoustic wave devices depends on (Ntagwirumugra et al., 2007): (1) wave propagation mode, fundamentals, and their harmonics; (2) the normalized thickness of ZnO film; (3) film texture; (4) film thickness; (5) the nature and dimension of the electrodes; and (6) the substrate materials. For example, the relationship between the ZnO thickness ratio and the k_t^2 (for FBAR device) is shown in Figure 8.12 (Takeuchi et al., 2002). Using a resonant (f_r) and an anti-resonant frequency (f_a) the k_t^2 is approximately given by:

$$k_t^2(\%) = 2(f_a - f_r)/f_a \qquad (8.4)$$

An increase in the k_t^2 is observed with an increase in the ZnO thickness ratio. In the case where the ZnO thickness ratio is larger than 70%, k_t^2 becomes a constant at 3.4%, which is 38% of the bulk ZnO effective coupling coefficient.

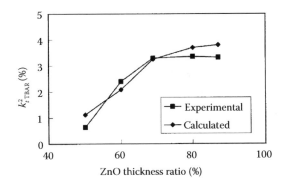

FIGURE 8.12

Relationship between the ZnO thickness ratio and effective coupling coefficient k_t^2. (From Takeuchi et al. *Vacuum*, 66, 463–466, 2002. With permission.)

The temperature coefficient of frequency (TCF) is an important parameter for ZnO FBAR and SAW applications for biosensors. There are different strategies to minimize the TCF or compensate for the temperature effect associated with ZnO-based devices. The common method is to combine a material with a positive (or negative) TCF value, with another one with a negative (or positive) TCF. A ZnO film has a negative TCF value; thus, an easy way to reduce the TCF is to use a substrate or interlayer with a positive TCF value, such as SiO_2 or quartz (Yoshino et al., 2002).

MEMS Processing of ZnO Films

ZnO films normally have excellent bonding to a range of substrate materials. However, caution is required for MEMS processing of ZnO films because they are quite reactive and sensitive to high temperature, as well as acids or water (Xu et al., 2003). In fact, ZnO will dissolve in deionized water with a solubility of about 2 mg/l (Zhou et al., 2006). Hence, any rinsing of ZnO films using DI water should be minimized. Acetone can be used for cleaning the samples, but Pirana, or other strong cleaning solutions, should be avoided. In addition, ZnO is easily hydrolyzed upon exposure to air. For MEMS processing with ZnO, it is necessary to pre-bake the film, remove the moisture, and improve the adhesion of photoresist. However, high temperature post-baking or annealing above 400°C should be avoided because ZnO recrystallization may occur and deteriorate the film.

Photoresist adheres well to clean and dry ZnO films, with adhesion being improved by (1) pre-baking; (2) coating with other materials, such as SiO_2; and (3) using an adhesion promoter. ZnO is soluble in most acids, and although etchants, such as HCl, H_3PO_4, HF, HNO_3, alkalis, ammonium chloride, and $NH_4Cl + NH_4OH + H_2O$, can be used for removing ZnO, the etch profile is typically difficult to control. Recommended ZnO film etching solutions also include (Zheng et al., 2007): (1) $H_3PO_4 + HAc + H_2O$ (1:1:50); (2) $FeCl_3 + 6H_2O$.

ZnO can be plasma etched using many gases, including oxygen. For dry etching of ZnO films with a photoresist mask, there are two types of gas systems which have been frequently used: (1) a hydrogen-based gas, such as $CH_4/H_2/Ar$, that can help with obtaining an anisotropic etch profile; (2) chlorine-based gases, such as Cl_2/Ar, BCl_3/Ar and $BCl_3/Cl_2/Ar$ plasma, but they are toxic (Pearton et al., 2004). A new plasma etching method using a remote Ar/H_2 plasma has been reported in which the hydrogen ions contribute to efficient and fast etching (Groenen et al., 2005). Inductively coupled plasma reactive ion etching has

(a)　　　　　　　　(b)

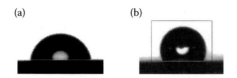

FIGURE 8.13
Contact angle of (a) untreated and (b) Teflon-treated ZnO film.

also been used to anisotropically etch ZnO films using HBr/Ar plasma with photoresist as the etch mask (Min et al., 2008). The etching of ZnO films in the HBr/Ar gas mixture is controlled by chemically assisted sputter etching.

For microfluidic applications, ZnO has the useful property that it is hydrophilic with a contact angle typically ranging from 50° to about 80° (see Figure 8.13a), with the value depending on the surface conditions and light exposure (Kenanakis et al., 2008). Ultraviolet irradiation of ZnO films results in a superhydrophilic surface (Sun et al., 2001). For efficient droplet pumping, a hydrophobic surface is normally needed, and methods for improving the hydrophobic properties of the ZnO films include (Hu et al., 2007; Badre et al., 2007; Mei et al., 2003): (1) spin coating PTFE (Teflon), (2) a monolayer of octadecyl thiol (ODT), (3) a monolayer of octadecylesilane (ODS, 97% Aldrich), and (4) an octadecyltrichrorosilane (OTS) self-assembled monolayer. After such treatment, the contact angle can be as high as 100° to 120° (see Figure 8.13b).

Functionalization of ZnO Surface for Biosensing

A critical issue in developing a high-performance biosensor is to determine a simple and reliable process for the functionalization of the ZnO surface through a covalent method to form a robust immobilization of appropriate probe molecules. Normally, Au is predeposited on the ZnO surface, and a cystamine surface atomic monolayer (SAM) forms on the Au surface to which antibodies are to be attached. Currently, little work has been performed on the direct surface functionalization of the ZnO films. Initial studies for immobilization of antibodies on the ZnO film surface have been realized using (Corso et al., 2008; Krishnamoorthy, 2006) (1) amine-terminated silane, 3-aminopropltryiethoxysilane, and glutaraldehyde as the secondary crosslinker to bind a protein; (2) 3-mercaptopropyl-trimethoxysilane in dry toluene; or (3) trimethoxysilane in dry toluene to immobilize the antibody. Although Au is not recognized as a good CMOS-compatible material that can be fully integrated into the fabrication process, the direct immobilzation on the ZnO film has its advantages in biosensing applications.

AlN Films

Currently, there is a concern that ZnO film is very reactive and unstable even in air or moisture. Therefore, the stability and reliability is potentially a major problem. Compared with ZnO, AlN shows a slightly lower PE coupling. The Rayleigh wave phase velocity in AlN is much higher than that in ZnO, which suggests that AlN is better for high-frequency

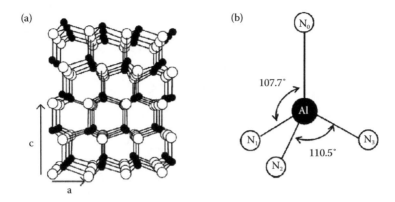

FIGURE 8.14
(a) Hexagonal structure of AlN and (b) tetrahedral structure, with one Al atom surrounded by four N atoms. (From Chiu et al., *Appl. Phys. Lett.*, 93, 163106, 2007. With permission.)

and high-sensitivity applications (Lee et al., 2004). AlN has a very large volume resistivity and is a hard material with a bulk hardness similar to quartz. Pure AlN is chemically stable with atmospheric gases at temperatures less than about 700°C. The combination of these physical and chemical properties is consequently promising in practical applications of AlN both in bulk and thin film forms. Using AlN could lead to the development of acoustic devices operating at higher frequencies, with improved sensitivity and performance (insertion loss and resistance) in harsh environments (Wingqvist et al., 2007). AlN thin films have other good properties, such as high thermal conductivity, good electrical isolation, a wide band gap (6.2 eV), and a thermal expansion coefficient, similar to that of GaAs. Therefore, AlN thin films have been applied not only to surface passivation of semiconductors and insulators but also to optical devices in the ultraviolet spectral region and acousto-optic devices.

The AlN crystal belongs to a hexagonal class (see Figure 8.14) or a distorted tetrahedron, with each Al atom surrounded by four N atoms (Chiu et al., 2007). The four Al–N bonds can be categorized into two types: three are equivalent Al–N$_{(x)}$ ($x = 1, 2, 3$) bonds, B$_1$, and one is a unique Al–N$_0$ bond, B$_2$, in the c-axis direction or the (002) orientation. Because B$_2$ is more ionic, it has a lower bonding energy than the other bonds. The highest value of k_t^2 and the PE stress constant are in the c-axis direction. Hence, when an acoustic wave device is excited in the film thickness direction, the AlN film will grow with c-axis orientation in the direction of film growth (normal to the bottom electrode) and enhance piezoelectricity.

AlN Film Deposition

AlN film can be deposited using CVD or PECVD (Sanchez et al., 2008), PLD (Tabbal et al., 2001; Tanosch et al., 2006; Ishihara et al., 2000; Liu et al., 2003), MBE (Kern et al., 1998), sputtering (Mortet et al., 2003, 2004; Auger et al., 2004; Clement et al., 2003), and FCVA (Ji et al., 2004). Of these technologies, MBE can grow a single-crystal epitaxial AlN film but with limitations that include low growth rate, expensive instrument setup, and a high process temperature. CVD, including MOCVD and PECVD, can be used to grow high-quality crystalline AlN films, but its high process temperature (about 500 to 1000°C) may be inappropriate for CMOS-compatible processes. Reactive sputtering methods can deposit a good crystalline AlN thin film at a relatively low temperature (between 25°C and

500°C), and these sputtered films normally show good epitaxial film structure (Ishihara et al., 2004; Engelmark et al., 2000). From an MEMS fabrication point of view, RF magnetron reactive sputtering is one of the best methods, with good reproducibility and compatibility with planar device fabrication technology. In this section, we will focus on the texture and acoustic wave properties of the sputtered AlN films.

Cheung and Ong (2004) have systematically studied the effect of substrate temperature, RF power, and substrate materials for the formation of a broad range of amorphous, poly-crystalline, and epitaxial AlN films. The growth dynamic or surface kinetic roughening of AlN films grown on Si (100) substrates by sputtering has been thoroughly studied, and a two-stage growth regime has been identified (Auger et al., 2005). In the first step, the growth dynamic is unstable with significant sticking probabilities of the impinging parti-cles. The films have a mixture of well-textured and randomly oriented crystals. In the sec-ond regime, the films are homogeneous and well textured, and the growth is dominated by the shadowing effect induced by the bombardment of impinging particles (Auger et al., 2005). Based on this, a two-step deposition technique has been proposed to increase film texture and reduce film stress by changing either gas pressure or plasma power during deposition (Cherng et al., 2008, 2009). For example, the first stage can be a low-power, high-temperature deposition that provides high mobility to the surface atoms. The second stage might be a high-power deposition at lower temperatures characterized by high deposition rates and low residual stress.

For film growth, conditions are more critical for the AlN films than those for ZnO films. Growing a thick AlN film is rather critical because of its tendency to present microcrack-ing. Oxygen and argon could have significant influences for AlN film growth during sput-tering and contamination due to residual oxygen or water can seriously interfere with the formation of the AlN film structure. Growth rate of the AlN film will decrease with increasing oxygen in the sputtering gas and their predominant polarity also changes from Al polarity to N polarity with increases in the oxygen concentration (Cherng et al., 2008; Vergara et al., 2004). Increased oxygen concentration in sputtering gas also increases Al–O bonding, as the bonding energy of Al–O (511 kJ/mol) is higher than that of Al–N (230 kcal/mol) (Akiyama et al., 2008), which is important as oxygen concentration significantly influ-ences the PE response of AlN films.

AlN Film Texture and Substrate Effect

Films with strong crystallinity can have good PE coefficients, high electromechanical cou-pling, and acoustic velocities approaching those of the single crystal AlN. The sputtering process parameters significantly affect the orientation of the deposited AlN films. Okano et al. (1992) identified that the c-axis orientation increases as the N_2 concentration in the mixture of Ar and N_2 decreases, whereas Naik et al. (1999) showed that the c-axis orienta-tion increases as the sputtering pressure is reduced. AlN films have been reported to show preferred (002) growth orientation on silicon, quartz, glass, $LiNbO_3$ (Caliendo et al., 2003; Lee et al., 2004), GaAs (Cheng et al., 1998), GaN/Sapphire (Kao et al., 2008; Xu et al., 2006), SiC (Takagaki et al., 2002), and ZnO layer (Lim et al., 2001).

Commonly used electrode materials for AlN SAW devices include Mo, Ti, Al, Au, Pt, Ni, and TiN. Al and Mo have low resistivity and high Q factors, with Mo being one of the most widely reported electrodes in the AlN film-based acoustic devices (Akiyama et al., 2005; Huang et al., 2004, 2005; Lee et al., 2003; Okamoto et al., 2008; Cherng et al., 2004). Ag, Al, Co, Cr, Cu Fe, Nb, Ni, Zn, and Zr have also been reported as electrodes for the AlN-based acoustic wave devices (Lee et al., 2004; Akiyama et al., 2004). For the AlN FBAR device, the bottom metal layer significantly affects the texture of AlN films and, hence, its electro-acoustic properties. AlN films deposited on the materials with fcc lattice structure show a high c-axis orientation, especially for Au and Pt (Tay et al., 2005). Ti has a hexagonal structure similar to that of AlN (Lee et al., 2004; Chou et al., 2006). W has a low acoustic attenuation, small mismatch in the coefficient of thermal expansion and high acoustic impedance with AlN, and is thus a good electrode material for AlN devices. Ni was often chosen because of its good surface smoothness, but the AlN film texture on Ni is not as good as that on the other fcc metals. Tantalum (Hirata et al., 2005) and iridium (Clement et al., 2009) have also been reported to be used as electrodes for AlN film growth. The thickness ratio of AlN and top electrodes has been reported to have a significant influence on PE effect of AlN films (Akiyama et al., 2004; Huang et al., 2005).

Sputtered AlN films normally show a (002) film texture, which results in longitudinal (or Rayleigh) wave modes and is therefore good for sensing in air or gas. However, as explained before, if liquid exists on the sensing surface, excessive damping and attenuation of the propagating wave occurs when the longitudinal mode couples into the liquid. This problem can be solved by generating a SH-SAW, which propagates on a piezo-material by an in-plane SH motion (Wingqvist et al., 2007), and dramatically reduces SAW coupling into a liquid medium (Mchale, 2003). However, the commonly observed (002) texture in the sputtered AlN films is unsuitable for generating SH-SAWs. Besides this, using a pure shear wave is not efficient in driving liquid droplets forward. A good approach to solving the problem is to develop AlN films in which the c-axis is inclined relative to the surface normal, thus allowing both longitudinal and shear wave modes to be generated (Webber, 2006). These two modes will have different frequencies and, thus, can be individually controlled for either pumping or sensing purposes. To the best of our knowledge, there are no reports of the application of both the functions (microfluidics and biosensing) on a c-axis inclined AlN-based SAW device in liquid conditions. The techniques for the deposition of the inclined AlN film include (1) using a tilted substrate (up to 45°) with a controlled position under the sputter-target; (2) using a high-energy nitrogen ion beam aimed at the desired angle with respect to the substrate surface normal (Yanagitani and Kiuchi, 2007). Obtaining the inclined AlN films strongly depends on the sputtering pressure, temperature, and the oblique incidence of particles (Yang et al., 2009). c-Axis–inclined AlN films have been deposited on silicon substrate and diamond substrate (Fardeheb-Mammeri et al., 2008).

During sputtering, the particle bombardment could induce large film stress (Iborra et al., 2004). Films with large compressive stress can cause buckling-induced delamination in the deposited films and fracture in the released devices. In Ar/N_2-based deposition system for AlN film deposition, the energy of Ar ions colliding with the substrate controls the preferred orientation of the AlN films; moreover, directionality and the energy of the ions determine the residual stress levels. The energy of the Ar bombardment can be adjusted by the substrate bias voltage during sputter deposition. Thermal annealing is a good method for posttreatment to reduce film stress and improve coating quality (Hung and Chung, 2009).

PE Properties of Sputtered AlN Films

There are two key issues for the PE properties of the AlN acoustic wave device: the electromechanical coupling coefficient and the quality factor Q. The quality of the AlN film, such as film texture and stress, strongly affects the resonant frequency. For the AlN-based acoustic wave device, parameters of Q factor, resonant frequency, and effective coupling constant are determined by AlN film quality, the electrode material quality, and electrode thickness, as well as film roughness (Lee et al., 2002). The use of high impedance electrodes, such as W or Mo, is effective in obtaining a high effective coupling coefficient.

AlN films have also been deposited on 128° LiNbO$_3$ substrate to enhance the SAW velocity and improve the temperature stability, that is, decrease the TCF (Kao et al., 2003; Wu et al., 2001, 2002). The acoustic velocity in a AlN/Si SAW device also depends on the orientation of the Si substrate; it is about 4700 m/s for Si (111) and 5100 m/s for Si (100) (Clement, 2003). In a similar manner to that for ZnO films, as the AlN film thickness decreases, the fundamental resonant frequency decreases, as can be observed from Figure 8.15a. Figure 8.15b shows the effective coupling coefficient as a function of the thickness ratio of electrode layer to PE layer for AlN thin film resonators (Chen and Wang, 2005). For an AlN thin film resonator, an increase in the electrode layer thickness initially increases k_{eff}^2 and reaches a maximum value near the thickness ratios of 0.03 and 0.12 for gold and aluminum electrodes, respectively. This increase in the effective coupling coefficient can be attributed to the improved match in the distribution of acoustic standing wave to the linear distribution of applied electric potential (Chen and Wang, 2005). With further increases in electrode thickness, k_{eff}^2 begins to drop since more of the resonator volume becomes occupied by non-PE electrode material (Chen and Wang, 2005). The use of a thin layer of gold for the electrode (which has higher acoustic impedance than Al) has a significant effect on k_{eff}^2. For the *c*-axis–inclined AlN films, the inclined angle can have a dramatic effect on the acoustic velocity and coupling coefficient for both the Rayleigh wave and shear wave as shown in Figure 8.16 (Chen and Wang, 2005).

Recently, there has been a lot of research work on the deposition of AlN on diamond to create SAW devices (Mortet et al., 2003; Kirsch et al., 2006; Le Brizoual et al., 2007; Paci et al., 2007; Elmazria et al., 2007; El Hakiki et al., 2007; Wu et al., 2009; Elmazria et al., 2003; Shih et al., 2009; Iriarte et al., 2003; Benedic et al., 2008; Lin et al., 2009). The drive for this is that much higher phase velocities can be achieved from 6 to 16 km/s (Wu et al., 2008). The phase velocity dispersion curves of the first five Rayleigh SAW modes of propagation in the IDT/(002) AlN/(111) diamond structure are shown in Figure 8.17, and the curves

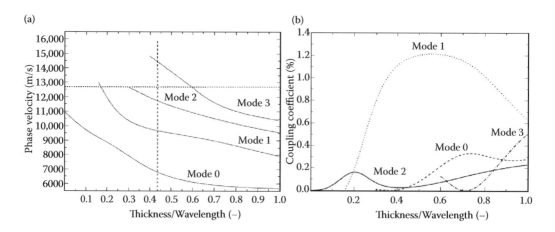

FIGURE 8.15
(a) Phase velocity for AlN film as a function of thickness/wavelength ratio for different acoustic wave modes (b). Effective coupling coefficient as a function of thickness ratio of electrode-to-PE layers for AlN thin film resonators. (From Clement et al., *Ultrasonics*, 42, 403–407, 2003. With permission.)

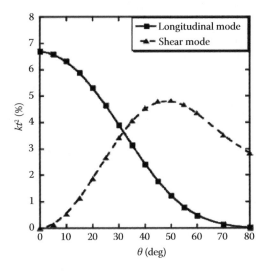

FIGURE 8.16
Calculated electromechanical coupling for both shear and longitudinal modes at different AlN crystal tilt, θ. For c-axis-inclined AlN films, inclined angle could have dramatic effect on acoustic velocity and coupling coefficient for both Rayleigh wave and shear wave. (From Chen, Q.M., and Wang, Q.M., *Appl. Phys. Lett.*, 86, 022904, 2005.)

are plotted as a function of the film thickness ratio h/λ. The phase velocity of each mode decreases as the film thickness ratio increases. For mode 0, the value of phase velocity is determined by the SAW velocity of (111) diamond, that is, 10.9 km/s at $h/\lambda = 0$. As the film thickness ratio h/λ increases, the phase velocity curve rapidly decreases. At $h/\lambda = 3$, the velocity of the (002) AlN/diamond is about 5.4 km/s. It can be observed that the harmonic peaks of modes 1, 2, 3, and 4 cutoff at the critical point where the phase velocity is equal to the shear bulk wave velocity in (111) diamond 12.3 km/s. For example, cutoff of mode 1 occurs at $h/\lambda = 0.172$, mode 2 at $h/\lambda = 0.295$, mode 3 at $h/\lambda = 0.594$, and mode 4 at $h/\lambda = 0.693$ (Wu et al., 2008).

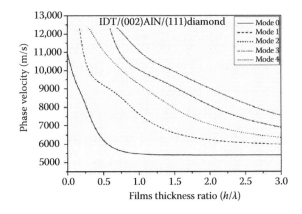

FIGURE 8.17
Phase velocities dispersion curves of first five Rayleigh SAW modes propagation in the IDT/_002_ AlN/_111_ diamond. The phase velocity dispersion curves of first five.

MEMS Processing of AlN Films

There are several reports on surface micromachining AlN (Hara et al., 2005). Germanium can be used as the sacrificial layer for the AlN films, instead of common amorphous silicon, SiO_2, or a metal. AlN can be etched in aqueous solutions, such as KOH, NaOH, HF/H_2O, HF/HNO_3, tetramethyl ammonium hydroxide (TMAH), and the etch rate is temperature- and crystal polarity–sensitive (Jasinki et al., 2003; Sheng et al., 1988; Tan et al., 1995). Cr can also be used to form both a good etch mask and electrode (Saravanan et al., 2006). AlN can be electrochemically etched in electrolytes, such as HPO_3 (60°C to 90°C) or KOH solutions, and the etch rate is strongly dependent on the coating quality (from tens of nm/min up to a few µm/min). The reaction is (Zhang and Edgar, 2005):

$$AlN + 6KOH \rightarrow Al(OH)_3 \downarrow + NH_3 \uparrow + 3K_2O \downarrow \qquad (8.5)$$

For dry etching process, AlN is normally etched using a chlorine-based plasma, such as chlorine and BCl_3, rather than a fluorine plasma because aluminum fluoride is stable and nonvolatile (Khan et al., 2002). Etching in a Cl-based plasma is normally isotropic, and the volatile reaction product is $AlCl_3$ at high temperature (above 180°C) or Al_2Cl_6 at a room temperature (Engelmark, 2003). SF_6/Ar plasma has also been used to etch AlN, and the etching process is believed to be a combination of the reactions of F and Al and sputtering of reactive a product (AlF_3), with highly anisotropic and smooth side walls.

Functionalization of AlN Surface for Biosensing

Recently, there have been some studies for the surface functionalization of AlN film for biosensing applications (Chiu et al., 2008). For example, by using silane, a new chemical layer can form on the AlN, and the functional groups on the silane surface can then be used as anchor points for the antibodies. A generic method for immobilization of gold nanoparticle bioconjugates onto AlN surfaces using aminosilane molecules as cross-linkers has been demonstrated for SAW sensor applications (Chiu et al., 2008). Electrostatic interaction between the positively charged surface amine groups and negatively charged DNA–Au nanoparticle conjugates allows the self-assembly of a probe nanoparticle monolayer onto the functionalized AlN surfaces under physiological conditions. Results showed that Au nanoparticles can play multiple roles in SAW sensing for probe molecule immobilization, signal amplification, and labeling (Chiu et al., 2008).

In reference (Cao et al., 2008), antibody immobilized AlN/sapphire was prepared using the process shown schematically in Figure 8.18. The AlN films were pretreated before silanization using two methods. In the first method, they were treated by exposure to an oxygen plasma. The second method treated the AlN surfaces by ultrasonication in 3:1 (in vol%) piranha solution, followed by rinsing in DI water. Piranha treatment was chosen because it is commonly used as a surface preparation method for silanization of other types of inorganic surfaces. Improved silane surfaces should create a more stable and ordered silane layer for the linkage of antibody, phages or other detecting ligands in the biosensor under development (Cao et al., 2008). The treated AlN samples were silanized with OTS. The ability to produce repeatable, homogeneous layers of selected chemical groups by silane derivatization of the AlN surface is considered to be a promising step in the development of a biosensor that uses surface immobilized phage or antibody ligands for analyte detection (Cao et al., 2008).

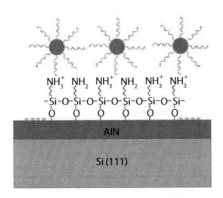

FIGURE 8.18
Schematic diagram of antibody immobilized AlN/sapphire. (From Cao et al., *Solids Surf. B*, 63, 176–182, 2008. With permission.)

Thin Film Acoustic Devices for Biosensor Applications

SAW Biosensor

A ZnO/Si SAW device has been successfully used in the detection of PSA antibody–antigen immunoreaction shown in Figure 8.19 (Lee et al., 2007). The resonant frequency of the ZnO SAW devices was found to shift to lower frequencies as the PSAs are specifically immobilized on the surface-modified ZnO SAW device. A linear dependence has been measured between the resonance frequency change and the PSA/ACT complex concentrations over the broad dynamic range of 2–10,000 ng/ml. However, as discussed before, a big challenge for SAW biosensors is how to realize detection in a liquid environment. Love mode SAW devices are promising technologies for biosensors in liquid environments because of their high-sensitivity and low-energy dissipation. The essential condition for a Love wave mode is that the shear wave velocity in the surface wave guide layer is smaller than that in the PE substrate. For example, ZnO has a shear wave velocity of 2578 m/s, whereas those of ST-cut

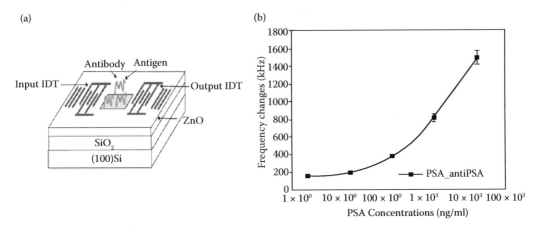

FIGURE 8.19
Illustration of the principle of ZnO-based SAW biosensor. (From Lee et al., ZnO surface acoustic wave biosensor, International Electron Devices Meeting, Washington, DC, Dec. 10–12, 2007. With permission.)

quartz and SiO$_2$ are 4996 and 3765 m/s, respectively. Therefore, it is reasonable to use ZnO as a guiding layer on substrates of ST-cut quartz to form the Love mode biosensors. The other potential substrate materials for Love-mode ZnO sensors include LiTaO$_3$, LiNbO$_3$, and sapphire. A ZnO Love mode device of ZnO/ST-cut quartz has a maximum sensitivity up to -18.77×10^{-8} m^2 s kg^{-1}, which is much higher than that of a SiO$_2$/quartz Love mode SAW device (Chu et al., 2003; Jian et al., 2004; Krishnamoorthy and Iliadis, 2006).

Most of the above-mentioned ZnO Love mode sensors are based on a bulk PE substrate (e.g., quartz, LiNbO$_3$ and LiTaO$_3$, etc.), which are expensive and incompatible with IC fabrication. In reference (Mchale et al., 2002), ZnO/SiO$_2$/Si SAW Love mode sensors with an acoustic wave velocity of 4814.4 m/s were studied, and the sensitivity of the devices was 8.64 μm^2/mg, which is about 2 to 5 times that of ZnO/LiTaO$_3$ (Powel, 2004) and SiO$_2$/quartz Love sensors (Du and Harding, 1998). Another promising approach for making a ZnO-based Love mode sensor is to use a polymer film (such as PMMA, polyimide, SU-8 or parylene C) on top of the ZnO layer as the guiding layer. However, this layered structure uses a polymer waveguide and has a relatively larger intrinsic attenuation than those with solid waveguide layers.

AlN SAW devices normally have higher phase velocities, for example, 5536 m/s for an AlN/Si SAW device (Assouar et al., 2002; Mortet et al., 2003). Currently, there are not so many reports on AlN-based SAW biosensors. The reason could be the difficulties in the deposition of thick AlN film for SAW devices, which normally have large film stress and poor adhesion with the substrate. AlN films have been reported to deposit on a LiNbO$_3$ substrate to form a highly sensitive Love mode sensing device (Kao et al., 2003, 2004).

Lamb Biosensor

In Lamb wave sensors, the wave propagation velocity in the membrane is lower than the acoustic wave velocity in the fluids on the surface. Therefore, the acoustic energy is not easily dissipated, and Lamb wave sensors can be used in liquid (Wenzel and White, 1990). A ZnO-based Lamb wave device has been used to monitor the growth of bacterium *Pseudomonas putida* in a bolus of toluene, as well as the reaction of antibodies in an immunoassay for an antigen present in breast cancer patients (White, 1997). Another Si/SiO$_2$/Si$_3$N$_4$/Cr/Au/ZnO Lamb wave device has been used for detecting human IgE based on the conventional cystamine SAM technology, with a sensitivity as high as 8.52×10^7 cm^2/g at a wave frequency of 9 MHz (Huang and Lee, 2008). In recent years, however, the Lamb wave biosensor has not been widely reported because (1) the sensitivity is not as high as that of the other devices due to the low operation frequency and (2) it is difficult to fabricate thin and fragile membrane structures. Duhamel et al. (2006) studied an AlN/Si-based Lamb wave biosensor, with a sensitivity of 326 cm^2/g. However, because of the thin membrane structure, temperature sensitivity is also significant, which makes temperature compensation necessary.

FBAR Biosensor

FBAR biosensors have recently attracted great attention because of their inherent advantages compared with SAW and QCM biosensors: high sensitivity, low insertion loss, high power handling capability, and small size (Bjurstrom et al., 2004; Kang et al., 2005). High-frequency ZnO FBAR sensors have good sensitivity and high energy densities owing to the trapping of the standing wave between the two electrodes, allowing device size to be scaled down to areas more than 3 orders of magnitude smaller than SAW and QCM devices. This makes the integration of FBAR arrays for parallel detection both feasible and low cost. Gabl et al. (2004) used a label-free FBAR gravimetric biosensor with a high operating frequency of 2 GHz based on a ZnO film to detect DNA and protein molecules. Its sensitivity of 2400 Hz cm^2/ng is about 2500 times higher than that of a conventional QCM device with a frequency of 20 MHz. A recent study using an Al/ZnO/Pt/Ti FBAR design gave a sensitivity of 3654 kHz cm^2/ng with a good thermal stability (Lin et al., 2008; Yan et al., 2007).

Conventional (0001) textured ZnO FBARs operate using a longitudinal wave and cannot be used for sensing in a liquid environment. In contrast, a (11–20) textured ZnO film exhibits pure shear modes waves that can propagate in a liquid with little damping effect. A ZnO shear mode FBAR device has been used in a water–glycerol solution, with a high operating frequency of 830 MHz and a sensitivity of 1000 Hz cm^2/ng (Link et al., 2007). Weber et al. (2006) fabricated a ZnO FBAR device that operated in a transversal shear mode, using a ZnO film with 16° off c-axis crystal orientation. For an avidin/anti-avidin system, the fabricated device had a high sensitivity of 585 Hz cm^2/ng and a mass detection limit of 2.3 ng/cm^2. This shear wave FBAR device has also been reported to have a stable TCF (Link et al., 2006).

Compared with ZnO films, AlN is a promising material for FBAR devices owing to its advantageous characteristics, including high BAW velocity, moderate electromechanical coupling constant, high electric resistivity, low dielectric loss, good chemical stability, good thermal stability, and a wide band gap (Chiu, 2007, 2008). PE AlN-based FBAR devices have already been successfully commercialized (Kim et al., 2001; Tadigadapa et al., 2009).

For liquid FBAR sensing, a good idea is to develop ZnO or AlN films in which the c-axis is inclined relative to the surface normal, thus allowing both longitudinal and shear wave modes to be generated (with one example shown in Figure 8.20a) (Weber, 2006). Another popular method is to use lateral field excitation (LFE) of the PE layer, requiring both signal and ground electrodes being in-plane and parallel on the exposed surface of the ZnO or AlN film. A laterally excited ZnO thickness shear mode resonator has been reported that

(a)

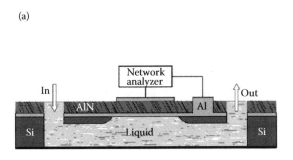

(b)

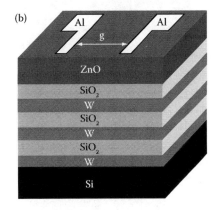

FIGURE 8.20
(a) Schematic illustration of a shear mode FBAR resonator together with a microfluidic transport system. (From Weber et al., *Sens. Actuators*, A128, 84–88, 2006. With permission.) (b) A laterally excited ZnO thickness shear mode resonator that is both extremely simple to fabricate and highly sensitive to surface perturbations. Resonator configuration consists of a laterally excited, solidly mounted ZnO thin film resonator that incorporates use of an acoustic mirror. (From Dickherber et al., *Sens. Actuators A*, 144, 7–12, 2008; Corso et al. *J. Appl. Phys.*, 101, 054514, 2007. With permission.)

is extremely simple to fabricate and highly sensitive to surface perturbations (see Figure 8.20b). The resonator configuration consists of a laterally excited, solidly mounted ZnO thin film resonator that incorporates the use of an acoustic mirror. The device operates stably in biologically equivalent environments such as NaCl in deionized water (Dickherber et al., 2008; Corso et al., 2007).

Although FBAR-based biosensor showed a high sensitivity and good resolution, there are several issues to be addressed. For example, they normally have high acoustic wave attenuation and low quality factors due to potential thin film material defects. Other issues include the sensor packaging and the effect of high frequency on biochemistry (Wingquist et al., 2007a, 2007b).

Thin Films for Microfluidic Applications

SAW Mixer and Pump

In a SAW device, the interaction between the longitudinal acoustic wave and liquid droplets can be used to create an acoustic streaming which can be used to establish a stable streaming pattern with a double vortex (see Figure 8.21a to d). This SAW streaming induces

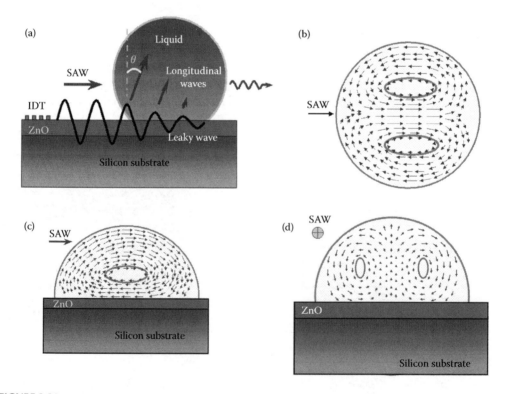

FIGURE 8.21
(a) Interaction between SAW and a liquid droplet on a ZnO based SAW device; (b) top view; (c) cross-section view; (d) front view of internal streaming inside the droplet on ZnO surface. (From Fu et al., *Sens. Actuators B*, 143, 606–619, 2010. With permission.)

an efficient mixing and agitation process within the droplets, which can be employed to produce good micromixers (Fu et al., 2008; Fu et al., 2010). When an RF voltage is applied to the IDTs on a ZnO film, the water droplet becomes deformed from its original shape (following the Rayleigh angle) with an increased leading edge contact angle and a decreased trailing edge contact angle. The large SAW pressure excites and stirs the droplet, causing it to vibrate along with the SAW. After surface hydrophobic treatment, the liquid droplets can be pumped forward with voltages as low as ~10 to 20 V (see Figure 8.22a). The movement of the droplet is a combination of rolling and sliding, which is also dependent on the power applied and the droplet size. Figure 8.22b shows the dependence of droplet speed as a function of RF signal voltage. The speed of the droplet shows an almost linear relationship with the applied driving voltage.

The SAW IDT design is important for efficient SAW streaming/pumping. The conventional bidirectional IDT may not be efficient for pumping because the wave propagates in two different directions with half the energy wasted. The simplest way to solve this problem is to use reflectors to mirror back some of the wave (see Figure 8.23a). More sophisticated IDT designs include (Nakamura et al., 2004; Lehtonen et al., 2004): (1) split IDTs (Figure 8.23b); (2) a single phase unidirectional transducer (SPUDT, Figure 8.23c) that shows internally tuned reflectors within the IDT to form a unidirectional SAW propagation from one side of the IDT; (3) focused or semicircular IDT designs to focus the acoustic

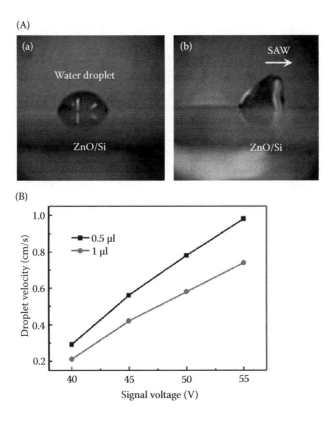

FIGURE 8.22
(A) A 2-μl water droplet (a) and its movement along with propagating acoustic wave (b), showing droplet is pushing upward and forward. (From Fu et al., *Sens. Actuators B*, 143, 606–619, 2010. With permission.) (B) Sezawa wave–driven droplet velocity as a function of applied voltage on SAW for a 5.5-μm ZnO SAW device.

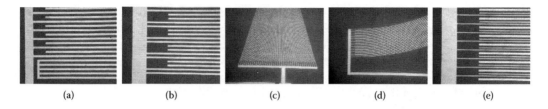

(a)   (b)   (c)   (d)   (e)

FIGURE 8.23
SAW IDT designs. (a) SAW IDT with reflector; (b) splitted IDT; (c) SPUDT IDT design; (d) angled IDT; (e) slanted IDT. (From Fu et al., *Sens. Actuators B*, 143, 606–619, 2010. With permission.)

energy and increase the pumping efficiency (see Figure 8.23d); (4) a slanted IDT (see Figure 8.23e) that has a broad range of resonant frequencies and can be used to alter the directions of streaming and droplet movement (Wu and Chang, 2005).

When a ZnO SAW device is immersed inside a large quantity of liquid in a tank and a voltage or power applied to the IDT, a steady flow pattern can be observed, with typical butterfly or quadrupolar streaming patterns, as illustrated in Figure 8.24a. The water is pushed from the IDT region to both sides of the SAW direction and flows back to the IDT via the bottom layer (see cross-sectional illustration in Figure 8.24b). On top of the IDT pattern, the liquid is pushed upward. The liquid near the IDT can be moved significantly, and the velocites near the IDT along the SAW direcition are quite large but decrease significantly away from the IDT because of the rapid decay of the strength of the SAW wave in the liquid. Increase in the applied voltage or SAW power can enlarge the size of the butterfly patterns.

As discussed before, ZnO is not inert and may react with reagents or liquid samples when it is used as a biosensor or for microfluidic manipulation. To solve this problem, an "island" ZnO SAW structure is proposed in reference (Du et al., 2009), which can avoid direct contact between the ZnO active layer and the fluid being pumped. In this design, the ZnO film is only beneath the SAW IDTs but not in the other areas. As the acoustic waves generated by the ZnO SAW device can continuously travel in the Si substrate without a

(a)   (b)

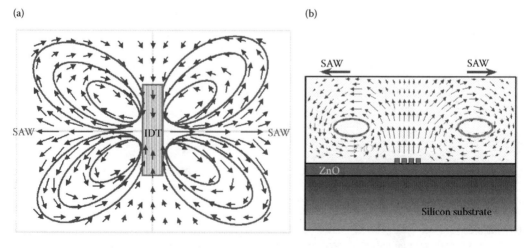

FIGURE 8.24
Water flow patterns on top of Al IDT: (a) top view (b) cross-section view.

ZnO film on top of the wave path, this offers much greater flexibility in the fabrication of highly integrated microfluidics. The SAW devices can be built on the isolated ZnO islands, whereas the other components, such as the microchannels, chamber, and sensors, can be directly fabricated on the Si substrate.

SAW Heating/Droplet Ejector

For SAW devices, a higher RF power generates faster streaming, hence a higher mixing and pumping efficiency. However, high RF power will also induce localized heating. The surface temperature of the ZnO SAW device increases with higher voltage amplitudes and the duration of the RF signal and decreases with the distance from the IDT (Fu et al., 2010). The maximum temperature can reach values of about 140°C for a signal voltage of 60 V (see Figure 8.25). It should be pointed out that the temperature was measured without any water on the device surface, and it would be expected that the temperature readings would be lower when water is present (at least lower than the boiling point). Significant acoustic heating is detrimental for many of the biosubstances that might be investigated and can also induce severe detection errors due to temperature-induced resonant frequency shift. For ZnO SAW-based liquid transportation and mixing, heating effects can be suppressed by using a pulsed RF signal to maintain the temperature below 40°C. A pulsed RF signal can also used to direct the droplet motion, as this offers more precise control of the distance moved and droplet positioning. Although acoustic heating has many negative effects for biosensing, controlled acoustic heating can be utilized as a remote heater for biomedical and life science applications, such as in polymeric chain reactions (PCRs) to amplify the DNA concentration for detection and in others to accelerate bioreaction processes.

When the RF power applied to the IDT of a ZnO SAW device is sufficiently high, tiny liquid droplets will be ejected from the surface (see Figure 8.26a), and this has been frequently reported for LiNbO$_3$ SAW devices (Chono et al., 2004). Ejection of small particles and liquids has many applications ranging from inkjet printing, fuel and oil ejection, and biotechnology. The authors have recently demonstrated that thin film ZnO-based SAW devices can eject the droplets, which are so tiny that an atomization process occurs as

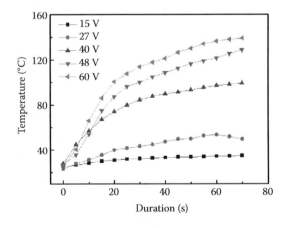

FIGURE 8.25
Temperature change as a function of time with RF signal voltage as a parameter. Temperature rises rapidly during the initial 20 s, and then increases slowly thereafter. (From Fu et al., *Sens. Actuators B*, 143, 606–619, 2010. With permission.)

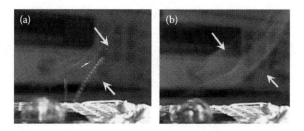

FIGURE 8.26
Surface droplet ejection (a) and atomization process (b) on a ZnO SAW device. (From Fu et al., *Sens. Actuators B*, 143, 606–619, 2010. With permission.)

shown in Figure 8.26b (Fu et al., 2010). In general, the ejected or atomized droplets from a SAW device have a large range of sizes and can only be ejected at a fixed Rayleigh angle.

SAW Particle Manipulation

Transportation and concentration of particles or biosubstances are one of the very important issues for microfluidic and biosensor applications. A SAW can be utilized to concentrate and transport nano/microparticles or yeast cells dispensed in a liquid droplet. A simple method to concentrate the particles within a droplet is to use an asymmetric distribution of SAW radiation along the width of the droplet (Li et al., 2007). Figure 8.27 shows the frame images of starch particles captured during the concentration process within a 20-µl droplet with an input RF power of 20 dBm. The induced flow circulation into the droplet due to acoustic streaming rapidly establishes a particle cluster toward the center of vortex patterns in the form of a conical shape, as depicted in Figure 8.27b. The particle concentration is attributed to shear force-induced particle migration due to the gradient in the azimuthal streaming velocity into the droplet. This results in particle motion from a higher shear force area at the droplet periphery to a lower shear force area at the bottom of the droplet center (Li et al., 2007). The shear velocity is large on the edge of the droplet and gradually decreases on approaching the center of the droplet. The particles circulate with the liquid in the droplet and simultaneously migrate from high to low shear velocity regions (Wood et al., 2008). The concentration effect is dependent on the RF power and amplitude of the SAW, as well as the properties of the particles. At very low or very high

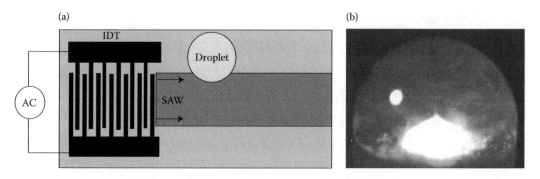

FIGURE 8.27
Illustration of asymmetric positioning of water droplet on SAW device in concentration experiments.

powers, the particles become dispersed. The particle size is also critical, and particles with certain sizes will be easily agglomerated, but particles that are smaller can flow inside the liquid. Therefore, it is possible to separate the particles according to their size using a SAW device (Shilton et al., 2008).

Membrane-Based Microfluidics Devices

Flexural plate waves or Lamb waves have also been proposed for pumping, agitating, and enhancing biochemical reactions (Nguyen and White, 1999), with the principle that fluid motion via the traveling flexural wave in a ZnO or AlN membrane can be used for the transport of liquids resulting in a steady flow of a few mm/s to cm/s in water (Moroney et al., 1991). The potential applications include a micro total analysis system (μTAS), cell manipulating systems, and drug delivery systems (Meng et al., 2000). However, because of the low frequency resulting from the thin membrane, the agitation is not significant as insufficient energy is coupled into the liquid.

A recent development using a ZnO membrane–based, acoustic wave–based device and a self-focusing acoustic transducer successfully demonstrated that liquid can be pumped by strong acoustic streaming (Zhu and Kim, 1998). These membrane-based acoustic wave devices have also been used to transport and trap particles and sort cells, with the principle that acoustic streaming produced at the interface of the membrane and fluid can actuate the particles in the liquid (Luginbuhl et al., 1997). There are also several reports of new designs using ZnO acoustic wave devices as droplet ejectors (Kwon et al., 2006). Annular Fresnel ring (with different opening angles) half-wave band electrodes have been used on the surface of a ZnO film as a self-focusing acoustic transducer. Directional liquid droplets with different ejection angles can be generated by changing the opening angle of the sectored electrodes, as shown in Figure 8.28 (Huang and Kim, 2001; Kwon et al., 2006).

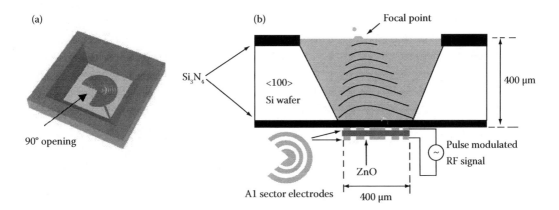

FIGURE 8.28
Annular Fresnel ring (with different opening angles) half-wave band electrodes were used on surface of a ZnO film as self-focusing acoustic transducer, and a directional liquid droplet with different ejection angles can be generated by changing the opening angle of sectored electrodes. (From Kown et al., *IEEE Autom. Sci. Eng.*, 3, 152–158, 2006. With permission.)

Future Trends for ZnO and AlN Devices for Lab-on-a-Chip

The elements required for operating detection as part of a lab-on-a-chip system include (1) transportation of liquids, such as blood or biofluids containing DNA/proteins into an area on which probe molecules have been predeposited; (2) mixing/reaction of the extracted DNA or proteins with oligonucleotide or the antibody binders; and (3) detection of an associated change in the physical, chemical, mechanical, or electrical signals. Thin film-based acoustic wave devices can be used to fabricate lab-on-chip biodetection systems, which combine the functions of microdroplet transportation, mixing, and biodetection.

ZnO- or AlN-based acoustic wave technologies can be integrated with other technologies, such as the SPR method (Homola et al., 1999). SPR sensor technology has been commercialized, and SPR biosensors have become a central tool for characterizing and qualifying biomolecular interactions. A combination of SAW microfluidics and SPR sensing would appear to be sensible for both microfluidic and detection functions. A potential problem is that the surface temperature change induced by acoustic excitation may cause changes in the refractive index, which is used for SPR sensor detection. A pulse mode SAW signals can be used to minimize this effect. ZnO- and AlN-based acoustic wave microfluidic devices can also be combined with liquid or gas chromatography that can be used to identify the protein or molecules by mass spectroscopy (Sokolowski et al., 2006). Integration of a SAW with optical methods enables the simultaneous qualification of biological soft layers formed on the sensor surface under different density, viscosity, thickness, and water content.

For digital microfluidics, there is a need to precisely and continuously generate liquid droplets. ZnO and AlN acoustic wave technology can be used for the ejection of liquid droplets, but it is rather difficult to precisely control the micro-droplet generation. A potential technology to overcome the drawbacks is to combine electrowetting-on-dielectrics (EWOD) (Lee et al., 2007) with SAW microfluidics. In the past 10 years, EWOD technology has been successfully developed to dispense and transport nanoliter to microliter biosamples in droplet form at the exact volume required (Fair, 2007). However, one of the weaknesses is that EWOD technology does not provide efficient micromixing and requires the integration of other technologies, for example, CMOS to realize bioreaction and biosensing. A novel idea is to integrate the thin film-based SAW devices with the EWOD device to form lab-on-a-chip equipped with well-developed functionalities of droplet generation, transportation by EWOD, mixing, and biosensing using SAW technology (Li et al., 2009).

Acoustic wave devices can easily be integrated with standard CMOS technology. Dual SAW or FBAR devices can be fabricated next to each other, so that the neighboring devices can be used as a sensor–reference combination. One of the devices without predeposited probe molecules can be used as a reference, whereas the other one with probe molecules can be used to sense. Using such a combination, the errors due to temperature drift or other interference on the sensing measurement can be minimized. Multisensor arrays can be easily prepared on a chip, and a judicious selection of different immobilized biobinders enables the simultaneous detection of multiple DNA or proteins, leading to accurate diagnosis of a disease or detection of multiple diseases in parallel. The creation of these cost-effective sensor arrays can increase the functionality in real time and provide parallel reading functions.

Currently, one limitation of acoustic wave device applications is that they require expensive electronic detection systems, such as network analyzers. A final product aimed at the end user market must be small, portable, and packaged into a highly integrated cost-effective system. The detection of a resonant frequency can be easily realized using standard oscillator circuits that can measure the sensor losses based on a portable device. The required purposely built electronics for acoustic wave sensing are being developed, but at present, they are still bulky and heavy. Fabrication of portable thin film-based acoustic wave detection devices is also promising and will enable the system size to be minimized along with reducing the power consumption. A wireless RF signal can be used to remotely power and control/monitor physical, chemical, and biological quantities by using acoustic wave devices, without requiring a directly wired power supply. Currently, for a lab-on-chip device, sample pretreatment, purification, and concentration, as well as a good interface between the user and the integrated sensing system, also need to be developed. A simple, robust, cheap packaging method is also critical for commercialization.

Summary

ZnO or AlN films have good PE properties and a high electromechanical coupling coefficient and are, hence, a promising technology for the fabrication of fully automated and digitized microsystems with low cost, fast response, reduced reagent requirement, and precision. In this chapter, recent development on preparation and application of ZnO and AlN films for acoustic wave-based microfluidics and biosensors is discussed. The microstructure, texture, and PE properties of the films are affected by sputtering conditions such as plasma power, gas pressure, substrate material, and temperature as well as film thickness. However, high-quality and strongly textured thin films can be prepared using RF magnetron sputtering. ZnO or AlN acoustic wave devices can be successfully used as biosensors based on a biomolecular recognition system. Among these biosensors, Love wave devices, SAW, and FBAR devices using inclined films are promising for applications in highly sensitive biodetection systems for both dry and liquid environments. The acoustic wave generated on the ZnO or AlN acoustic devices can also induce significant acoustic streaming that can be employed for mixing, pumping, ejection, and atomization of the fluid on the small scale depending on the wave mode, amplitude, and surface condition. An integrated lab-on-a-chip diagnostic system based on these thin film based acoustic wave technologies has great potential, and other functions such as droplet creation, cell sorting, and precise biodetection, can be obtained by integration with other advanced technologies.

Acknowledgments

Experimental support from Dr. Yifan Li, Dr. Xiaoye Du, Mr. Stuart Brodie, and Mr. Alghane Mansuor is acknowledged. The authors acknowledge financial support from the Institute of Integrated Systems, Edinburgh Research Partnership in Engineering and Mathematics (ERPem). They also acknowledge support from the Royal Academy of Engineering-Research Exchanges with China and India Awards, Royal Society-Research Grant, Royal Society of Edinburgh, Carnegie Trust Funding, and China–Scotland Higher Education Partnership from the British Council. AJF, WIM, and JKL acknowledge the support of the EPSRC under grants EP/F063865, EP/D051266, and EP/F06294. AJW acknowledges support from the EU (GOLEM STRP 033211) and BBSRC (RASOR BBC5115991). AJW, MD, and YQF acknowledge financial support from Innovative electronic Manufacturing Research Centre (IeMRC) coordinated by Loughborough University through the EPSRC funded flagship project SMART MICROSYSTEMS (FS/01/02/10).

References

Akiyama M, Kamohara T, Kano K. et al. 2008. *Appl. Phys. Lett.* 93: 021903.
Akiyama M, Nagao K, Ueno N. et al. 2004. *Vacuum.* 74: 699–703.
Akiyama M, Ueno N, Tateyama H. et al. 2005. *J. Mater. Sci.* 40: 1159–1162.
Armstrong GA and Crampm S. *Electro. Lett.* 1973. 9: 322–323.
Assouar MB, Elmazria O, Brizoual L et al. 2002. *Diam. Relat. Mater.* 11: 413–417.
Auger MA, Vazquez L, Sanchez O et al. 2005. *J. Appl. Phys.* 97: 123528.
Auld BA. 1973. Acoustic Fields and Waves in Solids, vol. II, John Wiley & Sons: New York, 319.
Badre C, Pauporte T, Turmine M, Lincot D. 2007. *Superlattices Microstruct.* 42: 99–103.
Ballantine DS, White RM, Martin SJ, Ricco AJ, Zellers ET, Frye GC, Wohltjen H. 1996. *Acoustic Wave Sensors, Theory, Design and Physical–Chemical Applications*, Academic Press: San Diego, CA.
Barie N and Rapp M. 2001. *Biosens. Bioelectron.* 16: 978.
Benedic F, Assouar MB, Kirsch P et al. 2008. *Diamond Relat. Mater.* 17: 804–808.
Benetti A, Cannata D, Di Pietrantonio F et al. 2006. *Thin Solid Films* 497: 304–308.
Bjurstrom J, Rosen D, Katardjiev I, Yanchev VM, Petrov I. 2004. *IEEE Trans. Ultrason. Ferroelectr. Freq. Control* 51: 1347.
Brizoual Le L, Sarry F, Elmazria O, Alnot P, Ballandras S, Patureaud T. 2008. *IEEE Trans. Ultrasonics Ferroelectr. Freq. Control* 55: 442–450.
Brizoual Le L, Elmazria O, Sarry F, El Hakiki M, Talbi A, Alnot P. 2006. *Ultrasonics* 45: 100–103.
Brizoual Le L and Elmazria O. 2007. *Diamond Relat. Mater.* 16: 987–990.
Buttry DA and Ward MD. 1992. *Chem. Rev.* 92: 1355.
Caliendo C, Imperatori P, Cianci E. 2003. *Thin Solid Films* 441: 32–37.
Cao T, Wang AF, Liang XM et al. 2008. *Colloids Surf. B* 63: 176–182.
Chen QM and Wang QM. 2005. *Appl. Phys. Lett.* 86: 022904.
Chen Y, Bagnall DM, Koh H, Park K, Hiraga K, Zhu Z, Yao T. 1998. *J. Appl. Phys.* 84: 3912.
Cheng CC, Chen YC, Horng RC et al. 1998. *J. Vac. Sci. Technol.* 16: 3335–3340.
Cherng JS, Lin CM, Chen TY. 2008. *Surf. Coat. Technol.* 202: 5684–5687.
Cherng JS and Chang DS. 2008. *Thin Solid Films* 516: 5293–5295.
Cherng JS, Chen TY, Lin CM. 2009. *Ferroelectric.* 380: 89–96.
Cheung TT and Ong CW. 2004. *Diamond Relat Mater.* 13: 1603–1608.
Chiu CS, Lee HM, Kuo CT et al. 2008. *Appl. Phys. Lett.* 93: 163106.
Chiu CS. 2008. *Appl. Phys. Lett.* 93: 163106.
Chiu KH, Chen JH, Chen HR et al. 2007. *Thin Solid Films* 515: 4819–4825.
Chono K, Shimizu N, Matsu Y, Kondoh J, Shiokawa S. 2004. *Jpn. J. Appl. Phys.* 43: 2987.
Chou K and Liu G. 2003. *J. Cryst. Growth* 243: 439–443.
Chou CH, Lin YC, Huang JH et al. 2006. *Integr. Ferroelectrics* 80: 407–413.
Chu SY, Chen TY, Water W. 2003. *J. Cryst. Growth.* 257: 280.
Chu SY, Water W, Liaw JT. 2003. *Ultrasonics* 41: 133.
Clement M, Vergara L, Sangrador J et al. 2003. *Ultrasonics* 42: 403–407.
Clement M, Iborra E, Sangrador J et al. 2003. *J. Appl. Phys.* 94: 1495–1500.
Clement M, Olivares J, Iborra E et al. 2009. *Thin Solid Films* 517: 4673–4678.
Corso CD, Dickherber A, Hunt WD. 2008. *Biosens. Bioelectron.* 24: 805–811.
Corso CD, Dickherber A, Hunt WD. 2007. *J. Appl. Phys.* 101: 054514.

Cote GL, Lec RM, Pishko MV. 2003. *IEEE Sens. J.* 3: 251–266.

Dang WL, Fu YQ, Luo JK, Flewitt AJ, Milne WI. 2007. *Superlattices Microstruct.* 42: 89–93.

Dickherber A, Corso CD, Hunt WD. 2008. *Sens. Actuators A* 144: 7–12.

Du J and Harding GL. 1998. *Sens. Actuators A* 65: 152–159.

Du XY. 2008. PhD thesis, University of Cambridge.

Du XY, Fu YQ, Tan SC, Luo JK et al. 2008. *Appl.Phys. Lett.* 93: 094105.

Du XY, Fu YQ, Tan SC, Luo JK et al. 2009. *J. Appl. Phys.* 105: 024508.

Duhamel R, Robert L, Jia H et al. 2006. *Ultrasonics* 44: e893–e897.

Durdag K. 2008. *Sens. Rev.* 28: 68–73.

Elmazria O, Mortet V, El Hakiki M et al. 2003. *IEEE Trans. Ultrasonic Ferroelectr. Freq. Control* 50: 710–715.

Engelmark, F, Iriarte GF, Katardjiev IV. 2002. *J. Vac. Sci. Technol. B* 20: 843–848.

Engelmark F, Fucntes G, Katardjiev IV et al. 2000. *J. Vac. Sci. Technol. A* 18: 1609–1612.

Fair RB. 2007. *Microfluid Nanofluidics* 3: 245–281.

Fardeheb-Mammeri M, Assouar B, Elazria O et al. 2008. *Diamond Relat. Mater.* 17: 1770–1774.

Franke T and Wixforth A. 2008. *Chem. Phys. Chem.* 9: 2140–2156.

Fu YQ, Luo JK, Du X, Flewitt AJ, Li Y, Walton A, Milne WI. 2010. *Sens. Actuators B* 143: 606–619.

Fu YQ, Du XY, Luo JK, Flewitt XY, Milne MI. 2008. *IEEE Sens.* 1–3: 478–83.

Fujimura N, Nishihara T, Goto S et al. 1993. *J. Cryst. Growth* 130: 269.

Gabl R, Feucht HD, Zeininger H, Eckstein G, Schreter M, Primig R, Pitzer D, Wersing W. 2004. *Biosens. Bioelectron.* 19: 615.

Galipeau DW, Sory PR, Vetelino KA, Mileham RD. 1997. *Smart Mater. Struct.* 6: 658.

Gizeli, E. 1997. *Smart Mater. Struct.* 6: 700.

Goldsmith S. 2006. *Surf. Coat. Technol.* 201: 3993–3999.

Gorla CR, Emanetoglu NW, Liang S, Mayo WE, Lu Y, Wraback M, Shen H. 1999. *J. Appl. Phys.* 85.

Grate WJ, Martin SJ, White RM. 1993. *Anal Chem.* 65: 940.

Groenen R, Creatore M, Van de Sander MCM. 2005. *Appl. Surf. Sci.* 241: 321–325.

Hachigo A, Nakahata H, Higaki K, Fujii S, Shikata S. 1994. *Appl. Phys. Lett.* 65: 2556.

Hakiki ME, Elmazria O, Alnot P. 2007. *IEEE Trans. Ultrasonics Ferroelectr. Freq. Control* 54: 676–681.

Hara M, Kuypers J, Abe T et al. 2005. *Sens. Actuators A* 117: 211–216.

Hirata S, Okamoto K, Inoue S et al. 2007. *J. Solid State Chem.* 180: 2335–2339.

Homola J, Yee SS, Gauglitz G. 1999. *Sens. Actuators B* 54: 3–15.

Hong HS and Chung GS. 2009. *J. Korean Phys. Soc.* 54: 1519–1525.

Hou X, Zhou F, Yu B, Liu F. 2007. *Mater. Sci. Eng. A* 452–453: 732–736.

Hoummady M, Campitelli A, Wlodarski W. 1997. *Smart Mater. Struct.* 6: 647.

Huang D and Kim E. 2001. *J. MEMS* 10: 442–449.

Huang IY and Lee MC. 2008. *Sens. Actuators B* 132: 340–348.

Huang CL, Tay KW, Wu L. 2005. *Solid State Electron.* 49: 219–225.

Huang CL Tay KW, Wu L. 2005. *Jpn. J. Appl. Phys.* 44: 1397–1402.

Iborra E. Clement M, Sangrador J et al. 2004. *IEEE Trans. Ultrasonics Ferroelectr. Freq. Control* 51: 352–358.

Iriarte GF. 2003. *J. Appl. Phys.* 93: 9604–9609.

Ishihara M, Li SJ, Yumoto H et al. 1998. *Thin Solid Films* 316: 152–157.

Ishihara M, Yamamoto K, Kokai F et al. 2000. *Vacuum* 59: 649–656.

Jacoby B and Vellekoop M. 1997. *Smart Mater. Struct.* 6: 668–679.

Jagadish C and Pearton SJ. 2006. *Zinc Oxide Bulk, Thin Films and Nanoctstructures: Processing, Properties and Applications*, Elsevier.

Jasinki J, Liliental-Weber Z, Paduano QS, Weyburne DW. 2003. *Appl. Phys. Lett.* 83: 2811.

Ji XH, Lau SP, Yu GQ et al. 2004. *J. Phys. D* 37: 1472–1477.

Jian SJ, Chu SY, Huang TY, Water W. 2004. *J. Vac. Sci. Technnol. A* 22: 2424–2430.

Jo YD and Koo SM. 2009. *Appl. Surf. Sci.* 255: 3480–3484.

Josse F, Bender F, Cernosek CW. 2001. *Anal. Chem.* 73: 5937.

Jung JP, Lee JB, Kim JS, Park JS. 2004. *Thin Solid Films* 444–448: 605–609.

Kadoka M and Miura T. 2002. *Jpn. J. Appl. Phys.* 41: 3281.

Kamalasanan MN and Chandra S. 1996. *Thin Solid Films.* 288: 112–115.

Kang YR, Kang SC, Park KK, Kim YK, Kim SW, Ju BK. 2005. *Sens. Actuators* A117: 62.

Kao KS, Cheng CC, Chen YC, Lee YH. 2003. *Appl. Phys.* A76: 1125–1127.

Kao HL, Chen WC, Chien WC. et al. 2008. *Jpn. J. Appl. Phys.* 47: 124–129.

Kao HL, Shih PJ, Lai CH. 1999. *Jpn. J. Appl. Phys.* 38: 1526–1529.

Kao KS, Cheng CC, Chen YC et al. 2004. *Appl. Surf. Sci.* 230: 334–339.

Kao KS, Cheng CC, Chen YC et al. 2003. *Appl. Phys. A* 76: 1125–1127.

Kenanakis G, Stratakis E, K. Vlachou K, Vernardou D, Koudoumas E, Natsarakis N. 2008. *Appl. Surf. Sci.* 254: 5695.

Kern RS, Rowland LB, Tanaka S et al. 1998. *J. Mater. Res.* 13: 1816–1822.

Khan FA et al. 2006. *Mater. Sci. Eng. B* 95: 51–54.

Kim EK, Lee TY, Hwang HS et al. 2006. *Superlattices Microstruct.* 39: 138.

Kim SH, Kim JH, Park DD, G Yoon. 2001. *J. Vac. Sci. Technol. B* 19: 1164–1168.

Kirsch P, Assouar MB, Elmazria O. et al. 2006. *Appl. Phys. Lett.* 88: 223504.

Kluth O, Schöpe G, Hüpkes J, Agashe C, Müller J, Rech B. 2003. *Thin Solid Films* 442: 80.

Koch MH, Hartmann AJ, and Lamb RN, Neuber M, Grunze M. 1997. *J. Phys. Chem. B* 101: 8231–8236.

Kovacs G, Lubic GW, Vellekoop MJ, Venema A. 1992. *Sens. Actuators A* 43: 38–43.

Kovacs G and Venema M. 1992. *Appl Phys Lett.* 61: 639.

Kown JW, Kamal-Bahl S, Kim ES. 2006. *IEEE Autom. Sci. Eng.* 3: 152–158.

Krishnamoorthy S and Iliadis AA. 2006. *Solid-State Electronics* 50: 1113.

Krishnamoorthy S, Bei T, Zoumakis E, Chrousos GP, Iliadis AA. 2006. *Biosens. Bioelectron.* 22: 707–714.

Kumar KSA and Chen SM. 2008. *Anal. Lett.* 41: 141–58.

Kuribayashi M and Kurosawa M. 2000. *Ultrasonics* 38: 15–19.

Kuznestsova LA and Coakley WT. 2007. *Biosens. Bioelectron.* 22: 1567–1577.

Kwon JW, Yu WH, Zou Q, Kim ES. 2006. *J. Micromech. Microeng.* 16: 2697–2704.

Lamara T, Belmahi M, Elmazria O, Le Brizoual L, Bougdira J, Remy M, Alnot P. 2004. *Diamond Relat Mater.* 13: 581–584.

Lamara T, Belmahi M, Elmazria O, Le Brizoual L, Bougdira J, Remy M, Alnot P. 2004. *Diamond Relat. Mater.* 13: 581–584.

Lange K, Rapp BE, Rapp M. 2008. *Anal. Bioanal. Chem.* 391: 1509–1519.

Lee CK, Cochran S, Abrar A, Kirk KJ, Placido F. 2004. *Ultrasonics* 42: 485–490.

Lee DS, Fu YQ, Maeng S, Luo J, Park NM, Kim SH, Jung MY, Milne WI. 2007. ZnO surface acoustic wave biosensor, International Electron Devices Meeting, Washington, DC, Dec. 10–12.

Lee JB, Jung JP,Lee MH, Park JS. 2004. *Thin Solid Films* 447–448: 610–614.

Lee Y, Kim Y, Kim H. 1998. *J. Mater. Res.* 13: 1260–1265.

Lee HC, Park JY, Lee KH et al. 2004. *J. Vac. Sci. Technol. B* 22: 1127–1133.

Lee JB, Lee MH, Park CK et al. 2004. *Thin Solid Films* 447: 296–301.

Lee SH, Yoon KH, Lee JK. 2002. *J Appl. Phys.* 92: 4062–4069.

Lee SH, Lee JK, Yoon KH. 2003. *J. Vac. Sci. Technol. A* 21: 1–5.

Lehtonen S, Plessky VP, Hartmann CS, Salomaa M. 2004. *IEEE Trans. Ultrasonic Ferroelectr. Freq. Control* 51: 1697–1703.

Li H, Friend JR, Yeo LY. 2007. *Biomed. Microdevices* 9: 647.

Li Y, Parkes W, Haworth LI, Ross AWS, Stevenson JTM, Walton AJ. 2008. *IEEE JMEMS* 17: 1481–1488.

Li Y, Flynn BW, Parkes W. et al. Conference of ISSDERC 2009, in press.

Lim WT, Son BK, Kang DH, Lee CH. 2001. *Thin Solid Films* 382: 56–60.

Lin RC, Chen YC, Chang WT, Cheng CC, Koo KS. 2008. *Sens. Actuators* A147: 425–429.

Lin ZX, Wu S, Ro RY. et al. 2009. *IEEE Trans. Ultrasonics Ferroelectr. Freq. Control* 56: 1246–1251.

Lindner G. 2008. *J. Phys. D* 41: 123002.

Link M, Webber J, Schreiter M, Wersing W, Elmazria O, Alnot P. 2007. *Sens. Actuators B* 121: 372.

Link M, Schreiter M, Weber J, Gabl R, Pitzer D, Primig R, Wersing W, Assouar MB, Elmazria O. 2006. *J. Vac. Sci. Technol. A* 24: 218–222.

Link M, Schreiter M, Weber J, Primig R, Pitzer D, Gabl R. 2006. *IEEE. Trans. Ultrasonics Ferroelectr. Freq. Control* 53: 492–496.

Liu ZF, Shan FK, Li YX, Shin BC, Yu YS. 2003. *J. Cryst. Growth* 259: 130.

Liu JM, Chong N, Chan HLW et al. 2003. *Appl. Phys. A* 76: 93–96.

Look DC, Reynolds DC, Litton CW, Jones RL, Eason DB, Cantwell G. 2002. *Appl. Phys. Lett.* 81: 1830.

Lucklum R and Hauptmann P. 2003. *Meas. Sci. Technol.* 14: 1854.

Luginbuhl P, Collins SD, Racine GA, Gretillat MA, De Rooij NF, Brooks KG, Setter N. 1997. *J. MEMS* 6: 337–346.

Luginbuhl PH, Collins SD, Racine G-A, Grktillat M-A, de Rooij NF, Brooks KG, Setter N. 1998. *Sens. Actuators A* 64: 4119.

Luo JK, Fu YQ, Li YF, Du XY, Flewitt AJ, Walton A, Milne WI. 2009. *J. Micromech. Microeng.* 19: 054001.

Maniv S and Zangvil A. 1978. *J. Appl. Phys.* 5: 2787–2792.

Marx KA. 2003. *Biomacromolecules* 4: 1099.

Matsuda T, Furuta M, Hiramatsu T et al. 2008. *J. Cryst. Growth* 310: 31.

Mchale FG. 2003. *Meas. Sci. Technol* 14: 1847.

Mchale G, Newton MI, Martin F. 2002. *J. Appl. Phys.* 91: 9701–9710.

Mei L, Zhai J, Liu H, Song Y, Jiang L, Zhu D. 2003. *J. Phys. Chem.* B 107: 9954.

Meng AH, Nguyen NT, White RM. 2000. *Biomed. Microdevices* 2: 169–174.

Min SR, Cho HN, Li YL, Chung CW. 2008. *Thin Solid Films* 516: 3521–3529.

Minami T, Sonohara H, Takata S, Sato H. 1994. *Jpn. J. Appl. Phys. B* 5: L743–L746.

Mitsuyu T, Ono S, Wasa K. 1980. *J. Appl. Phys.* 51: 2464

Miyamoto Y, Yangaitani T, Watanabe Y. 2006. *Acoust. Sci. Technol.* 27: 53–55.

Moroney RM, White RM, Howe RT. 1991. *Appl. Phys. Lett.* 59: 774–776.

Mortet V, Elmazria O, Nesladek M et al. 2003. *Phys. Status Solidi A* 199: 145–150.

Mortet V, Williams OA, Haenen K. 2008. *Phys. Status Solidi* 205: 1009–1020.

Mortet V, Vasin A, Jouan PY et al. *Surf. Coat. Technol.* 176: 88–92.

Mortet V, Nesladek M, Haenen K et al. 2004. *Diamond Relat. Mater.* 13: 1120–1124.

Muralt P. 2008. *J. Am. Ceram. Soc.* 91: 1385–1396.

Muralt P, Ledermann N, Baborowski J et al. 2005. *IEEE Trans. Ultrasonics Ferroelectr. Freq. Control* 52: 2276.

Murochim N, Sugimoto M, Matui Y, Kondoh J. 2007. *Jpn. J. Appl. Phys.* 46: 4754.

Muthukumar S, Gorla CR, Emanetoglu NW, Liang S, Lu Y. 20001. *J. Cryst. Growth* 225: 197.

Naik RS, Reif R, Lutsky JJ, Sodini CG. 1999. *J. Electrochem. Soc.* 146: 691.

Nakamura H, Yamada T, Ishizaki T, Nishimura K. 2004. *IEEE Trans. Ultrasonics Ferroelectr. Freq. Control* 49: 761–768.

Nakamura K, Shoji T, Kang H-B. 2000. *Jpn. J. Appl. Phys.* 6: L534–L536.

Narayan J, Dovidenko K, Sharma AK, Oktyabrsky S. 1998. *J. Appl. Phys.* 84: 2597.

Newton MI, Banerjee MK, Starke TKH, Bowan SM, McHale G. 1999. *Sens. Actuators* 76: 89.

Nguyen NT and White RT. 1999. *Sens. Actuators* 77: 229–236.

Nguyen NT and White RM. 2000. *IEEE Trans. Ultrasonics Ferroelectr. Freq. Control* 47: 1463.

Nguyen NT and Wu ZG. 2005. *J. Micromech. Microeng.* 15: 1.

Ntagwirumugra E, Gryba T, Zhang VY, Dogheche E, Lefebvre JE. 2007. *IEEE Trans. Ultrasonic Ferroelectr. Freq. Control* 54: 2011–2015.

Okamoto K, Inoue S, Nakano T. et al. 2008. *Thin Solid Films* 516: 4809–4812.

Okano H, Takahashi Y, Tanaka T, Shibata K, Nakano S. 1992. *Jpn. J. Appl. Phys.* 3: 3446.

Özgür U, Alivov YI, Liu C et al. 2005. *J. Appl. Phys.* 98: 041301.

Paci B, Generosi A, Albertini VR et al. 2007. *Sens. Actuators A* 137: 279–286.

Park WI, An SJ, Yi G-C and Jang HM. 2001. *J. Mater. Res.* 16: 1358.

Pearton SJ, Norton DP, Ip K, Heo YW. 2004. *J. Vac. Sci. Technol. B* 22: 932.

Pearton SJ, Norton DP, Ip K, Heo YW, Steiner T. 2005. *Prog. Mater. Sci.* 50: 293.

Peruzzi M, Pedarnig JD, Bauerle D, Schwingger W, Schaffler F. 2004. *Appl. Phys. A* 79: 1873–1877.

Petrov I, Orlinov V, Misiuk A. 1984. *Thin Solid Films* 120: 55.

Pham VS, Mai L, Yoon G. 2008. *Jpn. J. Appl. Phys.* 47: 6383–6385.

Powell DA, Kalatair-Zadeh K,Wlodaiski W. 2004. *Sens. Actuators A* 115: 456–461.

Renaudin A, Tabourier P, Zhang V, Camart JC, Druon C. 2006. *Sens. Actuators B*. 113: 387.

Rey-Mermet S, Bjurstrom J, Rosen D, Petrov I. 2004. *IEEE Trans. Ultrasonics Ferroelectr. Freq. Control* 51: 1347.

Rotter M, Kalameitsev AV, Govorov AO, Ruile W, Wixforth A. 1999. *Phys. Rev. Lett.* 82: 2171.

Ruby R. 2007. *IEEE Ultrasonics Symp. Proc.* 1–6: 1029–1040.

Sanchez G, Wu A, Tristant P et al. 2008. *Thin Solid Films* 516: 4868–4875.

Sano A, Matsui Y, Shiokawa S. 1998. *Jpn. J. Appl. Phys.* 37: 2979.

Saravanan S, Berenschot E, Krijnen G, Elwenspoek M. 2006. *Sens. Actuators A* 130–131: 340–345.

Sheng TY, Yu ZQ, Collins GJ. 1988. *Appl. Phys. Lett.* 52: 576.

Shih WC, Huang RC, Peng YK et al. 2009. *Ferroelectrics* 380: 20–29.

Shilton R, Tan MK, Yeo LY, Friend JR. 2008. *J. Appl. Phys.* 104: 014910.

Shinagawa T, Otomo S, Katayama J, Izaki M. 2007. *Electrochim. Acta* 53: 1170–1174.

Shiokawa S and Kondoh J. 2004. *Jpn. J. Appl. Phys.* 43: 2799–2802.

Shiokawa S, Matsui Y and Morizum T. 1989. *Jpn. J. Appl. Phys.* 28: 126.

Smith TP, Mecouch WJ, Miraglia PQ, Roskowski AM, Hartlieb PJ, Davis RF. 2003. *J. Cryst. Growth* 257: 255.

Sokolowski SS, Trudell DE, Byrness JE, Okandan M, Bauer JM, Manley RG, Freye-Mason GC. 2006. *IEEE Sens. J.* 6: 784–795.

Sritharan K, Strobl CJ, Schneider MF, Wixforth A. 2006. *Appl. Phys. Lett.* 88: 054102.

Strobl CJ, Guttenberg Z, Wixforth A. 2004. *IEEE Trans. Ultrasonics, Ferrelectr. Freq. Control* 51: 1432.

Sun RD, Nakajima A, Fujishima A, Watanabe T, Hashimoto K. 2001. *J. Phys. Chem.* B105: 1984–1990.

Sundaram KB and Khan A. 1997. *Thin Solid Films* 295: 87–91.

Tadigadapa S, Mateti K. 2009. *Meas. Sci. Technol.* 20: 092001.

Takagaki Y, Santos PV, Wiebicke E, Bramdt O, Schonheer HP, Ploog KH. 2000. *Appl. Phy. Lett.* 81: 14.

Takagaki Y, Santos PV, Wiebicke E et al. 2002. *Appl. Phys. Lett.* 81: 2538–2540.

Takeuchi M, Yamada H, Yoshino Y et al. 2002. *Vacuum* 66: 463–466.

Talbi A, Sarry F, Brizoual LL, Elmazria O, Alnot P. 2004. *IEEE Trans Ultrasonics Ferroelectr. Freq. Control* 51: 1421.

Tan SS, Ye M, Milnes AG. 1995. *Solid State Electron.* 38: 17.

Tanosch K. et al. 2006. *Sens. Actuators* A132: 658–663.

Tay KW, Huang CL, Wu L. 2004. *Jpn. J. Appl. Phys.* 43: 1122–1126.

Tay KW, Huang CL, Wu L et al. 2004. *Jpn. J. Appl. Phys.* 43: 5510–5515.

Tay KW, Huang CL, Wu L 2005. *J. Vac. Sci. Technol.* 23: 1474–1479.

Teles FRR and Fonseca LP. 2008. *Talanta* 77: 606–623.

Toegl A, Scribe J, Wixforth A, Strobl C, Gauer C, Guttenburg ZV. 2004. *Anal. Bioanal. Chem.* 379: 69.

Toegl A, Kirchner R, Gauer C, Wixforth A. 2003. *J. Biomed. Technol.* 14: 197.

Triboulet R and Perriere J. 2003. *Prog. Cryst. Growth Charact. Mater.* 47: 65–138.

Tseng WK, Lin JL, Sung WC, Chen SH, Lee GB. 2006. *J. Micromech. Microeng.* 16: 539.

Tvarozek V, Novotny I, Sutta P, Flickyngerova S, Schtereva K, Vavrinsky E. 2007. *Thin Solid Films* 515: 8756–8760.

Vellekoop MJ. 1998. *Ultasonics* 36: 7.

Vergara L, Clement M, Iborra E et al. 2004. *Diamond Relat. Mater.* 13: 839–842.

Wang JS and Lakin KM. 1983. *Appl. Phys. Lett.* 42: 352.

Wang M, Wang H, Chen W, Chui Y. and Wang L. 2006. *Mater. Chem. Phys.* 97: 219–225.

Wang YG, Lau SP, Lee HW, Yu SF et al. 2003. *J. Appl. Phys.* 94: 1597.

Weber J, Albers WM, Tuppurainen J, Link M, Gabl R, Wersing W, Schreiter M. 2006. *Sens. Actuators A* 128: 84–88.

Wenzel S and White R. 1990. *Sens. Actuators* A21–23: 700.

White RM. 1997. *Faraday Discuss.* 107: 1.

Wingquist G, Bjurstrom J, Liljeholm L et al. 2007. *Sens. Actuators* B123: 466–473.

Wingquist G, Bjurstrom J, Hellgren AC, Katardjiev I. 2007. *Sens. Actuators* B127: 248–252.

Wixforth A, Strobl C, Gauer C, Toegl A, Sciba J, Guttenberg ZV. 2004. *Anal. Biomed. Chem.* 379: 982.

Wixforth A. 2004. *Superlattices Microstruct.* 33: 389.

Wohltjen H. et al. 1997. *Acoustic Wave Sensor—Theory, Design, and Physico-Chemical Applications.* Academic Press, San Diego, 39.

Wood CD, Evens SD, Cumingham JE, O'Rorke R, Walti C, Davies AG. 2008. *Appl. Phys. Lett.* 92: 044104.

Wu L, Wu S, Song HT. 2001. *J. Vac. Sci. Technol.* A19: 167.

Wu MS, Shih W-C, Tsai W-H. 1998. *J. Phys. D* 31: 943–950.

Wu S, Ro R, Lin ZX, Lee MS. 2008. *J. Appl. Phys.* 104: 064919.

Wu S, Chen YC, Chang YS. 2002. *Jpn. J. Appl. Phys.* 41: 4605–4608.

Wu TT and Chang IH. 2005. *J. Appl. Phys.* 98: 024903.

Wu HP, Wu LZ, Du SY 2008. *J. Appl. Phys.* 103: 083546.

Wu S, Ro RY, Lin ZX et al. 2009. *Appl. Phys. Lett.* 94: 092903.

Xu T, Wu G, Zhang G, Hao Y. 2003. *Sens. Actuators* A104: 61.

Xu J, Thakur JS, Hu G et al. 2006. *Appl. Phys. A* 83: 411–415.

Yan Z, Zhu XY, Pang GKH. 2007. *Appl. Phys. Lett.* 90: 143503.

Yan Z, Song Z, Liu M et al. 2007. *Appl. Surf. Sci.* 253: 9372–9380.

Yanagitani T and Kiuchi M. 2007. *J. Appl. Phys.* 102: 044115.

Yanagitani T, Matsukawa M, Watanabe Y, Otani T. 2005. *J. Cryst. Growth* 276: 424.

Yanagitani T, Tomohiro S, Nohara T et al. 2004. *Jap. J. Appl. Phys.* 43: 3004.

Yang PF, Jian SR, Wu S et al. 2009. *Appl. Surf. Sci.* 255: 5984–5988.

Yoshino Y. 2009. *J. Appl. Phys.* 105: 061623.

Yoshino Y, Lnoue K, Takeuchi M, Makino T, Katayama Y, Hata T. 2000. *Vacuum* 59: 403–410.

Yoshino Y, Takeuchi M, Inoue K, Makino T, Arai S, Hata T. 2002. *Vacuum* 66: 467–472.

Zhang BP, Wakatsuki K, Binh NT, Usami N, Segawa Y. 2004. *Thin Solid Films* 449: 12–19.

Zhang D and Edgar JH. 2005. *Mater Sci. Eng.* 48: 1–46.

Zheng H, Du XL, Luo Q, Jia JF, Cu CZ, Xue QK. 2007. *Thin Solid Films* 515: 3969.

Zhou J, Xu N, Wang ZL. 2006. *Adv. Mater.* 18: 2432.

Zhu S, Su C, Lehoczky SL, Peters P, George MA. 2000. *J. Cryst. Growth* 211: 106–110.

Zhu X and Kim ES. 1998. *Sens. Actuators* A66: 355–360.

9

Medical Applications of Sputter-Deposited Shape Memory Alloy Thin Films

Yong Qing Fu, Wei Min Huang, and Shuichi Miyazaki

CONTENTS

Introduction 382
    Biomedical Application of TiNi Alloys 382
    Thin Film TiNi SMAs 384
Shape Memory Effect and Martensitic Transformation 387
    TiNi Phase Diagram 388
    Crystallography of Martensitic Transformation 389
    Transformation Strain 391
    Transformation Temperatures 393
    Shape Memory and SE 393
    Deformation Behavior 395
Film Fabrication and Characterization 397
    Film Deposition 397
    TiNi Film Characterization 400
        TiNi Binary Alloy Thin Films 401
        Ni-Rich TiNi Alloy Thin Films 406
        Ti-Rich TiNi Alloy 410
        TiNiX Ternary Alloy Thin Films 414
    Film Stress and Stress Evolution 420
    Frequency Response 424
    Adhesion and Interfacial Analysis 425
    Stability, Degradation, and Fatigue 425
    Film Thickness Effect 428
    Temperature Memory Effect 429
    Nanoscale Mechanical Evaluation 430
    Functionally Graded and Composite-Based Films 431
    Modeling 433
    Biocompatibility of Thin Films 433
Biological and MEMS Applications of TiNi Thin Films 434
    Comparison of Microactuation Mechanisms 434
    Freestanding Microactuators Based on Two-Way Shape Memory Effect 434
    TiNi Diaphragms, Micropump, and Microvalves 437
        Microdiaphragm Using R-Phase of Ti–Ni 441
        Microdiaphragm Using M-Phase of Ti–Ni–Pd 442
        Microdiaphragm Using M-Phase of Ti–Ni–Cu 443
    Microgrippers 444

Pulsation Sensor 446
TiNi-Based Microcage..449
Freestanding TiNi-Based Microcage...450
TiNi/DLC Microcage...452
Intravascular Medical Stent and Tube Devices..456
Covered Stent...456
Heart Valve..457
Fabrication of Superelastic Thin Film Tubes 458
Summary and Future...460
References...461

Introduction

Shape memory alloy (SMA) is a metal that can "remember" its geometry, that is, after a piece of SMA is deformed from its original shape, it regains its original geometry by itself upon heating (shape memory effect, SME) or, simply upon unloading (superelasticity, SE). These extraordinary properties are due to temperature-dependent reverse martensitic transformation from a low-symmetry phase (martensite) to a highly symmetric crystallographic structure (austenite) upon heating and a martensitic transformation in its opposite direction upon cooling. SME has been found in many materials, such as metals, ceramics, and polymers. Among all these materials, TiNi-based alloys, often called nitinol, have been extensively studied and have found many commercial applications (Miyazaki and Otsuka, 1989; Humbeeck, 1999; Hane, 2000; Otsuka and Ren, 2005).

Biomedical Application of TiNi Alloys

Nitinol was first discovered by Buehler et al. in 1963. It has inspired a long-standing interest in both material research and industrial development. Although many applications of nitinol have been developed for different industries, their real success only came after the introduction of microsurgery. Nitinol provides a perfect solution for problems presented by microsurgery because of its unique mechanical properties—"shape memory effect," "superelasticity," and the excellent biocompatibility. The SME is characterized by a reversible phase transition between martensite (low temperature phase, soft) and austenite (high temperature phase, hard). At low temperature, nitinol can be plastically deformed, and the deformation can be recovered by heating through a phase transition. If the nitinol is deformed at a temperature above the phase transition temperature, the stress-induced martensitic transition can be recovered spontaneously once the stress is removed. This is known as SE. These remarkable shape memory properties are not present in any other conventional materials. Both superelastic and thermal recovery SMAs can provide large deformation and force for robust surgical devices for biological applications. More importantly, the nitinol is biocompatible with low toxicity and high corrosion resistance, thus, it can be used for implants, for example, stent, staple, and sutures without any adverse long-term effects on patients. Nitinol is also nonferromagnetic and can thus be used as medical devices for magnetron resonance imaging (MRI) guided surgery and minimal invasive interventions (Melzer et al., 2006). A brief history of SMAs (bulk materials and SMA thin films) for medicine is summarized in Table 9.1.

TABLE 9.1

Historical Development of SMAs for Microsurgery

Year	Device	Reference
1963	Discovery of nitinol	Buehler and Riley, 1963
1971	Orthodontic braces	Otsuka and Wayman, 1998
1977	Simon vena cava filter	Simon et al., 1977
1981	Orthopedic staple	Dai and Chu, 1996
1983	Prosthetic joint	Miyazaki, 1998
1983	Nitinol stent	Dotter et al., 1983
1990	Thin film SMA	Walker and Mehregany, 1990; Busch et al., 1990
1990	Thin film microdevices	Johnson, 1991
1993	Laparoscopic hernia repair mesh	Himpens, 1993
1995	Laparoscopic clamp	Frank and Cuschieri, 1995a
1995	Thin film microgripper	Krulevitch et al., 1996a
1996	Hernia repair retractor	Rickers et al., 1998; Thanopoulos et al., 1998
1999	Thin film SMA microvalve	Johnson, 1999
1999	Laparoscopic suturing clip	Xu et al., 1999; Song et al., 2002; Ng et al., 2003
2000	Vascular ligation clip	Frank et al., 2000
2000	Gastric loop snare	Nakamura et al., 2000
2001	Drug-eluting stent	Sousa et al., 2001
2001	Thin film microwrapper	Gill et al., 2001
2001	Thin film microstents	Gupta, 2001
2004	Laparoscopic anastomosis ring	Nudelman et al., 2004, 2005; Song et al., 2005
2005	Thin film heart valve	Stepan et al., 2005
2007	Endoscopic bleeding control device	Kirschniak et al., 2007a,b
2008	Thin film microtube and stent	Buenconsejo et al., 2008; Zamponi et al., 2008

Stent is probably the best example of SMAs in medicine (see Figure 9.1), and also the most successful product in terms of commercial and life-saving achievements. For the past 20 years, it is a remarkable achievement for the nitinol stent to be developed from a simple form of coiled wire to today's multibillion dollars market in minimally invasive cardiovascular therapy to revascularize arteries (Buenconsejo et al., 2008). Nitinol stents have also been used in esophagus, gastrointestinal tract, ureter, tracheal airway, and vascular anastomosis device, prosthetic heart valves, and radiofrequency ablation catheter (Terzo, 2006; Kulkarni and Bellamy, 1999).

Endoscopic surgery uses rigid or flexible endoscope to gain access to operative fields to diagnose and treat diseases. Surgical operations are conducted by remote surgical manipulation within the closed body cavities under visual control via endoscope. A range of nitinol-based surgical instruments have been developed for endoscopic surgery to overcome the limited degrees of freedom caused by the approach of minimal invasiveness. The devices made of nitinol enable surgeons to achieve complex surgical tasks, such as tissue holding (tissue graspers and retractors), suturing (needle holder and suturing clip),

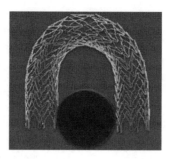

FIGURE 9.1
Nitinol stents showing kink resistance of a nitinol stent (images courtesy of Abbott Laboratories).

anastomosis (anastomosis ring), homeostasis (bleeding control clip), dissection (scissors), ablation (multiple radiofrequency electrodes), surgical materials delivery, and hernia repair. These include (1) curved surgical instruments—a variable curvature spatula for laparoscopic surgery (Figure 9.2; Cuschieri et al., 1991); (2) suturing devices—for tissue suturing in self-closing clips (Figure 9.3; Song et al., 2002; Ng et al., 2003); (3) bleeding control devices—SMA clip gastrointestinal lesion, perforation, and bleeding (see Figure 9.4; Ovesco Endoscopy GmbH, Tubingen, Germany; Raju and Gajula, 2004; Kirschniak et al., 2007).

The early applications of nitinol in orthopedic surgery were staples and clamps to treat adolescent scoliosis and bone fractures (Musialek et al., 1998). Recent development of porous nitinol has shown good biocompatibility and excellent bone ingrowths that could be used as ideal bone substitute (Rhalmi et al., 1999). In the urological field, an SMA ureter stent was used in 15 patients to treat ureter stricture with encouraging results (Chonan et al., 1997). The endovascular device with shape memory function might be a promising tool for treating ischemia stroke without the need for infusion of clot-dissolving drugs (Small et al., 2007). The current trend of surgical technologies is toward less invasiveness or non-scar diagnostics and treatment, and shape memory technology continues to find exciting applications.

Thin Film TiNi SMAs

For microelectromechanical system (MEMS) and biomedical applications, thin film–based SMAs possess many desirable properties, such as high-power density (up to 10 J/cm³), the

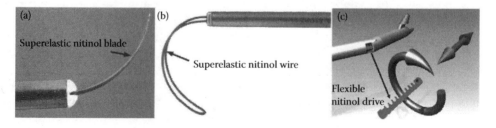

FIGURE 9.2
Variable-curvature devices for laparoscopic surgery. (a) Dissecting spatula, (b) suture passer, (c) flexible drive for an articulating needle holder. (From Cuschieri et al., *Surg. Endosc.*, 5, 179, 1991, reproduced with permission from Springer.)

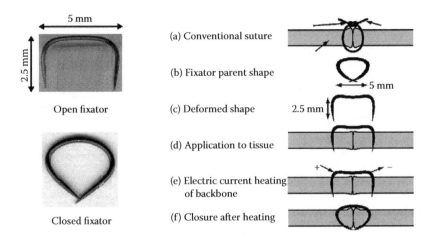

FIGURE 9.3
Prototype and working principle of a self-closing clip for MIS. (From Song et al., *Smart Mater. Struct.*, 11, 1–5, 2002, reproduced with permission from Springer.)

ability to recover large transformation stress and strain upon heating, SME, peudoelasticity (or SE), and biocompatibility (Miyazaki and Ishida, 1999; Wolf and Heuer, 1995; Khan et al., 1998). The work output per volume of SMA exceeds those of other microactuation mechanisms. The phase transformation in SMA thin film is accompanied by significant changes in mechanical, physical, chemical, electrical, and optical properties, such as yield stress, elastic modulus, hardness, damping, shape recovery, electrical resistivity, thermal conductivity, thermal expansion coefficient, surface roughness, vapor permeability, dielectric constant, and so on (Fu et al., 2001; Fu et al., 2004). These changes can be fully utilized in design and fabrication of microsensors and microactuators (Winzek et al., 2004; Miyazaki, 1990).

In the early 1990s, several trials were made to fabricate TiNi thin films by sputter deposition (Walker et al., 1990). Some of these results showed that conventional micromachining processes are applicable for making microstructures consisting of a silicon substrate and a TiNi thin film. If the films contain microdefects, which are characteristic in sputter-

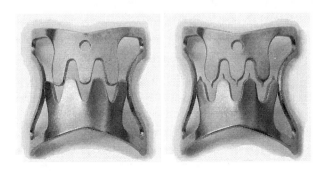

FIGURE 9.4
Over-the-scope clip system for gastrointestinal bleeding control. Left, atraumatic; right, traumatic versions. (From Kirschniak et al., *Gastrointest. Endosc.*, 66, 162–167, 2007, reproduced with permission from Elsevier.)

deposited films, and other elements such as oxygen and hydrogen, they will become brittle. Application of stress to such films will cause them to fracture. Without information about the characteristics of materials, any trial for the improvement in the sputtering process will be ineffective. Therefore, it was very important both to establish fabrication methods for high-quality thin films in enduring high stress applications and to develop mechanical testing methods to evaluate shape memory characteristics of thin films.

Mechanical behavior of TiNi thin films can be characterized by damping measurement, tensile tests, and thermomechanical tests. Crystal structures of the austenite (A), martensite (M), and R phases were determined to be B2, monoclinic and rhombohedral, respectively. The transformation and shape memory characteristics of TiNi thin films were shown to strongly depend on metallurgical factors and sputtering conditions. The former includes alloy composition, annealing temperature, aging temperature, and time, whereas the latter includes Ar pressure, sputtering power, substrate temperature, and so on (Ishida et al., 1995; Kajawara et al., 1996). Conventional mechanical properties such as yield stress, ductility, and fracture stress have been investigated by measuring stress–strain curves at various temperatures. The maximum elongation amounted to more than 40% in an equiatomic TiNi thin film. The yield and fracture stresses of the martensite can be as high as 600 and 800 MPa, respectively (Ishida et al., 1995). These mechanical properties provide good evidence to indicate that the sputter-deposited TiNi thin films possess sufficient ductility and stable shape memory characteristics for practical applications.

The R-phase transformation characteristics show perfect stability against cyclic deformation because of the small shape change that causes no slip deformation to occur, whereas the martensitic transformation temperatures increase and temperature hysteresis decreases during cycling because of the introduction of dislocations. However, no slip deformation occurs during cyclic deformation under 100 MPa so that perfect stability of SME is also observed in the martensitic transformation. Besides, with increasing the number of cycles under higher stresses, the shape memory characteristics associated with the martensitic transformation are stabilized by a training effect.

If a large recovery strain is required for a microactuator, we need to use the martensitic transformation, which has a larger temperature hysteresis of about 30 K in TiNi binary alloys. To improve the response, it is necessary to decrease the temperature hysteresis. Addition of Cu is effective in decreasing the transformation temperature hysteresis without decreasing transformation temperatures themselves. TiNiCu thin films with Cu contents varying from 0 to 18 at.% were investigated (Miyazaki et al., 1996; Meng et al., 2008; Ishida et al., 2008). The martensitic transformation temperatures of all the thin films were about 323 K, decreasing only slightly with increasing Cu content in the range within 9.5 at.%, while slightly increasing in the range beyond 9.5 at.%. The hysteresis associated with the transformation showed a strong dependence on Cu content, that is, it decreased from 27 to 10 K with increasing Cu content from 0 to 9.5 at.%. In the 9.5 at.% Cu thin film, a two-stage transformation appeared and it was determined as B2 → Orthorhombic → M-phase by the x-ray diffractometry. Perfect two-stage SME was observed correspondingly to these transformations. The addition of Cu caused the maximum recovery strain to decrease from 3.9% to 1.1% and the critical stress for slip to increase greatly from 55 to 350 MPa with increasing Cu content up to 18 at.% (Miyazaki and Ishida, 1999).

Additions of third elements, such as Pd, Au, Pt, Ag, Hf, etc., are effective for increasing transformation temperatures. In the case of sputter-deposited thin films, Pd and Hf have been added as a third element for this purpose (Quandt et al., 1996). However, Hf increases transformation hysteresis, whereas Pd is effective in decreasing the transformation hysteresis in addition to increasing transformation temperatures (Baldin et al., 2006; Lee et al., 2006). With this reason, Pd addition is more promising for applications. The TiNiPd ternary alloy thin films basically show the M-phase and O-phase transformations except the R-phase transformation in a narrow Pd-content region. The addition of Pd is effective in increasing the O-phase transformation temperatures, for example, the O_s (O-phase transformation start temperature) of a 21.8 at.% Pd thin film is higher than the M_s (M-phase transformation start temperature) of an equiatomic TiNi binary alloy thin film by about 50 K. It was found that Pd additions are also effective in decreasing transformation temperature hysteresis, for example, 16 K in a thin film with 22 at.% Pd content (Miyazaki and Ishida, 1999). The achievement of the small transformation temperature hysteresis in TiNiCu thin films or the high transformation temperatures in TiNiPd thin films is promising for achieving quick movement in microactuators made of TiNi base shape memory thin films.

Because TiNi films can provide large forces for actuation and large displacement, most applications of TiNi films in MEMS are focused on microactuators (Johnson, 1999; Tan and Miyazaki, 1997), such as cantilevers, diaphragms, micropumps, microvalves, microgrippers, springs, microspacers, micropositioners, micromirror actuators, etc. TiNi thin films are sensitive to environmental changes, such as thermal, stress, magnetic or electrical fields. Thus, they should be also ideal for applications in microsensors.

The main potential problems associated with the TiNi thin film in MEMS applications include: (1) Low energy efficiency, low dynamic response speed and large hysteresis. (2) Nonlinearity and complex thermomechanical behavior and ineffectiveness for precise and complex motion control and force tracking. (3) Potential degradation and fatigue problems. Even with the above disadvantages, the TiNi-based thin film is still considered a core technology for actuation of some MEMS devices, where large force and stroke are essential and in conditions of low duty cycles or intermittent operation, and in extreme environment, such as radioactive, space, biological, and corrosive conditions.

TiNi thin film with superelastic characteristics makes it particularly useful for implantable devices, such as aneurysm closures, miniature stents, and stent covers, and can be used to retrieve, filter, capture, or remove blood clots in small blood vessels (Johnson, 2009). Sieves and clot retrievers are other potential applications for TiNi thin film, especially in areas of the body distal from the heart where vessels are smaller, stiffer, and more muscular, as in the case of intracranial arteries and veins (Johnson, 2009). Thin film stents can be from 1 to 40 µm thick and fenestration feature size can be as small as 1 µm. As medical implantable devices made of TiNi alloys become smaller, designers can benefit from the combination of sputter deposition of TiNi and photolithography for manufacturing miniature medical devices. This chapter reviews the recent development and biomedical applications of sputter-deposited TiNi-based SMA thin films and fabrication of microsystems. In the next section, the mechanism of martensitic transformation and SME will be introduced.

Shape Memory Effect and Martensitic Transformation

SME and SE are associated with the crystallographically reversible nature of the martensitic transformation which appears in SMAs. Such crystallographically reversible martensitic transformation was specially named as "thermoelastic martensitic transformation." The name originates from the characteristic of the martensitic transformation in SMAs, that is, the total free energy change associated with the thermoelastic martensitic transformation mainly consists of two thermoelastic terms, chemical free energy and elastic energy, whereas the total free energy change associated with the conventional martensitic transformation, which appears in steels for instance, consists of the interfacial energy and plastic deformation in addition to the two thermoelastic terms. Therefore, the interface between transformed and untransformed regions moves smoothly according to the temperature variation so that the transformation temperature hysteresis is small, from several to several tens K, when compared with those of steels of several hundreds K. The characteristic that plastic deformation does not occur in the thermoelastic martensitic transformation is one of the necessary factors for the perfect shape recovery upon the reverse transformation in SMAs.

The martensitic transformation itself is not a new phenomenon. It was first found long time ago in steel (Nishiyama, 1978) which was heat-treated at a high temperature followed by rapid quenching: the martensitic transformation in most steels is not thermoelastic, hence the SME does not appear. Among several tens alloys showing the shape memory and superelastic behavior, the TiNi alloys have been successfully developed as practical materials for many applications. In this section, the basic characteristics such as the martensitic transformation and shape-memory/superelastic properties of the TiNi alloys are reviewed.

TiNi Phase Diagram

An equilibrium phase diagram of the TiNi system is shown in Figure 9.5, which describes a middle composition region including an equiatomic composition TiNi. Full information on the equilibrium phase diagram is given by Murray (1987). The TiNi locates around the equiatomic composition region, whereas Ti_2Ni and $TiNi_3$ intermetallic compounds locate at 33.3 at.% Ni and 75 at.% Ni, respectively. These three alloys are equilibrium phases. There is another phase, Ti_3Ni_4, which is not equilibrium but important for affecting both the transformation temperatures and shape memory behavior (Miyazaki, 1990). The

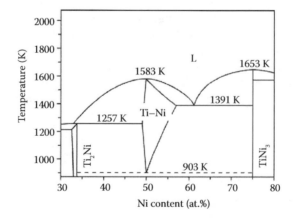

FIGURE 9.5
An equilibrium-phase diagram of TiNi system. (From Miyazaki, S., in Miyazaki et al., eds., *Thin Film Shape Memory Alloys: Fundamentals and Device Applications*, Cambridge University Press, UK, 2009, reproduced with permission from Cambridge University Press.)

TiNi single phase region terminates at 903 K in Figure 9.5; however, the region seems to extend to around room temperature in a narrow Ni content width according to empirical information.

Crystallography of Martensitic Transformation

The parent phase of the TiNi has a CsCl-type B2 superlattice, whereas the martensite phase is three-dimensionally close packed (monoclinic or B19′), as shown in Figure 9.6. The TiNi alloy also shows another phase transformation before the martensitic transformation according to heat-treatment and alloy composition. This transformation (rhombohedral phase or R-phase transformation) can be formed by elongating along any one of the $\langle 111 \rangle$ directions of the B2 structure as shown in Figure 9.7 and characterized by a small lattice distortion when compared with that of the martensitic transformation. The R-phase transformation usually appears before the martensitic transformation when the martensitic transformation start temperature M_s is lowered by some means than the R-phase transformation start temperature T_R. There are many factors that effectively depress M_s as follows (Miyazaki et al., 1986):

(1) Increasing Ni content
(2) Aging at intermediate temperatures
(3) Annealing at temperatures below the recrystallization temperature after cold working
(4) Thermal cycling
(5) Substitution of a third element

Among these factors, items (2)–(5) are effective to realize the R-phase transformation.

The martensitic transformation occurs in such a way that the interface between the martensite variant and parent phase becomes an undistorted and unrotated plane (invariant plane or habit plane) to minimize the strain energy. To form such a martensite variant (habit-plane variant), it is necessary to introduce a lattice invariant shear, such as twins, dislocations or stacking faults. The lattice invariant shear is generally twinning, which is reversible, in the SMAs.

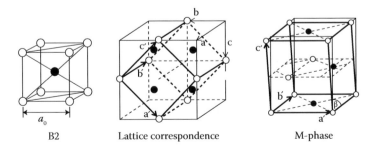

B2	Lattice correspondence	M-phase

FIGURE 9.6
Crystal structures of parent (B2) and martensite (B19′) phases and lattice correspondence between two phases. (From Miyazaki, S., in Miyazaki et al., eds., *Thin Film Shape Memory Alloys: Fundamentals and Device Applications*, Cambridge University Press, UK, 2009, reproduced with permission from Cambridge University Press.)

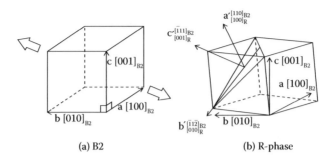

FIGURE 9.7
Crystal structure of R-phase, which is formed by elongation along one of ⟨111⟩ directions of B2 lattice.

Crystallographic characteristics of the martensitic transformation are now well under-stood by the phenomenological crystallographic theory (Miyazaki et al., 1990). This theory describes that the transformation consists of the following three operational processes: (1) a lattice deformation B creating the martensite structure from the parent phase, (2) a lattice invariant shear P_2 (twinning, slip, or faulting) and (3) a lattice rotation R. Thus, the total strain (or the shape strain) associated with the transformation is written in the fol-lowing matrix form:

$$P_1 = RP_2B \qquad (9.1)$$

This theory requires that the shape strain produced by the martensitic transformation is described by an invariant plane strain, that is, a plane of no distortion and no rotation, which is macroscopically homogeneous and consists of a shear strain parallel to the habit plane and a volume change (an expansion or contraction normal to the habit plane). Thus, the shape strain can also be represented as:

$$P_1 = I + m_1 d_1 p_1', \qquad (9.2)$$

where I is the (3×3) identity matrix, m_1 the magnitude of the shape strain, d_1 is a unit column vector in the direction of the shape strain, and p_1' is a unit row vector in the direc-tion normal to the invariant plane. If we know the lattice parameters of the parent and martensite phases, a lattice correspondence between the two phases and a lattice invariant shear, the matrix p_1' can be determined by solving Equation 9.1 under invariant plane strain condition. Then, all crystallographic parameters such as P_1, m_1, d_1 and orientation relation-ship are determined. The lattice invariant shear of the TiNi is the ⟨011⟩$_M$ Type II twinning (Miyazaki and Ishida, 1999).

There are generally 6, 12, or 24 martensite variants with each shape strain P_1. Each vari-ant requires formation of other variants to minimize the net strain of the grouped variants. This is called self-accommodation, hence the whole specimen shows no macroscopic shape change except surface relief corresponding to each variant by the martensitic transforma-tion upon cooling.

Transformation Strain

The strain induced by the martensitic transformation shows strong orientation dependence in TiNi alloys (Miyazaki and Wayman, 1988). It is conventionally assumed that the most favorable martensite variant grows to induce the maximum recoverable transformation strain ε_M^i in each grain: ε_M^i can be calculated by using the lattice constants of the parent phase and martensite phase. The lattice constants of the parent and martensite phases of a TiNi alloy are as follows: $a_0 = 0.3013$ nm for the parent phase and $a = 0.2889$ nm, $b = 0.4150$ nm, $c = 0.4619$ nm, and $\theta = 96°$ for the martensite phase, respectively.

Using the lattice constants of the parent phase and martensite phase, the transformation strain produced by lattice distortion due to the martensitic transformation can be calculated. If it is assumed that the most favorable martensite variants grow to induce the maximum transformation strain in each grain, the lattice distortion matrix T' is expressed in the coordinates of the martensite as follows using the lattice constants of the parent phase (a_0) and those of the martensite phase (a, b, c, β):

$$T' = \begin{bmatrix} \dfrac{a}{a_0} & 0 & \dfrac{c'\gamma}{\sqrt{2}a_0} \\[2ex] 0 & \dfrac{b}{\sqrt{2}a_0} & 0 \\[2ex] 0 & 0 & \dfrac{c'}{\sqrt{2}a_0} \end{bmatrix} \tag{9.3}$$

where $c' = c\sin\beta$ and $\gamma = 1/\tan\beta$.

Then, the lattice distortion matrix T, which is expressed in the coordinates of the parent phase, can be obtained as follows:

$$T = RT'R_t \tag{9.4}$$

where R is the coordinate transformation matrix from the martensite to the parent phase and R_t is the transpose of R. R corresponding to the most favorable martensite variant is expressed as follows:

$$R = \begin{bmatrix} -1 & 0 & 0 \\[2ex] 0 & \dfrac{1}{\sqrt{2}} & -\dfrac{1}{\sqrt{2}} \\[2ex] 0 & -\dfrac{1}{\sqrt{2}} & \dfrac{1}{\sqrt{2}} \end{bmatrix} \tag{9.5}$$

Any vector x in the coordinates of the parent phase is transformed to x' due to the martensitic transformation using the following equation

$$x' = Tx \tag{9.6}$$

The maximum transformation strain ε^i_M in each grain can be calculated as follows:

$$\varepsilon^i_M = \frac{|x'| - |x|}{|x|} \tag{9.7}$$

Figure 9.8a shows the calculated result of the transformation strain ε^i_M expressed by contour lines for each direction in a $[001] - [011] - [\bar{1}11]$ standard stereographic triangle. For example, the transformation strains along $[001]$, $[011]$, $[\bar{1}11]$ and $[\bar{3}11]$ are 3.0%, 8.4%, 9.9%, and 10.7%, respectively. By applying the similar calculation for the R-phase transformation, the transformation strain ε^i_R at a temperature 35 K lower than T_R can be shown in Figure 9.8b. The result indicates that the strain is the maximum along $[\bar{1}11]$ and that along $[001]$ is the minimum nearly equal to zero. The strain decreases with decreasing temperature from T_R, because the rhombohedral angle of the R-phase lattice shows temperature dependence.

By averaging ε^i_M for representative 36 orientations which locate periodically in a stereographic standard triangle, the transformation strain for a polycrystal can be estimated as follows if there is no specific texture and the axis density distributes uniformly (Tan and Miyazaki, 1997):

$$\bar{\varepsilon}^0_M = \left(\sum_{i=1}^{36} \varepsilon^i_M \right) \Big/ 36 \tag{9.8}$$

If there is texture, the axis density I^i is not uniform in each inverse pole figure so that it is necessary to consider I^i in the calculation of the transformation strain as follows (Miyazaki et al., 2000):

$$\bar{\varepsilon}_M = \left(\sum_{i=1}^{36} \varepsilon^i_M I^i \right) \Big/ 36 \tag{9.9}$$

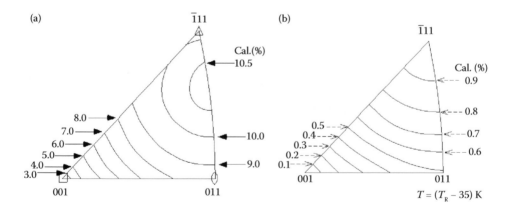

FIGURE 9.8
Orientation dependence of calculated strain induced by (a) martensitic transformation; (b) R-phase transformation. (From Miyazaki, S., in Miyazaki et al., eds., *Thin Film Shape Memory Alloys: Fundamentals and Device Applications*, Cambridge University Press, UK, 2009, reproduced with permission from Cambridge University Press.)

Transformation Temperatures

The martensitic transformation temperatures are conventionally determined by the electrical resistivity measurement or by the differential scanning calorimetry (DSC). Figure 9.9a and b shows example results of such measurements applied to an equiatomic TiNi alloy, which was solution-treated at 1273 K for 3.6 ks. When the specimen is cooled from the parent B2 phase, the martensitic transformation starts at M_s (the martensitic transformation start temperature) by evolving transformation heat, that is, the change in chemical enthalpy ΔH is negative and the reaction is exothermic as shown in the DSC curve upon cooling. The electrical resistivity shows a normal decrease upon cooling in the B2 phase region and increase of the decreasing rate at the onset of the transformation at M_s because of the crystal structural change. Upon further cooling, the martensitic transformation finishes at M_f (the martensitic transformation finish temperature).

Upon heating the specimen from the martensite phase, the martensite phase starts to reverse transform to the B2 phase at A_s (the reverse martensitic transformation start temperature) and finish at A_f (the reverse martensitic transformation finish temperature). The DSC curve upon heating shows an endothermic reaction, that is, ΔH is positive and transformation heat is absorbed. The M_s is shown in Figure 9.10 as a function of Ni content. In the composition range of the TiNi, the M_s decreases with increasing Ni content above 49.7 at.% Ni, whereas they are constant below 49.7 at.% Ni. A_f is about 30 K higher than M_s in all composition region. The reason for the constant M_s in the Ni-content region less than 49.7 at.% can be ascribed to the constant Ni content in the TiNi phase, because the Ti_2Ni appears in the Ni-content region less than 49.7 at.%, keeping the Ni content of the TiNi to be 49.7 at.%.

Shape Memory and SE

The mechanisms of SME and SE are explained using a two-dimensional crystal model shown in Figure 9.11. The crystal structure of the parent phase is shown in Figure 9.11a.

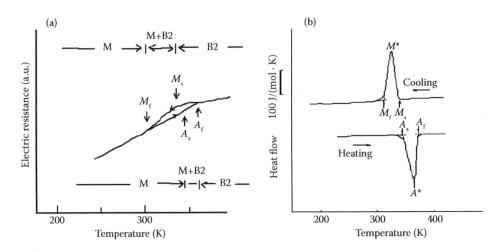

FIGURE 9.9
(a) Electrical resistance vs. temperature curve showing transformation temperatures of Ti50.0 at.% Ni alloy; (b) DSC curves showing transformation temperatures of Ti50.0 at.% Ni alloy. (From Miyazaki, S., in Miyazaki et al., eds., *Thin Film Shape Memory Alloys: Fundamentals and Device Applications*, Cambridge University Press, UK, 2009, reproduced with permission from Cambridge University Press.)

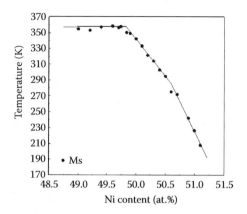

FIGURE 9.10
Ni-content dependence of M_s temperature. (From Miyazaki, S., in Miyazaki et al., eds., *Thin Film Shape Memory Alloys: Fundamentals and Device Applications*, 2009, reproduced with permission from Cambridge University Press.)

It perfectly transforms to the martensite upon cooling below M_f as shown in Figure 9.11b, where two martensite variants labeled A and B with the same crystal structure but different orientations are shown. Thermally induced martensite should be a habit plane variant because it will be formed in the parent phase and is necessary to connect the parent phase along the habit plane. However, the lattice invariant shear is not shown in A and B variants for simplicity. The lattices of both martensite variants are made by distorting the parent phase lattice upon the transformation, creating the same shear strain with opposite senses to each other. Therefore, the martensite morphology in Figure 9.11b is self-accommodated

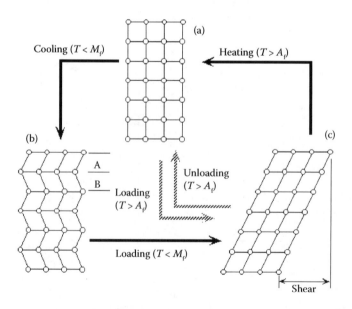

FIGURE 9.11
Schematic figure showing specimen shapes and crystal structures upon cooling, heating, loading, or unloading during shape memory and superelastic behavior.

to minimize the macroscopic net strain. In three-dimensional real crystal structures, the number of the martensite variants is generally 24 with different shear systems in a three-dimensional crystal.

By applying stress to the SMA below M_f, the A variant grows by the movement of the interface between A and B variants, which is usually a twinning plane. The interface moves easily under an extremely low stress so that the shape of the alloy changes to any shape. The selection of martensite variants is such that the most preferential variant which creates the maximum strain along the applied stress grows. In this case, the variant A grows: after replacing B with A, the martensite morphology consisting of a single variant A is obtained, generating a macroscopic shear deformation as shown in Figure 9.11c. The same specimen shape is maintained after unloading except for an elastic recovery. When the alloy is heated to the A_s point, the alloy starts to recover the original shape at the onset of the reverse martensitic transformation. Upon further heating above the A_f point, the reverse martensitic transformation finishes, resulting in a perfect shape recovery. This is the process of the SME.

The martensitic transformation generally occurs by cooling the specimen. However, an applied stress also induces the martensitic transformation even above the M_s point. The reason why the applied stress assists the transformation is that the martensitic transformation is achieved by distorting the lattice of the parent phase. Therefore, the shape of the alloy changes from Figure 9.11a directly to Figure 9.11c by the lattice distortion associated with the stress-induced martensitic transformation. If the deformation temperature is below the A_f point, the shape recovery is not perfect upon unloading. However, if it is above the A_f point, the alloy recovers the original shape upon unloading without following heating. This is the process of the SE. Because both SME and SE are associated with the same martensitic transformation, they show the same amount of shape recovery. The driving forces for the shape recovery in both phenomena originate from the recovery stress associated with the reverse martensitic transformation.

Deformation Behavior

The deformation behavior of SMAs is strongly temperature sensitive, because the deformation is associated with the martensitic transformation: this is different from plastic deformation by slip which occurs in conventional metals and alloys. Schematic stress–strain curves of a TiNi alloy obtained at various temperatures (T) are shown in Figure 9.12. In the temperature range of $T < M_f$, the specimen is fully transformed before applying stress so that the elastic deformation takes place in the martensite phase at first as shown in Figure 9.12a, where many martensite variants self-accommodate each other before loading. Upon further loading, twin planes in the martensite phase move to create an apparent plastic deformation. Therefore, the yield stress in Figure 9.12a corresponds to the critical stress for twinning deformation in the martensite phase. In the temperature range $M_f < T < M_s$, the parent and martensite phases coexist so that yielding occurs due to twinning in the martensite phase and/or stress-induced martensitic transformation in the parent phase. Both the yield stresses by twinning and stress-induced transformation in Figure 9.12b are lowest in this temperature range, because the former decreases with increasing temperature and the latter decreases with decreasing temperature until reaching this temperature region. The stress–strain curves in Figure 9.12a and b are essentially the same, except the yield stress is a little lower in Figure 9.12b than that in Figure 9.12a. In the temperature range of $M_s < T < A_s$, the parent phase elastically deforms at first and yielding occurs due to the stress-induced martensitic transformation. Therefore, the yield stress linearly

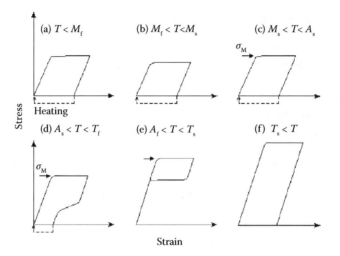

FIGURE 9.12
Schematic stress–strain curves at various temperatures in a TiNi alloy. (From Miyazaki, S., in Miyazaki et al., eds., *Thin Film Shape Memory Alloys: Fundamentals and Device Applications*, 2009, reproduced with permission from Cambridge University Press.)

increases with increasing temperature satisfying the Clausius–Clapeyron relationship. The stress-induced martensite phase remains after unloading, because the temperature is below A_s. The shape of the stress–strain curve of Figure 9.12c is similar to those of Figure 9.12a and b. In the temperature range $A_s < T < A_f$, the deformation induced by the stress-induced martensitic transformation recovers partially upon unloading as shown in Figure

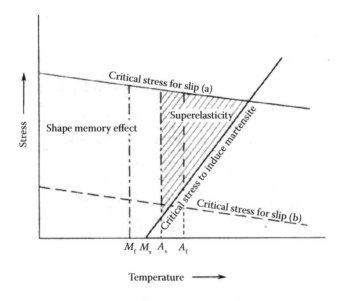

FIGURE 9.13
Schematic illustration of region of SME and SE: (a) critical stress for a high critical stress; (b) critical stress for a low critical stress. (From Miyazaki, S., in Miyazaki et al., eds., *Thin Film Shape Memory Alloys: Fundamentals and Device Applications*, 2009, reproduced with permission from Cambridge University Press.)

9.12d, resulting in partial SE and partial SME by following heating. In the temperature range $A_f < T < T_s$, perfect SE appears as shown in Figure 9.12e, where T_s stands for the critical temperature above which the martensitic transformation does not take place and deformation occurs by slip. If T is above T_s, plastic deformation occurs as in conventional metals and alloys as shown in Figure 9.12f.

The stress–strain relationship of SMA is different at different temperature range. Figure 9.13 illustrates the region SME and SE with the critical stress for slip and stress induced martensitic transformation. In principle, both SME and SE are observable in the same specimen, depending on the testing temperature, as long as the critical stress for slip is high enough. SME occurs below A_s, followed by heating above A_f, whereas SE occurs above A_f, where the martensites are completely unstable in the absence of stress.

Film Fabrication and Characterization

Film Deposition

TiNi-based films are the most frequently used thin film SMA materials and they are typically prepared using sputtering method. Laser ablation, ion beam deposition, arc plasma ion plating, plasma spray, and flash evaporation were also reported but with some intrinsic problems, such as nonuniformity in film thickness and composition, low deposition rate, and/or nonbatch processing, incompatibility with MEMS process, and so on. Figure 9.14 shows a schematic drawing of a most common radio frequency (r.f.) magnetron sputtering apparatus (Miyazaki and Ishida, 1999). Ar ions are accelerated into the target to sputter Ti and Ni atoms which are deposited onto the substrate to form a TiNi film. Transformation temperatures, shape memory behaviors, and SE of the sputtered TiNi films are sensitive to metallurgical factors (alloy composition, contamination, thermomechanical treatment, annealing and aging process, etc.), sputtering conditions (cosputtering with multitargets, target power, gas pressure, target-to-substrate distance, deposition temperature, substrate bias, etc.), and the application conditions (loading conditions, ambient temperature and environment, heat dissipation, heating/cooling rate, strain rate, etc.) (Ishida et al., 1996). Systematic studies on the detailed effects of all the above parameters are necessary. The sensitivity of TiNi films to all these factors seems an intrinsic disadvantage, but at the same time, this sensitivity provides tremendous flexibility in engineering a combination of properties for intended applications.

Precise control of Ti/Ni ratio in TiNi films is of essential importance, as has been documented because TiNi film studies started more than two decades ago. The intrinsic problems associated with sputtering of TiNi films include the difference in sputtering yields of titanium and nickel at a given sputtering power density, geometrical composition uniformity over substrate and along cross-section thickness of the coating, as well as wear, erosion, and roughening of targets during sputtering (Shih et al., 2001). To combat these problems, co-sputtering of TiNi target with another Ti target, or using two separate single element (Ti and Ni) targets, or adding titanium plates on TiNi target are widely used (Ohta et al., 2000). Substrate rotation, optimal configuration of target position and precise control of sputtering conditions, etc., are also helpful. Varying the target temperature can produce the compositional modification: sputtering with a heated TiNi target can limit the loss of Ti, thus improving the uniformity of film properties (Ho and Carman, 2000; Ho et al.,

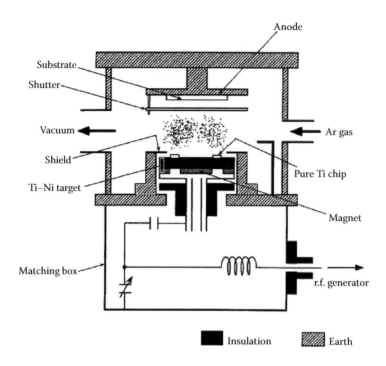

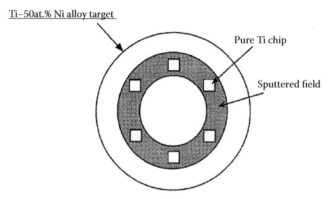

FIGURE 9.14
A schematic figure showing a radio frequency magnetron sputtering system. (From Miyazaki, S., Ishida, A., *Mater. Sci. Eng.*, 273–275, 106–133, 1999, with permission from Elsevier.)

2002). Good performance TiNi films can also be obtained by post-annealing of multilayer of Ti/Ni (Cho et al., 2006). Because contamination is a big problem for good mechanical properties of the sputtered TiNi films, it is important to limit the impurities, typically oxygen and carbon, to prevent the brittleness, deterioration, or even loss of SME. For this reason, the purity of Ar gas and targets is essential, and the base vacuum of the main chamber should be as high as possible (usually lower than 10^{-7} Torr). Pre-sputtering cleaning of targets before deposition effectively removes the surface oxides on targets, and thus constitutes one of the important steps in ensuring film purity. To deposit films without columnar structure (thus with good mechanical properties), a low processing pressure of Ar gas (0.5 to 5 mTorr) is essential. Application of bias voltage during sputtering could modify the film microstructure, texture, and stress, thus is also important, but few studies have been reported on this topic so far.

Important sputtering factors which will affect the quality of the films are r.f. power, Ar gas pressure, substrate–target distance, substrate temperature, and alloy composition of the target used. Figure 9.15 shows the fracture surface of as-deposited thin films. The film prepared at a low Ar gas pressure exhibits a flat and featureless structure, whereas films prepared at high Ar gas pressure exhibit a columnar structure. This columnar structure suggests that the films are porous. This structure seems to be caused by the restricted mobility of deposited atoms on the surface of the growing film. A high Ar gas pressure is likely to decrease the energy of the sputtered atoms by collision with Ar ions, resulting in a decrease in their surface diffusion. Furthermore, under a high Ar gas pressure, Ar ions adsorbed on the film surface can interfere with the surface diffusion of sputtered Ti and Ni atoms. Of the films prepared at a high Ar gas pressure, the fracture surface of the film prepared at an r.f. power of 600 W seems to be less porous than the other films.

Depending on processing conditions, TiNi films can be deposited at room temperature or high temperatures. TiNi films sputtered at room temperature are usually amorphous, thus post-sputtering annealing (usually higher than 450°C) is a must because SME only occurs in materials of crystalline form. However, martensitic transformation and SE of TiNi films are sensitive to post-annealing and/or aging temperature and duration (Lehnert et al., 2002; Surbled et al., 2001), thus post-sputtering annealing should be handled with care. It is suggested that the lowest possible annealing or aging temperature be used in a bid to conserve thermal processing budgets and more importantly minimize the reactions between film and substrate (Isalgue et al., 1999). Long-term post annealing and aging process should be avoided because it could trigger dramatic changes in film microstructure (i.e., precipitation), mechanical properties and SMEs. Films deposited at a relatively high temperature (about 400°C) is crystallized in situ, thus there is no need for post-annealing. Films can be deposited at relatively high temperatures (400 to 500°C) during sputtering to form crystallized phase, then at a relatively lower temperature (about 300°C) to maintain

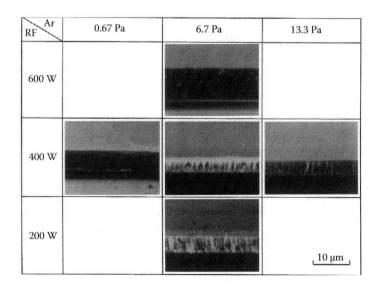

FIGURE 9.15
Cross-section microstructure of TiNi thin films formed under various sputtering conditions. (From Miyazaki, S., Ishida, A., *Mater. Sci. Eng.*, 273–275, 106–133, 1999, with permission from Elsevier.)

a crystalline growth during the later sputtering process. Films can also be deposited at a low temperature (about 300°C) to get partial crystallization, then annealed at a higher temperature (500°C) for a short time to promote further crystallization.

Recently a localized laser annealing method was used for TiNi films (Huang et al., 2002), where only certain areas of a film are annealed by laser beam to exhibit SME, and the other nonannealed areas remain amorphous, thus acting as a pullback spring during cooling process. This method opens a new way for fabrication of microdevices (Bellouard et al., 1999). The advantages of the localized laser annealing process include: (1) precision in selection of the areas to be annealed, down to micron meter scale; (2) noncontact and high efficiency; (3) free of restrictions on design and processing; (4) ease in integration in MEMS processes; (4) ease in cutting of the final structure using the laser beam. However, still some problems exist that include: (1) Energy loss. TiNi film surface is usually smooth and reflection loss of laser beam energy is a big problem. Possible solutions include selection of excimer laser beam, choice of suitable parameters (e.g. wavelength of laser), and surface treatment or roughening of film surface to improve laser adsorption. (2) Difficulty in duration control. Crystallization of film structure is a thermodynamic process, and it is necessary to maintain sufficient treatment time for crystallization to complete. However, overexposure easily causes surface damage of the thin films. (3) Need of protection environment, such as Ar gas or vacuum condition, which adds complexity and cost to the process.

TiNi Film Characterization

For freestanding TiNi films, conventional methods, such as DSC and tensile tests (stress–strain curves) are quite applicable to characterize the SME. The stress–strain and strain–temperature responses of freestanding films are commonly evaluated using tensile tests (Ishida et al., 1996; Ishida et al., 1999). Results show that the stress–strain–temperature relationship, elongation, fracture stress, and yield stress are at least comparable to (if not better than) those of bulk materials, because of the grain size effect (micron or submicron size in thin films as compared with tens of microns for bulk materials) (Fu et al., 2003; Matsunaga et al., 1999). The difficulties in tensile testing of TiNi thin films include: (1) obtaining freestanding films without predeformation; and (2) clamping tightly the films on tester grips. For MEMS applications, the TiNi films are usually deposited on Si or other substrates. One of the important issues in characterization of the TiNi films for MEMS applications is how to correctly evaluate the SME and mechanical properties of the constrained thin films on substrates. For this purpose, curvature and electrical resistivity measurements are widely used (Grummon et al., 1999). Some new methods based on MEMS techniques (Espinosa et al., 2003), such as bulge test (Moyne et al., 1999), TiNi/Si diaphragm (Makino et al., 1999, 2000), cantilever bending, or damping (Craciunescu and Wuttig 2000), are more appropriate for microactuator applications, which are compatible with small dimensions and high sensitivities. Nanoindentation testing with/or without changes in temperature could reveal the different elastic and plastic deformation behaviors of austenite and martensite, and is thus also promising for characterization of superelasicity, phase transformation, SME, and mechanical properties of the constrained thin films (Ni et al., 2002; Shaw et al., 2003; Ma and Komvopoulos, 2003). Indentation of TiNi-based films is strongly dependent on the materials resistance to dislocation. Because the dislocation is closely related to fatigue properties of films, indentation for materials characterization is particularly useful for MEMS applications, where optimization of fatigue performance is critical.

Recently, an AFM-based in situ testing method has been applied to characterize the phase transformation behavior of constrained films (Fu et al., 2004). Figure 9.16 shows two

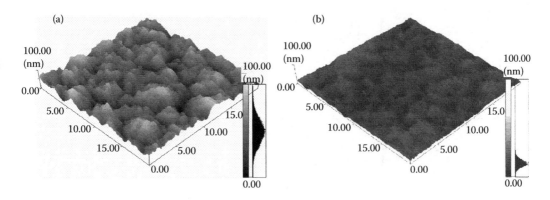

FIGURE 9.16
AFM surface morphologies of TiNiCu films (a) low temperature in martensite state and (b) high temperature in austenite state. (From Fu et al, *Sens. Actuat.* 112, 395–408, 2004, with permission from Elsevier.)

micrographs of AFM surface morphology of TiNi films on Si substrate at a low temperature (martensite) and a high temperature (austenite), respectively. The surface roughness of the martensite is much higher than that of the austenite. With the change in temperature, the surface roughness changes drastically during transformation between the martensite and austenite, thus clearly revealing the occurrence of phase transformation. The advantages of this method are its nondestructive nature and applicability to very small size films (down to nanometers). Moreover, the changes in optical reflection caused by the changes in the surface roughness and reflective index can also be used to characterize the transformation behaviors of TiNi films (Wu et al., 2006).

There are usually some discrepancies in transformation temperatures obtained from different characterization methods (Fu et al., 2003). The possible reasons include: (1) the phase transformation and mechanical behaviors of constrained TiNi films could be different from those of freestanding films, due to substrate effect, residual stress, strain rate effect, stress gradient effect, and temperature gradient effect; (2) the intrinsic nature of testing method (thus the changes in physical properties will not start at exactly the same temperatures); (3) differences in testing conditions, for example, heating/cooling rate; (4) nonuniformity of film composition over whole substrate and along cross-section thickness of coating. Therefore, it is necessary to identify whether the application is based on the freestanding film or constrained film/substrate system, so that a suitable method can be chosen.

In the following sections, we will discuss the characterization results of TiNi films as well as Ti-rich and Ni-rich films.

TiNi Binary Alloy Thin Films

As mentioned above, the as-sputtered TiNi thin films are amorphous if the substrate is not heated during deposition. As a consequence, they should be crystallized by heating at 973 K, which is higher than the crystallization temperature, followed by aging at 773 K for various times. The crystalline structures of the Ti–51.9 at.% Ni alloy thin film age-treated for 36 ks were determined at three different temperatures, that is, 300, 270, and 200 K, by x-ray diffraction. The parent (B2) phase, R-phase, and martensitic (M)0-phase exist independently at these temperatures, respectively, as shown in Figure 9.17. The crystal structure of the parent phase was determined to be B2, whereas those of the R-phase and M-phase were rhombohedral and monoclinic, respectively. The lattice parameters of each phase are

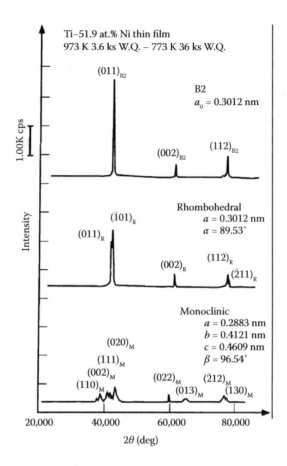

FIGURE 9.17
X-ray diffraction profiles of parent B2, R-phase, and monoclinic martensite phase in a Ti51.9 at.% Ni thin film. (From Miyazaki, S., Ishida, A., *Mater. Sci. Eng.*, 273–275, 106–133, 1999, with permission from Elsevier.)

shown on the right side of the corresponding diffraction profile. The lattice parameters of the three phases are essentially the same as those measured in bulk specimens, although they differ only slightly depending on the alloy content. The rhombohedral angle α shows a unique dependence on temperature. Figure 9.18a shows the temperature dependence of α in the Ti–51.9 at.% Ni thin film. The angle starts to decrease at R_s, the temperature for the R-phase transformation to start, and gradually decreases with decreasing temperature. The lattice constant a of the R-phase is almost constant irrespective of temperature.

Figure 9.18b shows the transformation strains measured in the Ti–51.9 at.% Ni, which was crystallized at 973 K for 3.6 ks followed by aging at 773 K for 3.6 ks. The recovery strain ε_A associated with the reverse martensitic transformation increases with increasing the applied constant stress applied to the thin film during thermal cycling until reaching a strain of about 2.6%. Then, the strain becomes a constant irrespective of the applied stress after reaching 2.6% at a critical stress of 300 MPa. The critical stress is the minimum stress required for the most preferentially oriented variant to grow almost fully in each grain. Therefore, stresses higher than 300 MPa are not effective in increasing ε_A. The strain ε_R associated with the R-phase transformation is also shown in Figure 9.18b. It also increases with increasing applied constant stress until reaching about 0.26%, which is one-tenth of ε_A. After reaching a strain of 0.26% at a stress of about 175 MPa, ε_R starts to decrease with

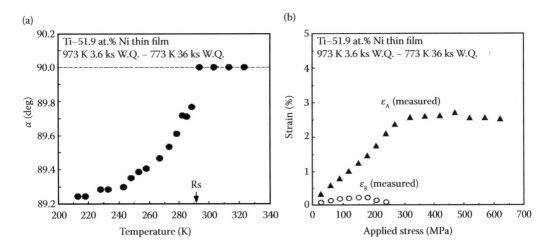

FIGURE 9.18

Rhombohedral angle α of R-phase as a function of temperatures. (a, b) Transformation strains measured in Ti–51.9 at.% Ni, which was crystallized at 973 K for 3.6 ks followed by aging at 773 K for 3.6 ks. (From Miyazaki, S., Ishida, A., *Mater. Sci. Eng.*, 273–275, 106–133, 1999, with permission from Elsevier.)

further increasing applied stress. The major reason for the increase in ε_R before the maximum point is that the most preferential variant grows with increasing the applied stress, whereas the major reason for the decrease in ε_R after reaching the maximum point is that the temperature range where the R-phase can exist becomes narrower with increasing the applied stress, so that the lattice distortion of the R-phase becomes less as shown in Figure 9.18b.

Table 9.2 shows the transformation strains ε_A, which were calculated on the basis of the lattice distortion from the B2 phase to the M phase, along some specific crystal orientations and the average strain of ε_A. The average strain is 8.42%, which is about three times that of the observed strain. The reason why the observed strain is so small is not attributable to the texture because the x-ray diffraction pattern of the B2 phase does not reveal a strong texture, although the (011) peak intensity is a little larger than that of a TiNi film with randomly oriented grains. The possible reason is the strong internal structure consisting of fine Ti_3Ni_4 precipitates and fine grains of submicron size because such internal structure will suppress the growth of the most preferentially oriented M variant. On the other hand, Figure 9.19a shows the recovery strain ε_A in a Ti–50.5 at.% Ni thin film that was solution-treated at 973 K for 3.6 ks. Because the solution-treated thin film does not contain

TABLE 9.2

Calculated Martensite Transformation Strains along Specific Orientations

Crystal Orientation	Calculated Martensitic Transformation Strain (%)
[0 0 1]	2.63
[0 1 1]	8.20
[1 1 1]	9.42
Average strain	8.42

Source: Miyazaki, S., Ishida, A., *Mater. Sci. Eng. A*, 273–275, 106–133, 1999, with permission from Elsevier.

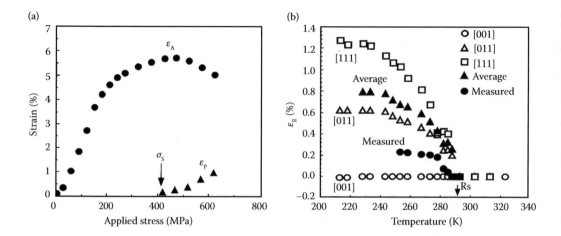

FIGURE 9.19

(a) Effect of applied stress on transformation strain and permanent strain in a Ti–50.5 at.% Ni film. (b) Transformation strains associated with R-phase as a function of temperature. (From Miyazaki, S., Ishida, A., *Mater. Sci. Eng.*, 273–275, 106–133, 1999, with permission from Elsevier.)

fine Ti$_3$Ni$_4$ precipitates, the most preferentially oriented martensite variant can grow easily under low stresses. The maximum ε_A observed in Figure 9.19a is 5.8% under a stress of 470 MPa, at around which macroscopic plastic strain ε_p appears.

To calculate the transformation strain ε_R, it is necessary to use the lattice constants of the R-phase. The length of each axis of the R-phase unit cell is almost constant irrespective of temperature and is the same as that of the B2 phase. Therefore, the transformation strain ε_R depends on the temperature. Figure 9.19b shows calculated strains along some specific orientations and also the average strain as a function of temperature, calculated average strain is also shown. The strain along each orientation increases with decreasing temperature in the temperature region below R_s: the strain along the orientation (111) shows the maximum and that along the orientation (001) the minimum. The observed strain is about one-half of the calculated average strain. Because the observed ε_A is one-third of the calculated average strain, the suppressing effect against the growth of the preferentially oriented variant is less in the R-phase than that in the M-phase. This can be understood in such a way that the transformation strains associated with the R-phase transformation is only one-tenth of that associated with the M transformation. Details of the calculation methods for the strains associated with the M-phase and R-phase transformations are explained in references (Miyazaki, 1988; Miyazaki and Weyman, 1988).

Superelastic Behavior

Figure 9.20 shows stress–strain curves of a Ti–50.3 at.% Ni film at different temperatures. Curves (a) and (b) show the stress–strain curves obtained below A_s so that the shape change remains after unloading. The residual strain disappears upon heating to above A_f, revealing the perfect SME. Curve (c) is obtained by deforming the film at a temperature between A_s and A_f so that it shows a partial shape recovery upon unloading and further shape recovery upon heating. Finally, curve (d) shows a perfect SE at a temperature above A_f. Because the SE is accompanied by a stress hysteresis, it is necessary to apply a high enough stress to observe such SE. In this case, the maximum stress applied to the film is higher than 600 MPa.

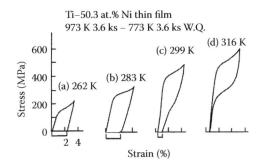

FIGURE 9.20
Stress–strain curves showing SME and SE in a Ti–50.3 at.% Ni thin film. (From Miyazaki, S., Ishida, A., *Mater. Sci. Eng.*, 273–275, 106–133, 1999, with permission from Elsevier.)

Texture and Transformation Strain Anisotropy

Specific texture developed in materials causes anisotropic characteristics to appear in mechanical, electrical, and magnetic behavior. Shape memory and mechanical properties of the TiNi films depends significantly on the orientation of the crystal grains. Deposition conditions, film composition, and post-deposition thermomechanical treatment could have important consequences on formation and evolution of the film texture. A strong film texture may lead to anisotropic SME because the recoverable strain and deformation behavior is highly dependent on the film crystallographic orientation (Shu et al., 1998; Liu et al., 2005; Gall et al., 1999).

Figure 9.21a and b shows pole figures obtained using diffraction from {110}, {200}, and {211} planes in Ti–52.2 at.% Ni and Ti–51.6 at.% Ni thin films, respectively. The Ti–52.2 at.% Ni thin film shows a considerably uniform orientation distribution of grains with a weak (302) fiber texture, the maximum axis density being only 3.9. On the other hand, the Ti–51.6 at.% Ni thin film shows a strong (110) fiber texture with a maximum axis density of 110. Because the poles of the fiber textures are both normal to film planes, the in-plane crystal orientation distribution is uniform so that transformation strain anisotropy is weak in both

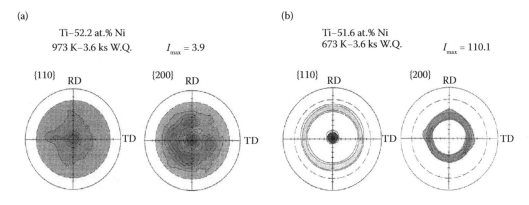

FIGURE 9.21
(a) {110} and {200} pole figures in a Ti–52.2 at.% Ni thin film which was crystallized at 973 K for 3.6 ks; (b) {110} and {200} pole figures in a Ti–51.6 at.% Ni thin films which were heat-treated at 673 K for 3.6 ks. Film was sputtered on substrate at 623 K. (From Miyazaki, S., Ishida, A., *Mater. Sci. Eng.*, 273–275, 106–133, 1999, with permission from Elsevier.)

film planes. Calculated and experimentally measured transformation strains are shown in Figure 9.21c and d for the Ti–52.2 at.% Ni and Ti–51.6 at.% Ni, respectively. The experimental results were obtained under various constant stresses by cooling and heating the films. The transformation strain increases with increasing stress. However, it is almost constant for each stress irrespective of direction. The calculated results were obtained by assuming that only the most favorable martensite variant grows in the entire grain, so that the calculated result gives the maximum recoverable strain, which is always larger than the experimental result. This isotropic nature in the transformation strain in the film plane is convenient for designing microactuators of TiNi thin films.

Some studies have been done to clarify the texture and the anisotropy in the deformation behavior in rolled TiNi thick plates (Inoue et al., 1996). However, few studies have investigated the texture and the anisotropy in shape memory behavior in sputter-deposited TiNi thin films with a thickness less than 10 μm. The post-annealed crystallized TiNi films normally have a strong texture along austenite A (110) (Miyazaki et al., 2000). At room temperature, martensite (200) and (022) peaks become dominant. Hassdorf et al. (2002) deposited a TiNiCu film on a SiO_2 substrate using molecular beam epitaxy (MBE) technology, and found the film has a distinct austenite (200) diffraction peak. The crystallites are oriented within ±3° along the film plane normal. The authors pointed out that an intermediate Ti_2Ni layer is crucial for the formation of (200) texture. Under tensile load, (100) orientation is characterized as "hard" because it demonstrates small uniaxial transformation strain levels and begins transforming at a significant higher stress (Miyazaki et al., 1984). The film with (100) texture has the highest transformation stress compared with (111) and (110) texture. The (111) orientation is characterized as "soft" because it demonstrates large uniaxial transformation strains and low critical transformation stress levels. The recoverable strain of TiNi film with A(111) texture is much higher than that of the commonly observed (110) texture. However, so far, (111) dominant texture in TiNi-based films is difficult to achieve. It clearly indicates an opportunity to improve SME by targeting special textures using a novel processing technique.

Ni-Rich TiNi Alloy Thin Films

Microstructure of Age-Treated Thin Films

Figure 9.22 shows the microstructures of Ti–51.3 at.% Ni thin films aged at various temperatures between 573 and 773 K for various times of 1, 10, and 100 h (3.6, 36, and 360 ks) after solution treatment at 973 K for 1 h. As can be seen in this figure, the size of the precipitates increases with increasing aging temperature and aging time for all the age-treated thin films, whereas the grain size is almost constant, about 1 μm. All the precipitates in the figure are confirmed to be a Ti_3Ni_4 phase by electron diffraction. The bright field image and diffraction pattern of the precipitates in the thin film aged at 673 K for 10 h are shown in Figure 9.23. The diffraction pattern is consistent with a mixture of (111) B2 zone and (111) Ti_3Ni_4 zones, and the same diffraction pattern is observed for all the age-treated thin films. The bright field image also shows characteristic morphology of Ti_3Ni_4 precipitates. That is, the lenticular shape precipitates are observed along the three directions of $[\bar{1}10]B2$, $[10\bar{1}]$ B2, and $[0\bar{1}1]B2$, which are the traces of $(11\bar{1})B2$, $(1\bar{1}1)B2$, and $(\bar{1}11)B2$ respectively. Another precipitate is located on the (111)B2 plane, which is parallel to the photograph. The sizes of the precipitates were measured to describe the fineness of the microstructure. Because the precipitates are formed on {111} planes of the B2 phase in a lenticular shape, the longitudinal length was chosen to represent the size of the precipitates. The sizes of the precipitates

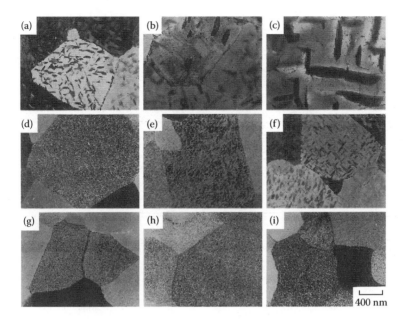

FIGURE 9.22
Transmission electron micrographs of Ti_3Ni_4 precipitates in Ti–51.3 at.% Ni thin films which were solution-treated at 973 K for 3.6 ks followed by age treatment at 773 K for (a) 3.6 ks; (b) 36 ks and (c) 360 ks, at 673 K for (d) 3.6 ks; (e) 36 ks and (f) 360 ks, and at 573 K for (g) 3.6 ks; (h) 36 ks and (i) 360 ks. (From Miyazaki, S., Ishida, A., *Mater. Sci. Eng.*, 273–275, 106–133, 1999, with permission from Elsevier.)

in the thin films aged at 573 and 623 K are not listed here because the precipitate contrast is too weak to measure the size.

Aging Effect

Figure 9.24a shows the effect of aging time on the transformation temperatures of the Ti–51.9 at.% Ni alloy thin films which were aged at 773 K for different durations after solution treatment at 973 K for 3.6 ks. The solid lines show the DSC curves measured upon cooling, whereas the dashed curves show those upon heating. Solution-treated film ($X = 0$) shows no transformation peak upon cooling in the DSC curve, indicating that the transformation temperatures are very low, hence again no reverse transformation peak upon heating. In age-treated thin films, there are two transformation peaks appearing on each solid

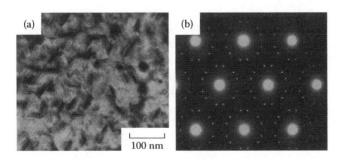

FIGURE 9.23
(a) Bright-field image and (b) electron diffraction pattern of Ti_3Ni_4 precipitates in a Ti–51.3 at.% Ni thin film which was age-treated at 673 K for 36 ks.

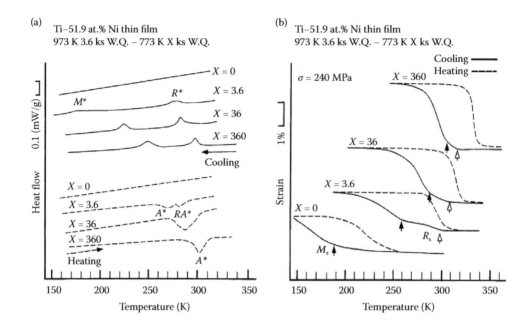

FIGURE 9.24

(a) Effect of aging time on transformation temperatures measured by DSC in the Ti–51.9 at.% Ni thin film. (From Miyazaki, S., Ishida, A., *Mater. Sci. Eng.*, 273–275, 106–133, 1999, with permission from Elsevier.) (b) Effect of aging time on the shape memory behavior in the Ti–51.9 at.% Ni thin film. (From Miyazaki, S., Ishida, A., *Mater. Sci. Eng.*, 273–275, 106–133, 1999, with permission from Elsevier.)

curve; the two peaks denoted by R^* and M^* correspond to the R-phase and martensitic transformations, respectively. Upon heating the age-treated films show only one reverse transformation peak A^* except for the film aged for 3.6 ks which shows transformation peaks A^* and RA^*. A^* points of the films aged for 36 and 360 ks represent the reverse transformation from M directly to B2, whereas A^* and RA^* of the film aged for 3.6 ks represent the reverse transformation from M to R and from R to B2, respectively. Both of the R^* and M^* show an aging effect which causes them to increase with increasing aging time. However, M^* increases more sensitively to the aging time than R^*. The increase in M^* and R^* can be explained by the decrease in the Ni content of the matrix of the film because the growth of the Ti_3Ni_4 precipitates will consume excess Ni in the matrix and the transformation temperatures increase with decreasing Ni content of the matrix.

The shape memory behavior of the thin films is shown in Figure 9.24b. Strains were measured upon cooling (solid lines) and heating (dashed lines) under 240 MPa in the Ti–51.9 at.% Ni thin films which were aged at 773 K for 0, 3.6, 36 and 360 ks, respectively. Two-stage shape change appears both at R_s and M_s in the age-treated thin films, whereas a single-stage shape change at M_s in the solution-treated thin film. All the R_s and M_s in Figure 9.24b are higher than those estimated by the DSC curves because the DSC curves were measured under no load, whereas the strain was measured under stress: the stress increases the transformation temperatures following the Clausius–Clapeyron relationship. Because M_s (or M^*) increases more effectively by aging than R_s (or R^*), the temperature difference between R_s and M_s becomes smaller with increasing aging time. The strain induced by the transformations increases with increasing aging time, indicating that as the Ti_3Ni_4

precipitates grow by aging they lose the suppressing force against the growth of the preferentially oriented martensite variants.

The aging effect was also investigated in the Ti–43.9 at.% Ni thin films. There is no aging effect observed in the transformation temperatures as shown by the DSC results in Figure 9.25a. Two-stage transformation behaviors are observed both upon cooling and heating. The appearance of the R-phase is usually attributed to a fine internal structure consisting of dislocations and/or precipitates in bulk specimens. However, the R-phase cannot be attributed to such internal structure in the Ti–43.9 at.% Ni thin film because there are neither dislocations nor Ni-rich Ti_3Ni_4 precipitates. The cause for the appearance of the R-phase is considered to be another fine internal structure consisting of Ti_2Ni compounds and small grains. The grain size of sputter-deposited TiNi thin films generally ranges from 0.5 μm to several microns, whereas the grain size of solution-treated bulk TiNi alloys is up to several tens of microns. This fine internal structure in the thin films also suppresses the martensitic transformation more effectively than the R-phase transformation.

Figure 9.25b shows the shape memory behavior in the thin films. Again no aging effect is observed in the shape memory behavior. The transformation temperatures and transformation strains do not change with aging time. The reason why there is no aging effect in the Ti–43.9 at.% Ni thin film is that in Ni-poor TiNi alloy, the Ti_3Ni_4 precipitates cannot be created, so that there is no variation in Ni content of the matrix. The strain-versus-temperature curves clearly show two-stage deformation behavior both upon cooling and heating, corresponding to the two-stage transformation behavior in Figure 9.25b.

M_s of both the Ti–51.9 at.% Ni and Ti–43.9 at.% Ni thin films are replotted against aging time in Figure 9.26, where M_s measured by both DSC and mechanical tests are included. Controlling transformation temperature is one of the important techniques to fabricate

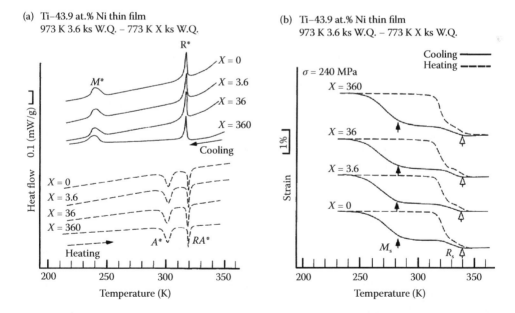

FIGURE 9.25
(a) Effect of aging time on transformation temperatures measured by DSC in the Ti–43.9 at.% Ni thin film. (From Miyazaki, S., Ishida, A., *Mater. Sci. Eng.*, 273–275, 106–133, 1999, with permission from Elsevier.) (b) Effect of aging time on shape memory behavior in Ti–43.9 at.% Ni thin film. (From Miyazaki, S., Ishida, A., *Mater. Sci. Eng.*, 273–275, 106–133, 1999, with permission from Elsevier.)

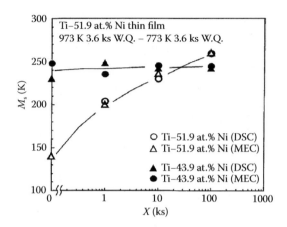

FIGURE 9.26
Effect of aging time on martensitic transformation start temperature M_s in Ti–51.9 at.% Ni and Ti–43.9 at.% Ni thin films. (From Miyazaki, S., Ishida, A., *Mater. Sci. Eng.*, 273–275, 106–133, 1999, with permission from Elsevier.)

SMA thin film microactuators suitable for various purposes. The M_s increases with increasing aging time in the Ti–51.9 at.% Ni, whereas there is no aging effect in the Ti–43.9 at.% Ni film. These alloys are considered to possess an advantageous characteristic for fabricating microactuators, that is, the Ni-rich alloy shows the aging effect so that the transformation temperatures are adjustable by heat treatment even if the alloy content of the thin film cannot be adjusted as one wishes, whereas the Ni-poor alloy does not show aging effect so that the transformation temperatures are less sensitive to the variation of heat treatment condition. Besides, the Ni content of the matrix is also constant irrespective of nominal composition because the formation of Ti$_2$Ni keeps the Ni content of the matrix to be of equilibrium. Hence the transformation temperatures are insensitive to nominal composition of the Ni-poor thin films.

However, because as-sputtered thin films are amorphous in Ni-poor (or Ti-rich) films if the heat-treatment is not sufficient to achieve an equilibrium condition, nonequilibrium condition can exist so that transformation temperatures and shape memory behavior will show sensitivity to heat treatment.

Ti-Rich TiNi Alloy

Nonequilibrium Phase and Composition

Because as-sputtered TiNi thin films are amorphous if the substrate temperature is not raised intentionally, the Ti-rich or Ni-rich TiNi thin films can contain excess Ti or Ni atoms, respectively, in the amorphous phase. Although equilibrium composition of TiNi varies depending on temperature, generally speaking, it only ranges from 49.5 at.% Ni to 50.5 at.% Ni, where the B2 single phase is stable above M_s. Therefore, both Ti-rich or Ni-rich TiNi thin films may reveal nonequilibrium phases during a crystallization process.

Figure 9.27a shows a high-resolution electron micrograph of a Ti–48.2 at.% Ni thin film which was heated at 745 K for 3.6 ks. The electron diffraction pattern taken from this area is shown in Figure 9.27b. The same internal structure can be observed in the Ti–48.2 at.%

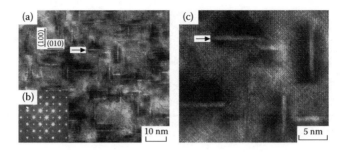

FIGURE 9.27
(a) High-resolution electron micrograph of a T-48.2 at.% Ni thin film heated at 745 K for 3.6 ks and (b) corresponding diffraction pattern. (c) Enlarged micrograph of a part of (a), showing details of plate precipitates. (From Miyazaki, S., Ishida, A., *Mater. Sci. Eng.*, 273–275, 106–133, 1999, with permission from Elsevier.)

Ni which was heated at 773 K for 0.3 ks (5 min) as shown in Figure 9.28a. The corresponding diffraction pattern in Figure 9.28b shows a (100) zone pattern of the B2 parent phase. This observation indicates that the nonequilibrium Ti-rich platelets can be formed at the initial stage of heating even at considerably high temperatures. Figure 9.29a and b shows a bright-field image and the corresponding diffraction pattern of the same alloy film which was heated at 773 K for 3.6 ks. Figure 9.29a reveals spherical precipitates which appear as Moiré patterns in addition to the Ti-rich platelets. These spherical precipitates can be distinguished from the Ti-rich platelets by taking a picture in random orientation, as shown in Figure 9.29c. The formation of the spherical precipitates produces extra spots in the diffraction pattern in addition to the streaks due to the platelets (Figure 9.29b). These extra spots could be indexed as a Ti_2Ni phase.

Figures 9.30a and b show bright-field images of a Ti–48.2 at.% Ni thin film annealed at 773 K for 36 ks. The corresponding electron beams are parallel to the (100) and (111) of B2, respectively. In both figures, the spherical precipitates are distinguished by Moiré patterns. Moiré fringes are parallel to the {110} planes of B2. The Ti_2Ni is an equilibrium phase. However, such uniform distribution of Ti_2Ni precipitates in grains is not of an equilibrium state. In case of Ti-rich TiNi bulk materials, the Ti_2Ni precipitates preferentially distribute along grain boundaries. Such equilibrium distribution of Ti_2Ni can be formed in the film when it is heated for a longer time or at higher temperatures. More detailed information can be found in the study of Zhang et al. (2006).

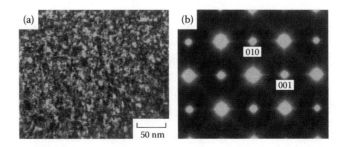

FIGURE 9.28
(a) Bright-field image and (b) the corresponding diffraction pattern of a Ti–48.2 at.% Ni thin film heated at 773 K for 0.3 ks. (From Miyazaki, S., Ishida, A., *Mater. Sci. Eng.*, 273–275, 106–133, 1999, with permission from Elsevier.)

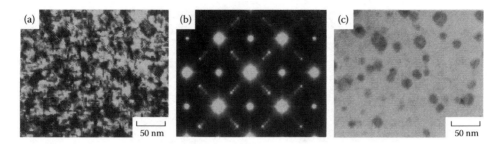

FIGURE 9.29
Microstructure of a Ti–48.2 at.% Ni thin film heated at 773 K for 3.6 ks; (a) bright-field image; (b) corresponding diffraction pattern; and (c) bright-field image taken in random orientation. (From Miyazaki, S., Ishida, A., *Mater. Sci. Eng.*, 273–275, 106–133, 1999, with permission from Elsevier.)

Strengthening Mechanism

As described above, the internal structure of the Ti-rich TiNi thin film evolves by means of changing the type of phases and their distribution. Therefore, it is expected that there will be an optimum heat treatment condition for shape memory characteristics. Figure 9.31 shows a typical result of a mechanical test in which a Ti–48.2 at.% Ni thin film was thermally cycled between 140 and 550 K under various constant stresses. The specimen was heat-treated at 745 K for 3.6 ks before the test. The test was performed in such a way that the magnitude of the applied stress was increased stepwise in each thermal cycle, starting from 30 MPa. One specimen was used throughout the whole test. It is revealed in Figure 9.31 that the recoverable strain (ε_A) increases with increasing stress, up to 5.5% at 240 MPa without noticeable plastic strain involved. Above this stress level, the plastic strain ε_p in each thermal cycle gradually increases to nearly 1% at 570 MPa. However, it should be noted that a recoverable strain of about 5% can still be obtained under such a high level of stress.

The critical stress σ_s, below, which any appreciable amount of σ_p could not be detected in the thermal cycle test, was measured in specimens heat-treated at various temperatures for 3.6 ks. The results are shown in Figure 9.32a, where σ_s is plotted as a function of heat-treatment temperature T_h. The critical stress σ_s rapidly increases with decreasing T_h below 820 K. Above 820 K, σ_s appears to be almost constant. This critical temperature of 820 K coincides with the heat-treatment temperature above which subnanometric nonequilibrium plate precipitates are no longer observable. This indicates that the formation of the

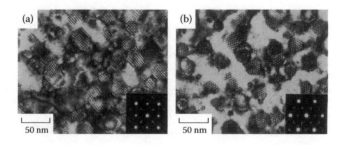

FIGURE 9.30
Bright-field images of a Ti–48.2 at.% Ni thin film heated at 773 K for 36 ks. Electron beams are parallel to (a) (100) and (b) (111), respectively. (From Miyazaki, S., Ishida, A., *Mater. Sci. Eng.*, 273–275, 106–133, 1999, with permission from Elsevier.)

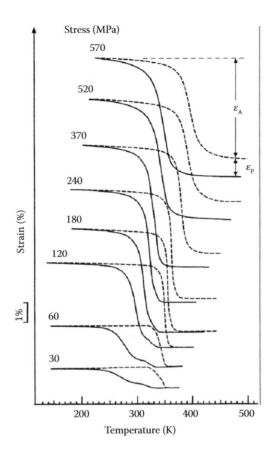

FIGURE 9.31
Strain–temperature curves under constant stresses for a Ti–48.2 at.% Ni thin film which was heated at 745 K for 3.6 ks. (From Miyazaki, S., Ishida, A., *Mater. Sci. Eng.*, 273–275, 106–133, 1999, with permission from Elsevier.)

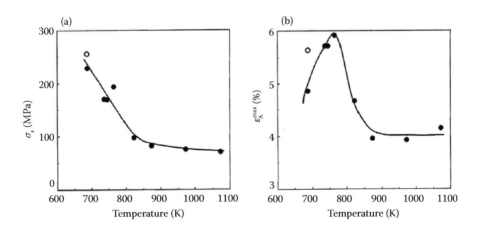

FIGURE 9.32
Variation in (a) critical stress for slip and (b) maximum recoverable strain as a function of heat-treatment temperature. (From Miyazaki, S., Ishida, A., *Mater. Sci. Eng.*, 273–275, 106–133, 1999, with permission from Elsevier.)

nonequilibrium plate precipitates is an important factor for the remarkable increase in σ_s below 820 K. The maximum value of σ_s, 260 MPa, was obtained in the specimen heat-treated at 687 K for 6.4 ks (open circle in Figure 9.32a).

The maximum recoverable strain ε_A^{max} for each heat treatment condition was obtained by the thermal cycling test and plotted as a function of T_h in Figure 9.32b. As shown in the figure, ε_A^{max} increases with decreasing T_h or increasing σ_s until T_h reaches down to 773 K. Below 773 K, however, ε_A^{max} decreases with further decreasing T_h. The ε_A^{max} decreases at 687 K, because the crystallization does not complete for this heat treatment. Heating at this temperature for 6.4 ks caused ε_A^{max} to increase as shown in Figure 9.32b because further precipitation of the plate precipitates and further crystallization occur.

TiNiX Ternary Alloy Thin Films

TiNiCu Films

Applications of microactuators require high frequency and fast response (narrow transformation temperature range and hysteresis). One of the challenges for the successful application of TiNi films is effective reduction of hysteresis and increase in operating frequency. The binary TiNi alloy films have a large temperature hysteresis of about 30°C, and TiNi films with small hysteresis are preferred for faster actuation. Addition of Cu in TiNi films is effective in reducing the hysteresis (Du and Fu, 2004). Compared with TiNi binary alloy, TiNiCu alloys also show less composition sensitivity in transformation temperatures, lower martensitic yield stress, and superior fatigue property, and so on, which make them more suitable for microactuator application (Chang and Grummon, 1997).

Figure 9.33 shows DSC curves measured in the TiNiCu thin films (Miyazaki and Ishida, 1999). The solid lines indicate the transformation upon cooling, whereas the dashed lines indicate the reverse transformation upon heating. The Ti–48.7 at.% Ni binary and the Ti–42.6Ni–5.0Cu (at.%) ternary alloys show single peak associated with the transformation from B2 (parent phase) to M (monoclinic martensite) upon cooling and associated with the reverse transformation from M to B2 upon heating, respectively. The sharpness of these peaks indicates that the distribution of alloy composition is uniform. The DSC curve of Ti–37.0Ni–9.5Cu (at.%) film shows two peaks. The first peak is very sharp and high, but the second one is very diffuse and almost invisible. However, when the ordinate of the curve is magnified, the second peak becomes visible. Based on the x-ray diffraction results, it is confirmed that the former transformation is associated with the transformation from B2 to O (orthorhombic martensite) upon cooling and the reverse transformation from O to B2 upon heating. The lattice parameters of these three phases (B2, O, M) are shown in Table 9.3. The Ti–26.6Ni–18.0Cu (at.%) shows only single-stage transformation which is associated with the transformation from B2 to O upon cooling and the corresponding reverse transformation from O to B2 upon heating, respectively. The transformation temperature from O to M is supposed to decrease significantly with an addition of Cu, so that it becomes unmeasurable.

Figure 9.34 shows the transformation temperatures of as a function of Cu content, M^* and O^* being the transformation peak temperatures of the B2 to M (or O to M) and B2 to O, respectively, while MA^* and OA^* the transformation peak temperatures of the corresponding reverse transformations, respectively. These temperatures are as high as those of bulk specimens, implying that the thin films contain few impurities. The M^* decreases slightly with increasing Cu content until 9.5 at.%. The 9.5 at.% Cu alloy shows a two-stage transformation, the first transformation temperature O^* being 314 K and the second one M^* being 270 K. By adding Cu furthermore, M^* decreases drastically, whereas O^* increases slightly.

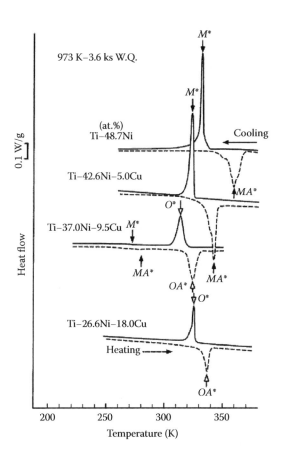

FIGURE 9.33
DSC curves showing transformation behavior in TiNiCu alloy thin films. (From Miyazaki, S., Ishida, A., *Mater. Sci. Eng.*, 273–275, 106–133, 1999, with permission from Elsevier.)

The transformation hysteresis, $(MA^*–M^*)$ or $(OA^*–O^*)$, shows a strong dependence on Cu content, as shown in Figure 9.34. A stronger Cu dependence of the hysteresis is observed in the single-stage transformation region than in the two-stage transformation region. The hysteresis decreases from 27 to 11 K with increasing Cu content from 0 to 9.5 at.%, and this property is comparable to that of bulk specimens.

Figure 9.35 shows the strain versus temperature ($\varepsilon–T$) curves for Ti–Ni–Cu alloy thin films measured during cooling and heating under a variety of constant stresses. The $\varepsilon–T$ curves measured under the same stresses (60, 120, 180 MPa) in each specimen are shown

TABLE 9.3

Lattice Parameters of Ti–37.0Ni–9.5Cu (at.%)

	a (nm)	b (nm)	c (nm)	α (°)	β (°)	γ (°)
B2	0.3032	0.3032	0.3032	90.00	90.00	90.00
Orthorhombic	0.2875	0.4198	0.4508	90.00	90.00	90.00
Monoclinic	0.3031	0.4254	0.4828	90.00	96.96	90.00

Source: Miyazaki, S., Ishida, A., *Mater. Sci. Eng. A*, 273–275, 106–133, 1999, with permission from Elsevier.

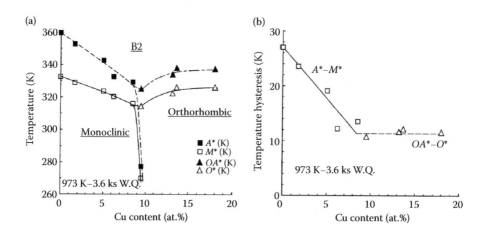

FIGURE 9.34

(a) Cu-content dependence of transformation temperatures (M^*, O^*, A^*, OA^*) in TiNiCu thin films. (b) Effect of Cu content on transformation temperature hysteresis in TiNiCu alloy thin films. (From Miyazaki, S., Ishida, A., *Mater. Sci. Eng.*, 273–275, 106–133, 1999, with permission from Elsevier.)

to clarify the effect of the Cu content on the deformation behavior. The 0 at.% Cu (binary) alloy thin film shows a single-stage shape change associated with the transformation from B2 to M upon cooling. The deformation starts at M_s and finishes at M_f; the strain induced here is estimated as ε_M, which generally consists of recoverable transformation strain and unrecoverable plastic strain. The elongated specimen contracts toward its original shape because of the reverse martensitic transformation upon heating; the recovery strain is estimated as ε_A. The unrecoverable strain ε_P is the permanent strain due to slip deformation which occurs during the transformation. Both the transformation strains ε_M and ε_A increase with increasing stress until the stress reaches a critical value under which the most preferential martensite variant will occupy the most part of the specimen.

The 5.0 at.% Cu specimen also shows a single-stage deformation associated with the transformation from B2 to M, similar to the 0 at.% Cu specimen. The strain and the shape of the ε–T curve are similar to those of the 0 at.% Cu specimen except the temperature hysteresis. This indicates that the addition of Cu is effective in reducing the hysteresis even though the structural change in the transformation is the same as that of the binary alloy. By adding further Cu, a two-stage deformation is observed for 9.5 at.% Cu. The first shape change is associated with the B2–O transformation, whereas the second shape change is associated with the O–M transformation. The first shape change occurs in a narrow temperature region, whereas the second in a broad temperature region. The temperature hysteresis of the first stage transformation is smaller than that of the 5 at.% Cu specimen. The ε–T curve of the 18.0 at.% Cu shows only a single-stage deformation again, although it is associated with the transformation B2–O. The strain induced by the transformation is very small.

The maximum of the recovery strain ε_A^{max} is shown as a function of Cu content in Figure 9.36a. Open squares show the ε_A^{max} associated with the B2–M transformation in the specimens with 0, 1.7, and 5.0 at.% Cu or the B2–O–M transformation in the 9.5 at.% Cu specimen. Closed triangles show the ε_A^{max} associated with the B2–O transformation in the Cu-rich specimens. The ε_A^{max} is almost constant regardless of Cu content if the Cu content is less than 9.5 at.%, whereas it decreases from 3.9% to 1.1% with increasing Cu content from

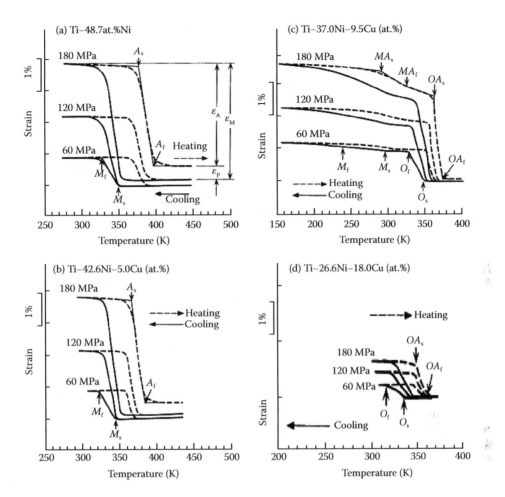

FIGURE 9.35
Strain versus temperature curves measured during cooling and heating under a variety of constant stresses in TiNiCu thin films. (From Miyazaki, S., Ishida, A., *Mater. Sci. Eng.*, 273–275, 106–133, 1999, with permission from Elsevier.)

9.5 at.% to 18.0 at.% in the Cu-rich region where the transformation only occurs from B2 to O. This Cu dependence of the ε_A^{max} in the thin films is similar to that in bulk specimens. However, the ε_A^{max} is a little smaller than that of the bulk specimens in the Cu-poor region. This is supposed to come from the grain size effect; that is, the grain size of thin films is smaller than that of bulk specimens.

The permanent strain ε_P due to slip deformation appears when the specimen is subjected to thermal cycling under a constant stress which is higher than the critical stress for slip. The critical stress for slip σ_s can be estimated by extrapolating the data of σ_P to zero strain in a diagram showing the σ_p versus constant applied stress relationship. Values of σ_s estimated in this way are shown in Figure 9.36b. It is found that σ_s increases with increasing Cu content. For example, σ_s of the 0 at.% Cu specimen is only 55 MPa and that of the 18 at.% Cu specimen increases to 350 MPa, showing that the addition of Cu is also effective to increase the stress for slip.

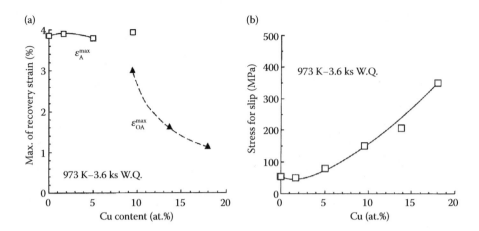

FIGURE 9.36

(a) Cu-content dependence of maximum recovery strain in TiNiCu thin films. (Miyazaki and Ishida, 1999, with permission from Elsevier.) (b) Cu-content dependence of the critical stress for slip in TiNiCu thin films. (From Miyazaki, S., Ishida, A., *Mater. Sci. Eng.*, 273–275, 106–133, 1999, with permission from Elsevier.)

Two factors are considered to be the causes for the effect of the addition of Cu on the critical stress for slip, that is, (1) solid-solution hardening due to the third element and (2) small transformation strain. Therefore, the addition of Cu is quite effective not only to decrease the temperature hysteresis but also to stabilize the SME.

TiNiPd Films

The working principle of TiNi microactuators renders them very sensitive to environment. The maximum transformation temperature of binary TiNi thin films is usually less than 100°C. However, a lot of MEMS applications require higher temperatures. For examples, in automobile applications, the transformation temperature required is up to 150°C, and in high-temperature gas chromatography the operation temperature is up to 180°C, and so on. Ternary system is a solution. By adding a varying amount of a third element, such as Pd, Hf, Zr, Pt, Au, and so on, into the binary alloys, one can easily adjust the transformation temperatures from 100°C to 600°C. TiNiPd and TiNiH$_f$ films are also effective in decreasing the temperature hysteresis, thus promising for quick movement at higher temperatures (Sawaguchi et al., 2002). The potential problem is that all these high temperature ternary thin films are high cost with poor SME and thermal stability as well as brittleness (Grummon, 2003). A small amount of Pd or Pt addition (less than 10 at.%) could reduce martensitic transformation temperatures rather than increase them (Fu and Du, 2003). Slight increase in Ni content in film can dramatically decrease the phase transformation temperatures. However, H$_f$ increases transformation hysteresis, whereas Pd is effective in decreasing the transformation hysteresis apart from increasing transformation temperatures. Because of this reason, Pd addition is more promising for applications. Figure 9.37a shows the effect of Pd content on the transformation temperatures (M_s, O_s, R_s) in the TiNiPd thin films which were annealed at 973 K for 3.6 ks, Ti content being kept between 50.0 and 51.0 at.%. M_s decreases slightly with increasing Pd content until about 6 at.%, then increases up to 390 K, which is 54 K higher than that of the binary TiNi film, with further increasing Pd content until 22 at.%. On the other hand, it is also found that the transformation temperature hysteresis is strongly affected by Pd content, that is, it decreases with

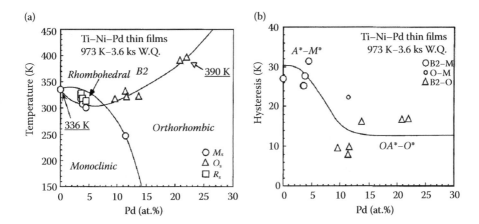

FIGURE 9.37
(a) Pd-content dependence of transformation temperatures in TiNiPd thin films; (b) Effect of Pd-content on transformation hystereses in TiNiPd thin films. (From Miyazaki, S., Ishida, A., *Mater. Sci. Eng.*, 273–275, 106–133, 1999, with permission from Elsevier.)

increasing Pd content down to about 10 K as shown in Figure 9.37b. This is an unexpected phenomenon, but both effects of Pd addition are useful for quick response in actuation.

Figure 9.38 shows the strain versus temperature relationships of a Ti–26.4Ni–21.8Pd (at.%) thin film. Upon thermal cycling, the shape changes occur in a higher temperature region than the binary TiNi and ternary TiNiCu alloys. TiNiPd thin films with different Pd contents were investigated. The transformation temperatures during shape change decrease with increasing Pd content until reaching 7 at.% Pd, then start to increase and become higher than those of the TiNi binary alloy when the Pd content is more than 17 at.%. The Ti–26.4Ni–21.8Pd (at.%) alloy thin film has not only higher transformation temperatures but also has a higher resistance against slip because an almost perfect shape recovery exhibits even under a stress of 200 MPa. The maximum recoverable strain is about 2.5%, and it is the smallest among TiNiCu, TiNiPd ternary and TiNi binary alloy films. The small transformation strain is also another reason for high critical stress for slip in addition to a

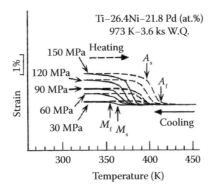

FIGURE 9.38
Strain versus temperature curves measured during cooling and heating under a variety of constant stresses in a TiNiPd thin films. (From Miyazaki, S., Ishida, A., *Mater. Sci. Eng.*, 273–275, 106–133, 1999, with permission from Elsevier.)

TABLE 9.4

Transformation and Shape Memory Characteristics of Ti–Ni, Ti–Ni–Cu, and Ti–Ni–Pd Alloy Thin Films

	Ti–Ni (M-Phase)	Ti–Ni–Cu (O-Phase)	Ti–Ni–Pd (O-Phase)
$M^*(O^*)$ (K)	332	313	385
$A^*(OA^*)$ (K)	359	324	401
Hys (K)	27	11	16
ε_A^{max} (%)	3.8	3.0	2.5
σ_S (MPa)	90	173	200

Source: Miyazaki, S., Ishida, A., *Mater. Sci. Eng. A*, 273–275, 106–133, 1999, with permission from Elsevier.

solid-solution hardening effect by the third element of Pd. The summary of the transformation and shape memory characteristics of these three alloy thin films is shown in Table 9.4. $M^*(O^*)$ and $A^*(OA^*)$ are abbreviations of the transformation peak temperatures for the martensitic (orthorhombic) and reverse-martensitic (reverse-orthorhombic) transformations, respectively, were measured by DSC. *Hys* is an abbreviation of the temperature hysteresis, that is, the temperature difference between $M^*(O^*)$ and $A^*(OA^*)$. ε_A^{max} and σ_s stand for the maximum recoverable transformation strain and the critical stress for slip, respectively.

Film Stress and Stress Evolution

Film stress and stress evolution in the films could pose potential problems in applications, as it may influence not only adhesion between film and substrate, but also deformation of MEMS structure, mechanics, and thermodynamics of transformation and SE effects, and so on (Craciunescu et al., 2003). Large residual stress could lead to either film cracking or decohesion under tension, or film delamination and buckling under compression. Deposition conditions, post-deposition thermomechanical treatment, and composition of the TiNi films could have important consequences with respect to the development of residual stress. These have been studied in detail and reported in Fu et al. (2003). In the crystalline TiNi films, large tensile stress is generated during heating due to the phase transformation from martensite to austenite, whereas during cooling, the martensitic transformation occurs and the tensile stress drops significantly because of the formation and alignment of twins. The stress generation and relaxation behaviors upon phase transformation are significantly affected by film composition, deposition, and/or annealing temperatures, which strongly control the formation and evolution of intrinsic stress, thermal stress, and phase transformation behaviors (Fu and Du, 2003).

Using the curvature method, stress change as a function of temperature can be measured in situ with change in temperature. The martensitic transformation temperatures and hysteresis, multistage transformation, and magnitude of shape recovery can be easily obtained from the stress–temperature curves (Fu and Du, 2002, 2003; Fu et al., 2003). Figure 9.39a shows a typical curve of the measured stress of a $Ti_{50}Ni_{46}Cu_4$ film as a function of temperature up to 100°C. The stress-versus-temperature plot shows a closed hysteresis loop shape. At room temperature, the stress is tensile with a low value. During heating, the tensile stress increases significantly because of the phase transformation from martensite to austenite. Above austenite transition start temperature (A_s), the stress increases linearly until the temperature reaches to austenite transition finish temperature (A_f). With

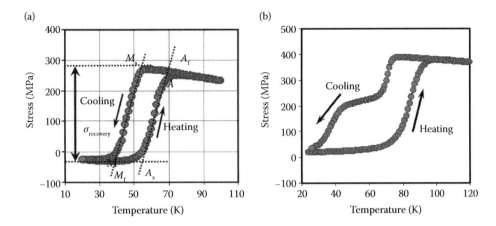

FIGURE 9.39
(a) Stress vs. temperature curve for a TiNiCu4 film showing the sequence of martensitic transformation; (b) stress vs. temperature curve for a $Ti_{50}Ni_{50}$ film showing sequence of martensitic transformation.

the further increase of temperature, the transformation completes and thermal stress generates, with the stress values decreasing linearly because of the difference in coefficient of thermal expansion (CTE) between the TiNiCu film ($\alpha_{TiNiCu} = 15.4 \times 10^{-6}/°C$) and Si substrate ($\alpha_{Si} = 3 \times 10^{-6}/°C$). The theoretical slope of stress versus temperature due to pure thermal effect can be calculated using the following equation

$$d\sigma/dT = (E_{TiNiCu}/(1 - \upsilon_{TiNiCu}))(\alpha_S - \alpha_{TiNiCu}) \tag{9.10}$$

in which E_{TiNiCu} is the Young's modulus of TiNiCu film (about 78 GPa according to nano-indentation results); υ_{TiNiCu} is the Poisson ratio of TiNiCu film (about 0.33). The calculated data of $d\sigma/dT$ is about 1.44 MPa/°C, which matches well with the experimental data of 1.38 MPa/°C. During cooling, tensile thermal stress develops in the TiNiCu films at a rate of 1.38 MPa/°C. When the temperature is just above martensitic transition start temperature (M_s), the residual stress reaches its maximum value. Cooling below M_s, the martensitic transformation occurs and the tensile stress decreases significantly because of the formation and alignment of twins (shear-induced phase transformation) (Duerig and Wayman, 1990).

A typical stress evolution versus temperature curve of a $Ti_{50}Ni_{50}$ film on Si is shown in Figure 9.39b. It shows a one-stage transformation corresponding to martensite (B19′) to austenite (B2) transformation during heating, and a two-stage transformation during cooling corresponding to transformations among martensite, R-phase, and austenite phases.

The stress evolution of an amorphous TiNiCu film during annealing up to 650°C is shown in Figure 9.40a (Fu et al., 2005). In the beginning, below 150°C (from a to b), a net compressive stress increases linearly, indicating that thermal stress is at play: compressive stress results because the film expands more than 4 times that of the substrate (CTE) of TiNiCu film, α_f, is about $15.4 \times 10^{-6}/K$ and that of Si substrate, α_{Si}, is $3 \times 10^{-6}/K$. However, above 120°C (i.e., after b), the tensile component prevails such that the net stress becomes less compressive as a result of densification with increasing temperature. Further heating to about 435°C (point c), crystallization of TiNiCu film occurs and densification ends. After c, heating-generated stress (compressive) prevails, resulting in an almost linear increase in net stress. From d to e, cooling-induced thermal stress (now tensile) increases linearly with

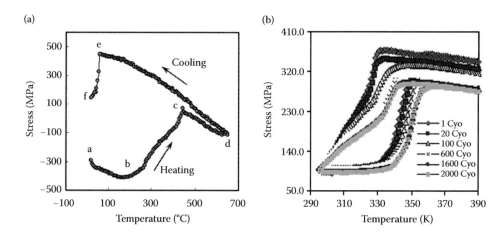

FIGURE 9.40
(a) Stress evolution of TiNiCu film annealed up to 650°C using curvature measurement method. (b) Hysteresis evolution of Ti52.5Ni film on Si substrate after thermal cycling in different cycles and become stable after 2000 cycles.

decreasing temperature. At e, martensitic transformation starts (M_s). With further decrease in temperature, significant decrease in stress occurs (from e to f). Figure 9.40a clearly shows that an appropriate annealing temperature is needed to promote the film crystallization, thus the phase transformation can occur above room temperature and the large thermal stress generated during cooling can be released significantly (Miyazaki and Ishida, 1999). Fu et al. (2004) studied the fatigue of the constrained TiNi films using the curvature method by investigating the changes in recovery stress during thermal cycling. Results show that the recovery stress of the TiNi films from curvature measurement decreases dramatically in the first tens of cycles and becomes stable after thousands of cycles (with one example shown in Figure 9.40b). This reduction of the recovery stress is believed to result from the dislocation movement, grain boundary sliding, void formation, or partial debonding at the film/substrate interfaces, nonrecoverable plastic deformation, changes in stress, and so on. Transformation temperatures also change dramatically during cycling. The repeated phase changes will alter the microstructure and hysteresis of the transformation and in turn lead to changes in transformation temperatures, recovery stresses, and strains.

The stress evolution could have significant effect on the film surface morphology evolution. Significant surface relief (or surface upheaval), caused by the martensitic transformation, is commonly observed in TiNi bulk materials and has recently also been reported in the sputtered TiNi thin films (He et al., 2004). During the martensitic transformation, the atomic displacement introduces stacking faults that lead to surface relief morphology on the film surface. A flat surface in austenite transforms to twinned martensite upon cooling and becomes rough, without a macroscopic shape change, and vice versa. Fu et al. (2006) reported a phenomenon of film surface morphology evolution between wrinkling and surface relief during heating/cooling in a sputtered TiNiCu thin film (see Figure 9.41). In situ optical microscopy observation upon heating revealed that the interweaving martensite plate structure disappeared. However, many radial surface wrinkles formed within the original martensitic structure. Further heating up to 300°C did not lead to much change in these wrinkling patterns. On subsequent cooling to room temperature, the twinned martensite plates or bands reformed in exactly the same wrinkling patterns as those before thermal cycling. After post annealing, a partially crystallized TiNiCu films at 650°C,

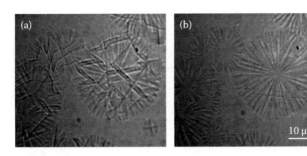

FIGURE 9.41
Surface morphology evolution with temperature for TiNiCu film (a) surface relief morphology, (b) surface wrinkles at 100°C. (From Fu et al., *J. Micromech. Microeng.*, 18, 035026, 2008, with permission to use from American Scientific Publisher, USA.)

optical microscopy (at room temperature) revealed an interconnected network structure of trenches on the film surface (see Figure 9.42) (Wu et al., 2006). In situ observation using optical microscopy, interferometry, and AFM during heating/cooling showed that these trenches gradually disappear upon heating, and the film surface becomes smooth and featureless. On subsequent cooling the trenches reappeared, with almost the identical surface morphology as present before heating, and the surface became slightly opaque and cloudy.

The formation of the shape memory trenches and wrinkling are due to the significant stress changes upon thermal cycling. It is well known that a TiO_2 and oxygen diffusion layer of tens of nanometers thick can easily form on the surface of the TiNi-based thin films, and this surface oxide layer could act as a rigid elastic layer on top of ductile martensite. During cooling, the difference between the thermal expansion coefficient of the oxide layer and TiNiCu thin film causes the oxide layer in compression, and theoretical calculation also verifies this conclusion. During cooling, the austenite transforms into martensite, along with the significant release of tensile stress. The relaxation of the in-plane compressive stress in the oxide layer on the martensite layer causes the out-of-plane wrinkling phenomenon by minimizing the total elastic energy in the film and the substrate.

Substrate effect is also significant in the stress generation and evolution because the difference in thermal expansion coefficients between substrate and TiNi films significantly affects the thermal stress. The film intrinsic stress is also critically dependent on the mismatch between film and substrate. So far, most studies have been focused on Si-based substrates for MEMS applications. TiNi deposited on other substrates (with different CTE) could result in different stress state (compress or tensile) and stress–temperature evolution behaviors, thus detailed studies of substrate effect on stress state, SME, phase transformation, and mechanical properties of TiNi films deserve more systematic effort (Winzek et al., 1999).

To minimize the residual stress in TiNi films, it is necessary to: (1) precisely control the Ti/Ni ratio; (2) deposit films at a possible lower pressure; (3) select a suitable deposition temperature or annealing temperature, with a compromise between thermal stress and intrinsic stress; (4) use interlayers (with possible compressive stress) to reduce large tensile stress in TiNi films; (5) perform post-annealing, ion beam post-modification, or in situ ion beam modification during sputtering to reduce intrinsic stress; (6) select suitable substrate to reduce thermal stress.

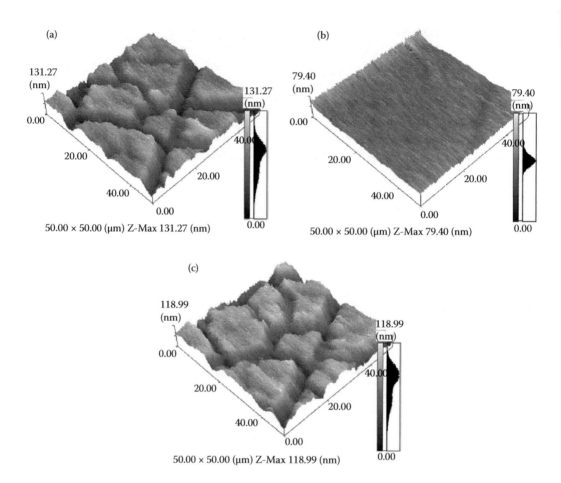

FIGURE 9.42
Reversible surface trench morphology upon thermal cycling. (From Wu et al., 2005, with permission to use from American Institute of Physics, USA.)

Frequency Response

Applications of microactuators require not only large recovery stress and large transformation deformation, but also high frequency and fast response (narrow transformation hysteresis). One of the challenges for the successful application of TiNi films is effective reduction of hysteresis to increase operating frequency. External heat is necessary for generating phase transformation and actuation, and the response speed of TiNi microactuators is mainly limited by their cooling capacities. The binary TiNi alloy films have a large temperature hysteresis of about 30°C. TiNi films with smaller hysteresis are preferred for faster actuation. The hysteresis could be slightly reduced by decreasing the cyclic temperature amplitude and/or increasing working stress. R-phase transformation usually has a much smaller temperature hysteresis, which is useful for MEMS applications (Tomozawa, 2006). However, the problem in R-phase transformation is that the strain and stress (or force) generated are too small to be of many practical uses. Addition of Cu in TiNi films is effective in reducing the hysteresis. Compared with TiNi binary alloy, TiNiCu alloys also show less composition sensitivity in transformation temperatures, lower martensitic yield stress, and superior fatigue property, and so on, which make them more suitable for micro-actuator application. However, the transformation temperatures of TiNiCu films decrease slightly, and the transformation becomes weaker with the increase in Cu contents, in terms of recovery stress, maximum recovery strain and heat generation, and so on. Also, the film becomes brittle when Cu content is more than 10 at.%.

Generally speaking, the constrained films have smaller hysteresis as compared with freestanding films, and the films with larger compressive stress could have much smaller (even almost zero) hysteresis compared with films with large tensile stress. Therefore, selection of a suitable substrate (with larger thermal expansion coefficient than TiNi film) could help generate large compressive stress, thus a smaller hysteresis. An alternative is to use an external heat sink. TiNi-based films can be deposited on a suitable substrate with good thermal conductivity, such as Cu plate, thus significantly improving thermal dissipation and working frequency. However, this brings in more critical issues, such as integration and compatibility with MEMS batch process, residual stress, and adhesion.

Adhesion and Interfacial Analysis

When TiNi films are deposited on Si substrate, there exist interfacial diffusion and chemical interactions at the interface, whereby titanium and nickel silicides may form during high-temperature deposition or post-deposition annealing. These interfacial reaction products could be complex, heterogeneous, and metastable (Stemmer et al., 1997; Wu et al., 2001). Because the thickness of TiNi film required in MEMS applications is usually less than a few microns, a relatively thin reaction layer could have significant adverse effect on adhesion and shape memory properties. TiNi film adheres well to silicon substrate provided it is clean and prechemically etched. TiNi films deposited on a glass substrate can be easily peeled off, which is quite useful to obtain freestanding films. In MEMS processes, there is a need for an electrically and thermally insulating or sacrificial layer. Thermally grown SiO_2 is often used as this sacrificial layer. However, the adhesion of TiNi films on SiO_2 layer (or on glass and polymer substrate) is poor owing to the formation of a thin intermixing layer and a fragile and brittle TiO_2 layer (Fu et al., 2003). Upon a significant deformation or during a complex interaction involving scratch, this layer is easy to be broken, thus peels off. Wolf et al. (1995) proposed a two-step deposition method to solve this problem: predeposition of 0.1 μm TiNi film on SiO_2 at 700°C to promote interdiffusion of elements, followed by bulk film deposition at room temperature. Fu et al. (2004) reported that the addition of Si_3N_4 interlayer between film and Si substrate did not cause much change in phase transformation behavior as well as adhesion properties. There is significant interdiffusion of elements and formation of Ti–N bond at the Si_3N_4/TiNi interlayer. If compared with poor adhesion of TiNi films on SiO_2 interlayer, Si_3N_4 interlayer seems to be a good choice for an electrically insulating and diffusion barrier layer in respect of adhesion properties. Adhesion of TiNi films on polysilicon and amorphous silicon layers is also quite good.

Stability, Degradation, and Fatigue

Stability and fatigue have always been concerns in development of TiNi thin films for applications. Fatigue of TiNi films is referred to as the nondurability and deterioration of the SME after many cycles. The repeated phase changes will alter the microstructure and hysteresis of the transformation and in turn will lead to changes in transformation temperatures, transformation stresses, and strains. The performance degradation and fatigue of thin films are influenced by a complex combination of internal (alloy composition, lattice structure, precipitation, defects, film/substrate interface) and external parameters (thermomechanical treatment, applied maximum stress, stress and strain rate, the amplitude of temperature cycling frequency) after long-term thermomechanical cycles.

Figure 9.43 shows the strain versus temperature curves as a function of the number of cyclic deformation associated with the R-phase transformation under 50 MPa in a Ti–43.9 at.% Ni solution-treated thin film. In the cooling process of the initial cycle ($N = 1$), the R-phase transformation starts at 333 K and finishes at 316 K, resulting in a shape change of 0.13% strain. In the heating process, the reverse R-phase transformation starts at 323 K and finishes at 336 K, resulting in a perfect shape recovery and small temperature hysteresis (H_R) of 4 K. Because of the small hysteresis, a quick response is expected in microactuators using such R-phase transformation. After cycling for 100 times, no significant change appears in the shape of the curves. The reason for the stability can be explained by the fact that the R-phase transformation strain is so small that slip deformation hardly occurs.

Figure 9.44 shows the effect of thermally induced cyclic deformation on the strain–temperature curve under a stress of 250 MPa in a solution-treated Ti–43.9 at.% Ni thin film. The curves of the cyclic deformation show a two-stage deformation; upon cooling, a shape change appears at R_s due to the R-phase transformation, and upon further cooling, a second shape change occurs at M_s because of the martensitic transformation as shown in the initial cyclic deformation curve. The strains ε_R and ε_M are 0.28% and 1.12%, respectively. Upon heating, the original shape of the specimen is almost recovered due to a two-stage deformation associated with the reverse-transformations occurring at A_s for the first stage and at RA_s for the second stage. The first stage is associated with the reverse martensitic transformation from the martensitic phase to the R-phase, whereas the second with the

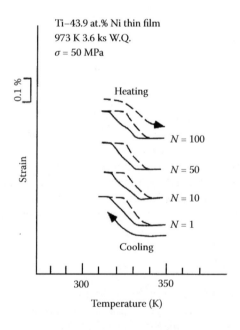

FIGURE 9.43
Effect of thermal cyclic deformation on strain vs. temperature curves associated with R-phase transformation for a solution-treated TiNi thin film; N indicates number of cycle. (From Miyazaki, S., Ishida, A., *Mater. Sci. Eng.*, 273–275, 106–133, 1999, with permission from Elsevier.)

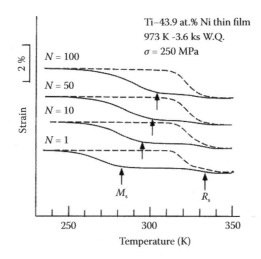

FIGURE 9.44
Effect of thermal cyclic deformation on strain vs. temperature curves associated with martensitic transformation for a solution-treated TiNi thin film; *N* indicates number of cycle; ks after solution-treatment at 973 K for 3.6 ks. (From Miyazaki, S., Ishida, A., *Mater. Sci. Eng.*, 273–275, 106–133, 1999, with permission from Elsevier.)

reverse R-phase transformation from the R-phase to the parent phase. Although there is an unrecoverable strain which is caused by slip deformation, it is only 0.03%.

With increasing the number of cycles, the R-phase transformation characteristics such as R_s, ε_R, and H_R are kept almost constant, whereas the martensitic transformation characteristics change apparently. For example, M_s rises and hence the temperature difference between R_s and M_s decreases. Besides, temperature hysteresis (H_M) decreases and martensitic transformation strain increases gradually. Such changes in the martensitic transformation can be considered to be caused by the internal stress field which is formed by the introduction of dislocations during cyclic deformation. The internal stress field overlaps with the external applied stress so that the martensitic transformation temperatures increase. However, the R-phase transformation characteristics show few changes during cyclic deformation because the R-phase transformation involving a small strain is not so sensitive to applied stress.

Fu et al. (2002) studied the fatigue of the constrained TiNi films using the changes of recovery stress during cycling and showed that the recovery stress of TiNi films from curvature measurement decreased dramatically in the first tens of cycles and became stable after thousands of cycles. This reduction of the recovery stress is believed to be resulted from the dislocation movement, grain boundary sliding, void formation, or partial debonding at the film/substrate interfaces, nonrecoverable plastic deformation, changes in stress, and so on. Transformation temperatures also changed dramatically during cycling. The repeated phase changes will alter the microstructure and hysteresis of the transformation and in turn lead to changes in transformation temperatures, stresses, and strains. All these changes in the martensitic transformation behavior become insensitive to thermal cycling after the number of cycles exceeds 50, indicating that training is effective in stabilizing the shape memory behavior. Such a steady state has been achieved by the work hardening during cyclic deformation. Therefore, it is concluded that the stabilization of the shape memory characteristics against thermal cycles under stress can be improved by training.

Film Thickness Effect

Effects of film thickness on crystallization and SME have been investigated by several groups recently (Ishida and Sato, 2003; Wan and Komvopoulos, 2005; Wang et al., 2008). TiNi films usually undergo a high temperature (between 400°C and 650°C) during deposition or post-annealing. At such a temperature, the surface oxidation and interfacial diffusion between the film and substrate could significantly affect the phase transformation behavior if the film is too thin. It is important to know how thin the TiNi based film can go or how small the TiNi structure can be without losing the SME. In the study of Fu et al. (2006), the stress–temperature evolution in the TiNi films with different thickness was measured using the curvature method (see Figure 9.45). The stress–temperature response of a 50-nm film is linear, that is, this film experiences only thermal effect (due to the difference in thermal expansion between film and substrate) with no apparent phase transformation. Thicker films (up to 4 μm thick) produce stress/temperature hysteresis loops upon thermal cycling, demonstrating the SME. With the increase in film thickness, the residual stress decreases sharply and then remains at low value, whereas the recovery stress increases significantly, and reaches a maximum at a film thickness of 820 nm before it gradually decreases with a further increase in film thickness.

Results revealed that a minimum thickness (about 100 nm) is necessary to guarantee an apparent SME in the TiNi films. Surface oxide and oxygen diffusion layer as well as interfacial diffusion layer are dominant in the films with a thickness of tens of nanometers. The combined constraining effects from both surface oxide and interfacial diffusion layers in a very thin film will be detrimental to the phase transformation. As the film thickness increases to above a few hundred nanometers, the effects of the surface oxide, oxygen diffusion layer, and interdiffusion layer become relatively insignificant. Therefore, phase transformation becomes significant and the recovery stress increases as thickness

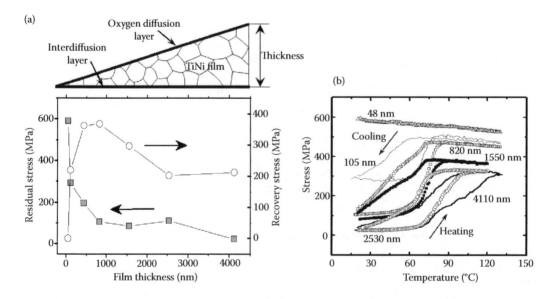

FIGURE 9.45

(a) Residual stress and recovery stress for films with different thickness; (b) stress–temperature evolution curves for TiNi films with different thickness. (From Fu et al., *Mater. Sci. Forum*, 437, 37–40, 2004; *Sens. Actuators A Phys.*, 112, 395–408, 2004, with permission to use from Elsevier Publisher, UK.)

increases. Because of the significant phase transformation effect, thermal and intrinsic stresses in the films are drastically relieved, resulting in a significant decrease in residual stress. With the further increase in film thickness, more and more grain boundaries form in the films. The grain boundaries are the weak points for generation of large distortion and twinning processes. Therefore, as the film thickness increases, the constraining effect from the neighboring grains becomes more and more significant, causing decreases in recovery stress.

Temperature Memory Effect

A new phenomenon, temperature memory effect (TME), has also been reported in the TiNi-based films (Wang et al., 2005). An incomplete thermal cycle upon heating in a SMA (arrested at a temperature between austenite transformation start and finish temperatures, A_s and A_f) induced a kinetic stop in the next complete thermal cycle (Zeng et al., 2004), and the kinetic stop temperature is a "memory" of the previous arrested temperature (see Figure 9.46) (Wang and Zu, 2005). If a number N of incomplete heating processes with different arrested temperatures are performed in a decreasing order, N temperatures can be memorized. TME can be fully eliminated by following a complete transformation heat cycle to above A_f. During the partial reverse transformation, only part of the martensite transforms into the parent phase, with the rest of the martensite, M1, remaining. With a further decrease in the temperature to below martensitic transformation finish temperature, the parent phase transforms back to martensite, and the newly formed martensite is called M2. M1 and M2 are different martensite variants with different elastic energies, which cause different transformation temperatures of M1 and M2 during the next heating process. On the contrary, if a partial austenite to martensite transformation is performed by an incomplete cycle on cooling, the next complete austenite to martensite transformation does not show any evidence of kinetic interruptions. TME can be found in both thermally and external stress–induced transformations.

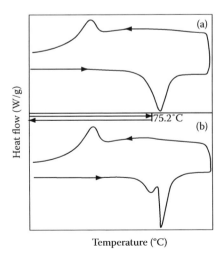

FIGURE 9.46
DSC results of (a) TiNiCu4 film and (b) temperature memory effect of same sample with a single incomplete cycle on heating at 75.2°C. (Fu, 2009, with permission from Interscience Publisher.)

Nanoscale Mechanical Evaluation

Nanoindentation test is a promising method for characterization of nanoscale psudoelasticity (PE) (Ma and Komvopoulos, 2003). The psudoelasticity behavior in TiNi-based thin films demonstrates their intrinsic capacity to undergo large deformations without permanent surface damage, or known as self-healing behavior. Nanoindentation testing with or without changes in temperature could reveal the different elastic and plastic deformation behaviors of austenite and martensite, thus is promising for characterization of SME and thermomechanical properties of the constrained thin films (Shaw et al., 2003; Cole et al., 2008). During loading and unloading in nanoindentation, there is a large force hysteresis, that is, large energy dissipation during loading/unloading in the TiNi-based thin films. During the reverse phase transformation, the martensite variants must overcome the internal stress generated during phase change to reverse back to the parent austenite matrix. Therefore, energy is dissipated as friction heat due to the existence of defects in austenite matrix and the martensite. The energy dissipation associated with the pseudoelastic behavior contributes to the high vibration damping capacity of the TiNi films.

Using a sharp tip, it is difficult to obtain pseudoelastic behavior because the plastic deformation due to dislocation movement is more dominant than the phase transformation (Zhang et al., 2005). Therefore, spherical-shape tips have been widely used recently to characterize the nanorange SE behavior of TiNi and thin films (Wood et al., 2008). Indentation using a spherical indenter could avoid large plastic deformation if the indentation force is not too high. During nanoindentation on SMA thin films using a spherical indenter, Yan et al. (2006) found that there exist two characteristic points, the bifurcating point and the returning point in one indentation loading/unloading curve, which are associated with the forward transformation stress and the reverse transformation stress. They proposed a method to determine the transformation stresses of SMA films-based on the measured bifurcating and returning forces.

The SME of those materials at the indented area has been quantitatively studied by AFM (Zhang et al., 2006a, 2006b; Cinchetti et al., 2005). The two-way shape recovery nature in indents and indent arrays on SMAs and their thin films explored an alternative approach for high-density data storage (Figure 9.47) and controllable reversible surface protrusions (Shaw et al., 2005).

Nanometer scale indentations in TiNi thin films (for example) less than 100 nm in depth can be fully recovered upon further heating because of thermally induced reverse martensitic transformation. Using a spherical indentation method, surface protrusions can be made on the surfaces, which will disappear upon heating. Reversible circular surface protrusions can be produced due to two-way SME (Zhang et al., 2006a). SMAs with shape relief ability can find more optical and mechanical applications in their greater load bearing capacity and/or better durability than normally used polymers. For example, information storage technology has undergone a revolution in past years, and magnetic storage is reaching fundamental limits of about 100 Gbit/in^2 (or 6500 nm^2 bit^{-1}) (Chikazume, 1997). This is because with the shrinkage of the size of magnetic domains, the fluctuation in temperature could easily cause the random changing of the moments of the magnetic domains, thus the loss of the stored data. Recently, the nanoindentation method has been proposed to be used for high-density mechanical storage applications (Shaw et al., 2005). The storage devices with capacity 1 Tbit/in^2 are achievable. The write–read or erase–rewrite operations can be performed with a nanoindenter or atomic force microscope. Information is written into the martensite TiNi thin film by nanoindentation with probe tips. The indents are then scanned, and the nanoindentation tip is heated for SME, thus erasing the data recorded.

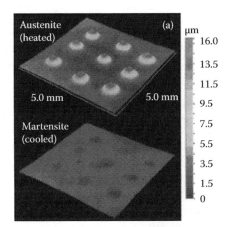
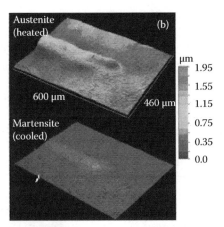
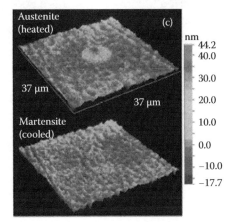

FIGURE 9.47
Three-dimensional profiles of reversible surface protrusions. (a) A 3 × 3 matrix of circular protrusions on surface of austenite phase of TiNi at high temperature which disappears when sample is cooled to martensite phase. (b) A protruding line on surface of austenite phase that nearly disappears in martensite phase. (c) A nanoscale reversible protrusion on surface a TiNi film. (From Zhang et al., *Acta Mater.*, 54, 1185–1198, 2006; Shaw et al., *Appl. Phys. Lett.*, 83, 257–259, 2003; *Adv. Mater.*, 17, 1123–1127, 2005, Reproduced with permission from Elsevier, AIP and Wiley-VCH GmbH & Co.)

Subsequent rewriting can be again performed by the indentation. For this application, the use of sharper probes than the relatively blunt or spherical diamond indenter could increase storage density. There are some drawbacks in this mechanical storage method: slow speed, strong dependence on film planarity (and roughness), and tip wear.

Functionally Graded and Composite-Based Films

To further improve the properties of TiNi films, multilayer, composite, or functionally graded TiNi-based films can be designed. So far, there are different design models for the functionally graded TiNi thin films. The first type is through the gradual change in composition (Ti/Ni ratio), crystalline structures, transformation temperatures, and/or residual stress through film thickness (Takabayashi et al., 1996). As the Ti or Ni content changes in the micron-thick film, the material properties could change from pseudo-elastic (similar to rubber) to shape memory. The seamless integration of pseudo-elastic with shape memory characteristics produces a two-way reversible actuation, because variations in the residual stress in thickness direction will enable biasing force to be built inside the thin films. These functionally graded TiNi films can be easily prepared by slightly changing the target powers during deposition. Another novel way is to vary the target temperature during sputtering, and the films produced by hot targets have compositions similar to that of the target, whereas films produced from cold target are Ti deficient. To successfully develop functionally graded TiNi thin films for MEMS application, it is necessary to characterize, model, and control the variations in composition, thermomechanical properties, and residual stress in these films.

The second type of functionally graded films involves new materials and functions other than TiNi films. Recently there are some reports (Fu et al., 2003) on the deposition of a functionally graded TiN/TiNi layer to fulfill this purpose. The presence of an adherent and hard TiN layer (300 nm) on TiNi film (3.5 µm) forms a good passivation layer (to eliminate the potential Ni release), and improves the overall hardness, load bearing capacity, and tribological properties without sacrificing the SME of the TiNi films. Also TiN layer is able to restore elastic strain energy during heating and to provide a driving force for martensitic transformation on subsequent cooling, forming a two-way SMA effect. To improve biocompatibility and adhesion of TiNi films, a functionally graded Ti/TiNi/Ti/Si graded layer could be used. A thin cover layer of Ti can improve biocompatibility (prevent potential Ni allergic reactions), whereas the Ti interlayer can be used to improve film adhesion. Using cosputtering with multitargets, or controlling the gases during sputtering, these graded film designs can be easily realized.

Some surface modification methods, such as irradiation of TiNi films by electrons, ions (Ar, N, He, Ni, or O ions), laser beams, or neutrals can be used (1) to modify the surface physical, mechanical, metallurgical, wear, corrosion, and biological properties for application in hostile and wear environment; and (2) to cause lattice damage and/or alter the phase transformation behaviors along thickness of film, forming novel two-way shape memory actuation (Goldberg et al., 1999, Grummon and Gotthardt 2000, Lagrange and Gotthard 2003). The problems of these surface treatments are high cost, possible ion induced surface damage, amorphous phase formation, or degradation of SMEs. Surface oxidation in TiNi bulk materials has often been reported to prevent the Ni ion releasing and improve the biocompatibility (Firstov et al., 2002; Tan and Crone, 2002). It is possible to have the same process for TiNi films with slight sacrificing in the SME.

Other functionally graded or composite designs include the combination of TiNi films with piezoelectric, ferromagnetic, or magnetostrictive thin films (Craciunescu and Wuttig, 2003; Zhu et al., 2006). Response time of the piezoelectricity mechanisms (PZT films) is fast, but the displacement is relatively small. TiNi film, on the other hand, has a larger force and displacement, but with slower response frequency. By coupling TiNi and PZT films to fabricate a new hybrid heterostructure composite or functionally graded film, it is possible to tune or tailor the static and dynamic properties of TiNi thin films, which may generate a larger displacement than conventional piezoelectric or magnetostrictive thin films and have an improved dynamic response compared with that of single layer TiNi films. Both PZT and TiNi films can be prepared by sputtering methods, or PZT film by sol–gel method and TiNi film by sputtering. Either TiNi or PZT films can be the bottom layer. However, the complexity of the fabrication processing, the interfacial diffusion and adhesion, and dynamic coupling of dissimilar components remain tough issues for these types of composite thin films.

Modeling

Numerical modeling and computational simulation of the behaviors of TiNi films and their microactuators, together with experimental characterization efforts, will lead to the optimization of technical factors, such as structural configuration, geometry, and processing procedures and further improvement in the overall performance of TiNi thin film-based microactuators (Auricchio et al., 1997). There are two levels of simulations. The first level is the simulation and modeling of thermomechanical behaviors of TiNi films, and the second is the design of geometry and structures as well as performance of TiNi microactuators. There are many models describing the constitutive behaviors based on thermodynamics and continuum mechanics (Bhattacharyya et al., 2000), but only a few have been used in engineering practice. It is difficult to obtain an accurate constitutive relationship for a particular TiNi film. The intrinsic hysteresis, nonlinearity, and history-dependent behaviors make it more difficult to accurately predict the response of a TiNi thin film microactuator. At present, only phenomenological models appear to be realistic for engineers (Ishida et al., 2007), and the transformation can be assumed as either a linear or a sine/cosine function (Huang, 1999; Gao and Huang, 2002; Huang and Zhu, 2002). As compared with bulk TiNi materials, there are several special issues in simulation of TiNi films: (1) smaller grain size in TiNi films and constraint effect on substrates; (2) large film biaxial stress after deposition and stress evolution during phase transformation process; and (3) possible textured structure in the thin films. Gabry et al. (2000), Lexcellent et al. (1998), and Bhattacharya and James (1999) reported different thermodynamic simulations for TiNi thin films. Jin and Weng (2000) developed a relaxed self-consistent model to simulate the thermomechanical behavior of TiNi films, and it is confirmed that thermally induced phase transformation has a narrower range of transformation temperatures in the films, and the work hardening characteristics are lower than the bulk material because of geometrical relaxation. For TiNi thin film–based microdevices, the nonuniform stress and temperature distribution could affect the precision of deformation and lead to inaccurate position control.

Biocompatibility of Thin Films

When the TiNi-based films are applied in biomedical fields, they must be capable of fulfilling functional requirements relating not only to mechanical reliability but also to chemical reliability (in vivo degradation, decomposition and dissolution and corrosion) and biological reliability (toxicity, antigenicity, etc.). Although TiNi has been recognized as a good material for biological applications, it is still not clear if release of small amounts of nickel and copper could cause allergy and inflammation of human organs (Es-Souni and Brandies, 2001).

Nickel is among the metals considered toxic and therefore not acceptable for medical implants. However, nitinol, the atoms of which are half nickel, has been demonstrated to be noncytotoxic along with stainless steel and titanium and is accepted by the medical community as biocompatible for intravascular uses. TiNi thin film, with a much larger exposed surface than bulk nitinol, might be more prone to toxicity, but experiments have demonstrated that thin film is also biocompatible. The presence of TiO_2 oxide layer on the TiNi film is beneficial to its corrosion resistance and biocompatibility. The sputtered TiNi thin films are easily contaminated with carbon and oxygen in air. With exposure to atmosphere, carbon and oxygen increase drastically at the surface, and at the same time diffuse deep into the film. The increase is very fast at the beginning but slows down with time after long-time exposure. This is beneficial for the compatibility of the TiNi films.

Biological and MEMS Applications of TiNi Thin Films

Comparison of Microactuation Mechanisms

Many types of materials and methods have been proposed for fabricating microactuators. Their actuation capacity can be characterized by the work per unit volume and cycling frequency. These characteristics are summarized in Table 9.5 (Miyazaki and Ishida, 1999). Figure 9.48 shows the work per volume as a function of cycling frequency for various actuators: that is, (1) TiNi SMA, (2) solid–liquid phase change (SL), (3) thermopneumatic (TP), (4) thermal expansion (TE), (5) electromagnetic (EM), (6) electrostatic (ES), (7) piezoelectric (PE), (8) muscle (M), and (9) microbubble (MB), which are also shown in Table 9.4. Among these actuators, only the first three can generate large forces over long displacements.

The work output per unit volume W can be defined as $W = Fu/v$, where F, u, and v are force, displacement, and volume, respectively. If an actuator material is deformed in the course of performing the work, the work output per unit volume equals the elastic strain energy, that is, $W = \sigma\varepsilon/2$, where σ and ε are stress and strain, respectively. However, for SMA, $W = \sigma\varepsilon$, which generate a constant force over the actuation. According to Figure 9.48, SMA films can generate the greatest work per volume up to a reasonably high cycling frequency.

Freestanding Microactuators Based on Two-Way Shape Memory Effect

Freestanding films usually show intrinsic "two-way" SME, with large displacement, but relatively small force in actuation. This is applicable in microsensors, microswitches, or micropositioners. The origin of the two-way SME observed in the TiNiCu films can be attributed to the difference in sputtering yields of titanium and nickel, which produces a compositional gradient through the film thickness (Gyobu et al., 2001; Gill et al., 2002). The film layer near the substrate is normally nickel rich, and no SME is observed, but the material may possess SE. As the Ti/Ni content changes through the film thickness, the material properties change from being superelastic to having a shape memory. A stress gradient is generated because of the changing microstructure and composition as a function of thickness, thus causing freestanding structures to bend upward. When heated, the film layer returns to a flat position because of the SME. Figure 9.49 shows some examples of simple structures which can be actuated by heating/cooling through the two-way SME (Fu et al., 2008).

TiNi alloys with Ni-rich content can show a two-way SME if aged under elastic constraint (Nishida and Honma, 1984). Because this effect enables a TiNi thin film to deform spontaneously upon thermal cycling without any bias force, it is ideal for miniaturizing and simplifying actuators. Because the two-way SME is related to the precipitation process and distribution of fine Ti_3Ni_4 plate precipitates in the matrix, this effect is sensitive to aging treatment conditions, such as temperature and time.

Ti–51.3 at.% Ni alloy thin films with a thickness of 8.5 μm were made on glass substrates by sputter deposition. They were peeled off from the glass substrates mechanically. Samples of 20 mm length and 1 mm width were cut out of the thin films. They were first solution-treated at 973 K for 3.6 ks followed by aging treatment at various temperatures between 573 and 773 K for three different times, that is, 3.6, 36, and 360 ks, under elastic constraint and without constraint, respectively. These heat treatments form a single parent phase of TiNi with a surplus of Ni atoms (solution treatment) and fine Ti_3Ni_4 precipitates

TABLE 9.5

Work per Unit Volume for Various Microactuators

Actuator Type	W/v (J m⁻³)	Equation	Comments
1. Ni–Ti SMA (SMA)	2.5×10^7	$\sigma \cdot \varepsilon$	Maximum one time output: $\sigma = 500$ MPa, $\varepsilon = 5\%$
	6.0×10^6	$\sigma \cdot \varepsilon$	Thousands of cycles: $\sigma = 300$ MPa, $\varepsilon = 2\%$
2. Solid–liquid phase change (SL)	4.7×10^6	$\dfrac{1}{3}\left(\dfrac{\Delta v}{v}\right)^2 k$	k = bulk modulus = 2.2 GPa (H_2O) 8% volume change (acetamide)
3. Thermo-pneumatic (TP)	1.2×10^6	$\dfrac{F \cdot \delta}{v}$	Measured values: $F = 20$N, $\delta = 50$ μm, $v = 4$mm $\times$ 4mm $\times$ 50 μm³
4. Thermal expansion (TE)	4.6×10^5	$\dfrac{1}{2}\dfrac{(E_s + E_f)}{2}(\Delta\alpha \cdot \Delta T)^2$	Ideal, nickel on silicon, s = substrate, f = film, $\Delta T = 200$ K
5. Electro-magnetic (EM)	4.0×10^5	$\dfrac{F \cdot \delta}{v} \quad F = \dfrac{-M_s^2 A}{2\mu}$	Ideal, variable reluctance: v = total gap volume, $M_s = 1$ V s m⁻²
	2.8×10^4	$\dfrac{F \cdot \delta'}{v}$	Measured values, variable reluctance: $F = 0.28$ mN, $\delta = 250$ μm, $v = 100 \times 100 \times 250$ μm³
	1.6×10^3	$\dfrac{T}{v}$	Measured values, external field: Torque = 0.185 nN m⁻¹, $v = 400 \times 40 \times 7$ μm³
6. Electrostatic (ES)	1.8×10^5	$\dfrac{F \cdot \delta}{A \cdot \text{gap}} \quad F = \dfrac{\varepsilon V^2 A}{2\delta^2}$	Ideal: $V = 100$ volts, δ = gap = 0.5 μm
	3.4×10^3	$\dfrac{F \cdot \delta}{v}$	Measured values, comb drive: $F = 0.2$ mN (60 volts), $v = 2 \times 2 \times 3000$ μm³ (total gap) $\delta = 2$ μm
	7.0×10^2	$\dfrac{F \cdot \delta}{v}$	Measured values, integrated force array: v = device volume, 120 V
7. Piezoelectric (PE)	1.2×10^5	$\dfrac{1}{2}(d_{33}E)^2 E_f$	Calculated, PZT: $E_f = 60$ GPa (bulk), $d_{33} = 500$ (bulk), $E = 40$ kv cm⁻¹
	1.8×10^2	$\dfrac{1}{2}(d_{33}E)^2 E_f$	Calculated, ZnO: $E_f = 160$ GPa (bulk), $d_{33} = 12$ (bulk), $E = 40$ kv cm⁻¹
8. Muscle (M)	1.8×10^4	$\dfrac{1}{2}(\sigma \cdot \varepsilon)$	Measured values: $\sigma = 350$ kPa, $\varepsilon = 10\%$
9. Microbubble (MB)	3.4×10^2	$\dfrac{F \cdot \delta}{v_b}$	Measured values: bubble diameter = 71 μm, $F = 0.9$ μN, $\delta = 71$ μm

Sources: Krulevitch et al., *J. MEMS*, 5, 270–282, 1996; Miyazaki, S., Ishida, A., *Mater. Sci. Eng. A*, 273–275, 106–133, 1999, with permission from Elsevier.

in the TiNi parent phase in the following age treatment. The constraint during the aging treatment produced preferentially oriented precipitates which have an intrinsic stress field around them, causing the two-way SME to appear. The constraint was given by winding the thin films on to a stainless steel pipe with an outer diameter of 7.5 mm. The two-way SME was evaluated by measuring the curvature radii of the thin film in both boiling and iced water.

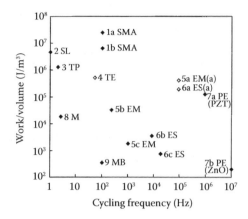

FIGURE 9.48
Work per volume versus cycling frequency for various microactuators. Ideal values (2) represent energy available for actuation. Other values (") are based on actual microactuator data. (From Miyazaki, S., Ishida, A., *Mater. Sci. Eng.*, 273–275, 106–133, 1999, with permission from Elsevier.)

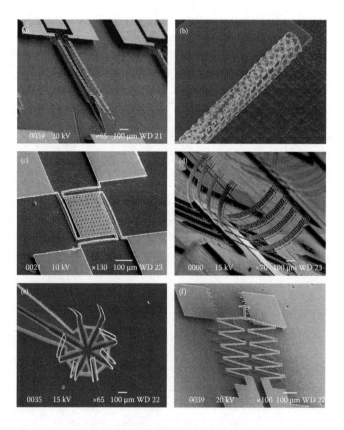

FIGURE 9.49
Free standing TiNi-based film structures: (a) a microtweezer structure which has both horizontal and vertical movement due to both shape memory and thermal effects; (b) microstent which can be opened by heating; (c) a micromirror structure which can be actuated by four arms when electrically heated; (d) microfinger which can operate both horizontally and laterally, and can be designed and integrated into a walking robotics; (e) microcage structure with fingers opening/closing by two-way effect; (f) microspring structures.

All the aging-treated thin films exhibited two-stage transformation behavior both upon cooling and heating, that is, the R-phase transformation in a higher temperature region and the martensitic transformation in a lower temperature region. The major part of the two-way SME was associated with the R-phase transformation. The two-way shape memory behavior is sensitive to aging conditions. For example, the film aged at 573 K for 3.6 ks and the film aged at 723 K for 3.6 ks bend in the same direction as the constrained direction in boiling water. However, in iced water, they show different behavior; the film aged at 573 K bends forward, but the film aged at 723 K bends backward and shows an opposite curvature. As described earlier, Ti_3Ni_4 plate precipitates are formed in the TiNi matrix during age-treatment. These precipitates form in a disk shape on {111} planes of the TiNi matrix and reduce the volume by 2.3% along ⟨111⟩ directions. When a film is aged under constraint, the precipitates form on one of the {111} planes selectively, relaxing the constraint stress by the volume change. If the film is aged at a low temperature for a short time, the precipitation of Ti_3Ni_4 is not sufficient for relaxing the constraint stress. In this case, when the constraint is removed, the film tends to go back to the original shape before the constraint-aging. However, even after the removal of the constraint, internal stress seems to remain locally between relaxed and unrelaxed regions in this film. This internal stress may determine a specific R-phase variant upon the transformation, so that the film shape approaches the constrained shape. However, if the constraint stress is fully relaxed after aging at a high temperature for a long time, such internal stress becomes small. Instead, the coherent strain around the precipitates becomes large. This stress field determines the specific R-phase variant so that the film shape returns to the original shape. This effect has been also found in bulk specimens by Nishida et al. (1984). They called it "all round shape memory effect" because this effect is so prominent that the film curvature reverses. However, "two-way shape memory effect" is more appropriate to reflect the nature of the phenomenon.

TiNi Diaphragms, Micropump, and Microvalves

MEMS-based micropumps and microvalves are attractive for many applications such as implantable drug delivery, chemical analysis, and analytical instruments, and so on. TiNi thin films are suitable for building microvalves and pumps (Shih et al., 2006). Control of fluid flow is essential to operation of all pneumatic and hydraulic systems from implantable insulin pumps to heating, ventilating, and air conditioning systems. The trend to miniaturization is driven by the needs for portability and improved performance. Miniaturization of fluidics systems requires miniaturization of all the components including microvalves and pumps. Microvalves are potentially useful in microfluidics, pumps, thermal switches, and a wide range of other applications. The main purpose of microvalves is to open and allow fluid to flow or close and prevent fluid to flow. Both shape memory microvalves (i.e., active valves) and superelastic microvalves (i.e., passive check valves) have been fabricated. The microvalve manufactured by the TiNi Alloy Company (Figure 9.50; Johnson, 2009) was the first miniature SMA-actuated pneumatic control device to be offered commercially. It consists of an actuator die with a poppet controlled by the 8 TiNi thin film strips, 3.5 μm thick and 250 μm wide, a silicon orifice die, a spacer, and a bias spring. All elements are assembled in a plastic package. The bias spring forces the poppet toward the orifice. Resistive heating of the SMA thin films supporting the poppet causes it to transform from the martensite phase to the parent phase. By this transformation, TiNi strips recover the original length, lifting the poppet against the bias force and opening the valve. This device has a poppet displacement of ~100 μm and bias force of 0.5 N. It is operated with an electric

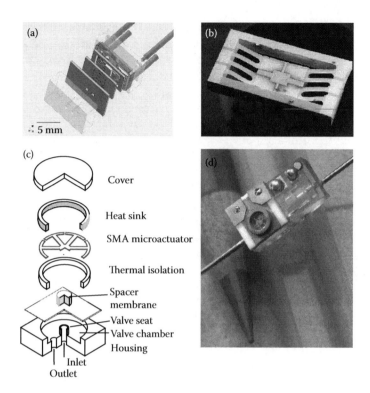

FIGURE 9.50
(a, b, d) Pictures of a TiNi pump; (c) schematic diagram of the pump's cross section. (Johnson, A.D., in Miyazaki et al., eds., *Thin Film Shape Memory Alloys: Fundamentals and Device Applications,* Cambridge University Press, UK, 2009, with permission to use from Cambridge University Press.)

current of 50–100 mA. The response time when operating in air is about 20 ms, and maximum flow is up to 2000 standard cm^3/min at 1.3 atm (Johnson, 2009).

There are different designs for TiNi film-based micropumps or microvalves, and most of them use TiNi membrane (or diaphragm, microbubble, etc.) for actuation with one example shown in Figure 9.51 (Reynaerts, 1997; Benard et al., 1998). Both freestanding TiNi films and constrained TiNi films are used. Although freestanding TiNi film has intrinsic two-way SME, to maximize this effect, extra process, such as 3-D hot-shaping of TiNi film (membrane) and externally biased structure (such as a polyimide layer, or a bonded Si cap or glass cap) are often applied. All of these extra processes could result in complicated structure and difficulty in MEMS processing (Kohl et al., 1999; Makino et al., 2001). Another concern is the effective thermal isolation between the heated TiNi films and the fluid being pumped. TiNi/Si bimorph membrane-based micropumps and valves are more commonly reported. The advantages of using TiNi/Si membrane as the driving diaphragm include (Xu et al., 2001): (1) large actuation force; (2) simplicity in process and no special bias structure needed because the silicon substrate can provide bias force; and (3) no isolating structure is needed because silicon structure can separate the working liquid from SMA film completely.

Two types of diaphragm-type microactuators were fabricated by Miyazaki et al. (2009), that is, a multilayer diaphragm comprising a SMA film and a SiO_2 layer and a single layer diaphragm comprising a SMA film as shown in Figure 9.52. The multilayer diaphragm microactuators were operated by the martensitic transformation induced in the Ti–Ni,

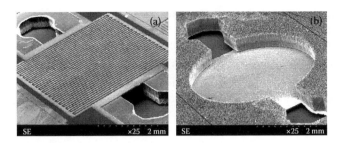

FIGURE 9.51
TiNi microvalve fabricated with TiNi electrode on silicon membrane structure (a) top view of membrane and TiNi electrode; (b) bottom view.

Ti–Ni–Cu, and Ti–Ni–Pd films, whereas the single layer diaphragm microactuators were operated by the R-phase transformation induced in the Ti–Ni films. Figure 9.52 illustrates the cross sections of the microactuator at room temperature and high temperature, respectively (Miyazaki et al., 2009). Because the diaphragm consists of two layers with different thermal expansion coefficients, an internal stress is generated in the diaphragm after heat treatment, that is, compression in the SiO_2 layer and tension in the SMA film layer. At room temperature, the Ti–Ni film layer is of martensite and can be easily deformed. The crystal lattice of the martensite (low temperature phase) is an orthorhombic structure, whereas that of the parent phase (high temperature phase) is a B2 structure (Miyazaki, 1990). Therefore, the diaphragm becomes convex as shown in Figure 9.52a to relax the internal stress. By heating to a temperature above the reverse transformation temperature of the SMA film layer, the diaphragm reverts to the initially memorized flat shape due to the SME. By cooling to a temperature below the martensitic transformation temperature, the diaphragm shape becomes convex again (Miyazaki et al., 2009).

As shown in Figure 9.52, the microactuator operates because of temperature variation. Therefore, the temperature dependence of the height at the center of the diaphragm is measured to investigate actuation process (Miyazaki et al., 2009). The height at the center of the diaphragm is abbreviated to h. The parameter h is measured at each fixed temperature during cooling and heating in a step-by-step way to characterize a quasi-static actuation. Dynamic actuation is investigated by using a three-dimensional shape analyzer equipped with a laser scanner. The microactuator is dynamically operated by thermal

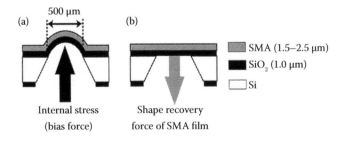

FIGURE 9.52
Schematic figures showing the cross section of a microactuator utilizing a SMA thin film deposited on a SiO_2/Si substrate at room temperature and a high temperature. (From Miyazaki, S., in Miyazaki et al., eds., *Thin Film Shape Memory Alloys: Fundamentals and Device Applications*, Cambridge University Press, UK, 2009, reproduced with permission from Cambridge University Press.)

cycling. The thermal cycling was conducted by applying a pulse current to the Ti–Ni film layer in the microactuator, that is, by means of joule heating and natural cooling. Height h was continuously measured during dynamic actuation. The displacement was estimated by measuring the difference between the maximum and minimum values of h, and it was used as one of the measures of dynamic actuation characteristics. The temperature of the microactuator was measured by a thermocouple microwelded to a part of the SMA film attached to the SiO_2/Si substrate. The working frequency and temperature of the microactuator were adjusted by changing the frequency and amplitude of the pulse current, respectively. The ratio of heating time to cooling time, that is, a duty ratio, was fixed at 5:95 for each working frequency. The measurement was conducted at an ambient atmosphere (23 to 25°C).

As for the second type of microactuator with a single layer diaphragm, Ti–Ni films were deposited on Si substrates by r.f. magnetron sputtering. The thicknesses of the Ti–Ni films were 2.0 μm. The Ti–Ni films on the substrates were heat-treated at 873 and 823 K for 0.6 ks, respectively, to memorize the initial flat shape. Diaphragm-type microactuators were fabricated again by using the conventional Si micromachining technique. Figure 9.53 illustrates the cross sections of a microactuator at low and high temperatures (Miyazaki et al., 2009). The shape of the diaphragm is square with a width of 500 μm. N_2 gas pressure of 40 kPa is used as a bias force for the microactuator. The microactuator is convex at room temperature because the Ti–Ni film is deformed by the N_2 gas pressure in a low-temperature phase such as M-phase or R-phase.

To investigate the displacement and the transformation temperatures of the microactuator, the height at the center of the diaphragm is measured as a function of temperature during heating and cooling at each fixed temperature in a step-by-step way. Figure 9.54 reveals the temperature dependence of the height at the center of the diaphragm. Upon cooling, the height starts to increase at $M_s(R_s)$ due to the start of the M-phase (R-phase) transformation and the increase in height at $M_f(R_f)$ because the M-phase (R-phase) transformation finishes. Upon heating, the height decreases with increasing temperature between $A_s(RA_s)$ and $A_f(RA_f)$ because of the progress of the reverse M-phase (R-phase) transformation. Displacement is defined as the difference between the maximum height and the minimum height ($h_{max}^s - h_{min}^s$), where the superscript "s" stands for "static" because each height is measured at fixed temperature. ΔH_M and ΔH_R represent the transforma-

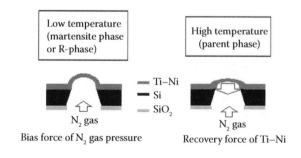

FIGURE 9.53
Schematic figures showing cross section of a microactuator consisting of a SMA thin film deposited on a Si substrate at room temperature and a high temperature. (From Miyazaki, S., in Miyazaki et al., eds., *Thin Film Shape Memory Alloys: Fundamentals and Device Applications*, Cambridge University Press, UK, 2009, reproduced with permission from Cambridge University Press.)

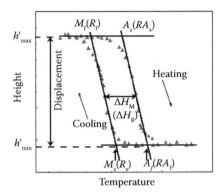

FIGURE 9.54

A schematic figure showing temperature dependence of height at the center of diaphragm. (From Miyazaki, S., in Miyazaki et al., eds., *Thin Film Shape Memory Alloys: Fundamentals and Device Applications*, Cambridge University Press, UK, 2009, reproduced with permission from Cambridge University Press.)

tion temperature hysteresis associated with the M-phase and R-phase transformations, respectively.

Microdiaphragm Using R-Phase of Ti–Ni

Figure 9.55 shows the change in height at the center of the diaphragm during heating and cooling in the microactuator using the M-phase transformation of the Ti–48.2Ni thin film or in that using the R-phase transformation of the Ti–47.3Ni under a N_2 gas pressure of 40 kPa (Tomozawa, 2005). The microactuator using R-phase transformation of the Ti–47.3Ni thin film is abbreviated to "Ti–Ni R-phase microactuator." The microactuator using the M-phase transformation of the Ti–48.2Ni thin film is abbreviated to "Ti–Ni M-phase microactuator." Open squares and circles, respectively, denote the results of the

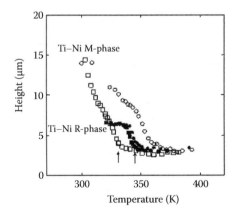

FIGURE 9.55

Temperature dependence of height at the center of diaphragm in Ti–Ni M-phase microactuator and TiNi R-phase microactuator under N_2 gas pressure of 40 kPa. (From Miyazaki, S., in Miyazaki et al., eds., *Thin Film Shape Memory Alloys: Fundamentals and Device Applications*, Cambridge University Press, UK, 2009, reproduced with permission from Cambridge University Press.)

cooling and heating processes in the Ti–Ni M-phase microactuator, whereas closed squares and circles, respectively, denote the cooling and heating processes in the Ti–Ni R-phase microactuator. Arrows indicate the M-phase and R-phase transformation start temperatures (M_s and R_s). The heights of the Ti–Ni M-phase and Ti–Ni R-phase microactuators reach almost the minimum values at the A_f temperature of 360 and 355 K, respectively. The minimum heights of these microactuators do not reach zero because of the elastic deformation of the parent phase by applied gas pressure. It can be seen that the displacement of the Ti–Ni R-phase microactuator is smaller than that of the Ti–Ni M-phase microactuator. However, the transformation temperature hysteresis of the Ti–Ni R-phase microactuator is only 3.2 K. This is significantly small when compared with the Ti–Ni M-phase microactuator (Miyazaki et al., 2009).

Microdiaphragm Using M-Phase of Ti–Ni–Pd

High transformation temperature is also effective in increasing actuation speed same as a narrow transformation hysteresis. Figure 9.56a shows the effect of Pd content on M_s in Ti–Ni–Pd thin films heat-treated at 973 K for 3.6 ks. As shown in Figure 9.56a, M_s decreases slightly with increasing Pd content up to 9 at.%. Then, M_s increases up to 560 K with further increasing Pd content to 36 at.% (Miyazaki et al., 2009).

Ti–48.2Ni and Ti–26.5Ni–22.7Pd SMA thin films were deposited on SiO_2/Si substrates by r.f. magnetron sputtering. The thicknesses of these thin films were 2.5 and 2.0 µm, respectively. The Ti–48.2Ni and Ti–26.5Ni–22.7Pd thin films on the substrates were heat-treated at 873 K for 0.6 ks to memorize the initial flat shape. Diaphragm-type microactuators were fabricated by using the Si micromachining technique.

Figure 9.56b shows the change in height at the center of the diaphragm during heating and cooling in the Ti–Ni M-phase microactuator and the Ti–Ni–Pd microactuator (Tomozawa, 2005). The height at the center of the diaphragm decreases with increasing temperature because the progress of the reverse transformation. The height reached almost

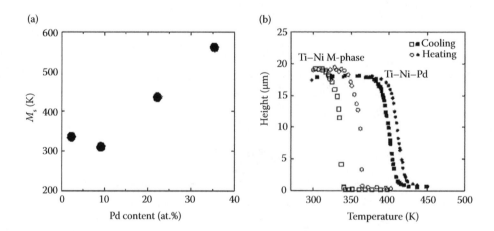

FIGURE 9.56
(a) Pd content dependence of M_s in Ti–Ni–Pd thin films heat-treated at 973 K for 3.6 ks; (b) temperature dependence of height at the center of diaphragm in TiNi M-phase microactuator and Ti–Ni–Pd microactuator deposited on SiO_2/Si substrates. (From Miyazaki, S., in Miyazaki et al., eds., *Thin Film Shape Memory Alloys: Fundamentals and Device Applications*, Cambridge University Press, UK, 2009, reproduced with permission from Cambridge University Press.)

zero at the A_f temperature of 370 K and 430 K for the Ti–Ni M-phase microactuator and the Ti–Ni–Pd microactuator, respectively. The Ti–Ni–Pd microactuator exhibits almost the same displacement as the Ti–Ni M-phase microactuator. M_s of the Ti–Ni–Pd microactuator is about 70 K higher than that of the Ti–Ni M-phase microactuator. Also, it is noted that the transformation temperature hysteresis of the Ti–Ni–Pd microactuator is smaller than that of the Ti–Ni M-phase microactuator (Miyazaki et al., 2009).

Microdiaphragm Using M-Phase of Ti–Ni–Cu

Figure 9.57a shows temperature dependence of h (height at the center of the diaphragm) during cooling and heating in the microactuator employing a Ti–38.0Ni–10.0Cu thin film that was heat-treated at 973 K for 0.6 ks (Miyazaki et al., 2009). Data obtained during the cooling and heating processes are denoted by open and closed circles, respectively. Upon cooling, h starts to increase at M_s and finishes at M_f, whereas h starts to decrease at A_s and finishes at A_f upon heating. The increase and decrease in h are due to the forward and reverse transformations, respectively, in the Ti–Ni–Cu layer of the microactuator. Therefore, the microactuator utilizing the Ti–Ni–Cu thin film is expected to exhibit a higher actuation speed than that utilizing the Ti–Ni binary thin film.

Figure 9.57b shows current amplitude dependence of the displacement at each working frequency (Miyazaki et al., 2009). As shown in the displacement–current curve for the working frequency of 10 Hz, the displacement increases with increasing current amplitude reaching a maximum, then becomes almost constant. When the current amplitude is small, the temperature of the Ti–Ni–Cu layer does not increase up to A_f, resulting in small displacement due to incomplete reverse transformation. By increasing the current amplitude, the temperature approaches A_f, leading to increase in displacement. The current amplitude necessary for generating a maximum displacement increases with increasing working frequency. This is because each heating time decreases with increasing working frequency under a fixed duty ratio condition.

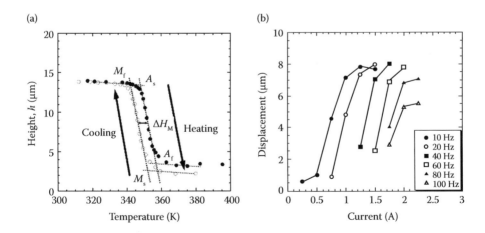

FIGURE 9.57
(a) Temperature dependence of height of a microactuator utilizing the Ti38.0Ni10.0Cu thin film that was heat-treated at 973 K for 0.6 ks; displacement as a function of current amplitude for each working frequency. (From Miyazaki, S., in Miyazaki et al., eds., *Thin Film Shape Memory Alloys: Fundamentals and Device Applications*, Cambridge University Press, UK, 2009, reproduced with permission from Cambridge University Press.)

The maximum displacement at each working frequency is plotted in Figure 9.58 (Miyazaki et al., 2009). For comparison, the result of the microactuator utilizing the Ti–Ni thin film is also included. The microactuator utilizing the Ti–Ni and Ti–Ni–Cu thin films are abbreviated to Ti–Ni microactuator and Ti–Ni–Cu microactuator, respectively. The displacement of the Ti–Ni microactuator is almost the same as that of the Ti–Ni–Cu microactuator at working frequency below 20 Hz. However, it decreases by increasing working frequency up to 50 Hz. The displacement of the Ti–Ni–Cu microactuator does not decrease until the working frequency reaches 60 Hz. Above 60 Hz of working frequency, it gradually decreases. However, the microactuator operates even at 100 Hz. As shown in Figure 9.58, the displacement of the Ti–Ni–Cu microactuator is even larger than that of the microactuator using the M-phase transformation within the working frequency range from 1 Hz to 100 Hz. Thus, a high-speed microactuator with large displacement was successfully fabricated by utilizing the Ti–Ni–Cu thin film.

The working frequency of the microactuators utilizing the Ti–Ni–Pd and Ti–Ni–Cu thin films reached 100 Hz and that of the microactuator using the R-phase transformation reached 125 Hz. Because the Ti–Ni–Pd and Ti–Ni–Cu show the shape memory behavior associated with the martensitic transformation, the displacements of the microactuators utilizing these two alloy films are almost equal to that of the Ti–Ni M-phase microactuator. However, the displacement of the Ti–Ni R-phase microactuator is one-third of that of the Ti–Ni M-phase microactuator. We can choose either of the microactuators depending on the requirements of response speed and magnitude of displacement.

Microgrippers

Wireless capsule endoscope (WCE) is a new diagnostic tool in searching for the cause of obscure gastrointestinal bleeding. A WCE contains video imaging, self-illumination, image transmission modules, and a battery (Iddan et al., 2000; Waye, 2003). The indwelling camera takes images and uses wireless radio transmission to send the images to a receiving recorder device that the patient wears around the waist. However, there are two drawbacks in the current WCE: (1) lack of ability for biopsy; and (2) difficulty in identifying

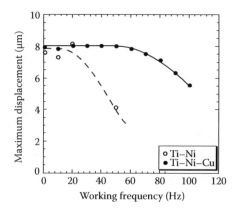

FIGURE 9.58

Comparison of maximum displacements expressed as a function of working frequency for two types of microactuators. (From Miyazaki, S., in Miyazaki et al., eds., *Thin Film Shape Memory Alloys: Fundamentals and Device Applications*, Cambridge University Press, UK, 2009, reproduced with permission from Cambridge University Press.)

the precise location of pathology. Without tissue diagnosis, it is often difficult to differentiate inflammatory lesions from tumor infiltration. The former may require only medical treatment, whereas the latter may need surgical solution. Therefore, there are two potential microactuator applications in capsule endoscopy: (1) microgripper for biopsy or tissue sampling (Sugawara et al., 2006); (2) microclipper or pin tagging device, to firmly attach to the tissue. SMA thin film-based microactuators are promising for these applications.

Grasping and manipulating small or micro-objects with high accuracy is required for a wide range of important applications, such as the assembly in microsystems, endoscopes for microsurgery, and drug injection micromanipulators for cells. There are some basic requirements for microgrippers, for example, large gripping force, sufficient opening distance for assembling works, and so on. TiNi films are promising in these applications. So far, two types of TiNi film-based microgripper designs are available.

The popular design is out-of-plane bending mode, mostly with two integrated TiNi/Si cantilever (or other substrate, such as SU-8 or polyimide, etc.) with opposite actuation directions (see Figure 9.59) (Seidemann et al., 2002; Lee et al., 1996). This SMA cantilever structure was heated to different temperatures (from room temperature to 423 K), results show that there is actually the SME and the tip displacement is quite large (up to 60 μm). This type of cantilever structure can be further fabricated as a microgripper, as shown in Figure 9.60, which can be actuated at relatively low temperatures with internal integrated heaters forming by polysilicon patterns. These grippers can be used as the end-manipulator for microassembly for industry, minimally invasive surgery for medical application, and handling of small particles in hazardous environment for military application.

Takeuchi and Shimoyama (2000) reported a novel microelectrode with TiNi clipping structure, which can be used for minimally invasive microelectrodes to clip a nerve cord or other living organisms. The TiNi film is actuated when a current is applied to the electrode. The clipping force of the electrode to the nerve is enhanced by a hook structure and two C-shaped probes as shown in Figure 9.61a and b. Another gripper design is in-plane mode, in which the deformation of two arms (using freestanding TiNi films or TiNi/Si beams) is within a plane realized by compliant structure design (Fu and Du, 2003). Wang et al. (2002) reported a microtweezer structure, in which residual stress in TiNi film is used as a bias force load. This can eliminate the need for providing bias force for device operation. However, the force from the deformation of the freestanding films is not large enough to grasp large objects. The other problem in this type of design is how to prevent

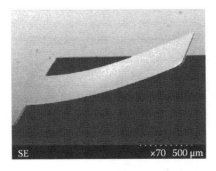

FIGURE 9.59
Cantilever structure with a thickness of 15 μm fabricated by conventional MEMS process. (From Fu et al., *Surf. Coat. Technol.*, 145, 107–112, 2001, with permission from Elsevier.)

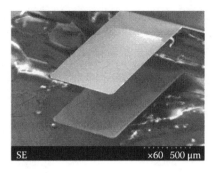

FIGURE 9.60
Bending of cantilever structure deposited with TiNi films during heating. (From Fu et al., *Surf. Coat. Technol.*, 145, 107–112, 2001, with permission from Elsevier.)

out-of-plane bending, beam deformation, and fracture during operation caused by intrinsic film stress.

Pulsation Sensor

Free tissue transfer operations have been improved as the result of advances in microsurgery technique. The microsurgery technique has also been applied to important organ graft operations such as liver transplantation. However, there is a serious problem of thrombus formation near an anastomotic site of a blood vessel. Tissue failure occurs in 5–10% after the free tissue transfer operations. The failures are caused by poor blood circulation due to thrombosis occurred mainly within the first 24 h after operation. Adequate and reliable monitoring techniques of thrombus formation are required (Machens et al., 1994). Micromechanism for attaching a miniaturized blood stream sensor to a blood vessel is required. After the use for blood stream monitoring, it is desirable to be detached from the blood vessel easily. Because of large deformation stroke and large generated force, SMA film actuator is suitable to use as a holding actuator. The function of two-step actuation of holding and releasing with integrated microheaters which can heat up the SMA locally has been designed as shown in Figure 9.62 (Sugawara et al., 2006). The detailed design of the pulsation sensor for monitoring of bloodstream obstruction caused by thrombus forma-

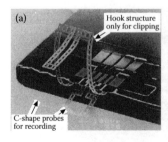
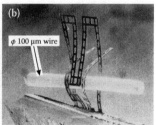

FIGURE 9.61
(a) A TiNi electrode with hook structure is returned to its memorized shape when it is heated, whereas two C-shape probes for recording are not heated; (b) microelectrode clipping a wire (100 μm) after hook structure is heated. (From Takeuchi, S., Shimoyama, I., *J. MEMS*, 9, 24–31, 2000, with permission from IEEE.)

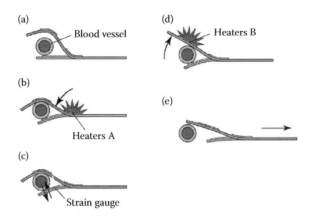

FIGURE 9.62
Concept of actuation: (a) setting; (b) hold actuation; (c) pulse monitoring; (d) release actuation; and (e) pull out. (From Mineta et al., *Sens. Actuators A Phys.*, 143, 14–19, 2008, with permission from Elsevier.)

tion is shown in Figure 9.63. The arms and a base part are made from a TiNiCu SMA film which is flash-evaporated on a flat substrate.

Two pairs of microheater circuit pattern of platinum film are formed on the root (heater A) and the halfway point (heater B) on the outer arm. Platinum strain gauge circuits are also formed on the cantilever in a same platinum film layer. Minimum line and space width of the strain gauge were 50 and 50 μm, respectively. The outer arm is bent at the root and the halfway point before setting. A blood vessel can be caught between the outer arm and inner cantilever, when heater A is turned on so that the outer arm deforms and closes. The strain gauges on the cantilever transduce the periodical diameter variation of the blood vessel by arterial pulsation into a voltage waveform. The measured waveform is displayed on a monitor through an external computer system. After use for pulsation monitoring,

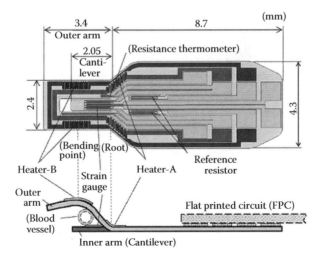

FIGURE 9.63
Structure of micropulsation sensor. (From Mineta et al., *Sens. Actuators A Phys.*, 143, 14–19, 2008, with permission from Elsevier.)

heater B is turned on and the outer arm opens to be a flat shape so that it can release the blood vessel safely. The temperature of the heaters exceeds 65°C, which is equal to the deformation temperature of the SMA film, within several seconds by the electric heating. It seems a short time enough for actual use in the body without serious biological damage.

A laboratory rat is chosen for the evaluation of pulsation monitoring. A femoral artery of a laboratory rat was held between the outer arm and the cantilever of the sensor to evaluate real-time blood pulsation waveform. The outer diameter of the examined artery was about 1 mm. Change in blood pulsation waveform was measured when bloodstream was obstructed by clamping of the artery from outside intermittently as shown in Figure 9.64 (Mineta et al., 2008). The result of the waveform measurement is shown in Figure 9.65. When the blood flowed normally, periodical output voltage with amplitude of about 3.5 mV was obtained. Not only swelling but also shrinking of the artery was observed during each pulse cycle. Frequency of the waveform well agreed with a pulse period of a rate of 180 pulses/min. On the other hand, amplitude of the output voltage decreased to 1 mV when the bloodstream was obstructed by a mechanical clamping from outside the artery. As the results of the examination, it is confirmed that the developed sensor is sensitive enough to distinguish the bloodstream obstruction from the normal arterial blood pulsation.

The sensor could detect static deflections with a sensitivity of 0.1 mV/μm or larger with the sensing cantilever of the SMA film. The sensor could also detect the waveform of the pulsation when the dynamic diameter change of the held tube was 15 μm or larger. In addition, the sensor was successfully applied to an in vivo examination using a femoral artery of a laboratory rat. When the bloodstream of the artery of the rat was obstructed, decrease in amplitude of pulsation waveform was detected clearly. The sensor was fabricated based on simple photofabrication processes, which provide a possibility of inexpensive disposable devices.

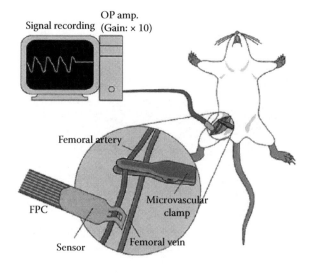

FIGURE 9.64
Scheme of laboratory rat examination. (From Mineta et al., *Sens. Actuators A Phys.*, 143, 14–19, 2008, with permission from Elsevier.)

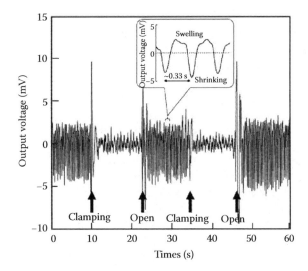

FIGURE 9.65
Detection of artery pulsation of laboratory rat under normal blood stream and obstructed blood stream conditions. (From Mineta et al., *Sens. Actuators A Phys.*, 143, 14–19, 2008, with permission from Elsevier.)

TiNi-Based Microcage

A biopsy is the removal of tissues or cells from the body and determination of any abnormality, such as cancer, infection, inflammation, or swelling. Microgrippers are such important microtools for the applications in biopsy, tissue sampling, cell manipulation, nerve repair, and minimally invasive surgery (Pan et al., 2007; Cecil et al., 2007; Volland et al., 2002; Wierzbicki et al., 2006; Luo et al., 2005). The requirements for the microgrippers for such applications include easy operation, low actuation temperature, low operation voltage, and low power consumption. A microgripper actuated by high temperature or high voltage will damage or even kill living cells or tissues. To manipulate the tissue, cells, or other biological objects, there are different types of microactuation mechanisms. Optical mechanism is mainly for cell manipulation application. A highly collimated light source, such as laser, can exert a focused radiation pressure that is substantial enough to manipulate large particles. Because the optical micromanipulation requires no physical contact, cells or tissues can be manipulated within enclosed glass chambers under sterile conditions. Optical scissors or optical tweezers are two examples of the optical micromanipulation (Reichle et al., 2000; Ericsson et al., 2000). However, photodamage incurred during manipulation could cause cell injury and death (Neuman et al., 1999). Microgrippers based on electrostatic, piezoelectric, electrophoresis, or dielectrophoretic manipulation have widely been studied (Volland, 2002; Kim et al., 1992; Millet et al., 2004). For example, dielectrophoresis can be used to trap, move, separate, or concentrate cells/particles based on the interaction between a polarized cell and nonuniform electric field (Gascoyn and Vykoukal, 2002). However, interaction with sample electrically is needed for electrokinetic micromanipulation, which may bring negative influence on the cell or tissue. Deriving the gripping ability of a microgripper by way of thermal expansion is one of the most common technologies for micromanipulation. The principle is based on that thermal expansion (upon heating) and contraction (upon cooling) of a material could provide actuation functions. However, the problems with this type of actuation include relatively small displacement and high working temperature. Some compliant mechanisms are normally designed and applied to amplify the displacement in thermal actuators (Chronis and Lee, 2005; Luo et al., 2005). In this section, the design, analysis, fabrication, and characterization of freestanding TiNiCu microcage and TiNi/DLC bimorph microcage are discussed.

Freestanding TiNi-Based Microcage

Films of $Ti_{50}Ni_{47}Cu_3$ alloy were deposited on 100 mm diameter Si(100) wafers by magnetron sputtering in an argon gas environment at a pressure of 0.8 mTorr from a $Ti_{55}Ni_{45}$ target (using a 400-W r.f. electric field) and a 99.99% pure Cu target (using a 2 W dc electric field). Film thickness is 3.5 µm. After the deposition, the films were annealed at a temperature of 550°C in a vacuum at 1×10^{-7} Torr. Microactuators were fabricated by photolithographically patterning 4.8 µm thick layers of AZ4562 photoresist on top of the TiNiCu films. HF/ HNO_3/H_2O (1:1:20) solution was employed to etch the TiNiCu films and form the microactuator patterns. With the remaining photoresist as the mask, the silicon substrate beneath the TiNiCu/SiN patterns was isotropically etched by SF_6 plasma using an r.f. reactive ion etch (rf-RIE) system with an SF_6 plasma (power of 100 W, 80 sccm, 100 mTorr) until the freestanding TiNiCu structures were released (Fu et al., 2007).

The freestanding TiNi films possess an intrinsic two-way SME with large displacements: the film curls up at room temperature, but becomes flat when heated and curls up once more when cooled back to room temperature (Fu et al., 2007). Microactuators made from these freestanding TiNi films can provide large deflections from simple structures and MEMS processes.

The actuation performance of the released freestanding microcages was evaluated by either heating the structure on a hot plate up to a maximum temperature of 100°C or by passing a current through the patterns and resistively heating the film in air. In the latter case, the current was provided by a Keithley 224A voltage/current power supply generating a square-wave voltage signal and this allowed actuation as a function of frequency to be analyzed (Fu et al., 2007). The displacement of the microgrppers was recorded on a video camera attached to a metallurgical microscope.

A microcage design consisting of thin TiNiCu beams patterned into microfingers is shown in Figure 9.66 (Fu et al., 2007). After release from the Si substrate, the fingers of the microcage curl up to form a cage structure due to the gradient stress that can be used to confine an object at room temperature. The microfingers uncurl when heated above 55°C and become flat at a temperature above 80°C. Upon cooling, the structure returns to its original curled shape. Figure 9.66b plots the experimentally measured changes in the horizontal and vertical displacement of the microcage fingertips as a function of substrate temperature when heating with a hot plate (Fu et al., 2007). Horizontal and vertical displacements of hundreds of micrometers are achievable at temperatures less than 100°C. It should be noted that negative values of vertical displacement indicate that the cage fingers bend downward upon actuation. The fabricated microcage has been thermally cycled between 20°C and 100°C for more than 100 cycles, and optical microscopy observation did not reveal apparent degradation.

The microcage can be actuated by passing a current through the TiNi microfingers. Figure 9.67a shows the horizontal displacement of the fingers achieved by varying applied power (Fu et al., 2007). Significant displacements are observed for input powers between 1.5 and 5 mW as the SMA is heated up through the transition temperature. Above 5 mW, the increase rate of tip displacement gradually decreases until up to a power of 7 mW, above which the displacement slightly decreases. Excessive heating through the

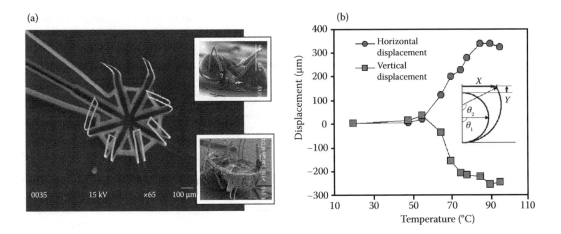

FIGURE 9.66
A TiNiCu bending-up microcage structure and examples of capturing of (a) an ant and (b) an aphid. (From Fu et al., 2007, reproduced with permission from IOP Publisher, UK.) Vertical and horizontal displacement of TiNiCu fingers in microcage as a function of substrate temperature where negative displacements denote a downward displacement. (From Fu et al, *Smart. Mater. Struct.* 16, 2651–2657, 2007.)

application of very high powers (>20 mW) resulted in visible changes in the color of the TiNiCu—an indication of overheating and surface oxidation. The microcage can be used to capture microscale objects (Fu et al., 2007). Figure 9.67b shows the measured tip displacement produced by passing a current through the metallic layers as a function of the voltage amplitude and frequency of the square wave signal applied (Fu et al., 2007). For frequencies below ~100 Hz, the tip displacement increases with applied voltage. However, above ~100 Hz, the displacement decreases with increasing frequency for all applied voltages, indicating that about 10 ms is required to cool the microstructure due to the thermal capacity of the system. This places a maximum operating frequency of about 100 Hz for this microcage design. The realization of high-frequency microactuators utilizing TiNi-based

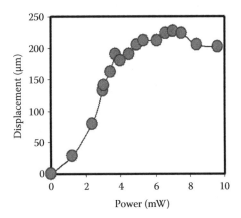

FIGURE 9.67
(a) Horizontal displacement of fingers of microcage as a function of input power applied; (b) horizontal displacement of fingers of microcage as a function of voltage and frequency of the applied actuation square wave. (From Fu et al, *Smart. Mater. Struct.* 16, 2651–2657, 2007. Reproduced with permission from IOP Publisher, UK.)

thin films has been a challenge. The frequency reported in thin film TiNi-based devices, such as microactuators and micropumps (Seguin et al., 1999; Benard et al., 1998; Markino et al., 2000) generally have maximum operating frequencies in the range from 1 to 100 Hz. It should also be noted that the frequency is strongly dependent on the medium in which the device is placed, as well as mass and dimension of the structure. Actuation in liquid, or thinner beams, and smaller structure dimension may permit higher operating frequencies to be achieved due to easier thermal dissipation into the liquid.

The microcage structure has been tested up to 18,000 cycles (with a fixed frequency of 20 Hz). With a low applied power less than 5 mW, upon up to a few thousands cycles, there are slight decreases in the horizontal displacement, as well as the original positions, but does not change much afterward even up to 18,000 cycles (Fu et al., 2007). The initial changes can be attributed to the training process, a common phenomenon for SMA. For the TiNi-based films, at the initial actuation stage, the repeated phase changes will alter the microstructure and hysteresis of the transformation and in turn lead to changes in transformation temperatures, transformation stresses and strains. Recovery stress of TiNi films was found to decrease dramatically in the first tens of cycles, and became stable after hundreds of cycles. However, at a power above 5 mW, the maximum displacement of cantilever tip gradually decreases. There is a gradual shift in the room temperature position of the microfingers, and the tips of microfingers do not return to their original position after 18,000 cycles. The reason is attributed to the fatigue and degradation problem, which may be attributed to the defects in the film. With the power increased to above 8 mW, there is a significant shift of finger tip, especially at the beginning of working cycles. This is attributed to the thermal degradation due to the excessive heating effect. It is apparent that the current or power applied on these microcages has a dramatic effect on the stability of fatigue properties. This issue should be addressed before application of the freestanding TiNiCu microactuators.

TiNi/DLC Microcage

A schematic bimorph microfinger TiNi/DLC structure is shown in Figure 9.68. The DLC film has a large compressive stress, and the TiNi film at room temperature (i.e., in martensite state) normally shows small tensile stress. When the DLC is used as the bottom layer and TiNi as the top layer of the bimorph structure, significant up-bending of the fingers of the microcage could occur when it is released from the Si substrate. The radius of curvature, R, of the bimorph TiNi/DLC structure (shown in Figure 9.68a and b) after release

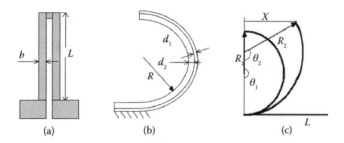

FIGURE 9.68
Schematic drawing of bimorph TiNi/DLC microfinger structures: (a) top view; (b) cross-section view after bending up; (c) illustration of bending angular and displacement. (From Fu et al., *J. Micromech. Microeng.*, 18, 035026, 2008, Reproduced with permission from IOP Publisher, UK.)

from Si substrate can be controlled by changing the thickness ratio of the two layers, or by changing the stress state in both the TiNi and DLC layers (Tsui et al., 1997; Fu et al., 2008):

$$\frac{1}{R} = \frac{6 \cdot \varepsilon_{eq}(1+m)^2}{d[3(1+m)^2 + (1+mn)(m^2 + (mn)^{-1})]} = \varepsilon_{eq} \cdot M \tag{9.11}$$

where M is a dimension-related parameter and ε_{eq} is the equivalent strain. Because the as-deposited TiNi film has a very low tensile stress, it is assumed that strain change in the bimorph structure is dominated by the DLC layer. Assuming that stress is uniaxial (due to the bimorph is slender), the equivalent strain ε_{eq} in the DLC layer can be simply calculated using the as-deposited stress σ_d and the Young's modulus E_d of the DLC layer, that is, $\varepsilon_{eq} = \sigma_d/E_d$. In Equation 9.11, $d = d_1 + d_2$, in which d_1 and d_2 are the thicknesses of the DLC and TiNi layer, respectively, and n (= E_1/E_2) and m (= d_1/d_2) are the ratios of the Young's modulus and the layer thickness of the two layers. M is a constant for the fixed materials and structural configuration. Equation 9.11 implies that once the materials and the layer thickness are fixed, the radius of curvature can be adjusted by varying the stress and strain of both the top TiNi layer and bottom DLC layer.

During thermal cycling, the opening/closing performance of the microcage is mainly determined by: (1) thermal effect: temperature change and the difference in the CTEs of the two materials, and (2) SME. First, the curvature changes due to pure thermal effect are analyzed. If the temperature of the bimorph finger increases from T_1 to T_2 because of the difference of the CTE between the TiNi and DLC, the thermal expansion mismatch leads to the TiNi layer expanding more than the DLC layer, thus opening the microcage and changing the radius of curvature from R_1 to R_2. The thermal strain, ε_{th}, generated through resistive Joule heating of the bimorph layer is expressed as: $\varepsilon_{eq} = (\alpha_d - \alpha_{TiNi}) \cdot \Delta T$, where α_d and α_{TiNi} are the CTEs of the DLC and TiNi, respectively. The radius of the curvature R, bending angle θ (in degree) and the length of the finger, L, have the following relationship (see Figure 9.68c):

$$\theta = \frac{180° \cdot L}{\pi \cdot R} \tag{9.12}$$

Combining Equations 9.11 and 9.12, the angle change from θ_1 (which refers to the initial degree of bending at room temperature) to θ_2 (a new position) due to the pure thermal effect from a temperature T_1 to a temperature T_2 ($\Delta T = T_2 - T_1$) can be expressed by

$$\Delta\theta = \theta_2 - \theta_1 = \frac{180° \cdot L}{\pi}\left(\frac{1}{R_2} - \frac{1}{R_1}\right) = \frac{180° \cdot L}{\pi}\Delta\varepsilon_{thermal} \cdot M = \frac{180° \cdot L}{\pi}\Delta\alpha \cdot \Delta T \cdot M \tag{9.13}$$

According to the design, the finger lengths are 50, 100, and 150 μm. The thickness of the DLC layer is 100 nm, and the thickness of the TiNi layer is 800 nm. The stress of the as-deposited DLC film was determined to be 5 GPa. In calculation, the elastic modulus and thermal expansion coefficient of the TiNi film is a variable as a function of temperature, based on the rule of mixtures depending on the percentage of martensite/austenite at a given temperature. The bending angle decreases slightly with the increase in temperature during heating, indicating the microfingers slightly open owing to bimorph thermal effect. A hysteresis is observed during the thermal cycle due to differences in forward and martensitic transformations upon heating/cooling (i.e., different contents of martensite and austenite at a certain temperature during thermal cycling).

A rough estimation according to Equation 9.13 indicates that if the thickness ratio of TiNi/DLC is 1, there will be a maximum bending effect. However, the thickness of TiNi should be larger than a few hundred nanometers, below which the SME will be too weak for an efficient actuation (Fu et al., 2006). When the film is too thin, surface oxide and film/substrate interfacial diffusion layers exert dominant constraining effect that renders high residual stress and low recovery capabilities (Ishida et al., 2003). The surface oxide and interdiffusion layer restricts the phase transformation, alters the chemical stoichiometry of the remaining TiNi film, which effectively reduces the volume of the material available for phase transformation. On the other hand, there is also a limit to the DLC thickness. When the thickness of DLC is above 100 nm, the DLC layer may peel off from the Si substrate because of intrinsic stress. This has severely restricted the usage of DLC of a few hundred nanometers thick.

Microcages of five, six, and seven fingers were designed. The width of the fingers and the gap between the beams were 4 μm. The fingers were connected to each other with bond pads. The central part of the microcage was large enough so that it remained attached to the substrate after the fingers were released from the substrate. A DLC film of 100 nm was deposited on Si substrate using a filtered cathodic vacuum arc (FCVA) method with a graphite source. The compressive stress of the film was 5 GPa as determined via curvature measurement. A TiNi film of 800 nm thick was deposited on top of the DLC layer by magnetron sputtering in an argon gas environment at a pressure of 0.8 mTorr from a $Ti_{50}Ni_{50}$ target (using a 400-W r.f. power) and a 99.99% pure Ti target (using a 70-W dc power). Post-annealing of the TiNi/DLC bimorph layer was performed at 480°C for 30 min in a high vacuum condition for crystallization. The DLC/TiNi microcage was fabricated by photolithographically patterning of 4.8 μm thick AZ4562 photoresist on top of the TiNi films. An $HF/HNO_3/H_2O$ (1:1:20) solution was employed to etch the TiNi films to form the microcage patterns. The exposed DLC underlayer was etched off in oxygen plasma at a flow rate of 80 sccm and a power of 100 W. A deep reactive ion etching machine was used to isotropically etch the silicon substrate with SF_6 plasma at a flow rate of 70 sccm and pressure of 72 mTorr. The coil and platen powers were set at 50 and 100 W, respectively. A time-controlled etching was performed to release the fingers leaving the middle parts of the microcage remained attached to the Si substrate. The actuation performance of the released microgrippers was evaluated using a peltier device (with a temperature range from 5°C to 100°C). The displacements of the TiNi pattern were measured using a video camera from the top view.

An SEM morphology of the fabricated TiNi/DLC microcages on a 4-inch silicon wafer is shown in Figure 9.69a (Fu et al., 2008). The microcages have different finger numbers and beam lengths. After released from the Si substrate, the microcages show significant curling up of the microfingers, depending on the beam lengths. The fabricated seven-finger microcages with different beam lengths. As designed, with increase in beam length, the microfinger patterns of the microcages change from fully open, under-closed to over-closed (Fu et al., 2008).

Figure 9.70 shows the top-view optical images of the deformation behavior of a five-finger microcage upon heating (Fu et al., 2008). Actuation of the microcage is mainly determined by SME. With temperature increased above martensitic start transformation temperature (about 50 to 60°C), martensite (loose structure) changes to austenite (a dense structure), causing the closing of microcages, and capturing an object. Further increase in temperature above 100°C causes the slight opening of the microfingers due to thermal effects.

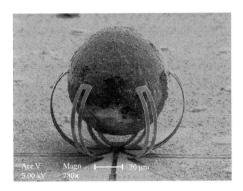

FIGURE 9.69
SEM picture of microcage capturing a micropolymer ball. (From Fu et al., *J. Micromech. Microeng.*, 18, 035026, 2008. Reproduced with permission from IOP Publisher, UK.)

Upon cooling, the microcage fingers quickly open due to the martensitic transformation. As one example for the real application, Figure 9.69 shows an SEM picture of the microcage capturing a micropolymer ball with a diameter of 50 µm (Fu et al., 2008).

Based on the calculation results of curvature angular change for the beams with different lengths shown in Figure 9.71b, the microfinger displacement in the horizontal direction can be estimated from the simplified relationship: $\sin(180 - \theta) = x/R = (x \cdot \theta)/L$, and the results are shown in Figure 9.71a (Fu et al., 2008). Beam length has a dramatic influence on the opening displacement in the x-direction. Figure 9.15b plots the experimentally measured changes in the horizontal displacement of a microcage fingertip (beam length of 150 µm) as a function of substrate temperature. Horizontal displacements of 50 to 60 µm can be achieved at temperatures lower than 80°C. The theoretical calculated results are comparable with the results as shown in Figure 9.71b. However, there is a discrepancy between the estimated and the measured results. Several reasons are possible for this discrepancy: (1) In theoretical calculation, the stress–temperature results measured from a film on a 4-in. Si wafer was used. However, the real stress–temperature relationship could be different from that on TiNi/DLC bimorph structure. (2) In measurement, the temperature of the fingers of the microcage should be lower than those measured on the surface of the peltier device. (3) During the fabrication of DLC/TiNi microcages, a post-annealing crystallization process was used which could have relaxed some of the DLC stress. Also, the plasma releasing of microfinger from silicon substrate could deteriorate the SME of

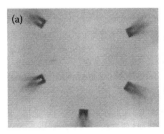
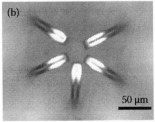

FIGURE 9.70
Optical microscopy images showing the closing of a five-finger microcage during heating (during cooling, process is reversed, beam length of 100 µm): (a) 20°C, (b) 100°C. (From Fu et al., *J. Micromech. Microeng.*, 18, 035026, 2008. Reproduced with permission from IOP Publisher, UK.)

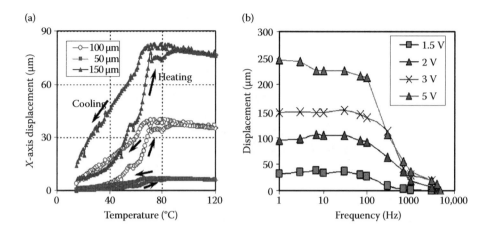

FIGURE 9.71
Horizontal displacement as a function of temperature for microfinger (a) with different finger lengths; and (b) experimental results and calculated results with a finger length of 150 μm. (From Fu et al., *J. Micromech. Microeng.*, 18, 035026, 2008. Reproduced with permission from IOP Publisher, UK.)

TiNi film due to the plasma damage on the surface of the material. These effects should be considered when designing the microcages for practical usages.

Intravascular Medical Stent and Tube Devices

Today's TiNi stents are normally made using bulk nitinol tubes, even though these drawn tubes are relatively large and not flexible to be delivered by intravascular microcatheters to brain lesions (Johnson, 2009). TiNi stents are collapsed into small diameter catheters (e.g., as small as 1 mm) and guided along the vascular system to the appropriate location using imaging hardware. Once at the site such as an occluded artery, the stent is forced out of the catheter with a push rod and exposed to the surrounding body temperature. The surrounding temperature causes the stent to fully deploy and open the occluded artery. Nitinol tubes with wall thickness as small as 50 μm have been achieved by etching and electropolishing techniques. However, such techniques are unsuitable to achieve wall thickness much smaller than 50 μm. Sputter deposition techniques can produce TiNi film as thin as 1 μm. The medical industry represents a growing demand for smaller and thinner stents that can be surgically implanted or delivered via catheter into small diameter, highly tortuous blood vessels (Johnson, 2009).

Covered Stent

Although traditional stents consist of nonocclusive metal scaffolds, the treatment of many disease processes requires the use of a "covered stent." These stents are able to open vessels and provide a circumferentially occlusive boundary between the stent and vessel. Thus, covered stents are ideal for reestablishing the integrity of aneurysmal vessels or for minimizing the risk of in-stent stenosis (Cambria, 2004). The potential applications of such covered stents include the treatment of coronary artery disease, aortic and central nervous system vascular aneurysms, carotid artery or pulmonary artery stenoses, and even treatment of ruptured vessels (Cambria, 2004). In the palliation of congenital heart disease, specifically, the appropriate covered stent would be of tremendous value in stenting the ductus arteriosus, coarctation of the aorta, or in the stenting of pulmonary veins, an intervention often plagued by in-stent stenosis (Mohanchandra and Carman, 2009).

In both in vivo and in vitro testing of the TiNi, thin film-covered stents were conducted by Mohanchandra and Carman (2009). The in vitro tests demonstrate the feasibility of successful stent deployment and the stent immobility under pulsatile flow of 1.5 L/min. For in vivo testing of the covered stent a swine animal model was used. All arterial plantations were performed in the descending aorta. Venous implants were performed in either the superior vena cava or inferior vena cava and evaluated at different time intervals. After animal euthanization, stent-containing vessels were harvested, as well as specimens from major organs (heart, lungs, liver, stomach, kidney, pancreas, and spleen). No significant in-stent neointimal hyperplasia was found on thin film TiNi covered stents placed in the arterial circulation. Moderate-to-severe neointimal proliferation was seen in all venous stent implants after 3 weeks. Notably, several of the stent covers were found to have defects that were likely caused during deployment (Mohanchandra and Carman, 2009). In the arterial circulation, the thin film nitinol cover did prevent in-growth of neointima and supported growth of endothelial cells over the first month after implantation. In the venous system, there was angiographic evidence of less in-stent stenosis in the first 3 weeks after implantation (when compared with an uncovered stent). However, by 4 and 6 weeks, all venous stents (covered and uncovered) had significant in-stent stenosis from neointimal growth (Mohanchandra and Carman, 2009). The vastly different thermodynamic environments encountered in the arterial versus the venous circulation likely contributed significantly to this differential result. The pulsatile arterial circulation, reaching peak flow velocities of approximately 1 m/s, is likely to have had a significant influence on the type and extent of neointimal proliferation when compared with the continuous low flow state present in the venous circulation. It is likely that the covered stents placed in the venous circulation prevented direct growth of the vessel wall through the stent but not onto and around the device (Mohanchandra and Carman, 2009). It may be possible to obtain improved results by covering both the outside and inside of the stent with thin film nitinol. Because thin film nitinol seems to promote a very thin layer of endothelialization, an inner covering may improve our results by shielding the lumen of the vessel from exposure to the bulk nitinol or stainless steel present in the stent scaffolding. As thin film nitinol is much smoother and contains many less contaminants than bulk nitinol, this inner covering could allow for a more favorable biological response when compared with bulk nitinol (Mohanchandra and Carman, 2009).

Heart Valve

One medical device recently proposed for thin film TiNi is a heart valve (Stepan et al., 2005). The TiNi film in the valve is used as the heart leaflets for a surgically placed heart valve replacing the mechanical or bioprosthetic heart valves currently on the market. First, the TiNi film may provide increased longevity compared to current bioprosthetic valves (i.e., average 10-year lifespan). Second, the TiNi thin film valve may not require anticoagulation therapy necessary in mechanical valves (Mohanchandra and Carman, 2009). For percutaneously placed heart valves, the TiNi leaflets could be substantially thinner than bioprosthetic allowing the heart valve to be collapsed into a substantially smaller catheter for delivery. This is extremely important in pediatric patients. The surgically placed TiNi prosthetic heart valve (see Figure 9.72) was designed and constructed by inserting an elliptically shaped piece of shape memory TiNi thin film into a Teflon scaffold made of two Teflon tubes with different diameters (Mohanchandra and Carman, 2009). After

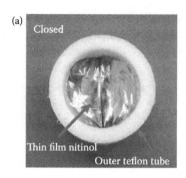
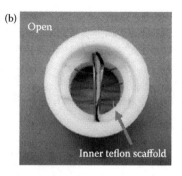

FIGURE 9.72

Closed (a) and open (b) positions of a TiNi thin film heart valve. (From Stepan et al., *J. Biomech. Eng. ASME Trans.*, 127, 915–918, 2005, with permission to use from ASME.)

deposition and fabrication of a TiNi leaflet, the leaflet was wrapped around the anchoring bar, made of TiNi wire, and fixed in place by the insertion of the smaller tube into the inferior portion of the large tube. Figure 9.72 shows the closed and open positions of the heart valve (Mohanchandra and Carman, 2009).

Fabrication of Superelastic Thin Film Tubes

Figure 9.73 shows a schematic of the deposition system used to fabricate Ti–Ni microtubes (Buenconsejo et al., 2008). A rotating jig is placed inside a sputter-deposition chamber and a Cu wire is fixed such that its length is parallel to the surface of the alloy target. The rotation of the wire is controlled by a motor. Cu wire was rotated at constant rotation speeds during the deposition process. The composition of the alloy target is Ti–50 at.% Ni and pure Ti chips were placed on the surface to control the composition. The composition of deposited Ti–Ni was determined by electron probe microanalysis to be Ti–52 at.% Ni. After deposition, the Cu wire was completely dissolved in a Nitric acid solution thus producing a tube hole. The microtubes were sealed in an Ar-filled quartz tube and then crystallized

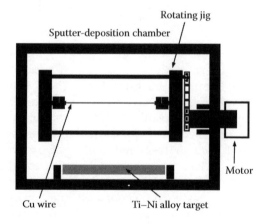

FIGURE 9.73

A schematic of rotating jig placed inside sputter-deposition chamber. (From Buenconsejo et al., *Acta Mater.*, 56, 2063–2072, 2008, with permission from Elsevier.)

by heat treatment at 873 K for 3.6 ks followed by water-quenching without breaking the quartz tube (Buenconsejo et al., 2008).

Figure 9.74 shows the fracture surfaces observed by SEM for Ti–Ni microtubes fabricated by deposition on a rotating wire at different rotation speeds, followed by crystallization at 873 K for 3.6 ks (Buenconsejo et al., 2008). The wall thickness for all the microtubes was uniform, with a thickness of about 6 μm. It was established that the deposition rate decreases with increasing β angle. The effect of rotating the Cu wire was to create a similar deposition condition and thus a uniform deposition rate around the substrate surface. Examination of the enlarged images of microtube cross sections (Figure 9.74) revealed that the morphologies are different with respect to the rotation speed (Buenconsejo et al., 2008). For example in the microtube deposited at 0.6 rpm, columnar grains were observed. Although the microtubes deposited at 15 rpm and 30 rpm did not contain any columnar grains, the deposition time on the oblique surface area in one cycle decreases with increasing rotation speed, causing the columnar grains not to be formed for the microtubes deposited at 15 and 30 rpm. The microtube fabricated at 0.6 rpm has a low fracture stress of 450 MPa. Whereas the microtubes fabricated at higher rotation speeds of 15 and 30 rpm exhibited high fracture stress above 800 MPa because no columnar grains were formed (Buenconsejo et al., 2008). The martensitic transformation temperatures and the recovery strains were not significantly affected with the rotation speed. The M_s and A_f slightly varied from 160 to 170 K and 250 to 260 K, respectively. Similarly ε_a^{max} was about 3.0% for all the specimens. The stress–strain curves revealed superelastic behavior at test temperatures between 223 K and 303 K. A high σ_M and a high fracture stress are suitable for practical applications as biomedical devices, such as microstents and microcatheters.

Figure 9.75a shows the strain–temperature curves of Ti–Ni microtubes fabricated by the rotating wire method at 0.6, 15, and 30 rpm (Buenconsejo et al., 2008). The strain–temperature curves were obtained during thermal cycling between 160 and 390 K, under various constant stresses. The martensitic transformation temperatures (M_s, M_f, A_s, and A_f) shape recovery strain (ε_a) and plastic strain (ε_p) were obtained as shown in Figure 9.75a. The tensile elongation during cooling and its recovery during heating confirm that the Ti–Ni microtubes exhibit the SME. The M_s and A_f extrapolated at zero applied stress for each specimen are plotted as a function of rotation speed in Figure 9.75a. The M_s and A_f slightly varied from 160 to 170 K and from 250 to 260 K, respectively, indicating that M_s and A_f are insensitive to the rotation speed. Similarly, the maximum recoverable strain (ε_a^{max}) is plotted as a function of rotation speed in Figure 9.75b. It is seen that the ε_a^{max} of microtubes exhibits a similar value about 3% (Buenconsejo et al., 2008). These results suggest that the martensitic transformation temperatures and the maximum recoverable strain of the Ti–Ni microtubes deposited by the rotating wire at various rotation speeds are not significantly affected by the rotation speed.

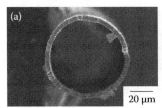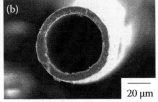

FIGURE 9.74
Fabricated TiNi microtube. (a) Ration speed of 0.6 rpm; (b) rotation speed of 15 rpm. (From Buenconsejo et al., *Acta Mater.*, 56, 2063–2072, 2008, with permission from Elsevier.)

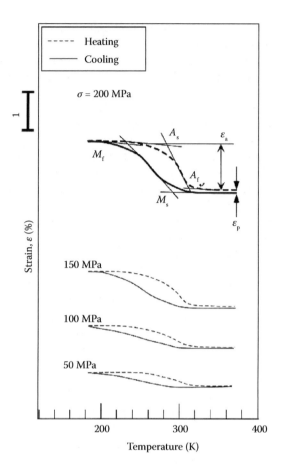

FIGURE 9.75

Stress–strain curves measured at various test temperatures for a TiNi microtube deposited on a rotating wire at 15 rpm. (From Buenconsejo et al., *Acta Mater.*, 56, 2063–2072, 2008, with permission from Elsevier.)

Summary and Future

Sputter-deposited TiNi and TiNi*X* (*X*=Cu, Pd) thin films have been successfully produced and show stable SME and thermomechanical properties which are equivalent to those of bulk materials. Worldwide research programs in universities and industry have produced many publications, prototypes, and patents on SMA thin film. TiNi thin film is a high-quality material with excellent physical properties. It has been shown to be highly biocompatible and has a long fatigue life. Intrinsic properties are equivalent or better than bulk nitinol. Development of TiNi-based SMA thin films and microactuators witnessed a considerable progress in recent years. Some important issues pertaining to the preparation of high-performance shape memory TiNi films using sputtering methods and their MEMS applications were reviewed in this chapter. Successful application of TiNi thin films in MEMS requires consideration of the following issues: preparation and characterization, residual stress and adhesion, frequency improvement, fatigue and stability, and patterning and modeling of behavior. Development of a variety of characterization methods is needed to evaluate the actuator characteristics of the TiNi thin films in service in micro-mechanical systems. Systematic investigation on the interaction between TiNi films and substrates is also demanded to achieve tight bonding of the films onto the substrates without much chemical reaction between them. With further development of fabrication and characterization techniques, it is clear that a variety of micromechanical systems utilizing microactuators of TiNi thin films will be developed and present important technical impacts in the quite near future. At microscale, TiNi actuators out-perform other actuation mechanisms in work/volume (or power/weight) ratio, large deflection and force, but with a relatively low frequency (less than 100 Hz) and efficiency, as well as nonlinear behavior. More functional and complex designs based on TiNi film devices are needed with multi degree-of-freedom and compact structure. TiNi film–based microactuators will find potential applications in medicine, aerospace, automotive, and consumer products. Miniature TiNi-actuated devices based on sputtered TiNi films are ready for the huge commercial market, especially for medical microdevices and implantable applications.

References

Auricchio F, Taylor RL, Lubliner J. 1997. Shape-memory alloys: macromodelling and numerical simulations of the superelastic behavior. *Comput. Methods Appl. Mech. Eng.* 146: 281–312.

Baldwin E, Thomas B, Lee JW, Rabiei A. 2005. Processing TiPdNi base thin-film shape memory alloys using ion beam assisted deposition, *Surf. Coat. Technol.* 200: 2571–2579.

Bellouard Y, Lehnert T, Bidaux JE, Sidler T, Clavel R, Gottardt R, Bellouard Y. 1999. Local annealing of complex mechanical devices: a new approach for developing monolithic micro-devices. *Mater. Sci. Eng. A* 273–275: 795–798.

Benard WL, Kahn H, Heuer AH and Huff MA. 1998. Thin-film shape-memory alloy actuated micropumps, *J. MEMS* 7: 245–251.

Bhattacharya K and James RD. 1999. A theory of thin films of martensitic materials with applications to microactuators, *J. Mech. Phys. Solids* 47: 531–576.

Bhattacharyya A, Faulkner MG, Amalraj JJ. 2000. Finite element modeling of cyclic thermal response of shape memory alloy wires with variable material properties. *Comput. Mater. Sci.* 17: 93–104.

Buehler W, Gilfrich J, Riley R. 1963. Effect of low-temperature phase changes on the mechanical properties of alloys near composition Ti–Ni J. *Appl. Phys.* 34: 1475–1477.

Buenconsejo PJ, Kanau I, Kim HY and Miyazaki S. 2008. High-strength superelastic Ti–Ni microtubes fabricated by sputter deposition. *Acta Mater.* 56: 2063–2072.

Busch JD, Johnson AD, Lee CH, and Stevenson DA. 1990. Shape-memory properties in Ni-Ti sputter-deposited film. *J. Appl. Phys.* 68: 6224–6228.

Cambria RP. 2004. Stenting for carotid-artery stenosis. *New Engl J Med.* 351: 1565–1567.

Cecil J, Powell D, Vasquez D. 2007. Assembly and manipulation of micro devices—a state of the art survey. *Robot. Comput. Integr. Manuf.* 23: 580–588.

Chang L and Grummon DS. 1997. Structure evolution in sputtered thin films of Ti–x(Ni,Cu)$(1 - x)$: 1. Diffusive transformations. *Philos. Mag. A* 76: 163–191.

Chikazume S. 1997. *Physics of Ferromagnetism*. Oxford University Press, Oxford, UK.

Cho H, Kim HY, Miyazaki S. 2006. Alloying process of sputter-deposited Ti/Ni multilayer thin films. *Mater. Sci. Eng. A* 438: 699–702.

Chonan S, Jiang ZW, Tani J, Orikasa S, Tanahashi Y, Takagi T, Tanaka M, Tanikawa J. 1997. Development of an Artificial Urethral Valve using SMA Actuators, *Smart Mater. Struct.* 6: 410–414.

Chronis N and Lee LP. 2005. Electrothermally activated SU-8 microgripper for single cell manipulation in solution. *J. MEMS* 14: 857–863.

Cinchetti M, Gloskovskii A, Nepjiko S, Schonhense G, Rochholz H, Kreiter M. 2005. Photoemission electron microscopy as a tool for the investigation of optical near fields, *Phys. Rev. Lett.* 95: 047601.

Cole DP, Bruck HA, Roytburd AL. 2008. Nanoindentation studies of graded shape memory alloy thin films processed using diffusion modification, *J. Appl. Phys.* 103: 064315.

Craciunescu CM and Wuttig M. 2003. New ferromagnetic and functionally graded shape memory alloys. *J. Optoelectr. Adv. Mater.* 5: 139–146.

Craciunescu C, Li J, Wuttig M. 2003. Thermoelastic stress-induced thin film martensites. *Scr. Mater.* 48: 65–70.

Craciunescu C and Wuttig M. 2000. Extraordinary damping of Ni–Ti double layer films. *Thin Solid Films* 378: 173–175.

Cuschieri A. 1991. Variable curvature shape-memory spatula for laparoscopic surgery. *Surg. Endosc.* 5: 179.

Dai K and Chu Y. 1996. Studies and applications of NiTi shape memory alloys in the medical field in China. *Biomed. Mater. Eng.* 6: 233–240.

Dotter CT, Buschmann RW, McKinney MK, Rosch J. 1983. Transluminal expandable nitinol coil stent grafting: preliminary report. *Radiology* 147: 259–260.

Du HJ and Fu YQ. 2004. Deposition and characterization of Ti1-x(Ni,Cu)x shape memory alloy thin films. *Surf. Coat. Technol.* 176: 182–187.

Duerig TW and Wayman CM. 1990. *Engineering Aspects of Shape-Memory Alloys*. In Durerig TW, Melton KN, Stockel D, Wayman CM (eds.). Butterworth-Heinemann, London, 3.

Ericsson M, Hanstorp D, Hagberg P, Enger J, Nystrom T. 2000. Sorting out bacterial viability with optical tweezers. *J. Bacteriol.* 182: 5551–5555.

Espinosa HD, Prorok BC, Fischer M. 2003. A methodology for determining mechanical properties of freestanding thin films and MEMS materials. *J. Mech. Phys. Solids* 51: 46–67.

Es-Souni M and Brandies HF. 2001. On the transformation behaviour, mechanical properties and bio-compatibility of two TiNi-based shape memory alloys: NiTi42 and NiTi42Cu7. *Biomaterials* 22: 2153.

Firstov GS, Vitchev RG, Kumar H, Blanpain B, Van Humbeeck J. 2002. Surface oxidation of TiNi shape memory alloy. *Biomaterials* 23: 4863–4871.

Frank T, Willets G, Cuschieri A. 1995. Detachable clamps for minimal access surgery. *Proc. Inst. Mech. Eng. Part H* 209: 117–120.

Frank TW, Xu A, Cuschieri A. 2000. Instruments based on shape memory alloy properties for mini-mal access surgery, interventional radiology and flexible endoscopy. *Minim. Invasive Ther. Allied Technol.* 9: 89–98.

Fu YQ and Du HJ. 2002. Relaxation and recovery of stress during martensite transformation for sput-tered shape memory TiNi film. *Surf. Coat. Technol.* 153: 100–105.

Fu YQ and Du HJ. 2003. Effects of film composition and annealing on residual stress evolution for shape memory TiNi film. *Mater. Sci. Eng. A* 342: 236–244.

Fu YQ and Du HJ. 2003. Fabrication of micromachined TiNi-based microgripper with complaint structure, SPIE Vol. 5116, 2003, pp 38–47. *Smart Sensors, Actuators, and MEMS*, 19–21 May, 2003, Gran Canaria, Spain. SPIE-Int. Soc. Opt. Eng, USA.

Fu YQ and Du HJ. 2003. RF magnetron sputtered TiNiCu shape memory alloy thin film. *Mater. Sci. Eng. A*, 339: 10.

Fu YQ, Du HJ, Zhang S. 2002. Curvature method as a tool for shape memory effect. In *Surface Engineering: Science and Technology II symposium at TMS 2002 Annual Meeting*, Kumar A, Chung YW, Moore JJ, Doll GL, Yahi K, Misra DS (eds.), TMS, pp 293–303, Feb. 17–21, 2002, Seattle, WA, USA.

Fu YQ, Du HJ, Zhang S. 2003. Adhesion and interfacial structure of magnetron sputtered TiNi films on Si/SiO₂ substrate. *Thin Solid Films* 444: 85–90.

Fu YQ, Du HJ, Zhang S. 2003. Deposition of TiN layer on TiNi thin films to improve surface proper-ties. *Surf. Coat. Technol.* 167: 129–136.

Fu YQ, Du HJ, Zhang S. 2003. Functionally graded TiN/TiNi shape memory alloy films. *Mater. Lett.* 57: 2995–2999.

Fu YQ, Du HJ, Zhang S, Ong SE. 2004. Effects of silicon nitride interlayer on phase transformation and adhesion of TiNi films. *Thin Solid Films* 476: 352–357.

Fu YQ, Du HJ, Zhang S, Gu YW. 2005. Stress and surface morphology of TiNiCu thin films: effect of annealing temperature. *Surf. Coat. Technol.* 198: 389–394.

Fu YQ and Du HJ. 2003. Magnetron sputtered Ti50Ni40Pt10 shape memory alloy thin films. *J. Mater. Sci. Lett.* 22: 531–533.

Fu YQ, Du HJ, Gao S, Yi S. 2003. Mechanical properties of sputtered TiNiCu shape memory alloy thin films. *Mater. Sci. Forum* 437: 37–40.

Fu YQ, Du HJ, Huang W, Zhang S, Hu M. 2004. TiNi-based thin films in MEMS applications: a review. *Sens. Actuators: A. Physical* 112: 395–408.

Fu YQ, Luo JK, Flewitt AJ, Ong SE, Zhang S, Du HJ, Milne WI. 2008. Shape memory microcage of TiNi/DLC films for biological applications. *J. Micromech. Microeng.* 18: 035026.

Fu YQ, Luo JK, Ong SE, Zhang S, Flewitt AJ, Milne WI. 2008. TiNi/DLC shape memory microcage for biological applications. *J. Micromech. Microeng.* 18: 035026.

Fu YQ, Zhang S, Wu MJ, Huang WM, Du HJ, Luo JK, Flewitt AJ, Milne WI. 2006. On the lower thickness boundary of sputtered TiNi films for shape memory application. *Thin Solid Films* 515: 80–86.

Fu YQ, Sanjabi S, Barber ZH, Clyne TW, Huang WM, Cai MD, Luo, JK, Flewitt AJ, Milne WI. 2006. Evolution of surface morphology in TiNiCu shape memory thin films. *Appl. Phys. Lett.* 89: 171922.

Fu YQ, Huang WM, Du HJ, Huang X, Tan JP, Gao XY. 2001. Characterization of TiNi shape-memory alloy thin films for MEMS applications. *Surf. Coat. Technol.* 145: 107–112.

Fu YQ, Luo JK, Flewitt AJ, Ong SE, Zhang S, Du HJ, Milne WI. 2007. Microactuators of free-standing TiNiCu Films, *Smart. Mater. Struct.* 16, 2651–2657.

Gabry B, Lexcellent C, No VH, Miyazaki S. 2000. Thermodynamic modeling of the recovery strains of sputter-deposited shape memory alloys Ti–Ni and Ti–Ni–Cu thin films. *Thin Solid Films* 372: 118–133.

Gall K and Sehitoglu H. 1999. The role of texture in tension-compression asymmetry in polycrystalline NiTi. *Int. J. Plast.* 15: 69–92.

Gao XY and Huang WM. 2002. Transformation start stress in non-textured shape memory alloys. *Smart Mater. Struct.* 11: 256–268.

Gascoyne PRC and Vykoukal J. 2002. Particle separation by dielectrophoresis. *Electrophoresis* 23: 1973–1983.

Gill JJ, Chang DT, Momoda LA, Carman GP. 2001. Manufacturing issues of thin film TiNi microwrapper. *Sens. Actuators A* 93: 148–156.

Gill JJ, Ho K, Carman GP. 2002. Three-dimensional thin-film shape memory alloy microactuator with two-way effect. *J. MEMS.* 11: 68–77.

Goldberg F and Knystautas EJ. 1999. The effects of ion irradiation on TiNi shape memory alloy thin films. *Thin Solid Films* 342: 67–73.

Grummon DS and Gotthardt R. 2000. Latent strain in titanium-nickel thin films modified by irradiation of the plastically-deformed martensite phase with 5 MeV Ni^{2+}. *Acta Mater.* 48: 635–646.

Grummon DS. 2003. Thin-film shape-memory materials for high-temperature applications. *JOM* 55: 24–32.

Grummon DS, Zhang JP, Pence TJ. 1999. Relaxation and recovery of extrinsic stress in sputtered titanium-nickel thin films on (100)-Si. *Mater. Sci. Eng. A* 273–275: 722–726.

Gupta V, Johnson AD, Martynov V. 2001. Sputtered shape memory alloy thin film for medical applications—planar and 3D structures, 4th Pacific Rim International Conference on Advanced Materials and Processing (PRICM4), Honolulu, Hawaii, PRICM 4, Vols. I and II, pp 2347–2349. Dec. 11–15.

Gyobu A, Kawamura Y, Horikawa H, Saburi T. 1999. Two-way shape memory effect of sputter-deposited Ti-rich Ti–Ni alloy films. *Mater. Sci. Eng. A* 273–275: 749–753.

Gyobu A, Kawamura Y, Saburi T, Asai M. 2001. Two-way shape memory effect of sputter-deposited Ti-rich Ti–Ni alloy films. *Mater. Sci. Eng. A* 312: 227–231.

Hassdorf R, Feydt J, Pascal P, Thienhaus S, Boese M, Sterzl T, Winzek B, Noske M. 2002. Phase formation and structural sequence of highly-oriented MBE-grown NiTiCu shape memory thin films. *Mater. Trans.* 43: 933–938.

He Q, Huang WM, Hong MH, Wu MJ, Fu YQ, Chong TC, Chellet F, Du HJ. 2004. Characterization of sputtering deposited NiTi shape memory thin films using a temperature controllable atomic force microscope. *Smart Mater. Struct.* 13: 977.

Himpens JM. 1993. Laparoscopic inguinal hernioplasty repair with a conventional vs. a new self-expandable mesh. *Surg. Endosc.* 7: 315–318.

Ho KK and Carman GP. 2000. Sputter deposition of TiNi thin film shape memory alloy using a heated target. *Thin Solid Films.* 370: 18–29.

Ho KK, Mohanchandra KP, Carman GP. 2002. Examination of the sputtering profile of TiNi under target heating conditions. *Thin Solid Films* 413: 1–7.

Huang WM. 1999. Modified Shape Memory Alloy (SMA) model for SMA wire based actuator design. *J. Intell. Mater. Sys. Struct.* 10: 221–231.

Huang WM and Zhu JJ. 2002. To predict the behavior of shape memory alloys under proportional load. *Mech. Mater.* 34: 547–561.

Huang WM, He Q, Hong MH, Xie Q, Fu YQ, Du HJ. 2002. On the fabrication of TiNi shape memory alloy micro devices using laser. *Photonics Asia 2002*, 14–18 October 2002, Shanghai, China, SPIE Vol. 4915, 234–240.

Huang WM, Liu QY, He LM. 2004. Micro NiTi–Si cantilever with three stable positions. *Sens. Actuators A* 114: 118–122.

Humbeeck JV. 1999. Non-medical applications of shape-memory alloys. *Mater. Sci. Eng. A* 273–275: 134–148.

Iddan G, Meron G, Glukhovsky A, Swain P. 2000. Wireless capsule endoscopy. *Nature* 405: 417.

Inoue H, Miwa N, Inakazu N. 1996. Texture and shape memory strain in TiNi alloy sheets. *Acta Mater.* 44: 4825.

Isalgue A, Torra V, Seguin J-L, Bendahan M, Amigo JM, Esteve-Cano V. 1999. Shape memory TiNi thin films deposited at low temperature. *Mater. Sci. Eng. A* 273–275: 717–721.

Ishida A, Takei A, Sato M, Miyazaki S. 1996. Stress–strain curves of sputtered thin films of Ti–Ni. *Thin Solid Films* 281–282: 337–339.

Ishida A, Sato M and Miyazaki S, Ishida A. 1999. Mechanical properties of Ti–Ni shape memory thin films formed by sputtering. *Mater. Sci. Eng. A* 273–275: 754–757.

Ishida A and Sato M. 2003. Thickness effect on shape memory behavior of Ti–50.0at.%Ni thin film. *Acta Mater.* 51: 5571–5578.

Ishida A, Sato M, Takei A, Miyazaki S. 1995. Effect of heat treatment on shape memory behavior of Ti-rich Ti–Ni thin films. *Mater. Trans., JIM* 36: 1349.

Ishida A, Sato M, Takei A, Nomura K, Miyazaki S. 1996. Effect of aging on shape memory behavior of Ti–51.3 at pct Ni thin films. *Metall. Mater. Trans. A* 27: 3753–3759.

Ishida A, Sato M, Ogawa K. 2008. Microstructure and shape memory behavior of annealed Ti–36.8 at.% Ni–11.6 at.% Cu thin film. *Mater. Sci. Eng. A* 481: 91–94.

Ishida A, Sato M, Yoshikawa W, et al. 2007. Graphical design for thin-film SMA microactuators. *Smart Mater. Struct.* 16: 1672–1677.

James RD and Hane KF. 2000. Martensitic transformations and shape-memory materials. *Acta Mater.* 48: 197–222.

Jin YM and Weng GJ. 2000. Micromechanics study of thermo mechanical characteristics of polycrystal shape-memory alloy films. *Thin Solid Films* 376: 198–207.

Johnson AD. 1991. Vacuum-deposited TiNi shape memory film: characterization and applications in microdevices. *J. Micromechan. Microeng.* 1: 34–41.

Johnson AD. 1999. Thin film shape-memory technology: a tool for MEMS. *Micromach. Devices* 4: 12.

Johnson AD. 2009. Chapters 3 and 10: applications of TiNi thin film shape memory alloys. In *Thin Film Shape Memory Alloys: Fundamentals and Device Applications*, Miyazaki S, Fu YQ, Huang WM (eds.). Cambridge University Press, UK.

Kahn H, Huff MA, Heuer AH. 1998. The TiNi shape-memory alloy and its applications for MEMS, *J. Micromech. Microeng.* 8: 213–221.

Kajiwara S, Kikuchi T, Ogawa K, Matsunaga T, Miyazaki S. 1996. Strengthening of Ti–Ni shape-memory films by coherent subnanometric plate precipitates. *Philos. Mag. Lett.* 74: 137.

Kim CJ, Pisano AP, Muller RS. 1992. Silicon-processed overhanging microgripper. *J. Microelectromech. Syst.* 1: 31–36.

Kirschniak A, Kratt T, Stuker D, Braun A, Schurr MO, Kronigsrainer A. 2007. A new endoscopic over-the-scope clip system for treatment of lesions and bleeding in the GI tract: first clinical experience. *Gastrointest. Endosc.* 66: 162–167.

Ko ST, Airan M, Frank T, Cuschieri A. 1996. Percutaneous endoscopic external ring (PEER) hernio-plasty. *Surg. Endosc.* 10: 690–693.

Kohl M, Dittmann D, Quandt E, Winzek B, Miyazaki S and Allen DM. 1999. Shape memory micro-valves based on thin films or rolled sheets. *Mater. Sci. Eng. A* 273–275: 784–788.

Kohl M, Skrobanek KD, Miyazaki S and Ishida A. 1999. Development of stress-optimised shape memory microvalves. *Sensors and Actuators A* 72: 243–250.

Krulevitch P, Lee AP, Ramsey PB, Trevino JC, Hamilton J, Northrup MA. 1996. Mixed-sputter deposition of Ni–Ti–Cu shape memory films. *J. MEMS* 5: 270–282.

Kulkarni RP, Bellamy EA. 1999. A new thermo-expandable shape-memory nickel-titanium alloy stent for the management of ureteric strictures. *BIU International* 83:755–759.

Lagrange TB and Gotthard R. 2003. Microstructrual evolution and thermo-mechanical response of Ni ion irradiated TiNiSMA thin films. *J. Optoelectr. Adv. Mater.* 5: 313–318.

Lee AP, Ciarlo DR, Krulevitch PA, Lehew S, Trevino J, Northrup MA. 1996. A practical microgripper by fine alignment, eutectic bonding and SMA actuation. *Sens. Actuators A* 54: 755–759.

Lee JW, Thomas B, Rabiei A. 2006. Microstructural study of titanium–palladium–nickel base thin film shape memory alloys. *Thin Solid Film* 500: 309–315.

Lehnert T, Crevoiserat S, Gotthardt R. 2002. Transformation properties and microstructure of sputter-deposited Ni–Ti shape memory alloy thin films. *J. Mater. Sci.* 37: 1523–1533.

Lexcellent C, Moyne S, Ishida A, Miyazaki S. 1998. Deformation behaviour associated with the stress-induced martensitic transformation in Ti–Ni thin films and their thermodynamical modeling. *Thin Solid Films* 324: 184–189.

Liu YS, Xu D, Jiang BH, Yuang ZY, Van Houtte P. 2005. The effect of crystallizing procedure on micro-structure and characteristics of sputter-deposited TiNi shape memory thin films. *J. Micromech. Microeng.* 15: 575–579.

Luo JK, Flewitt AJ, Spearing SM, Fleck NA, Milne WI. 2005. Comparison of microtweezers based on three lateral thermal actuator configurations. *J. Micromech. Microeng.* 15: 1294–1302.

Ma XG and Komvopoulos K. 2003. Nanoscale pseudoelastic behavior of indented titanium–nickel films. *Appl. Phys. Lett.* 83: 3773–3775.

Machens H, Mailaender P, Rieck B, Berger A. 1994. Techniques of postoperative blood flow monitoring after free tissue transfer: an overview. *Microsurgery* 15: 778–786.

Makino E, Mitsuya T, Shibata T. 2000. Micromachining of NiTi shape memory thin film for fabrication of micropump. *Sens. Actuators* 79: 128–135.

Makino E, Mitsuya T, Shibata T. 2001. Fabrication of TiNi shape memory micropump. *Sens. Actuators A* 88: 256–262.

Makino E, Shibata T, Kato K. 1999. Dynamic thermo-mechanical properties of evaporated TiNi shape memory thin film. *Sens. Actuators A* 78: 163–167.

Matsunaga T, Kajiwara S, Ogawa K, Kikuchi T and Miyazaki S, Ishida A. 1999. High strength Ti–Ni-based shape memory thin films. *Mater. Sci. Eng. A* 273–275: 745–748.

Melzer A, Michitsch S, Konak S. 2004. Nitinol in magnetic resonance imaging. *Minim. Invasive Ther. Allied Technol.* 13: 261–271.

Meng XL, Sato M, Ishida A. 2008. Structure of martensite in Ti-rich Ti–Ni–Cu thin films annealed at different temperatures. *Acta Mater.* 56: 3394–3402.

Meng XL, Sato M, Ishida A. 2008. Transmission electron microscopy study of the microstructure of B19 martensite in sputter-deposited $Ti_{50.2}Ni_{30}Cu_{19.8}$ thin films. *Scr. Mater.* 59: 451–454.

Millet O, Bernardoni P, Regnier S, Bidaud P, Tsitsiris E, Collard D, Buchaillot L. 2004. Electrostatic actuated micro gripper using an amplification mechanism. *Sens. Actuators A* 114: 371–378.

Mineta T, Kida N, Nomura S, Makino E, Sugawara T, Toh S, Shibata T. 2008. Pulsation sensor integrated with microvascular holding actuator for thrombosis monitoring. *Sens. Actuators A Phys.* 143: 14–19.

Miyazaki S and Wayman CM. 1988. The R-phase transition and associated shape memory mechanism in TiNi single crystals. *Acta Metall.* 36: 181.

Miyazaki S. 1990. *Engineering Aspects of Shape Memory Alloys*, Duerig TW, et al. (eds.). Butterworth-Heinemann Ltd., London UK 394.

Miyazaki S and Ishida A. 1999. Martensitic transformation and shape memory behavior in sputter-deposited TiNi-base thin films. *Mater. Sci. Eng. A* 273–275: 106–133.

Miyazaki S, Kimura S, Otsuka K. 1988. Shape memory effect and pseudoelectricity associated with the R-phase transition in Ti-50.5 at in single crystals. *Philos. Mag. A* 57: 467.

Miyazaki S, Kimura S, Otsuka K, Suzuki Y. 1984. Shape memory effect and pseudoelectricity in a TiNi single crystals. *Scr. Metall.* 18: 883.

Miyazaki S, Hashinaga T, Ishida A. 1996. Martensitic transformations in sputter-deposited Ti–Ni–Cu shape memory alloy thin films. *Thin Solid Films* 281–282: 364.

Miyazaki S, No VH, Kitamura K, Khantachawwana A, Hosoda H. 2000. Texture of Ti–Ni rolled thin plates and sputter-deposited thin films. *Int. J. Plast.* 16: 1135–1154.

Miyazaki S. 1998. Medical and dental applications of shape memory alloys, Chapter 12. In *Shape Memory Materials*, Otsuka K and Wayman C (eds.). Cambridge University Press, Cambridge, UK.

Miyazaki S and Otsuka K. 1989. Development of Shape Memory Alloys. *ISIJ Int.* 29: 353–377.

Miyazaki S. 2009, Chapter 2: Martensitic transformation in shape memory alloys. In *Thin Film Shape Memory Alloys: Fundamentals and Device Applications*, Miyazaki S, Fu YQ, Huang WM (eds.). Cambridge University Press, UK.

Miyazaki S, Tomozawa M, Kim HY. 2009. Binary and ternary alloy film diaphragm microactuators, Chapter 12. In *Thin Film Shape Memory Alloys: Fundamentals and Device Applications*, Miyazaki S, Fu YQ, Huang WM (eds.). Cambridge University Press, UK.

Moyne S, Poilane C, Kitamura K, Miyazaki S, Delobelle P, Lexcellent C. 1999. Analysis of the thermo mechanical behavior of Ti–Ni shape memory alloy thin films by bulging and nanoindentation procedures. *Mater. Sci. Eng. A* 273–275: 727–732.

Mohanchandra KP and Carman GP. 2009. TiNi thin films devices, Chapter 13. In *Thin Film Shape Memory Alloys: Fundamentals and Device Applications*, Miyazaki S, Fu YQ, Huang WM (eds.). Cambridge University Press, UK.

Musialek J, Filip P, Nieslanik J. 1998. Titanium–nickel shape memory clamps in small bone surgery. *Arch. Orthop. Trauma Surg.* 117: 341–344.

Murray JL. 1987. *Phase Diagrams of Binary Titanium Alloys, Monograph Series on Alloy Phase Diagrams*. ASM International. Metals Park, OH, USA.

Nakamura T, Fukui H, Ishii Y. 2000. Shape memory alloy loop snare for endoscopic photodynamic therapy of early gastric cancer. *Endoscopy* 32: 609–613.

Neuman KC, Hadd EH, Liou GF, Bergman K, Block SM. 1999. Characterization of photodamage to Escherichia coli in optical traps. *Biophys. J.* 77: 2856–2863.

Ng Y, Song C, McLean D, Shimi SM, et al. 2003. Optimized deployment of heat-activated surgical staples using thermography. *Appl. Phys. Lett.* 83: 1884–1886.

Ni W, ChengYT, Grummon DS. 2002. Recovery of microindents in a nickel–titanium shape-memory alloy: a "self-healing" effect. *Appl. Phys. Lett.* 80: 3310–3312.

Nishida M and Honma T. 1984. All round shape memory effect in Ni rich TiNi alloys generated by constrained aging. *Scr. Metall.* 18: 1293.

Nishiyama Z. 1978. *Martensitic Transformation*. Academic Press Inc., USA.

Ohta A, Bhansali S, Kishimoto I, Umeda A. 2000. Novel fabrication technique of TiNi shape memory alloy film using separate Ti and Ni targets. *Sens. Actuators A* 86: 165–170.

Otsuka K and Ren X. 2005. Physical metallurgy of Ti–Ni-based shape memory alloys. *Prog. Mater. Sci.* 50: 511–678.

Otsuka K and Wayman C. 1989. *Shape Memory Materials.* Cambridge University Press, Cambridge, UK.

Pan CS and Hsu WY. 1997. An electro-thermally and laterally driven polysilicon microactuator. *J. Micromech. Microeng.* 7: 7–13.

Quandt E, Halene C, Holleck H, Feit K, Kohl M, Schloßmacher P, Skokan A, Skrobanek KD. 1996. Sputter deposition of NiTi, NiTiPd and TiPd films displaying the two-way shape-memory effect. *Sens. Actuators A* 53: 434–439.

Raju GS and Gajula L. 2004. Endoclips for GI endoscopy. *Gastrointest. Endosc.* 59: 267–279.

Reichle C, Schnelle T, Müller T, Leya T, Fuhr G. 2000. A new microsystem for automated electrorotation measurements using laser tweezers. *Biochim. Biophys. Acta* 1459: 218–229.

Reynaerts D, Peirs J, Van Brussel H. 1997. An implantable drug-delivery system based on shape memory alloy micro-actuation. *Sens. Actuators A* 61: 455–462.

Rhalmi S, Odin M, Assad M, et al. 1999. Hard, soft tissue and in vitro cell response to porous nickel-titanium: a biocompatibility evaluation. *Biomed. Mater. Eng.* 9: 151–162.

Sawaguchi T, Sato M, Ishida A. 2002. Microstructure and shape memory behavior of Ti–51.2 (Pd27.0Ni21.8) and Ti–49.5(Pd28.5Ni22.0) thin films. *Mater. Sci. Eng. A* 332: 47–55.

Seguin JL, Bendahan M, Isalgue A, Esteve-Cano V, Carchano H, Torra V. 1999. Low temperature crystallised Ti-rich NiTi shape memory alloy films for microactuators. *Sens. Actuators* 74: 65–69.

Seidemann V, Butefisch S, Buttgenbach S. 2002. Fabrication and investigation of in-plane compliant SU8 structures for MEMS and their application to micro valves and micro grippers. *Sens. Actuators A* 97–98: 457–461.

Shaw GA, Stone DD, Johnson AD, Ellis AB, Crone WC. 2003. Shape memory effect in nanoindentation of nickel–titanium thin films. *Appl. Phys. Lett.* 83: 257–259.

Shaw GA, Trethewey JS, Johnson AD, Drugan WJ, Crone WC. 2005. Thermomechanical high-density data storage in a metallic material via the shape-memory effect. *Adv. Mater.* 17: 1123–1127.

Shih CL, Lai BK, Kahn H, Philips SM, Heuer AH. 2001. A robust co-sputtering fabrication procedure for TiNi shape memory alloys for MEMS. *J. MEMS* 10: 69–79.

Shin DD, Lee DG, Mohanchandra KP, et al. 2006. Thin film NiTi microthermostat array. *Sens. Actuators A* 130: 37–41.

Shu YC and Bhattacharya K. 1998. The influence of texture on the shape-memory effect in polycrystals. *Acta Mater.* 46: 5457–5473.

Simon M, Kaplan R, Salzman E, Freiman DA. 1977. Vena cava filter using thermal shape memory alloy. *Radiology.* 125: 87–94.

Small W, Wilson TS, Buckley PR, Benett WJ, Loge JA, Hartman J, Maitland DJ. 2007. Prototype fabrication and preliminary in vitro testing of a shape memory endovascular thrombectomy device. *IEEE Trans. Biomed. Eng.* 54: 1657–1666.

Snow S and Jacobsen SC. 2006. Microfabrication processes on cylindrical substrates—Part I: Material deposition and removal. *Microelectron. Eng.* 83: 2534–2542.

Snow S and Jacobsen SC. 2007. Microfabrication processes on cylindrical substrates—Part II: Lithography and connections. *Microelectron. Eng.* 84: 11–20.

Song C, Campbell P, Frank T, Cuschieri A. 2002. Thermal modelling of shape memory alloy fixator for medical application. *Smart Mater. Struct.* 11: 1–5.

Song C, Frank T, Cuschieri A. 2005. Shape memory alloy clip for compression colonic anastomosis. *J. Biomech. Eng. Trans. ASME* 127: 351–354.

Sousa JE, Costa MA, Abizaid A. 2001. Lack of neointimal proliferation after implantation of sirolimus-coated stents in human coronary arteries: a quantitative coronary angiography and three-dimensional intravascular ultrasound study. *Circulation* 103: 192–195.

Stemmer S, Duscher G, Scheu C, Heuer AH, Ruhle M. 1997. The reaction between a TiNi shape memory thin film and silicon. *J. Mater. Res.* 12: 1734–1740.

Stepan LL, Levi DS, Carman GP. 2005. A thin film Nitinol heart valve. *J. Biomech. Eng. ASME Trans.* 127: 915–918.

Sugawara T, Hirota K, Watanabe M, Mineta T, Makino E, Toh S, Shibata T. 2006. Shape memory thin film actuator for holding a fine blood vessel. *Sens. Actuators A* 130/131: 461–467.

Surbled P, Clerc C, Pioufle BL, Afaka M, Fujita H. 2001. Effect of the composition and thermal annealing on the transformation temperatures of sputtered TiNi shape memory alloy thin films. *Thin Solid Films* 401: 52–59.

Takabayashi S, Tanino E, Fukumoto S, Mimatsu Y, Yamashita S, Ichikawa Y. 1996. Functionally gradient TiNi films fabricated by sputtering. *Jpn. J. Appl. Phys.* 35: 200–204.

Takeuchi S and Shimoyama I. 2000. A three-dimensional shape memory alloy microelectrode with clipping structure for insect neural recording. *J. MEMS* 9: 24–31.

Tan L and Crone WC. 2002. Surface characterization of TiNi modified by plasma source ion implantation. *Acta Mater.* 50: 4449–4460.

Tan SM and Miyazaki S. 1997. Ti-content and annealing temperature dependence of deformation characteristics of TiXNi(92-X)Cu-8 shape memory alloys. *Acta Mater.* 46: 2729.

Terzo G. 2008. Capital market crusaders; activist investors strike out, and corporate America strikes back. *The Investments Dealers' Digest: IDD*, 74(48), 10.

Tomozawa M, Kim HY, Miyazaki S. 2006. Microactuators using R-phase transformation of sputter-deposited Ti–47.3Ni shape memory alloy thin films. *J. Intel. Mater. Syst. Struct.* 17: 1049–1058.

Tomozawa M, Okutsu K, Kim HY, Miyazaki S. 2005. Characterization of high-speed microactuator utilizing shape memory alloy thin films. *Mater. Sci. Forum* 475–479: 2037–2042.

Tsui YC and Clyne TW. 1997. An analytical model for predicting residual stresses in progressively deposited coatings: 1. Planar geometry. *Thin Solid Films* 306: 23.

Volland BE. 2002. Electrostatically driven microgripper. *Microelectron. Eng.* 61: 1015.

Volland BE, Heerlein H, Rangelow IW. 2002. Electrostatically driven microgripper, *Microelectron. Eng.* 61–62: 1015–1023.

Walker JA, Gabriel KJ, Mehregany M. 1990. Thin film processing of shape memory alloy. *Sens. Actuators A* 21–23: 243.

Wan D and Komvopoulos K. 2005. Thickness effect on thermally induced phase transformations in sputtered titanium–nickel shape-memory films. *J. Mater Res.* 20: 1606.

Wang RX, Zohar Y, Wong M. 2002. Residual stress-loaded titanium–nickel shape-memory alloy thin-film micro-actuators. *J. Micromech. Microeng.* 12: 323–327.

Wang X, Rein M, Vlassak JJ. 2008. Crystallization kinetics of amorphous equiatomic NiTi thin films: effect of film thickness. *J. Appl. Phys.* 103: 023501.

Wang ZG and Zu XT. 2005. Incomplete transformation induced multiple-step transformation in TiNi shape memory alloys. *Scr. Mater.* 53: 335.

Wang ZG, Zu XT, Fu YQ, Wang LM. 2005. Temperature memory effect in TiNi-based shape memory alloys. *Thermochim. Acta* 428: 199.

Waye JD. 2003. Small-bowel endoscopy. *Endoscopy* 35: 15.

Wierzbicki R, Houston K, Heerlein H, Barth W, Debski T, Eisinberg A, Menciassi A, Carrozza MC, Dario P. 2006. Design and fabrication of an electrostatically driven microgripper for blood vessel manipulation. *Microelectron. Eng.* 83: 1651–1654.

Winzek B and Quandt E. 1999. Shape-memory Ti–Ni–X-films (X = Cu, Pd) under constraint. *Z Metallkd.* 90: 796–802.

Winzek B, Schmitz S, Rumpf H, Sterzl T, Hassdorf R, Thienhaus S, Feydt J, Moske M, Quandt E. 2004. Recent developments in shape memory thin film technology. *Mater. Sci. Eng. A* 378: 40–46.

Wolf RH and Heuer AH. 1995. TiNi shape-memory alloy and its applications for MEMS. *J. MEMS* 4: 206–212.

Wood AJM, Sanjabi S, Fu YQ. 2008. Nanoindentation of binary and ternary Ni–Ti-based shape memory alloy thin films. *Surf. Coat. Technol.* 202: 3115–3120.

Wu MJ and Huang WM. 2006. In situ characterization of NiTi based shape memory thin films by optical measurement. *Smart Mater. Struct.* 15: N29–N35.

Wu SK, Chen JZ, Wu YJ, Wang JY, Yu MN, Chen FR, Kai JJ. 2001. Interfacial microstructures of rf-sputtered TiNi shape memory alloy thin films on (100) silicon, *Philos. Mag. A* 81: 1939–1949.

Xu D, Wang L, Ding GF, Zhou Y, Yu AB, Cai BC. 2001. Characteristics and fabrication of TiNi/Si diaphragm micropump. *Sens. Actuators A* 93: 87–92.

Xu W, Frank TG, Stockham G, Cuschieri A. 1999. Shape memory alloy fixator for suturing tissue in minimal access surgery. *Ann. Biomed. Eng.* 27: 663–669.

Yan W, Sun Q, Feng XQ, Qian L. 2006. Determination of transformation stresses of shape memory alloy thin films: a method based on spherical indentation. *Appl. Phys. Lett.* 88: 241912.

Zamponi C, Rumpf H, Schmutz C, Quandt E. 2008. Structuring of sputtered superelastic NiTi thin films by photolithography and etching. *Mater. Sci. Eng. A* 481–482: 623–625.

Zeng YJ, Cui LS, Schrooten J. 2004. Temperature memory effect of a nickel-titanium shape memory alloy. *Appl. Phys. Lett.* 84: 31.

Zhang JX, Sato M, Ishida A. 2006. Deformation mechanism of martensite in Ti-rich Ti–Ni shape memory alloy thin films. *Acta Mater.* 54: 1185–1198.

Zhang YJ, Cheng YT, Grummon DS. 2005. Finite element modeling of indentation-induced superelastic effect using a three-dimensional constitutive model for shape memory materials with plasticity. *J. Appl. Phys.* 98: 033505.

Zhang Y, Cheng Y-T, Grummon DS. 2006a. Shape memory surfaces. *Appl. Phys. Lett.* 89: 041912.

Zhang Y, Cheng Y-T, Grummon DS. 2006b. Two-way indent depth recovery in a NiTi shape memory alloy. *Appl. Phys. Lett.* 88: 131904.

Zhu TJ, Zhao XB, Lu L. 2006. Pb(Zr0.52Ti0.48)O-3/TiNi multilayered heterostructures on Si substrates for smart systems. *Thin Solid Films* 515: 1445–1449.

10

Bioactive Coatings for Implanted Devices

Subbu Venkatraman, Xia Yun, Huang Yingying, Debasish Mondal, and Liu Kerh Lin

CONTENTS

Introduction and Brief Historic Survey 471
Bioactive Coatings Type 1: Controlled Bioactive Elution..472
    Applications 472
    Cardiovascular Coating..472
        Cardiovascular Stent Coatings 473
        Other Stent Coatings and Bioactives 475
        Drug-Eluting Balloons..477
    Other Bioactive-Eluting Implants: Orthopedic Applications 478
Bioactive Coatings II: Surface Modification for Cellular Interactions..............................479
    Platelet Interactions...480
    Endothelialization of Biomaterial Surfaces 482
    Topological Modification 483
    Chemical Modification 483
    Micropatterning...484
Status and Prognosis..485
References..485

Introduction and Brief Historic Survey

One of the earliest successful bioactive coatings was that of a heparin-modified surface of a polymer blood oxygenator component trademarked as Carmeda Affinity Blood Oxygenator Trillium Affinity NT Blood Oxygenator, which received FDA approval in 1997. This bioactive surface was based on a poly(ethylene oxide)-coupled heparin immobilization on a hollow porous membrane used as part of an oxygenator used in bypass surgery, for instance. Since then, several types of heparin-modified surfaces have been introduced in various devices, including chronic dialysis catheter (Bridges, 2007), stent coatings (Michael et al., 2003), blood oxygenators (Okkema et al., 1991) as well as other components of the adult perfusion circuit. The FDA Web site lists an extensive array of such devices. In our opinion, heparin modification of surfaces is the most successful coating technology so far for indwelling or implanted medical devices.

The other area of bioactive coating research involves hard-tissue implants, such as an artificial hip or knee joint. Here, the issue is acceleration of healing to reduce immobilization time for surgery patients. Thus, the role of the coating is to induce bone cell attachment and proliferation on the implant surface. The first commercialization was a calcium phosphate coating for titanium-based hip joints (Epinette et al., 2004), whereas cervical disks have also been coated (Helmut et al., 2004). Other coatings have been used to minimize frictional resistance and wear debris; such coatings are not considered strictly bioactive.

Coatings that elute bioactive compounds locally to enhance efficacy have also been the focus of research for several decades. Stemming from the unprecedented success of drug-eluting stents (DES), research has intensified in this area (Venkatraman and Boey, 2007). Other applications include coatings that elute bone morphogenic protein (BMP) in osteo implants (Sohier et al., 2010), antifouling or antibiotic coatings, and coated micro- and nanoparticles that have controlled the release of a bioactive. In this chapter, we discuss both types of bioactive surfaces, the ones that involve elution of a bioactive compound and the ones that involve immobilization of bioactive molecules.

Bioactive Coatings Type 1: Controlled Bioactive Elution

These coatings may be on metallic devices (osteo implants, stents) or part of a fully poly-meric device (biodegradable stents).

Applications

Invariably, the major objective of a drug-eluting coating on an implant is to localize and sustain the release of a bioactive, thereby enhancing its bioavailability and minimizing systemic side effects. The idea is simple, yet surprisingly this concept did not enjoy com-mercial success until the advent of the drug-eluting coronary stents in 2002. Attempts to improve the performance of osteo implants using BMP have not enjoyed a similar level of success, however. Also, although incorporation of antibiotics into bone cement has been successful, coating of the device (such as an artificial hip joint shaft) to release an antibi-otic has not yet been clinically successful (Pioletti et al., 2008). Similarly, bisphosphonate (BP)-releasing coatings are the subject of intensive investigation at present (Roussiere et al., 2005), but clinically not yet proven to be effective. Therefore, in what follows, we will focus on drug- and bioactive-eluting stents.

Cardiovascular Coating

The use of the so-called bare metal stents results in an unacceptable rate of restenosis in coronary arteries. To overcome this problem, stents that elute antiproliferative drugs were first approved in the US in April 2003. The first such stent was a sirolimus-eluting stent (SES, Cypher®) developed by the Cordis division of Johnson and Johnson; the sec-ond one to win approval was a paclitaxel-eluting stent (PES, Taxus®) developed by Boston Scientific and approved in March 2004. The market acceptance of these stents was spec-tacular, with the DES displacing about 90% of the implantations previously done with BMS in 2006 (Venkatraman and Boey, 2007). Such successes led to several other com-panies developing DES. Approved stents include Endeavor®, developed by Medtronic/ Abbott Labs and approved in February 2008 and Xience™ developed by Guidant/Abbott Vascular and approved in July 2008. Other DES approved ex-US includes the Infinnium® stent (Sahajanand Medical Technologies) as well as the Axxion® (Biosensors Int) stainless steel stent. Clearly, in spite of potential problems associated with the use of DES, such stents continue to be implanted in coronary disease patients, although their share of the market vis-à-vis the bare metals tent has dwindled somewhat.

Cardiovascular Stent Coatings

The Cypher stent is a 316 stainless steel, with a three-layer coating as shown schematically in Figure 10.1.

The PEVAC (Poly (ethylene-co-vinyl acetate)) is a biostable copolymer of ethylene and vinyl acetate, whereas the PBMA (Poly (butyl methacrylate)) is the biostable poly butyl methacrylate polymer. The layer in contact with the stainless steel is a parylene primer layer that is applied to enhance the adhesion of the top two layers. The total thickness is 12.6 μm (2 μm Parylene C base coat; 10 μm main coat of PEVAC, PBMA, and sirolimus; and a 0.6 μm top coat of PBMA). The drug is sirolimus and is dispersed in the middle layer at a loading of about 111 μg/stent for a 3-mm-diameter, 13-mm-long stent, data published in the FDA Web site. The approved product used relatively slow-release kinetics, with the entire drug content being delivered in about 90 days in vitro (Venkatraman and Boey, 2007). Although the reservoir/membrane structure should enable the so-called zero-order kinetics of release of drug, this is not observed in practice, most likely because of the drug redistribution into the top layer, effectively making this a matrix system.

Clinically, this stent performed well, as reported in several studies (Sousa et al., 2001, 2003; Fröbert et al., 2009). In larger studies (19,004 patients in Sweden), the overall restenosis rate appears to be about 5% for Cypher.

The Taxus stent has a biostable coating as well, made of a rubbery polymer, styrene-*b*-isobutylene-*b*-styrene (SIBS) terpolymer (Ranade et al., 2004). Paclitaxel is dispersed in this coating (thickness about 16 μm) at a loading of about 79 μg for a 3-mm-diameter, 12-mm-long stainless steel stent, as shown in the FDA Web site. There is no primer coating and no top coat of drug-free polymer. Although diffusion of the paclitaxel drug through the rubbery matrix should be relatively fast, this coating retains the drug for up to 180 days (Venkatraman and Boey, 2007) because of the compatibility (solubility) of the drug in this particular polymer.

Clinical studies on a large scale show restenosis rates comparable to the Cypher stent at 2 years.

The Endeavor stent is based on a cobalt–chromium alloy and presents a lower profile. The coating is made of phosphorylcholine (PC) head group, which is a phospholipid, that is co-polymerized with some acrylate monomers. The PC head group forms are present in most of the phospholipids in the cell membrane of a red blood cell, as shown in Figure 10.2.

This PC head group is polymerized with a mixture of lauryl methacrylate, hydroxy-propyl methacrylate and trimethoxysilylpropyl methacrylate (crosslinker) to yield the PC polymer. It is not clear whether the polymer is in fact crosslinked because the FDA document indicates that the polymer is applied via coating from ethanol solutions.

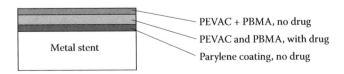

FIGURE 10.1
Schematic representation of the cross-section of the coating on the Cypher stent.

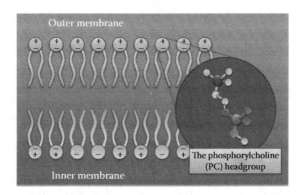

FIGURE 10.2
Schematic representation of the PC molecules self-assembled in a membrane; this material is used as coating for targeted local delivery of zotarolimus to the artery.

There is a base layer of PC polymer, then a drug-containing layer of the PC polymer, and a third layer of drug-free PC polymer. The total thickness is about 4.3 μm, with a base coat of 1 μm. The drug is a sirolimus derivative, known as zotarolimus, and is dispersed in the PC coating at a loading of about 150 μg in a 3-mm-diameter, 15-mm-long stent. Although not much information is available regarding the release kinetics, it is expected to be similar to that of sirolimus release from the Cypher stent.

In clinical studies, as reported by Medtronic, a comparative study involving approximately 500–600 patients per cohort, it was found that the target lesion revascularization rate (TLR, related to restenosis) was about 7.5% for Endeavor at 5 years, compared with 11.9% (Cypher) and 9.1% (Taxus). However, the large Swedish study mentioned above reported that Endeavor had a statistically higher restenosis rate compared with Cypher at 2 years.

The Xience V stent has a base coating of poly(*n*-butyl acrylate) with a drug-containing layer of a fluoropolymer, poly(vinylidene fluoride-*co*-hexafluoropropylene) or PVDF-HFP. The poly(*n*-butyl acrylate) is a base coating (~1 μm), while a thicker (7.6 μm) PVDF-HFP coating containing drug is added on top with no top-coat. The drug is everolimus and loaded at about 150 μg for a 3-mm-diameter, 15-mm-long stent.

The release profile consists of a burst of about 25% released in the first day, followed by 75% release in a month and complete (100%) release in 4 months (Sheiban et al., 2008). In clinical trials using this stent (e.g., in the SPIRIT III trial involving a total of 1002 patients, randomized to Xience V (*n* = 669) vs. Taxus (*n* = 333)), a restenosis rate of 2.6% was reported for Xience as compared with 5% for Taxus (Sheiban et al., 2008). Longer-term and larger cohort study data are not yet available for this stent, but are expected to be similar to the others reported above.

Biosensors International has developed a biodegradable coating with incorporation of another sirolimus derivative, which is given the name Biolimus®. This is the first successful clinical trial using a biodegradable coating on a stainless steel stent. The Biolimus is loaded or dispersed into a poly(L-lactide) polymer, which is coated from solution onto the abluminal side of the stent. The polymer is said to degrade completely in vivo in about 6–8 months (Grube and Buellefeld, 2006). Clinical study results were favorable (Windecker et al., 2008) showing "noninferiority" to the Cypher stent in 2-year follow-up. Although not explicitly stated, the PLA polymer appears to be of low molecular mass, and the thickness is probably about 5–7 μm; together, these ensure fairly rapid absorption of the coating in vivo.

Our group at Nanyang Technological University (NTU), has also been developing a coated stent, based on a Co–Cr stent that has won CE approval (Huang et al., 2009) as a bare metal stent. We have also employed a PLGA-based coating that is completely biodegradable and incorporates two drugs, sirolimus and an antithrombotic, triflusal (Huang et al., 2010). As shown in Figure 10.3, the co-elution of the two drugs does improve restenosis rates favorably in a 30-day pig model compared with stents eluting only sirolimus. We postulate that this improvement is related to the minimization of thrombosis by the dual drug-eluting stent that helps to also minimize eventual stenosis. There is some evidence in the literature attesting to thrombi acting as scaffolds for eventual stenosis (Lowe et al., 2001).

In summary, it should be noted that the whole concept of localized delivery of bioactives using coatings on a device has gathered momentum only after the success of the first DES for the coronary artery in 2003. The consequent introduction of several DES is testimony to its continuing use. Nevertheless, it is now accepted that the use of these types of drugs (cytostatic in the case of sirolimus and derivatives; cytotoxic in the case of paclitaxel) leads to delayed endothelialization, and, hence, to fatal thrombosis in some cases (Chen et al., 2005; Venkatraman and Boey, 2007; Kukreja et al., 2008). This happens because of the nonselective nature of the drugs that affect not only the smooth muscle cells involved in restenosis but also the endothelial cells that usually cover the stent completely. If endothelialization is delayed or incomplete, the exposed metal/polymer surface can initiate what is called "late-stage" thrombosis (which could happen anytime after 6 months) which can be fatal. Conversely, apprehension regarding late-stage thrombosis has led to continuation of antiplatelet therapy beyond the usual 1-year period, such therapy has its own set of undesirable side effects. Hence it is imperative that the next generation of coated stents does not cause delayed endothelialization. This may be achieved using selective drugs or compounds, or alternatively encouraging endothelial cell attachment and proliferation. Both approaches are the focus of intensive research, as described in the following sections.

Other Stent Coatings and Bioactives

There is considerable literature on coating materials for stents, as well as on different bioactive compounds incorporated into such coatings. Most of these studies are in the preclinical phase. We highlight some of the more interesting advances below.

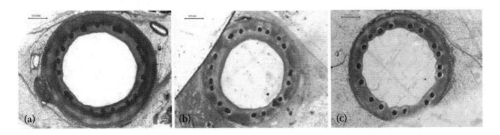

FIGURE 10.3
Overview of stented artery at 4 weeks showing the comparison in neointimal area in fBMS (a), stent with sirolimus only (b) and stent with sirolimus and triflusal (c) groups (bar = 500 μm).

Various biodegradable polymers have been employed as carrier coatings, including collagen (Chen et al., 2005) with sirolimus and a PLGA grafted with polyvinyl alcohol (Wested et al., 2006) to increase water uptake and, hence, degradation rate. The graft copolymer did not increase degradation rate but appeared to give a slightly more linear release rate of paclitaxel dissolved in the coating. The clinical significance of this linearity of rate is unclear, however.

A different approach was to use a degradable polymer based on poly(salicylic acid) and poly(adipic acid) (Jabara et al., 2008). This polymer degrades into salicylic and adipic acids, which are deemed as acceptable degradation products. The in vitro degradation time is 4–6 weeks, and the pig study was carried out over 4 weeks. The stent coated with just the polymer (PSA) did not reduce restenosis compared with BMS; however, incorporation of sirolimus in the coating did. Nevertheless, a tendency of the PSA-coated stent to lower inflammatory scores was noted. Whether suppression of the inflammatory response is beneficial is not clear because there is a chance that this may delay the healing process further. It was also not possible, from the study design, to determine whether acute thrombosis was reduced with the salicylate coating.

As of this writing, there is a bewildering range of coatings available for DES. Many polymers may be coated either directly on the metal or on a parylene-coated metal surface with reasonable adhesion and resistance to cracking under balloon expansion. What appears to be lacking, however, is a range of new, more selective antiproliferation compounds. The issue of endothelialization is still the key to the continued use of DES, and although biodegradable coatings help in this regard (by ensuring complete release of drug into tissue), the drugs themselves are hydrophobic and are not cleared rapidly from tissue.

The search for alternatives to sirolimus (and limus compounds) and paclitaxel continues. An early candidate was heparin, although this was more to reduce thrombosis than restenosis. Combining an antiproliferative in a heparin-polymer yielded some interesting results (Leea et al., 2007). In this case, heparin was hydrophobically modified using polyacrylic acid and *N*-hydroxy succinimide. The resulting polymer was dissolved in cyclohexane. A base coat of polyurethane was sprayed onto a stainless steel stent and then dipped in the cyclohexane solution of the modified heparin. The resulting coating showed some antiplatelet activity in vitro, confirming, to some degree, the retained bioactivity of heparin (in spite of dissolution in an organic solvent). The drug used was echinomycin, a potent anticancer drug, not known for its selectivity. The 30-day pig study indicated reduction in stenosis for the 5% echinomycin loading in the coating, although this is evident more through histological micrographs than any calculated % stenosis values. Disappointingly, the stent with a top-coated heparin polymer alone (no echinomycin) appeared to not have been used as one of the controls; hence, it is difficult to draw any conclusions regarding minimization of thrombosis by the heparin.

An interesting compound that has been studied for its antiproliferative and antithrombotic effects is curcumin, obtained from turmeric, which belongs to the ginger family. The curcumin is hydrophobic and dissolves in organic solvents. A solution with PLGA was spray-coated to a home-made stainless steel stent (Pan et al., 2006). The resulting coating appeared to be robust and withstood the balloon expansion of the stent quite well. In vitro activated partial thromplastin time (APTT) studies showed an increased time for the curcumin-containing samples approaching 45 to 50 s, although it is not clear that sufficient curcumin would have been released in this period (and in the 3 min of prior incubation). An in vitro study (Nguyen et al., 2004) showed that PLLA films containing curcumin inhibited SMC proliferation (but not attachment).

A recent rabbit iliac artery implantation of curcumin-eluting stents has been reported (Jang et al., 2009). The 30-day study showed some antirestenotic effects of both a low (50 μg) and a high dose (500 μg) of curcumin. The higher dose of curcumin led to % restenosis of about 18% vs. about 30% for the bare metal stent, which is encouraging. It is not clear how the curcumin was released in a sustained manner (as is claimed for the higher dose) because the curcumin is loaded onto the stent by dip-coating with no polymeric carrier. Nevertheless, the results warrant further investigation into this compound, which is claimed to have antiproliferative as well as antithrombotic effects.

Therapeutic genes addressing cardiovascular diseases have also been studied for stent-based delivery. Several targets for restenosis are available (Sanghong and Keith, 1998), including proteins that are cytostatic and cytotoxic, as well as overproduction of enzymes such as NO synthase (endothelial cell-derived) which appear to have both antiaggregation (platelets) as well as antiproliferation (SMC) activity. Stent-based delivery of plasmid DNA (pDNA) was demonstrated in 2000 (Klugherz et al., 2000) both in vitro and in vivo, using an emulsion coating of pDNA in PLGA solution (chloroform). About 1 mg of pDNA was present per stent. The PLGA type (i.e., ratio of GA to LA) is not mentioned, but it is presumably a 50:50 PLGA of molecular mass about 50,000 Da. There is a burst release of pDNA followed by sustained release over a week. Expression of green fluorescent protein in local tissue is shown via fluorescence quantification. Surprisingly, the pDNA appears to transfect cells locally, even though in cell culture the extent of transfection is low.

Sustained release of both pDNA and complexed pDNA (which is better at transfecting cells) is critical for the success of a stent-based system. We have been studying the release of such pDNA in our laboratory (Ramgopal et al., 2007; Ramgopal et al., 2009). Not all biodegradable polymers may be used as carriers; for example, rapidly degrading PLGA is not suitable (Ramgopal et al., 2008), either due to lowered pH or due to a coating by the oligomers around the pDNA. Sustained delivery of bioactive pDNA is achievable for up to 20 days using certain formulations. Beyond this time frame, the complexed or naked pDNA appear to aggregate excessively and/or become decomplexed.

Our group has also developed noncardiovascular stents that elute bioactives. One of these is a tracheal stent that elutes mitomycin to prevent restenosis, and another is a ureteric stent that elutes antibiotics locally. Both of these prototypes have undergone animal testing with successful outcomes and await further refinement.

In summary, a variety of alternatives to cytotoxic/cytostatic drugs has been explored for stent-based delivery. None has made it to clinical trials yet, although curcumin-eluting stents are now being studied in man. Until there is demonstrated evidence of selectivity in terms of SMC inhibition without delayed endothelialization, new compounds are unlikely to be accepted in the marketplace. There is considerable promise for gene-eluting stents because the genes are, by definition, selective in their action.

Drug-Eluting Balloons

Given the issue of delayed endothelialization with DES, another concept is gaining attention. These are coated angioplasty balloons that can deliver the same drugs (paclitaxel, sirolimus). Drug-eluting balloons (DEBs) have some advantages over DES:

(1) They can be used to treat in-stent restenosis (ISR).

(2) The drug is released into tissue in about a minute or less, and is probably cleared from the tissue in 1 or 2 weeks.

(3) There is no sustained delivery of the drugs over many months, as is the case with some DES.

(4) In all likelihood, the use of a DEB will not produce delayed endothelialization, hence antiplatelet therapy may be stopped sooner.

(5) DEBs may offer the possibility of better lesion coverage.

Several companies are working on introducing DEBs to the market (Waksman and Pakala, 2009). The ones in advanced stages include Elutax® developed by Aachen Resonance in Germany, Sequent® Please developed by Braun Melsungen AG, and DIOR® developed by Eurocor AG. All of the balloons appear to be simply coated with drug solutions, perhaps when expanded, and then deflated to entrap solid drug in pockets. A slight variation on this theme is the addition of the main component of x-ray contrast medium, iopromide, to act as a "matrix" for the paclitaxel. This hydrophilic matrix (used in the Sequent Please balloon) apparently allows for more complete delivery of the drug from the balloon into tissue (Scheller et al., 2004) and, consequently, better results in inhibiting restenosis in a porcine coronary artery model compared with paclitaxel trapped on roughened balloon surfaces (Cremers et al., 2009).

Clinical studies with DEBs have been very encouraging. One study compared the coated balloon to a paclitaxel-eluting stent (Unverdorben et al., 2009), and found late loss at 12 months to be significantly lower for the balloon compared to the stent. Adverse events were also significantly fewer in the DEB cohort. Paclitaxel appears to be the drug of choice in these DEBs, primarily because of the long retention time in tissue of paclitaxel after administration (Mori et al., 2006).

The predominant use of DEBs is for treatment of ISR, as double-stenting in the same area is not advisable. ISR rates (as mentioned before) for DES are about 8–10%, and DEBs have taken over this segment of the market. With improved methods of delivery and more clinical data, it is likely that DEBs will continue to make further inroads into the DES segment.

Other Bioactive-Eluting Implants: Orthopedic Applications

As mentioned in the "Introduction," there are very few coated implants, other than stents, that release bioactive compounds in vivo. The field of bioactive coatings for osteo implants (Figure 10.4) has been covered well in a 2008 review (Pioletti et al., 2008).

Of the various options, the first is a coating of a carrier film containing the bioactive molecule, and this carrier film may be a calcium phosphate or a polymer. The second and third options involve incorporation of drug into the body of the implant and will not concern us here.

Of the bioactives that have been studied, the most clinically relevant ones appear to be bisphosphonates, or BP and bone morphogenic protein, or BMP. BP are excellent molecules for inhibition of osteoclasts and thus help in minimizing bone resorption. Clinically, their administration is done primarily to prevent or minimize bone loss in osteoporosis, Paget's disease, bone lytic tumors, and periodontal disease. However, their use in coated osteoimplants is being increasingly recognized.

BPs target the catabolic phase of bone remodeling, where the osteoclasts are active in removing callus. BMP is involved in the anabolic phase, where tissue regeneration occurs. However, the required physiological dose of BMP required to inhibit osteoclasts is high and so is the cost. Therefore, BPs appear to be the agent of choice in osteoimplants.

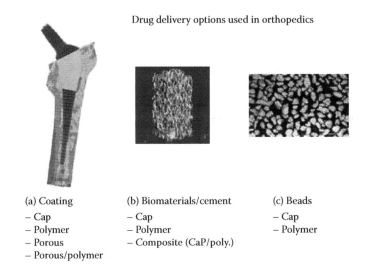

Drug delivery options used in orthopedics

(a) Coating
  – Cap
  – Polymer
  – Porous
  – Porous/polymer

(b) Biomaterials/cement
  – Cap
  – Polymer
  – Composite (CaP/poly.)

(c) Beads
  – Cap
  – Polymer

FIGURE 10.4
Drug delivery options used in orthopedics: (a) drug coating on an implant, (b) drug incorporation in a scaffold or cement, and (c) drug incorporation in beads, as described by Pioletti et al. (*Current Drug Delivery*, 5, 59–63, 2008; with permission).

BP are generally delivered from a CaP coating. In particular, calcium-deficient apatites (CDA) have been used to complex with BP such as zoledronate (Roussiere et al., 2005). Release is controlled by disassociation of the complex. The efficacy of the BPs has been demonstrated in an in vivo study involving rats (Peter et al., 2005). Here, a titanium implant was inserted into the femur, and bone density was followed as a function of distance from the implants. The implants were first coated with hydroxyl apatite sing plasma and then soaked in zoledronate solutions of varying concentrations to obtain a range of BP loadings, ranging from 0.2 to 16 μg. Bone density correlated well with loading, clearly demonstrating the efficacy of local delivery of BP.

rhBMP was delivered locally from a carrier and tested in a canine total hip arthroplasty (THP) model (Bragdon et al., 2003). The localized delivery did enhance bone formation near the implant. Such an approach does appear promising, but the cost and the dose needed may prove to be prohibitive.

In summary, the local delivery of BPs from a CaP coating appears to be the closest to clinical examination, although there are no reports to date of such trials.

Bioactive Coatings II: Surface Modification for Cellular Interactions

Drug or other bioactive elution from coatings has been commercially successful. However, that approach has a temporal limitation in that the effect lasts only as long as the drug is being eluted. To make the "coating" more permanent, researchers have been exploring the use of surface modification techniques. Most of these attempts have been focused on improving biocompatibility, particularly blood compatibility and osteointegration.

Platelet Interactions

By far, prevention of thrombus formation has been the focus of researchers over the past four decades. A variety of approaches have been tried, with very little success. Early attempts focused on making the surface more hydrophilic, particularly with the use of attached polyethylene glycol (PEG) molecules. Other approaches have included hydrogel coatings and plasma treatment; most of these approaches have been reviewed by Sefton and Gemmel (2004). Nevertheless, in spite of more than 30 years of research, the only successful approach has been to use tethered heparin.

Heparin is a well-studied polysaccharide from the glycosaminoglycan family. It exerts its anticoagulant activity via binding to antithrombin III. Heparin and its partially depolymerized form (low molecular weight heparin) are currently used for anticoagulation.

As mentioned earlier, heparinized coatings (strictly speaking, heparin immobilization on surfaces) have enjoyed commercial success, specifically in blood oxygenators and dialysis catheters. In both cases tethered heparin has been employed. We now briefly discuss the various methods for attaching heparin chemically onto surfaces.

Because of the presence of several active functional groups in heparin, such as amine, carboxyl, as well as hydroxyl groups, several chemical attachment options are available. For example, for attachment to polyethylene, the following sequence has been proposed. First, introduce carboxyl groups on PE using acrylic acid–enhanced plasma. Then react this surface with bis 2-aminopropyl polyethylene glycol to attach PEG molecules on the PE surface. Once this PEG molecule is attached, it can be used as a tether to attach heparin, using the dangling amino group on the PEG molecules. The attachment of heparin via a PEG tether allows for adjustment of the length of the tether unit (PEG) by simply using PEGs of different molecular mass, whereas PEG itself can also act to repel adhesion proteins on the surface.

As shown in Figure 10.5, heparin consists of a pentasaccharide sequence (Murugesan et al., 2008) that is believed to be essential for binding to antithrombin (AT).

It is this unit that must not be changed as a result of any covalent attachment technique that is used. The first such report of surface modification involved the use of a polyethyleneimine primer surface (Larsson et al., 1983). First, heparin with MW of about 12,000 was partially degraded in nitrous acid, and this introduced reactive aldehyde groups at the terminal residues. The chosen biomaterial is then made to be negatively charged using plasma or other chemical techniques. For example, polyethylene can be treated with sulfuric acid and potassium permanganate to introduce sulfate groups. Then the negatively charged surface is treated with polyethyleneimine to irreversibly adsorb the positively

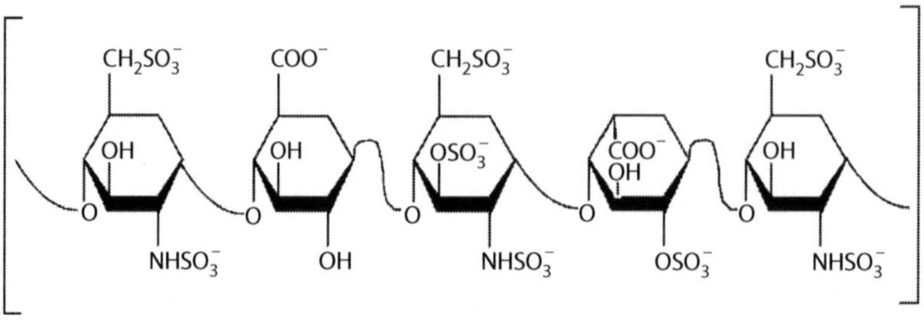

FIGURE 10.5
Chemical structure of the pentasaccharide sequence of heparin; this is considered the active sequence that predominates in binding to AT.

charged PEI. The heparin is then attached to the PEI surface by reductive amination using sodium cyanoborohydride. This procedure enhances the stability of the heparinized surface compared with simple ionic attachment without the reductive amination (Larsson et al. 1983).

The above sequence of steps is believed to be the methodology used to generate the Carmeda® Bioactive Surface (Figure 10.6) that was approved for use on blood oxygenators and on dialysis catheters. This was developed by Carmeda AB (Sweden) and licensed to Medtronic Corporation, and has been the "gold standard" for nonthrombogenic surfaces for several years. Its structure is shown schematically in Figure 10.6.

The same company, Medtronic, introduced another heparinized surface, which they termed the Trillium™ Biosurface, which is a technology licensed from Biointeractions plc (UK). This technology utilizes the PEG tether described above to attach heparin molecules (undegraded) via a multipoint attachment. The surface has a priming layer which allows for attachment of hydrophilic entities to the (usually hydrophobic) biomaterial surface. The functional layer is also sulfonated to introduce negative charges to mimic an endothelial surface as shown in Figure 10.7.

Several clinical studies have attested to the nonthrombogenicity of these surfaces. In one study (Palanzo et al., 2001) which compared the two surfaces, sixty patients undergoing non-emergency revascularization were enrolled. Both devices were used in the procedure, divided into 2 cohorts. The net blood platelet drop counts for the Carmeda and the Trillium groups were 3.6 ± 15.8% and 6.2 ± 10.2%, respectively. The two surfaces were not statistically different in this respect and were deemed to perform satisfactorily in this procedure.

The Carmeda Bioactive coating has been applied to stents as well. The Cordis company's Hepacoat stent was approved by the FDA in 2000. An extensive study of 1288 patients (1366 procedures) comparing the Hepacoat® stent vs. a bare metal stent was reported in 2004 (Gupta et al., 2004). Angiographic measurement of subacute thrombosis (SAT) was one of the study outcomes. SAT was seen in 25 (2.44%) of 1024 procedures in the bare-metal stent group and in 1 (0.29%) of 342 procedures in the heparin-coated stent group, a statistically significant difference. The benefit of using Hepacoat was substantiated in another study (Mehran et al., 2003) where aspirin administration with Hepacoat stenting in 200 patients was found to be safe and did not cause any major adverse events except in 2.5% of the patients, and thrombosis rate (1%) was similar to that seen with antiplatelet therapy (in addition to aspirin).

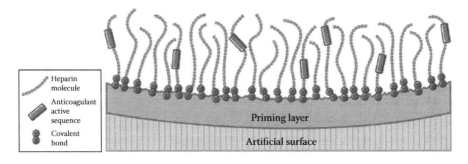

FIGURE 10.6
Generalized schema of the construction of a Carmeda Bioactive Surface, as depicted on the Medtronic Corporation Web site.

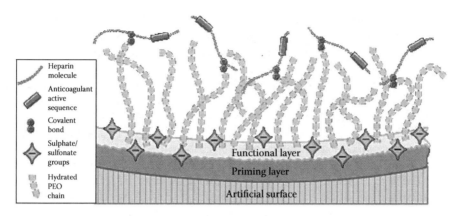

FIGURE 10.7
Generalized schema of the construction of a Trillium Biosurface, as depicted on the Medtronic Corporation Web site.

The Carmeda coating has also been applied to vascular grafts. The Gore Viabahn Endoprosthesis (W.L. Gore & Associates) is a Carmeda-coated stent graft and is approved for use in the treatment of lower limb artery disease. This is a PTFE-based graft that has been surface modified using an approach similar to that mentioned above for PE. The PROPATEN® graft has been approved by the FDA in 2006 and can be used in cardiovascular disease generally. It has been proven superior to noncoated synthetic grafts in clinical studies.

The same coating has also been applied to ventricularly assist devices successfully. The device is marketed by Berlin Heart GmbH, under the name of Excor® and Incor® and is being readied for approval in the US.

Taken together, the Hepacoat stent (although it really addresses only sub-acute thrombosis, or SAT) and the LVADs (left ventricular assist device) would establish the first successful long-term usefulness of the heparinization approach.

The Durafloll coating (Baxter) relies on initial sulfation of the surface to generate negative charges, followed by attachment or coating with a positively charged surfactant (containing quarternary ammonium groups). These positively charged molecules then ionically bind to heparin, preserving their bioactivity substantially. This coating has also been successfully applied to oxygenator surfaces.

These are the true success stories of nonthrombogenic surface generation. Longer-term blood-contacting devices such as stents and heart valves may require a different solution, namely, the generation of a functioning endothelium. Those attempts are described next.

Endothelialization of Biomaterial Surfaces

If the blood-contacting surface of an implant can be completely covered by endothelial cells, the blood then treats the device the same way as it does a blood vessel: no platelets adhere and cause clotting. Part of the reason for this is the negative charge on the endothelial surface that seems to repel platelets. Simply making a surface negative helps, but does not provide long-term protection. Thus, in the following sections, we describe the various approaches to accelerating endothelialization of surfaces.

The fundamental problem with most polymers in biomedical application is poor endothelial cell adhesion due to lack of cell recognition sites. This has led to a broad spectrum of surface modification methods to promote endothelial cell adhesion. Generally, these are classified into three categories: topological modification, chemical modification, and patterning (Goddard and Hotchkiss, 2007).

Topological Modification

(1) Creating surface roughness or porosity by means of base hydrolysis (Wang and Cai, 2007)

(2) Micro/nano grade salt/sugar leaching (Mattioli-Belmonte, Vozzi et al., 2008; Sin, Miao et al., 2010).

Chemical Modification

According to modification intention, there are three categories:

(1) Impartation of functional groups

The essence of these studies is to introduce functional groups on the biomedical polymeric surface by means of plasma treatment or wet chemical reaction to improve EC adhesion (Favia and d'Agostino, 1998). Many types of gaseous plasmas have been used, including NH_3 (Chu et al., 1999; Lu and Sipehia, 2001; Pu et al., 2002; Wan et al., 2003), Ar (Chen et al., 2007), air (Pratt et al., 1989), oxygen (Ryu et al., 2005), helium (De et al., 2005), and H_2O (Pompe et al., 2007). Functional groups such as hydroxyl (–OH) and amine (–NH$_2$) were imparted onto the polymeric surface to improve endothelial cell compatibility. It was believed that those functional groups changed the wettability of the polymeric surface and sequentially influenced cell adhesion.

Plasma polymerization and grafting are the alternative ways to introduce functional groups on a surface, such as lactic acid grafting (Hsu and Chen, 2000) and acrylamide polymerization (Croll et al., 2004).

Wet chemical reaction: Primary amines have been introduced to PLA and PLGA by aminolysis using 1,6-hexanediamine (Eisenbarth et al., 2007).

Impartation of functional groups improves cell attachment marginally by increasing hydrophilicity or protein adsorption. Bioactive molecules including extracellular matrix proteins and adhesion ligands were immobilized/incorporated on biomaterials for specific cell adhesion.

(2) Immobilization of extra-cellular matrix materials

It has become evident that certain molecules in the basement membrane (basal lamina) are responsible for adhesion of the endothelial cells (EC) and thus essential for endothelial integrity. Researchers attempted to immobilize them covalently on polymeric surface with the aim of better endothelial cell adhesion (74). One of the most widely studied of these is fibronectin (Sheiban et al., 2008), which accounts for approximately 15% of the protein synthesized and secreted by EC. Another commonly studied protein is collagen (Yang et al., 2003; Cheng and Teoh, 2004; De et al., 2005; Feugier et al., 2005); its denatured form, gelatin

(Zhu et al., 2002; Zhu et al., 2003; Ma et al., 2005); and laminin (Chandy et al., 2000).

(3) Incorporation of cell adhesion peptides and ligands

Cell adhesion, both in the body and on synthetic substrates, is mediated by cell adhesion ligands interaction with cell-surface receptor. These cell adhesion ligands can be oligopeptides, saccharides, or glycolipids (Alberts et al., 2002). Immobilization of them could improve cell–surface interaction. Certain short amino acid sequences appear to bind to receptors on cell surfaces and mediate cell adhesion, for example, RGD in fibronectin (Massia and Hubbell, 1991; Hersel et al., 2003; Gabriel et al., 2006; Larsen et al., 2006; Tugulu et al., 2007), YIGSR (Massia and Hubbell, 1990; Jun and West, 2004) and IKVAV (Lin et al., 2006) in laminin, and REDV (Hubbell et al., 1991; Hodde et al., 2002).

Micropatterning

Micropatterns printed on substrate were found to regulate/control EC adhesion and function (Christopher et al., 1998; Ito, 1999; Kumar et al., 2003; Gauvreau and Laroche, 2005; Satomi et al., 2007; Yamamoto et al., 2007).

We have provided the above review of methods to illustrate the fact that this area of research is quite an active one. However, it is fair to say that none of these approaches have been proven to work for accelerating in situ endothelialization. As we have reviewed in an earlier paper (Venkatraman et al., 2008), seeding of graft surfaces before implantation appears to be the most clinically successful approach to date. For example, Williams et al. (1985) found that it was necessary to precoat the vascular graft material (Dacron, PTFE) with proteins, such as fibronectin, to enhance the stability of the attached ECs ex vivo. The RGD peptide sequence found in these plasma proteins appears to enhance EC attachment and stability, although it is not as selective as the REDV sequence. EC were taken from the jugular or cephalic vein, and fibronectin-modified surfaces seeded with a seeding density of 3000 cells/cm^2, requiring 9–10 days after seeding to achieve full surface coverage ex vivo. Such ex vivo seeded grafts were found to perform much better than unseeded grafts clinically, improving long-term patency rates (70% patency at 7 years comparable to saphenous vein grafts) substantially (Meinhart et al., 1997). This approach is extremely promising as an interim improvement while we await the completely tissue-engineered graft.

Faster endothelialization of stents is also critical to its long-term acceptance. As mentioned above, DES delay endothelialization of the stent, resulting in prolonged therapy with systemic antiplatelet agents (expensive and with possible adverse side effects such as bleeding). To overcome this, one elegant technique is to anchor an antibody that captures floating endothelial progenitor cells (EPCs) from the bloodstream. In clinical trials, the Genous® stent, which is not drug-eluting, was reported to have fared as well as the paclitaxel-eluting stent. The e-HEALING clinical study is a multicenter, worldwide study with 5000 enrolled patients treated with the Genous stent. The study protocol recommends that patients receive 1 month of clopidogrel treatment after the procedure. The data from 3200 patients showed a TLR rate of 5%, a SAT rate of 0.4%, a late stent thrombosis (LST) rate of 0.3%, and MACE rate of 8.5%. The data support the use of Genous as an alternative to DES, in light of the relatively minimal dual antiplatelet therapy requirements of the stent, according to company news reports.

Status and Prognosis

In summary, we believe that the short-term success of bioactive coatings will involve either immobilization of bioactive molecules or elution. Localized elution will enhance the efficacy of the bioactive, especially if it can be sustained for a few days. Elution from a biodegradable substrate is clearly warranted in certain devices such as stents. For long-term implants such as valves and vascular grafts, immobilization followed by ex vivo seeding of cells to produce a semi-tissue engineered surface is the approach that has an immediate acceptance. In the osteo world, coatings that provide lubricity are already well accepted; bioactive eluting coatings will be the next to find acceptance, especially those that elute inhibitors of osteoclasts.

References

Albert B, Johnson A, Alexander J, Lewis J, Raff M, Roberts K and Walter P. 2002. *Molecular biology of the cell*, 4th ed. Garland Publishers, New York, NY.

Bragdon CR, Doherty AM, Rubash HE, Jasty M, Li XJ, Seeherman H and Harris WH. 2003. The efficacy of BMP-2 to induce bone ingrowth in a total hip replacement model. *Clinical Orthopaedics and Related Research* 417: 50–61.

Bridges C. 2007. New heparin coating reduces thrombosis and fibrin sheath formation in HD catheters. *Nephrol News Issues* 21: 32.

Klugherz BD, Jones PL, Cui X, Chen W, Meneveau NF, DeFelice S, Connolly J, Wilensky RL and Levy RJ. 2000. Gene delivery from a DNA controlledrelease stent in porcine coronary arteries. *Nature Biotechnology* 18: 1181–1184.

Chandy T, Das GS, Wilson RF and Rao GH. 2000. Use of plasma glow for surface-engineering biomolecules to enhance bloodcompatibility of Dacron and PTFE vascular prosthesis. *Biomaterials* 21: 699–712.

Chen JY, Tian RL, Leng YX, Yang P, Wang J, Wan GJ, Zhao AS, Sun H and Huang N. 2007. Effect of Ar plasma etching of Ti–O film surfaces on biological behavior of endothelial cell. *Surface and Coatings Technology* 201: 6901–6905.

Chen M, Liang H, Chiu YL, Chang Y, Wei HJ and Sung HW. 2005. A novel drug-eluting stent spray-coated with multi-layers of collagen and sirolimus. *Journal of Controlled Release* 108: 178–189.

Cheng ZY and Teoh SH. 2004. Surface modification of ultra thin poly(ε-caprolactone) films using acrylic acid and collagen. *Biomaterials* 25: 1991–2001.

Christopher SC, Milan M, Sui H, George MW and Donald EI. 1998. Micropatterned surfaces for control of cell shape, position, and function. *Biotechnology Progress* 14: 356–363.

Chu CFL, Lu A, Liszkowski M and Sipehia R. 1999. Enhanced growth of animal and human endothelial cells on biodegradable polymers. *Biochimica et Biophysica Acta* 1472: 479–485.

Cremers B, Biederman M, Mahnkopf D, Böhm M and Scheller B. 2009. Comparison of two different paclitaxel-coated balloon catheters in the porcine coronary restenosis model. *Clinical Research in Cardiology* 98: 325–330.

Croll TI, O'Connor AJ, Stevens GW and Cooper-White JJ. 2004. Controllable surface modification of poly(lactic-*co*-glycolic acid) (PLGA) by hydrolysis or aminolysis I: physical, chemical and theoretical aspects. *Biomacromolecules* 5: 463–473.

De S, Sharma R, Trigwell S, Laska B, Ali N, Mazumder MK and Mehta JL. 2005. Plasma treatment of polyurethane coating for improving endothelial cell growth and adhesion. *Journal of Biomaterials Science, Polymer Edition* 16: 973–989.

Eisenbarth E, Velten D and Breme J. 2007. Biomimetic implant coatings. *Biomolecular Engineering* 24: 27–32.

Epinette JA, Manley MT and Duthoit E. 2004. Long-term results with the HA-coated Arc2F in primary hip surgery. In: *Fifteen years of clinical experience with hydroxyapatite coatings in joint arthroplasty.* JA Epinette and MT Manley (ed.). Springer-Verlag, France, pp 313–324.

Favia P and d'Agostino R. 1998. Plasma treatments and plasma deposition of polymers for biomedical applications. *Surface and Coatings Technology* 98: 1102–1106.

Feugier P, Black RA, Hunt JA and How TV. 2005. Attachment, morphology and adherence of human endothelial cells to vascular prosthesis materials under the action of shear stress. *Biomaterials* 26: 1457–1466.

Fröbert O, Lagerqvist B, Carlsson J, Lindbäck J, Stenestrand U and James SK. 2009. Differences in restenosis rate with different drug-eluting stents in patients with and without diabetes mellitus. *Journal of the American College of Cardiology* 53: 1660–1667.

Gabriel M, van Nieuw Amerongen GP, Van Hinsbergh VWM, Van Nieuw Amerongen AV, and Zentner A. 2006. Direct grafting of RGD-motif-containing peptide on the surface of polycaprolactone films. *Journal of Biomaterials Science, Polymer Edition* 17: 567–577.

Gauvreau V and Laroche G. 2005. Micropattern printing of adhesion, spreading, and migration peptides on poly(tetrafluoroethylene) films to promote endothelialization. *Bioconjugate Chemistry* 16: 1088-1097.

Goddard JM and Hotchkiss JH. 2007. Polymer surface modification for the attachment of bioactive compounds. *Progress in Polymer Science* 32: 698–725.

Grube E and Buellefeld L. 2006. BioMatrix® Biolimus A9®-eluting coronary stent: a next-generation drug-eluting stent for coronary artery disease. *Expert Review of Medical Devices* 3: 731–741.

Gupta V, Aravamuthan BR, Baskerville S, Smith SK, Gupta V, Lauer MA and Fischell TA. 2004. Reduction of subacute stent thrombosis (SAT) using heparin-coated stents ina large-scale, real world registry. *Invasive Cardiology* 16: 304–310.

Helmut DL, Paul CM and Luiz P. 2004. Choosing a cervical disc replacement. *The Spine Journal* 4: S294–S302.

Hersel U, Dahmen C and Kessler H. 2003. RGD modified polymers: biomaterials for stimulated cell adhesion and beyond. *Biomaterials* 24: 4385–4415.

Hodde J, Record R, Tullius R and Badylak S. 2002. Fibronectin peptides mediate HMEC adhesion to porcine-derived extracellular matrix. *Biomaterials* 23: 1841–1848.

Hsu S and Chen WC. 2000. Improved cell adhesion by plasma-induced grafting of -lactide onto polyurethane surface. *Biomaterials* 21: 359–367.

Huang Y, Venkatraman S, Boey FYC, Umashankar PR, Mohanty M and Arumugam S. 2009. The short-term effect on restenosis and thrombosis of a cobalt–chromium stent eluting two drugs in a porcine coronary artery model. *Journal of Interventional Cardiology* 22: 466–478.

Huang Y, Venkatraman SS, Boey FYC, Lahti EM, Umashankar PR, Mohanty M, Arumugam S, Khanolkar L and Vaishnav S. 2010. In vitro and in vivo performance of a dual drug-eluting stent (DDES). *Biomaterials.*

Hubbell JA, Massia SP, Desai NP and Drumheller PD. 1991. Endothelial cell-selective materials for tissue engineering in the vascular graft via a new receptor. *Nature Biotechnology* 9: 568–572.

Ito Y. 1999. Surface micropatterning to regulate cell functions. *Biomaterials* 20: 2333–2342.

Jabara R, Chronos N and Robinson K. 2008. Novel bioabsorbable salicylate-based polymer as a drug-eluting stent coating. *Catheterization and Cardiovascular Interventions* 72: 186–194.

Jang HS, Nam HY, Kim JM, Hahm DH, Nam SH, Kim KL, Joo JR, Suh W, Park JS, Kim DK and Gwon HC. 2009. Effects of curcumin for preventing restenosis in a hypercholesterolemic rabbit iliac artery stent model. *Catheterization and Cardiovascular Interventions* 74: 6881–6888.

Jun HW and West J. 2004. Development of a YIGSR-peptide–modified polyurethaneurea to enhance endothelialization. *Journal of Biomaterials Science, Polymer Edition* 15: 73–94.

Kukreja N, Onuma S, Daemen J and Serruys PW. 2008. The future of drug-eluting stents. *Pharmacological Research* 57: 171–180.

Kumar G, Wang YC, Co C and Ho CC. 2003. Spatially controlled cell engineering on biomaterials using polyelectrolytes. *Langmuir* 19: 10550–10556.

Larsen CC, Kligman F, Kottke-Marchant K and Marchant RE. 2006. The effect of RGD fluorosurfactant polymer modification of ePTFE on endothelial cell adhesion, growth, and function. *Biomaterials* 27: 4846–4855.

Larsson R, Larm O and Olsson, R. 1983. The search for thromboresistance using immobilized heparin. *Annals of the New York Academy of Sciences* 516: 102–115.

Lee Y, Park JH, Moon HT, Lee DY, Yun JH and Byun Y. 2007. The short-term effects on restenosis and thrombosis of echinomycin-eluting stents topcoated with a hydrophobic heparin-containing polymer. *Biomaterials* 28: 1523–1530.

Lin X, Takahashi K, Liu Y and Zamora PO. 2006. Enhancement of cell attachment and tissue integration by a IKVAV containing multi-domain peptide. *Biochimica et Biophysica Acta* 1760: 1403–1410.

Lowe HC, Chesterman CN and Khachigian LM. 2001. Does thrombus contribute to in-stent restenosis in the porcine coronary stent model? *Journal of Thrombosis and Haemostasis* 5: 1117–1118.

Lu A and Sipehia R. 2001. Antithrombotic and fibrinolytic system of human endothelial cells seeded on PTFE: the effects of surface modification of PTFE by ammonia plasma treatment and ECM protein coatings. *Biomaterials* 22: 1439–1446.

Ma Z, He W, Yong T and Ramakrishna S. 2005. Grafting of gelatin on electrospun poly(caprolactone) nanofibers to improve endothelial cell spreading and proliferation and to control cell orientation. *Tissue Engineering* 11: 1149–1158.

Massia SP and Hubbell JA. 1990. Convalent surface immobilization of Arg-Gly-Asp- and Tyr-Ile-Gly-Ser-Arg-containing peptides to obtain well-defined cell-adhesive substrates. *Analytical Biochemistry* 187: 292–301.

Massia SP and Hubbell JA. 1991. An RGD spacing of 440 nm is sufficient for integrin alpha V beta 3-mediated fibroblast spreading and 140 nm for focal contact and stress fiber formation. *The Journal of Cell Biology* 114: 1089–1100.

Mattioli-Belmonte M, Vozzi G, Kyriakidou K, Pulieri E, Lucarini G, Vinci B, Pugnaloni A, Biagini G and Ahluwalia A. 2008. Rapid-prototyped and salt-leached PLGA scaffolds condition cell morpho-functional behavior. *Journal of Biomedical Materials Research Part A* 85A: 466–476.

Mehran R, Aymong ED, Fischell T, Whitworth HJ, Siegel R, Thomas W, Wong SC and Narasimaiah R. 2003. Safety of an aspirin-aloneregimen after intracoronary stenting with a heparin-coated stent: final results of the HOPE (HEPACOAT and an Antithrombotic Regimen of Aspirin Alone) study. *Circulation* 108: 1078–1083.

Meinhart J, Deustch M and Zilla P. 1997. Eight years of clinical endothelial cell transplantation: closing the gap between prosthetic grafts and vein grafts. *ASAIO Journal* 43: M515–M521.

Michael H, Thomas FMK, Uldis K, Andrejs E, Kari S, Helmut DG, Eberhard G, Robert G, Antonio S, Hans GR, Peter S and Raimund E. 2003. Heparin-coated stent placement for the treatment of stenoses in small coronary arteries of symptomatic patients. *Circulation* 107: 1265–1270.

Mori T, Kinoshita Y, Watanabe A, Yamaguchi T, Hosokawa K and Honjo H. 2006. Retention of paclitaxel in cancer cells for 1 week in vivo and in vitro. *Cancer Chemotherapy & Pharmacology* 58: 665–672.

Murugesan S, Xie J and Linhardt RJ. 2008. Immobilization of heparin: approaches and applications. *Current Topics in Medicinal Chemistry* 8: 80–100.

Nguyen KT, Shaikh N, Shukla KP, Su SH, Eberhart RC and Tang L. 2004. Molecular responses of vascular smooth muscle cells and phagocytes to curcumin-eluting bioresorbable stent materials. *Biomaterials* 25: 5333–5346.

Okkema AZ, Yu X-H and Cooper SL. 1991. Physical and blood contacting characteristics of propyl sulphonate grafted biomer. *Biomaterials* 12: 3–12.

Palanzo DA, Zarro DL, Montesano RM, Manley NJ, Quinn M, Elmore BA, Gustafson PA and Castagna JM. 2001. Effect of Carmeda® BioActive Surface coating versus Trillium™ Biopassive Surface coating of the oxygenator on circulating platelet count drop during cardiopulmonary bypass. *Perfusion* 16: 279–283.

Pan CJ, Tang JJ, Weng YJ, Wang J and Huang N. 2006. Preparation, characterization and anticoagulation of curcumin-eluting controlled biodegradable coating stents. *Journal of Controlled Release* 116: 42–49.

Peter B, Pioletti DP, Laib S, Bujoli B, Pilet P, Janvier. P, Guicheux J, Zambelli PY, Bouler JM and Gauthier O. 2005. Calcium phosphate drug delivery system: influence of local zoledronate release on bone implant osteointegration. *Bone* 36: 52–60.

Pioletti, DP, Gauthier O, Stadelmann VA, Bujoli B, Guicheux J, Zambelli PY and Bouler JM. 2008. Orthopedic implant used as drug delivery system: clinical situation and state of the research. *Current Drug Delivery* 5: 59–63.

Pompe T, Keller K, Mothes G, Nitschke M, Teese M, Zimmermann R and Werner C. 2007. Surface modification of poly(hydroxybutyrate) films to control cell-matrix adhesion. *Biomaterials* 28: 28–37.

Pratt KJ, Williams SK and Jarrell BE. 1989. Enhanced adherence of human adult endothelial cells to plasma discharge modified polyethylene terephthalate. *Journal of Biomedical Materials Research* 23: 1131–1147.

Pu FR, Williams RL, Markkula TK and Hunt JA. 2002. Effects of plasma treated PET and PTFE on expression of adhesion molecules by human endothelial cells in vitro. *Biomaterials* 23: 2411–2428.

Ramgopal Y, Mondal D, Venkatraman, SS and Godbey WT. 2007. Sustained release of complexed and naked pDNA from polymer films. *Journal of Biomedical Materials Research Part B: Applied Biomaterials* 85B: 496–503.

Ramgopal Y, Mondal D, Venkatraman, SS, Godbey WT and Yuen GY. 2009. Controlled release of complexed DNA from polycaprolactone film: Comparison of lipoplex and polyplex release. *Journal of Biomedical Materials Research Part B: Applied Biomaterials* 89: 439–447.

Ramgopal Y, Venkatraman SS and Godbey WT. 2008. In vitro release of complexed pDNA from biodegradable polymer films. *Journal of Applied Polymer Science* 108: 659–664.

Ranade S, Miller KM, Richard RE, Chan AK, Allen MJ and Helmus MN. 2004. Physical characterization of controlled release of paclitaxel from the TAXUS Express™ drug-eluting stent. *Journal of Biomedical Materials Research Part A* 71: 625–634.

Roussiere H, Montavon G, Laïb S, Janvier P, Alonso B, Fayon F, Petit M, Massiot D, Bouler JM and Bujoli B. 2005. Hybrid materials applied to biotechnologies: coating of calcium phosphates for the design of implants active against bone resorption disorders. *Journal of Materials Chemistry* 15: 3869–3875.

Ryu GH, Yang WS, Roh HW, Lee IS, Kim JK, Lee GH, Lee DH, Park BJ, Lee MS and Park JC. 2005. Plasma surface modification of poly(D,L-lactic-*co*-glycolic acid) (65/35) film for tissue engineering. *Surface and Coatings Technology* 193: 60–64.

Sanghong B and Keith LM. 1998. Gene therapy for restenosis: getting nearer the heart of the matter. *Circulation Research* 82: 295–305.

Satomi T, Nagasaki Y, Kobayashi H, Otsuka H and Kataoka K. 2007. Density control of poly(ethylene glycol) layer to regulate cellular attachment. *Langmuir* 23: 6698–6703.

Scheller B, Speck U, Abramjuk, C. Bernhardt U, Böhm M and Nickenig G. 2004. Paclitaxel balloon coating, a novel method for prevention and therapy of restenosis. *Circulation* 110: 810–814.

Sefton MV and Gemmel CH. 2004. Non-thrmobogenic treatments and strategies. In: *Biomaterials Science: An introduction to materials in medicine*. Ratner B, Hoffman AS, Schoen FJ, Lemons JE (eds). Academic Press, San Diego, CA, pp 456–469.

Sheiban I, Villata G, Bollati M, Sillano D, Lotrionte M and Biondi-Zoccai G. 2008. Next-generation drug-eluting stents in coronary artery disease: focus on everolimus-eluting stent (Xience V®). *Vascular Health and Risk Management* 4: 31–38.

Sin D, Miao X, Liu G, Wei F, Chadwick G, Yan C and Friis T. 2010. Polyurethane (PU) scaffolds prepared by solvent casting/particulate leaching (SCPL) combined with centrifugation. *Materials Science and Engineering: C* 30: 78–85.

Sohier J, Daculsi G, Sourice S, de Groot K and Layrolle P. 2010. Porous beta tricalcium phosphate scaffolds used as a BMP-2 delivery system for bone tissue engineering. *Journal of Biomedical Materials Research Part A* 92: 1105–1114.

Sousa JE, Costa MA, Abizaid AC, Rensing BJ and Abizaid AS. 2001. Sustained suppression of neointimal proliferation by sirolimus-eluting stents. *Circulation* 104: 2007–2011.

Sousa JE, Costa MA, Sousa AGMR, Abizaid AC, Seixas AC, Abizaid AS, Feres F and Mattos LA. 2003. Two-year angiographic and intravascular ultrasound follow-up after implantation of sirolimus-eluting stents in human coronary arteries. *Circulation* 107: 381–383.

Tugulu S, Silacci P, Stergiopulos N and Klok HA. 2007. RGD—functionalized polymer brushes as substrates for the integrin specific adhesion of human umbilical vein endothelial cells. *Biomaterials* 28: 2536–2546.

Unverdorben M, Vallbracht C, Cremers B, Heuer H and Hengstenberg C. 2009. Paclitaxel-coated balloon catheter versus paclitaxel-coated stent for the treatment of coronary in-stent restenosis. *Circulation* 119: 2986–2994.

Venkatraman S and Boey F. 2007. Release profiles in drug-eluting stents: issues and uncertainties. *Journal of Controlled Release* 120: 149–160.

Venkatraman S, Boey F and Lao LL. 2008. Implanted cardiovascular polymers: natural, synthetic and bio-inspired. *Progress in Polymer Science* 13: 853–874.

Waksma R and Pakala R. 2009. Drug eluting balloon: the comeback kid? *Circulation: Cardiovascular Interventions* 2: 352–358.

Wan Y, Yang J, Bei J and Wang S. 2003. Cell adhesion on gaseous plasma modified poly-(-lactide) surface under shear stress field. *Biomaterials* 24: 3757–3764.

Wang YQ and Cai JY. 2007. Enhanced cell affinity of poly(L-lactic acid) modified by base hydrolysis: Wettability and surface roughness at nanometer scale. *Current Applied Physics* 7: e108–e111.

Westedt U, Wittmar M, Hellwig M, Hanefeld P, Greiner A, Schaper AK and Kissel T. 2006. Paclitaxel releasing films consisting of poly(vinyl alcohol)-graft-poly(lactide-*co*-glycolide) and their potential as biodegradable stent coatings. *Journal of Controlled Release* 111: 235–246.

Williams SK, Jarrell BE, Friend L, Radmski JS, Carabasi RA, Koolpe E, Mueller SN, Thornton SC, Marinucci T and Levine E. 1985. Adult human endothelial cell compatibility with prosthetic graft material. *Journal of Surgical Research* 38: 618–629.

Windecker S, Serruys PW, Wandel S, Buszman P, Trznadel S, Linke A, Lenk K, Ischinger T, Klauss V, Eberli F, Corti R, Wijns W, Morice MC, di Mario C, Davies S, van Geuns RJ, Eerdmans P, van Es GA, Meier B and Jüni P. 2008. Biolimus-eluting stent with biodegradable polymer versus sirolimus-eluting stent with durable polymer for coronary revascularisation (LEADERS): a randomized non-inferiority trial. *Lancet* 372: 1163–1173.

Yamamoto S, Tanaka M, Sunami H, Ito E, Yamashita S, Morita Y and Shimomura M. 2007. Effect of honeycomb-patterned surface topography on the adhesion and signal transduction of porcine aortic endothelial cells. *Langmuir* 23: 8114–8120.

Yang J, Wan Y, Yang J, Bei J and Wang S. 2003. Plasma-treated, collagen-anchored polylactone: Its cell affinity evaluation under shear or shear-free conditions. *Journal of Biomedical Materials Research Part A* 67: 1139–1147.

Zhu Y, Gao C, He T and Shen J. 2003. Endothelium regeneration on luminla surface of polyurethane vascular scaffold modified with diamine and covalently grafted with gelatin. *Biomaterials* 25: 423–430.

Zhu YB, Gao CY, Liu XY and Shen JC. (2002). Surface modification of polycaprolactone with poly(methacrylic acid) and gelatin covalent immobilization for promoting its cytocompatibility. *Biomaterials* 23: 4889–4895.

Index

Note: Page numbers with italicized f's and t's refer to figures and tables.

A

Abbott Vascular, 269
Abrasives, 314
Acid-etching, 314
Acoustic wave devices, 336–373
  AIN films, 343–344, 356–362
  biosensors, 336–340
  bulk materials, 341–343
  fabrication requirements, 353
  frequency shift, 339
  membrane-based microfluidic devices, 371
  microfluidics, 340–341
  microstrocture requirements, 353
  overview, 336
  thin films, 341–343
    for biosensing, 363–366
    for microfluidic applications, 364–366
  ZnO films, 343–356
Acrylate-based materials, 239–240
Activated partial thromboplastin time
    (APTT), 476
Active coatings, 276–280
  intra-built cavity, 279
  intra-built holes, 279
  microporous membrane, 280
  multiple-layer reservoir, 278
  nanoporous membrane, 280
  single layer reservoir, 276–277
Activity coefficient, 219–226
Adherent platelets, 71–72
  morphology of, 72f
  SEM micrographs of, 73f
Adhesion strength, 14–17
Affinity chromatography, 117
African green monkey kidney fibroblast COS7
    cell line, 76–77
AGI-1067, 284
Aging effect, 407–410
AIN films, 356–362. *See also* Acoustic wave
    devices; ZnO film
  antibody immobilized, 363f
  for biosensing, 362
  crystal structure, 357f

  film texture effect, 358–359
  lab-on-a-chip system, 372–373
  MEMS processing, 362
  properties, 342t, 357
  Rayleigh wave phase velocity, 356–357
  sputtered, PE properties of, 359–361
  substrate effect, 358–359
Airbrush spraying, 281–282
Albumin/fibrinogen ratios, 61, 63–64
Aldehyde, 238
Alginate, 238, 243
Alkaline phosphatase (ALP), 29–30
Alkali treatment, 315
Alloys, 6–7
Alumina, 2t, 314
Aminobenzoic acid, 175
Amorphous calcium phosphate (ACP), 23,
    317–319
Amorphous carbon, 45–100. *See also*
    Carbon-based materials
  antibacterial behavior, 92–95
  biomedical applications of, 95–99
    contact lenses, 99
    coronary stent, 97–98
    guide wires, 98–99
    oral implants, 98
    orthopedic implants, 95–97
  bonding characterization, 52–55
    Raman spectroscopy, 52–55
    x-ray photoelectron spectroscopy, 52
  bonding in, 46
  classes, 59
  cytocompatibility, 76–92
    bone marrow cells, 89–90
    bovine retinal pericytes, 88
    cell culturing, 76–77
    endocrine cells, 90
    endothelial cells, 77–81
    epithelial colorectal adenocarcinoma
      cells, 89
    fibroblasts, 82–85
    glial cells, 89
    in vivo studies, 90–92
    macrophages, 81–82

Amorphous carbon (*continued*)
  neuronal cells, 90
  osteoblasts, 85–88
 electronic properties, 46
 growth mechanism, 46–51
  film evolution, 47
  film structure, 47
  penetration, 46–47
  phase formation, 47
  site occupation, 47
  sputtering, 47
  stopping, 47
  surface composition, 47
 hemocompatibility, 59–76
  doping effects, 66–76
  platelet-rich plasma assay, 59–61
  post-deposition treatment effects, 71–76
 hydrogenated, 61–66, 69–71
 overview, 45–46
 surface energy, 55–57
 surface tension components, 57–59
 tetrahedral, 66, 71, 91–92
 unhydrogenated, 61–66
Amorphous diamond. *See* Amorphous carbon
Angelini Lamina-flo, 98
Angelini Valvuloplasty ring, 98
Angioplasties, 292
Animal trials, 30–31
Annealing, post-sputtering, 399–400
Annealing temperatures, post-deposition, 71–76
Annular Fresnel ring, 371
Anodic oxidation, 315
Aqueous two-phase systems (ATPS), 217–218
Atherosclerosis, 260
Auger analysis, 46
Austenite, 382, 384
Axxion stent, 270, 276–277

B

Basal plane, 113
Berman-Simon P-T phase diagram, 48*f*
Beta-thromboglobulin, 69
Beta-tricalcium phosphate (b-TCP), 23
Binary alloy thin films, 401–406
 superelasticity, 404
 texture, 405–406
 transformation strain anisotropy, 405–406
Binding energy, 52
Bioabsorbable vascular solution sten, 271–272
Bioactive coatings, 471–485
 cardiovascular coating, 472–478
 chemical modification, 483–484

controlled bioactive elution, 472–479
 endothelization of biomaterial surfaces,
  482–483
 micropatterning, 484
 platelet interactions, 480–482
 surface modification, 479–484
 topological modification, 483
Bioactive-eluting implants, 478–479
Bioactive glasses, 315
Bioactive surface coatings, 315–324
 chemical treatments, 324
 electrochemical deposition method, 321–324
 grit-blasting with calcium phosphate
  abrasives, 320
 plasma-sprayed hydroxyapatite coatings,
  316–320
 precipitation method, 320
 sputtering techniques, 324
Bioactivity, 316
Biocorrodible metallic stents, 272
Biodegradable coating, 235
Biodegradation, 32
BioDiamond Stent, 98
BiodiVsio Stent, 275
BioFreedom stent, 274*f*
Biolimus, 284
Biolimus A9 stent, 267, 285
BioLinx, 265–266
Biomaterials, 1–2
 biocompatibility of, 304–305
 endothelization of surfaces, 482–483
 metallic, 2–3
Biomimetic coating, 5*t*, 320–321
Biophosphonates, 478
Biosensing, 344
Biosensors, 165–170
 acoustic wave, 336–340
 AIN films in, 362
 film bulk acoustic resonator, 364–366
 Lamb, 364
 surface acoustic wave, 363–364
 ZnO films in, 356
Biosensors International, 474
Bjerrum length, 232
Block copolymers, 263–264
Blood plasma, 26*t*
Boltzmann constant, 51, 203
Bone marrow cells, 89–90
Bone morphogenic proteins (BMPs), 478
Bone-to-implant contact (BIC), 308
Boron-doped diamond, 151–155
Bovine retinal pericytes, 88
Bovine serum albumin (BSA), 204, 231*t*

Brick layer model, 141*f*
Brushite, 321
Buckminsterfullerene (C₆₀), 116
Buffer layer, 350
Bulk acoustic wave (BAW), 336

C

Calcineurin inhibitors, 284, 286
Calcium acetate monohydrate, 8*t*
Calcium-deficient apatites (CDA), 479
Calcium diethoxide, 8*t*
Calcium hydroxide, 8*t*
Calcium nitrate tetrahydrate, 8*t*
Calcium oxide (CaO), 9, 317
Calcium phosphates, 315, 320–324
    ceramics, 325
    deposition by precipitation, 320–321
    electrochemical deposition method, 321–324
    grit-blasting with, 320
    sputtering techniques, 324
Calcium precursor, 8*t*
Capacitance, 145–150
    cross-section two-layer model, 148–149
    impedance and, 144–145
    one-layer model, 146–148
Ca/P peak ratio, 11
Capsules, 199
Carbodiimide, 238
Carbofilm coatings, 98, 276
Carbon
    fibers, 114
    film, 115
    phase diagram, 48*f*
    Raman spectra of, 53
Carbonate (CO₃²⁻), 12
Carbon-based materials, 111–127
    biomedical applications, 117–127, 118–126
        cardiovascular applications, 121–122
        cellular uptake, 118–119
        drug delivery, 119–120, 123–124
        guide wires, 122
        MRI contrast agents, 125–126
        orthopedic applications, 121
        suppression of reactive oxygen species, 124–125
        therapeutic applications, 117–118
    carbon black, 114
    carbon fibers, 114
    carbon film, 115
    carbon nanotubes, 115
    diamond-like carbon, 115, 120–124
    diamonds, 120–124

fullerenes, 116, 123–124
glassy carbon, 114
graphene, 116–117
highly oriented pyrolytic graphite, 113–114
impedance spectroscopy, 135–185
    capacitance, 145–150
    on diamond-based materials, 150–165
    equivalent circuits, 143–145
    on non-diamond-based materials, 172–185
non-diamond-based, 172–185
    catalysts, 178–179
    cells detection, 172–174
    diamond-like carbon thin films, 182–185
    DNA hybridization sensor, 174–175
    enzyme detection, 175–178
    lithium-ion battery, 179–181
    supercapacitors, 181–182
overview, 111–112
pyrolytic graphite, 112–113
synthesis of, 112–117
Carbon black, 114
Carbon nanotubes, 115–116
    biomedical applications of, 117–200
    cellular uptake, 118–119
    for drug delivery, 119–120
    multiwalled, 115–116
    single-walled, 115–116, 118–119
    therapeutic applications, 117–118
Carbonstent, 98
Cardio Carbon Company, 98
Cardiovascular coating, 472–478
    cardiovascular stent coatings, 473–475
    drug-eluting balloons, 477–478
Cardiovascular stent coating, 473–475
Carmeda Bioactive coating, 481–482
Catalysts, 178–179
CD41a antigen, 122
CD42b antigen, 122
CD62p antigen, 61, 122
CD63 antigen, 61, 122
Cell model polyelectrolyte solutions, 232
Cells
    attachment, 27–28
    culturing, 76–77
    detection, 172–174
    differentiation, 29–30
    morphology, 28–29
    proliferation, 29–30
Cellulose, 239, 247*t*
Centerline approximation, 208
Chemical potential, 210, 230, 231, 233–234
Chemical vapor deposition (CVD), 155–160, 344
Chitin, 239

Chitosan, 239
Cilostazol, 284
Circuits, 143–145
  double resistor and capacitor parallel in
    series, 145
  resistor and capacitor in parallel, 144
Citric acid-modified phosphate buffer solution
  (CPBS), 23
Clausius-Clapeyron relationship, 396
Closed-loop control system, 198*f*
Coating materials, 238–240
  acrylate-based materials, 239–240
  alginate, 238
  cellulose, 239
  chitosan, 239
  collagen, 238
  gelatin, 238
  polyesters, 240
  polyethylene glycol, 240
  polyvinyl-based polymers, 239
Coatings
  active, 276–280
  bioactive, 471–485
  bioactive surface, 315–324
  cross-linked systems, 245
  hydroxyapatite. *See* Hydroxyapatite coating
  release-controlled, 259–294
Coating techniques, 240–243
  compression coating, 241
  electrospinning, 242
  fluid bed, 240–241
  hot-melt, 241–242
  plasticizer dry coating, 241
  precipitation method, 242–243
  release-controlled coatings, 280–283
    dip coating, 280–281
    ink-jet technology, 282–283
    spray coating, 281–282
  supercritical fluid coating, 242
Co-Cr alloys, 2*t*, 7
Coefficient of thermal expansion (CTE), 21, 421
Cole-Cole plot, 143–145, 157, 158*f*, 159*f*, 161–163, 184*f*
Collagen, 238, 281
Collectin proteins, 117
Complementary metal-oxide semiconductor
  (CMOS), 339
Complement C3a, 69
Composite-based films, 431–432
Compression coating, 241
Conductivity models, 140–143
Conor Medsystems stent, 279, 289
Constant phase elements (CPEs), 166
Contact angle, 56

Contact lenses, 99
Contrast agents, 125–126
Controlled release, 283–291
  diffusion-controlled release, 288–290
  dissolution/degradation, 290–291
  local drugs, 284–287
Coordinate transformation matrix, 391
Coronary stents, 97–98, 260
Cortical bone, 2*t*
COS7 cell line, 76–77
CoStar stent, 274*f*
Counterion, 232
Covered stent, 452–453
Crack density, 17
Crack patterns, 17
Cross-linked systems
  coatings, 245
  normalized diffusion coefficient, 212
Curcumin, 476
Cyclic deformation, 426–427
CYPHER stent, 260, 261–263, 275, 278, 288, 289
Cytocompatibility, 76–92
  bone marrow cells, 89–90
  bovine retinal pericytes, 88
  cell culturing, 76–77
  endocrine cells, 90
  endothelial cells, 77–81
  epithelial colorectal adenocarcinoma cells,
    89
  fibroblasts, 82–85
  glial cells, 89
  in vivo studies, 90–92
  macrophages, 81–82
  neuronal cells, 90
  osteoblasts, 85–88

D

Debye behavior, 157
Debye-Huckel constant, 228
Deep groove matrix-free delivery system, 291
Deformation behavior, 395–397
Degradation kinetics, 236–237
Deinococcus geothermalis, 93
Dental implants
  animal models, 306–307
  surface treatments, 313*t*
Deposition, 5*t*, 47
Devax Axxess Biolimus A9 stent, 267
Diamond, 120–124
  biomedical applications of, 120–124
  cardiovascular applications, 121–122
  orthopedic applications, 121

phase diagram, 48*f*
Raman spectra of, 53
Diamond-based materials, 150–165. *See also*
    Carbon-based materials
    applications, 165–172
        biosensors, 165–170
        diamond electrodes, 170–171
        ultraviolet sensors, 172
    boron-doped diamond, 151–155
    impedance spectroscopy, 150–165
    nanocrystalline diamond, 160–165
    polycrystalline diamond, 155–160
Diamond electrodes, 170–171
Diamond-like carbon, 115. *See also* Carbon-
    based materials
    biomedical applications of, 120–124
    biomedical coating materials, 182–185
    cardiovascular applications, 121–122
    electrochemical equivalent circuit, 183*f*
    guide wires, 122
    orthopedic applications, 121
Diamond Rota Gliding, 97
Diaphragms, 437–444
Dicalcium phosphate (DCP), 23
Dicalcium phosphate dihydrate (DCPD), 321
Dicalcium phosphate hydrate (DCPH), 23
Diffusion activation energy, 50, 51
Diffusion coefficient, 209
    normalized, 212
    of solute, 214
Diffusion-controlled systems, 199–235
    aqueous two-phase systems, 217–218
    charged solution partitioning in hydrogel,
        230–235
    in degrading coatings, 236–237
    diffusion coefficient, 209
    diffusivity control theory, 202–203
    equilibrium condition of partition, 217
    excess function/activity coefficient, 219–226
        nonrandom, two-liquid model, 221–222
        UNIQUAC functional-group activity
            coefficients, 225–226
        universal quasi-chemical theory, 223–225
        Wilson model, 220–221
    frictional resistance, 203–204
    hindrance effect, 203*f*
    hydrodynamic dragging factor, 208
    matrix-based, 199
    membrane-based, 199, 200*f*
    multiple-layer reservoir, 289–290
    nonporous perspective, 210–214
        free volume, 211–214
        temperature effect, 214

partition coefficient, 199
    partition/solubility oriented, 215–217
    polymer solution, 226–229
        Flory-Huggin's model, 227
        free-volume contribution, 229
        UNIQUAC-based description, 227–229
    porous perspective, 203–210
    single-layer reservoir, 288–289
Diffusivity control theory, 202–203
Dip coating, 280–281
Displacement threshold, 48
Dissolution, 22–25
Dissolution/degradation-controlled release,
    290–291
DNA hybridization sensor, 174–175
Doping, 66–76
D peak, 53–55
Drug cocktails, 123
Drug delivery, 195–249
    carbon nanotubes for, 119–120
    with coating, 243–249
    coating materials, 238–240
        acrylate-based materials, 239–240
        alginate, 238
        cellulose, 239
        chitosan, 239
        collagen, 238
        gelatin, 238
        polyesters, 240
        polyethylene glycol, 240
        polyvinyl-based polymers, 239
    coating techniques, 240–243
        compression coating, 241
        electrospinning, 242
        fluid bed, 240–241
        hot-melt, 241–242
        plasticizer dry coating, 241
        precipitation method, 242–243
        supercritical fluid coating, 242
    coating technology, 196–197
    deep groove matrix-free system, 290–291
    fullerenes for, 119–120
    honeycombed matrix delivery system,
        290–291
    phases, 196
    pulsatile release profile, 197–198
    release rate control, 199–238
        coating technology, 196–197
        diffusion, 199–203
        erosion controlled, 235–237
        osmotic pressure controlled, 237–238
        porous perspective, 203–235
    sustained release profile, 197

Drug-eluting balloons (DEBs), 477–478
Drug-eluting stents (DES), 260–261, 292–294,
        472, 475
Dual-layer coating, 244
DurafloII coating, 481

E

Echinomycin, 476
Edge planes, 113
Effective diffusion coefficient, 211
Electrochemical deposition, 321–324
Electrochemical impedance, 136, 172–174
Electro-magnetic actuators, 435*t*
Electron, kinetic energy of, 52
Electron dispersive x-ray spectroscopy (EDS/
        EDX), 13
Electronic circuits, 143–145
Electron spectroscopy for chemical analysis
        (ESCA), 10
Electrophoretic deposition, 5*t*
Electrospinning, 242
Electrostatic actuators, 435*t*
Electrowetting-on-dielectrics (EWOD), 372
Endeavour stents, 262*t*, 264–265, 472, 473
Endocrine cells, 90
Endohedral metallofullerenes, 125
Endothelial cells, 77–81, 484
Enzyme, detection, 175–178
Epitaxial growth, 350–351
Epithelial colorectal adenocarcinoma cells, 89
Erodible polymer matrix, 266–269. *See also*
        Matrix materials
    polylactide, 266–268
    poly(lactide-co-glycolide), 268
    polymer blends, 268–269
Erosion-controlled release, 235–237
Escherichia coli, 94
Ethylene vinyl acetate, 239
Eudragit, 239–240, 246–247, 248
Everolimus, 271–272, 284, 285
EXCEL stent, 267–268
Excess function, 219–226
Extracellular matrix (ECM), 483

F

Ferromagnetic thin films, 432
Fibrinogen, 63–64, 67–68
Fibroblasts, 82–85
Fick's first law, 200, 204, 211
Film bulk acoustic resonator (FBAR), 338*f*, 339,
        364–366

Film structure, 47
Filtered cathodic vacuum arc (FCVA), 51
Filtered vacuum arc deposition (FVAD), 344
FK506-binding protein 12 (FKBP12), 284
Flexural plate wave, 337, 371
Flory characteristic ratio, 214
Flory-Huggin's model, 227
Flory thermodynamic interaction parameter, 213
Fluid bed coating, 240–241
Fluoropolymer, 264
Folic acid, 284
Formaldehyde, 238
Fourier transform infrared (FTIR), 11–12, 62
Fracture toughness, 19
Free drugs, partition coefficient of, 234
Free energy, 55
Freestanding microactuators, 434–437
Free volume, 211–214
Free-volume contribution, 229
Frequency, 136
Frictional resistance, 203–204
Fugacity, 216
Fullerenes, 116. *See also* Carbon-based materials
    biomedical applications of, 123–127
    as drug delivery agents, 123–124
    endohedral metallofullerenes, 125
    as MRI contrast agents, 125–126
    suppression of reactive oxygen species,
        124–125
Functional groups, impartation of, 483
Functionally graded films, 431–432

G

Gallium arsenide, 342
Gelatin, 238
Genous Bio-engineered R stent, 270–271
Genous endothelial progenitor cell capture
        stent, 294
Gibbs free energy, 215–216
    excess
        combinatorial, 227
        electrostatic contribution to, 228
        partial molar, 227
    infinitesimal expression, 233
    of solution, 217, 219–220
Glass transition temperature, 213
Glassy carbon, 114
Glial cells, 89
Glow discharge optical emission spectroscopy
        (GDOES), 13
Glucose, 197–198
Glutaraldehyde, 238

Glycocalix, 276–277
Glycogen, 197–198
Gorham process, 275
G peak, 53–55
Grain boundary relaxation constant, 142
Grain interior rate constant, 141
Graphene, 116–117
Graphene nanosheets, 181–182
Graphene-ZnO composite films, 181–182
Graphite
    D peak, 53–55
    G peak, 53–55
    nanocrystalline, 54
    phase diagram, 48*f*
    Raman spectra of, 53
Grit-blasting, 314, 320
Grooves, intra-built, 273–274
Gruentzig, Andreas, 260
Guide wires, 98–99, 122
Guluronic acid, 238

H

Hamaker constant, 208–209
Heart valve, 457–458
Hemholtz energy, 215
Hemocompatibility, 59–76
    doping effects, 66–76
    hydrogenated amorphous carbon, 61–66
    platelet-rich plasma assay, 59–61
    post-deposition treatment effects, 71–76
    unhydrogenated amorphous carbon, 61–66
Hepacoat stent, 481
Heparin, 476, 480*f*
Heptane, 213
Heterodeposition, 47
Highly oriented pyrolytic graphite (HOPG),
        113–114
Hindrance effect, 203*f*
HIV-1 virus, 176–177
Hole-and-hinge structure, 273, 274*f*
Homodeposition, 47
Honeycombed matrix delivery system, 290–291
Hormones, 197–198
Hot-filament chemical vapor deposition
        (HFCVPD), 155–160
Hot isostatic pressing, 5*t*
Hot-melt coating, 241–242
Human blood plasma, 26*t*
Human microvascular endothelial cells
        (HMEC), 77–81
Human osteosarcoma MG63 cell line, 76–77
Human serum albumin (HSA), 63–64

Hydrodynamic dragging factor, 208
Hydrodynamic radius, 203
Hydrogel, 214
    components, 238
    solute partitioning in, 230–235
Hydrogel membrane, 218–219
Hydrogenated amorphous carbon, 61–66, 69–71
Hydrophobicity, 56
Hydroxyapatite, 2*t*, 3–6
    bioactivity, 4
    chemical properties, 3
    crystal structure, 4*f*
    mechanical properties, 3–4
Hydroxyapatite coating, 3–6, 5*t*, 6–33
    cell response to, 27–30
        cell attachment, 27–28
        cell morphology, 28–29
        cell proliferation/differentiation, 29–30
    chemical/physical properties, 8–14
        interfacial analysis, 13–14
        phase composition, 8–9
        surface chemistry/composition, 10–12
        surface morphology, 12
    deposition, high-temperature, 5*t*
    deposition, low-temperature, 5*t*
    fabrication methods, 4, 5*t*
    fluoridated, 32–33
    in vitro tests, 22–27
        in acellular simulated body fluid, 25–27
        dissolution behavior, 22–25
    in vivo animal trials, 30–31
    macro-/microporous surfaces, 32
    mechanical properties, 14–31
        adhesion strength, 14–17
        interfacial shear strength, 17–18
        residual stress, 19–22
        scratch test, 18–19
        toughness, 19
    metallic substrates, 6–7
    overview, 6
    plasma-sprayed, 316–320
    precursors, 7–8
    recent trends, 32–33
    sol-gel derived, 6–33
Hydroxypropyl methacrylate (HPMA), 277
Hydroxypropyl methylcellulose (HPMC), 239,
        247–248

I

Ideal gas law, 216
Igaki-Tamai stent, 271
Impedance, 136–140

Impedance spectroscopy, 135–185
　　capacitance, 145–150
　　　　cross-section two-layer model, 148–149
　　　　in-plane two-layer model, 150
　　　　one-layer model, 146–148
　　on diamond-based materials, 150–165
　　　　boron-doped diamond, 151–155
　　　　nanocrystalline diamond, 160–165
　　　　polycrystalline diamond, 155–160
　　equivalent circuits, 143–145
　　　　double resistor and capacitor parallel in
　　　　　　series, 145
　　　　resistor and capacitor in parallel, 144
　　in-plane two-layer model, 150
　　on non-diamond-based materials, 172–185
　　　　catalysts, 178–179
　　　　cells detection, 172–174
　　　　diamond-like carbon thin films, 182–185
　　　　DNA hybridization sensor, 174–175
　　　　enzyme detection, 175–178
　　　　lithium-ion battery, 179–181
　　　　supercapacitors, 181–182
　　overview, 135–136
　　theory, 136–150
　　　　conductivity models, 140–143
　　　　equivalent circuits, 143–145
Implant Design AG, 97
Implant retrieval analysis, 310
Implants
　　biocompatible, 95
　　orthopedic, 95–97
Implant surfaces, 301–326
　　bioactive surface coatings, 315–324
　　　　chemical treatments, 324
　　　　electrochemical deposition method,
　　　　　　321–324
　　　　grit-blasting with calcium phosphate
　　　　　　abrasives, 320
　　　　plasma-sprayed hydroxyapatite coatings,
　　　　　　316–320
　　　　precipitation method, 320
　　　　sputtering techniques, 324
　　biocompatibility of biomaterials, 304–305
　　bone-implant interface, 303–304
　　clinical evaluation, 309–310
　　implant retrieval analysis, 310
　　in vitro testing, 304–305
　　in vivo testing, 306–309
　　osteoinductivity, 324–325
　　overview, 303–304
　　surface treatments, 310–315
　　　　acid-etching, 314
　　　　alkali treatment, 315

　　　　anodic oxidation, 315
　　　　antibacterial properties, 325
　　　　laser texturing, 314
　　　　roughening by grit-blasting, 314
Infinnium stent, 268, 269*t*
Ink-jet technology, 282–283
Inorganic-based matrix, 269–271. *See also* Matrix
　　　　materials
　　Axxion paclitaxel-eluting stent, 270
　　biocorrodible metallic stents, 272
　　Genous Bio-engineered R stent, 270–271
　　Janus CarboStent, 270
　　polylactic acid stent, 271–272
　　tacrolimus-eluting stent, 269
　　Yukon drug-eluting stent, 270
In-stent restenosis (ISR), 477–478
Insulin, 197–198
Interatomic bonding, 52
Interfacial analysis, 13–14
Interfacial energy, 55
Interfacial shear strength, 17–18
Interfacial tensions, 56
Interlayer, 350
Intra-built cavity, 279, 291
Intra-built holes, 279, 290
In vitro tests, 22–27, 305–306
In vivo animal trials, 30–31
In vivo tests, 22–25
Ion-beam assisted deposition (IBAD), 323*f*, 324
Ion exchange, 237
Ionic strength, 228
Iron, 271

J

Janus Carbostent, 270, 274*f*, 275, 291
Jet spray process, 283
Jomed International, 269

K

Kaltera (drug), 177
Kinetic energy (KE), 52
Knock-on penetrations, 50, 50*f*
Kollicoat® SR30D, 239, 244

L

L605 CoCr alloy, 272
Lab-on-a-chip system, 372–373
Lactate dehydrogenase (LDH), 81
Lamb wave, 338*f*, 371
Lamb wave biosensor, 337–339, 364

Laser annealing, 400
LaserLok Silhouette implant, 314
Laser texturing, 314
Lattice distortion matrix, 391
Lekton Magic coronary stent, 272
Lifshtz-van der Walls/acid-base (van Oss)
    approach, 58, 67
Liquid-vapor interfacial tension, 56
Lithium-ion battery, 179–181
Lithium niobate, 342
Lithium tantalate, 342
Load-displacement curve, 20*f*
Local composition models, 220
Love mode wave, 338*f*
Low electronic grade diamond, 159
Low-energy subsurface implantation, 46
Low temperature isotropic (LTI) carbon, 66

M

Macrophages, 32, 81–82
Magnesium, 7, 271, 272
Magnesium alloys, 2*t*, 7
Magnetic resonance imaging (MRI), contrast
    agents, 125–126
Magnetostrictive thin films, 432
Mannuronic acid, 238
Martensite, 382, 384
Martensitic transformation, 387–388, 389–390,
    393, 410*f*
Matrix-based systems, 199
Matrix-free ink-jet printing, 283
Matrix materials, 261–272
    block copolymers, 263–264
    erodible, 266–269
    fluoropolymer, 264
    inorganic-based, 269–271
        Axxion paclitaxel-eluting stent, 270
        biocorrodible metallic stents, 272
        Genous Bio-engineered R stent, 270–271
        Janus CarboStent, 270
        polylactic acid stent, 271–272
        tacrolimus-eluting stent, 269
        Yukon drug-eluting stent, 270
    non-erodible, 262–266
    phospholipid polymer, 264–266
    polylactide, 266–268
    poly(lactide-co-glycolide), 268
    polymer-based, 261–269
    polymer blends, 262–263, 268–269
Maximum transformation matrix, 392
Maxwell-Stefan theory, 210
MedStent, 290

Medsystems stent, 279
Medtronic, 481
Meiothermus silvanus, 93
Membrane-based systems, 199, 200*f*
Mesh size, 213
Metallic biomaterials, 2–3
Metals, 6–7
2-Methacryloyloxyethyl phosphorylcholine
    (MPC), 265
MG63 cell line, 76–77
Microactuators, 434–437
Microbubble, 435*t*
Microcage, 449–455
    freestanding TiNi-based, 450–452
    TiNi-based, 449–450
    TiNi/DLC, 452–455
Microdiaphragms, 437–444
Microelectromechanical systems (MEMS), 342,
    384
Microfluidics, 340–341. *See also* Acoustic wave
        devices
    membrane-based, 371
    requirements for, 344
    surface acoustic wave devices, 366–371
        heating/droplet ejector, 369–370
        mixer/pump, 366–368
        particle manipulation, 370–371
    thin films for, 366–371
    ZnO films, 356
Microgrippers, 444–446
Micropatterning, 484
Microporous membrane, 280
Micropumps, 437–444
Microtubes, 458–459
Microvalves, 437–444
Microwave plasma-enhanced chemical vapor
        deposition (MPECVPD), 155–160
Modified Thornton zone models, 347
Molarity of species, 228
Molar volume, 216
Monetite, 321–322
MTT (Tetrazolium) assay, 80–81
Multiple-layer reservoir, 278, 289–290
Multiwalled nanotubes (MWNTs), 115–116
Muscle actuators, 435*t*

N

Nanocrystalline diamond, 160–165
Nanocrystalline graphite, 54
Nanoindentation, 20*f*, 430
Nanoporous membrane, 280
Nanosyringe, 118

Nanotubes, 115–116
  biomedical applications of, 117–200
  cellular uptake, 118–119
  for drug delivery, 119–120
  multiwalled, 115–116
  single-walled, 115–116, 118–119
  therapeutic applications, 117–118
Nanyang Technologies University, 475
NEVO stents, 268
Ni-rich thin films, 406–410
  aging effect, 407–410
  microstructure of age-treated thin films, 406–407
Nitinol alloy. *See* TiNi alloys
Non-diamond-based materials, 172–185. *See also* Diamond-based materials
  catalysts, 178–179
  cells detection, 172–174
  diamond-like carbon thin films, 182–185
  DNA hybridization sensor, 174–175
  enzyme detection, 175–178
  lithium-ion battery, 179–181
  supercapacitors, 181–182
Non-erodible polymeric matrix, 262–266. *See also* Matrix materials
  block copolymers, 263–264
  fluoropolymer, 264
  phospholipid polymer, 264–266
  polymer blends, 262–263
NOR-I stent, 272
Nyquist plot, 167*f*, 169*f*

O

O/Ca peak ratio, 11
Octacalcium phosphate (OCP), 23, 321–322, 323*f*
Ohm's law, 136
Open-loop control system, 198*f*
Oral implants, 98
Orthopedic implants, 95–97
  surface description, 313*t*
Osmotic pressure, 230, 237–238
Osseointegration, 302
Osteoblasts, 28*f*, 29–30, 85–88
Osteocalcin, 29–30
Osteoinductivity, 324–325
Oxygen ion bombardment, 351

P

Paclitaxel, 284, 286, 287*f*, 289, 476
Paclitaxel-embedded buckysomes (PEBs), 123

Parallel circuits, 144
Partition coefficient, 199, 217
  curve, 235*f*
  of free drugs, 234
  protein-polymer interaction, 232
  of solute, 230
Parylene C, 275, 278
Parylene N, 275
Passive coating, 275–276
Passive diffusion, 210
PC1036 hydrogel, 265
PC-1036 polymer, 277
PC2028 hydrogel, 265
Pectin, 243
Pemirolast, 284
Penetration, 46–47, 50*f*
Pharmaceutical phase, 196
Pharmacodynamics phase, 196
Pharmacokinetics phase, 196
Phase composition, 8–9, 23
Phase diagram, 388–389
Phase formation, 47
Phonons, 49
Phosphate precursor, 8*t*
Phospholipid polymer, 264–266
Phosphorylcholine, 265, 473
Photoresist, 355
Piezeoelectric actuators, 435*t*
Piezeoelectric thin films, 342, 432
Pimecrolimus, 286
Planck's constant, 52
Plasmachem, 98
Plasma etching, 355–356
Plasma immersion ion implantation (PIII), 61
Plasma-sprayed hydroxyapatite coatings, 316–320
Plasticizer dry coating, 241, 244
Platelet-rich plasma assay, 59–76
Platelets
  interactions, 480–482
  morphologies, 60*f*
Poisson's ratio, 19, 20
Poly-2-hydroxymethyl methacrylate (PHEMA), 245, 246*f*
Polyaniline-polyacrylate (PANI-PAA), 167
Polycrystalline diamond, 155–160
Polyesters, 240
Poly(ethylene carbonate) (PEC), 281
Polyethylene-*co*-vinyl acetate (PEVA), 261, 262–263, 289, 473
Polyethylene glycol (PEG), 240, 249, 480–482
Polylactic acid, 240, 248, 266
Polylactic acid stent, 271–272

Poly lactic-*co*-glycolic acid (PLGA), 240, 244, 248, 266
Polylactide, 266–268
Poly(lactide-co-glycolide), 268
Polymer-based matrix, 261–269
   erodible polymer matrix, 266–269
   non-erodible, 262–266
      block copolymers, 263–264
      fluoropolymer, 264
      phospholipid polymer, 264–266
      polymer blends, 262–263
Polymers, 3
   blends, 262–263
   degradation kinetics, 236
   mesh size, 213
Polymer solution, 226–229
   Flory-Huggin's model, 227
   free-volume contribution, 229
   UNIQUAC-based description, 227–229
Polymethyl methacrylate (PMMA), 2*t*, 61, 63, 239
Poly(*n*-butyl methacrylate) (PBMA), 262, 263*f*, 289
Polytetrafluoroethylene (PTFE), 56
Polyvinyl acetate (PVAc), 239, 244
Polyvinyl-based polymers, 239
Polyvinylidene fluoride, 342
Polyvinyl pyrrolidinone (PVP), 239, 265
Poole-Frenkel mechanism, 165
Post-deposition annealing temperature, 71–76
Precipitation method, 242–243, 320–321
Precursors, 7–8
Probucol, 284
Prograf, 286
Prosphorylcholine-based copolymers, 277, 278*f*
Proteins
   chemical potential, 218
   net charge, 232
   partition in aqueous two-phase system, 217–218
   partition in hydrogel membrane, 218–219
Pseudopodia, 64
Pseudoxanthomonas taiwanensis, 93
Pull-out shear test, 14–17
Pull-out tensile test, 14–17
Pulsatile release profile, 197–198
Pulsation sensor, 444–447
Pulsed laser deposition, 5*t*, 344
Pyrolytic graphite, 113
PZT films, 342, 432

Q

QCM, 337, 338*f*
Quantal exocytosis, 90
Quartz, 342

R

Radiofrequency magnetron sputtering, 324, 344–345, 398*f*
Raman spectroscopy, 52–55
Randles model, 177
Rapamycin, 265, 284
RAPTORRAIL® Rapid Exchange, 262
Rayleigh angle, 340
Rayleigh wave, 338*f*, 340
Reactive oxygen species, 124–125
Relaxation, 50*f*, 51
Relaxation rates, 141–142
Release-controlled coatings, 259–294
   active coatings, 276–280
      intra-built cavity, 279
      intra-built holes, 279
      microporous membrane, 280
      multiple-layer reservoir, 278
      nanoporous membrane, 280
      single layer reservoir, 276–277
   coating techniques, 280–283
      dip coating, 280–281
      ink-jet technology, 282–283
      spray coating, 281–282
   controlled release, 283–291
      diffusion-controlled release, 288–290
      dissolution/degradation, 290–291
      local drugs, 284–287
   matrix materials, 261–272
      inorganic-based matrix, 269–271
      polymer-based matrix, 261–269
   passive coating, 275–276
   perspectives, 292–294
   structures, 272–275
   top coat, 280
Release rate control, 199–238
   coating technology in, 196–197
   diffusion, 199–203
   erosion controlled, 235–237
   nonporous perspective, 210–214
      free volume, 211–214
      temperature effect, 214
   osmotic pressure controlled, 237–238
   porous perspective, 203–235
Renken equation, 204
Residual stress, 19–22
Resistance, 136, 144–145
Restenosis, 283
REVA stent, 271
Reverse martensitic transformation, 393
Rhodamine 6G, 281–282
R-phase transformation, 389

S

Sapphire, 342
Scanning electron microscopy (SEM), 12, 20*f*
Scratch test, 18–19
Self-texture, 349–350
Series circuits, 145
Shape memory alloys (SMAs), 382. *See also* TiNi
    alloys
   biomedical applications of, 382–384
   deformation behavior, 395–397
   historical development, 383*t*
   nanoindentation, 430
   thin films, 384–387
   work per unit volume, 435*t*
Shape memory effect (SME), 382, 387–388
   critical stress and, 396*f*
   superelasticity and, 393–395
   two-way, 430–431, 434–437
Shear strength, interfacial, 17–18
Short interfering RNA (siRNA), 118, 120
SIBS polymer, 263–264
Silicon carbide, 342
Simulated body fluids (SBFs), 25–27
Single-crystalline diamond, 151–155
Single layer reservoir, 276–277, 288–289
Single-stranded probe DNA (ss-DNA), 166
Single-walled nanotubes (SWNTs), 115–116
Sirolimus, 284, 290, 476
Sirolimus analogues, 284, 287*f*
Sirolimus-eluting stent (SES), 472
Snell's law of refraction, 340
Sol-gel deposition, 5*t*
Sol-gel derived hydroxyapatite coatings, 5*t*,
    6–33
   cell response to, 27–30
     cell attachment, 27–28
     cell morphology, 28–29
     cell proliferation/differentiation, 29–30
   chemical/physical properties, 8–14
     interfacial analysis, 13–14
     phase composition, 8–9
     surface chemistry/composition, 10–12
     surface morphology, 12
   fluoridated, 32–33
   in vitro tests, 22–27
     in acellular simulated body fluid, 25–27
     dissolution behavior, 22–25
   in vivo animal trials, 30–31
   macro-/microporous surfaces, 32
   mechanical properties, 14–31
     adhesion strength, 14–17
     interfacial shear strength, 17–18
     residual stress, 19–22
     scratch test, 18–19
     toughness, 19
   metallic substrates, 6–7
   overview, 6
   precursors, 7–8
   recent trends, 32–33
Sol-gel process, 6
Solid electrolyte interface (SEI), 179–180
Solid-liquid interfacial tension, 56
Solid-liquid phase change actuators, 435*t*
Solid-vapor interfacial tensions, 56
Solubilities, 23
Solubility product, 24
Solutes
   diffusion coefficient, 211, 214
   partitioning in hydrogel, 230–235
Solution
   chemical potential, 210
   Gibbs free energy of, 217, 219–220
   polymer solution, 226–229
Sorin Biomedica, 98
sp^2 carbon, 112*f*
Spectroscopic ellipsometry (SE), 63
Spherical spike, temperature profile of, 50
Spray coating, 281–282
   airbrush, 281–282
   ultrasonic, 281
Sputter coating, 5*t*, 324
Sputtering, 397–399
Sputtering yield, 47
Stainless steel, 2*t*
Staphylococcus aureus, 92–93
Staphylococcus epidermis, 92–93
Steady-state flux, 214
Stents, 97–98
   Axxion paclitaxel-eluting, 270
   biocorrodible metallic, 272
   cardiovascular, 473–475
   coatings, 473–477
   covered, 456–457
   drug-eluting, 260–261
   Genous Bio-engineered R, 270–271
   polylactic acid, 271–272
   structures, 272–275
   Yukon drug-eluting, 270
Steric effect, 230
Steric hindrance, 203–204
Stokes-Einstein equation, 203
Stokes force, 206
Strut, 272–273
Styrene-*b*-isobutylene-*b*-styrene (SIBS), 288, 473
Subplantation, 46, 48

basic processes in, 50*f*
densification by, 49*f*
SunMedical Technology Research Corporation, 98
Supercapacitors, 181–182
Supercritical fluid coating, 242
Superelasticity (SE), 382, 393–395, 396*f*, 404
Supralimus-Core stent, 269
Surface acoustic waves (SAW), 336
  biosensors, 363–364
  heating/droplet ejector, 369–370
  IDT design, 367–368
  microfluidics, 340–341
  mixer/pump, 366–368
  particle manipulation, 370–371
Surface chemistry, 10–12
Surface composition, 47
Surface energy, 55–57
Surface hydrophobicity, 56
Surface morphology, 12
Surface tension, 57–59
  Fowkes' concept, 57
  Lifshtz-van der Walls/acid-base (van Oss) approach, 58
  Owens-Wendt-Kaelbe, 58
Surface treatments, 310–315
  acid-etching, 314
  alkali treatment, 315
  anodic oxidation, 315
  antibacterial properties, 325
  laser texturing, 314
  osteoinductivity and, 324–325
  roughening by grit-blasting, 314
Surfactant proteins, 117
Sustained release profile, 197

T

Tablets, 199
Tacrolimus, 286
Tacrolimus-eluting stent, 269
TAXUS stent, 262, 263, 276–277, 288–289, 473
Telzir (drug), 177
Temperature coefficient frequency (TCF), 355
Temperature memory effect (TME), 429
TERT gene, 120
Tetracalcium phosphate (TCP), 9, 23, 317–318
Tetrahedral amorphous carbon, 66, 71, 91–92
Thermal management grade diamond, 159
Thermal spikes, 47, 50
Thermal spraying, 5*t*
Thermal stress, 21
Thermodynamics, 215

Thermoelastic martensitic transformation, 387–388
Thermo-pneumatic actuators, 435*t*
Thin films, 341–343
  for acoustic wave devices, 341–343
  age-treated, 406–407
  binary alloy, 401–406
    superelasticity, 404
    texture, 405–406
    transformation strain anisotropy, 405–406
  biocompatibility of, 433
  biological/MEMS applications of, 434–459
    covered stent, 452–453
    diaphragms, 437–444
    freestanding TiNi-based microcage, 450–452
    heart valve, 457–458
    microactuators, 434–437
    microgrippers, 444–446
    micropumps, 437–444
    microvalves, 437–444
    pulsation sensor, 444–447
    superelastic thin film tubes, 458–459
    TiNi-based microcage, 449–450
    TiNi/DLC microcage, 452–455
  biosensor applications, 363–366
  microfluidic applications, 366–371
  microtubes, 458–459
  Ni-rich, 406–410
    aging effect, 407–410
    microstructure of age-treated thin films, 406–407
  shape memory alloys, 384–387
  TiNiX ternary alloy, 414–420
    TiNiCu films, 414–418
    TiNiPd films, 418–420
Time-of-flight secondary mass emission spectrometry (ToF-SIMS), 13
TiNi alloys, 381–461
  adhesion, 425
  binary alloy thin films, 401–406
    superelasticity, 404
    texture, 405–406
    transformation strain anisotropy, 405–406
  biocompatibility of, 433
  biological/MEMS applications of thin films, 434–459
    covered stent, 452–453
    diaphragms, 437–444
    freestanding TiNi-based microcage, 450–452
    heart valve, 457–458
    microactuators, 434–437
    microgrippers, 444–446

TiNi alloys (*continued*)
    micropumps, 437–444
    microvalves, 437–444
    pulsation sensor, 444–447
    superelastic thin film tubes, 458–459
    TiNi-based microcage, 449–450
    TiNi/DLC microcage, 452–455
  biomedical applications of, 382–384
  composite-based films, 431–432
  crystallography of martensitic
       transformation, 389–390
  deformation behavior, 395–397
  degradation, 425–427
  fatigue, 425–427
  film
    characterization, 400–420
    deposition, 398–400
    stress, 420–423
    thickness effect, 428–429
  frequency response, 424–425
  functionally graded films, 431–432
  interfacial analysis, 425
  martensitic transformation, 387–390
  modeling, 433
  nanoscale mechanical evaluation, 430–431
  Ni-rich thin films, 406–410
    aging effect, 407–410
    microstructure of age-treated thin films,
      406–407
  phase diagram, 388–389
  reversible surface trench morphology, 424*f*
  shape memory effect, 387–388, 393–395
  sputtering, 397–399
  stability, 425–427
  stress evolution, 420–423
  stress-strain curves, 396*f*
  superelasticity, 393–395
  temperature memory effect, 429
  thermal cyclic deformation, 426–427
  thin films, 384
  TiNiX ternary alloy thin films, 414–420
    TiNiCu films, 414–418
    TiNiPd films, 418–420
  Ti-rich alloys, 410–414
    bright-field images, 412*f*
    electron diffraction pattern, 410–411
    nonequilibrium phase and composition,
      410–411
    strain-temperature curves, 413*f*
    strengthening mechanism, 412–414
  transformation strain, 391–392
  transformation temperatures, 393
TiNiCu films, 414–418, 421–422, 443–444

TiNiPd films, 418–420, 441–442
Ti-Ni R phase microactuator, 441–442
TiNiX ternary alloy thin films, 414–420
  TiNiCu films, 414–418
  TiNiPd films, 418–420
Ti-rich alloys, 410–414
  bright-field images, 412*f*
  electron diffraction pattern, 410–411
  nonequilibrium phase and composition,
    410–411
  strain-temperature curves, 413*f*
  strengthening mechanism, 412–414
Tissue culture polystyrene (TCPS), 88
Titanium, 7
Titanium alloy, 7
Titanium carbide, 61
Titanium nitride, 61
Top coat, 280
Trace elements, 33
Transferrin, 271
Transformation strain, 391–392, 405–406
Transformation temperatures, 393
Translumina Yukon CC stent, 270
Translute polymer, 288
Trhombin-antithrombin three complex
    (TAT), 69
Trimethoxysilylpropyl methacrylate
    (TSMA), 277
Tris-buffered physiological saline (TPS), 23
Troglitazone, 284
Tubular slotted structure, 272, 273*f*
Two-liquid model, non-random, 221–222
Type V platelets, 71

U

Ultra-high-molecular-weight polyethylene
    (UHMWPE), 96–97, 121
Ultrasonic spraying, 281
Ultraviolet sensors, 172
Unhydrogenated amorphous carbon, 61–66
UNIQUAC functional-group activity
    coefficients, 225–226
UNIQUAC-NRF model, 228
Universal quasi-chemical (UNIQUAC) theory,
    223–225, 227–229

V

Valsartan, 284
Van der Waals interaction, 208–209
Vapor-grown carbon fiber (VGCF), 182
Volume degree of swelling, 212

W

Wilson model, 220–221
Wireless capsule endoscope (WCE), 444
Wolff's law, 7
Work per unit volume, 434, 435*t*

X

Xience V stent, 262*t*, 264, 474
X-ray diffraction (XRD), 10, 20
X-ray photon electroscopy (XPS), 10, 11*f*, 11*t*, 52

Y

Young contact angle, 56
Young-Laplace equation, 56
Young's equation, 56–57
Young's modulus, 18, 421
Yukon drug-eluting stent, 270

Z

ZnO film, 342, 344–356. *See also* Acoustic wave
    devices; AIN films

for biosensing, 356
crystalline structure model, 348*f*
crystalline structure-Wurtzite structure, 349*f*
deposition, 344–349
lab-on-a-chip system, 372–373
MEMS processing, 355–356
microfluidic applications, 356
properties, 342*t*
sputtered, PE properties of, 352–355
    film thickness effect, 352–354
    substrate effect, 352
temperature coefficient frequency, 355
texture, 349–351
    buffer layer, 350
    epitaxial growth, 350–351
    interlayer, 350
    oxygen ion bombardment, 351
    self-texture, 349–350
    wave mode, 349–350
thickness ratio, 354
velocity on substrates, 345*t*
Zoledronate, 479
ZoMaxx stent, 277
Zotarolimus, 264–265, 284, 285